Your *Plus Code* to Success.

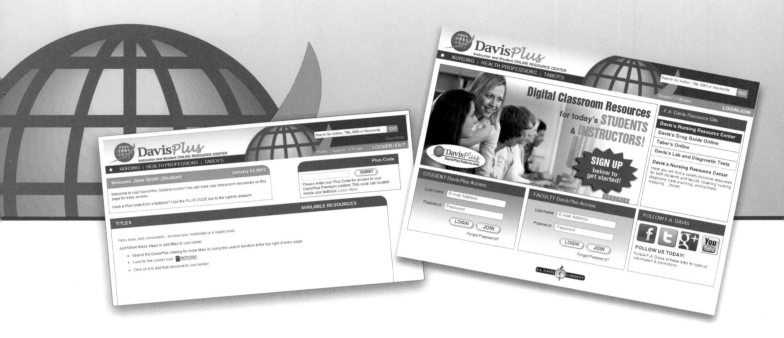

Unlock your book's premium resources using your *Plus* Code

1. **Scratch off** the shiny surface below to access your unique *Plus* Code.

2. **Go to:** davispl.us/durhamcode

3. **Look for** the 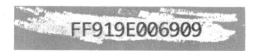 button and redeem your code.

   Note: You will be asked to sign up or log-in to Davis*Plus* before activating your code. (It's FREE.)

FF919E006909

Book cannot be returned for a refund once this code is scratched off.

Instructors: You don't need a *Plus* Code to access content.
Adopters have free access to all resources, including premium.

Each *Plus* Code may only be redeemed one time. If your code has already been used, visit **Davis*Plus*.FADavis.com** to purchase access. Follow the same instructions above and click the (**Purchase Access**) button.

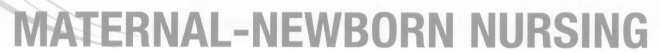

MATERNAL-NEWBORN NURSING

The Critical Components of Nursing Care

Second Edition

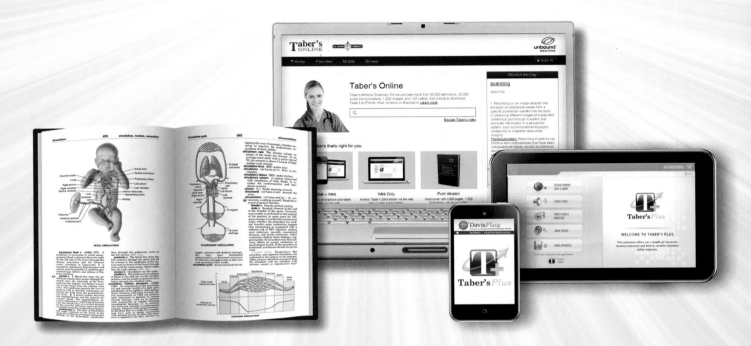

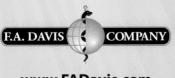

MATERNAL-NEWBORN NURSING

The Critical Components of Nursing Care

Second Edition

Roberta F. Durham, RN, PhD
Professor
Department of Nursing and Health Sciences
California State University, East Bay
Hayward, California
Professor Alumnus
Samuel Merritt University
Oakland, California

Linda Chapman, RN, PhD
Professor Emeritus
Samuel Merritt University
Oakland, California

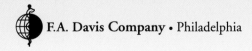
F.A. Davis Company • Philadelphia

F. A. Davis Company
1915 Arch Street
Philadelphia, PA 19103
www.fadavis.com

Copyright © 2014 by F. A. Davis Company

Printed in the United States of America

Last digit indicates print number: 10 9 8 7 6 5 4 3 2 1

Publisher, Nursing: Lisa D. Houck
Developmental Editor: Sarah M. Granlund
Director of Content Development: Darlene D. Pedersen
Project Editor: Christina L. Snyder
Design and Illustration Manager: Carolyn O'Brien
Cover Photo: Courtesy of Baby Jane-Hope Hallowell

As new scientific information becomes available through basic and clinical research, recommended treatments and drug therapies undergo changes. The author(s) and publisher have done everything possible to make this book accurate, up to date, and in accord with accepted standards at the time of publication. The author(s), editors, and publisher are not responsible for errors or omissions or for consequences from application of the book, and make no warranty, expressed or implied, in regard to the contents of the book. Any practice described in this book should be applied by the reader in accordance with professional standards of care used in regard to the unique circumstances that may apply in each situation. The reader is advised always to check product information (package inserts) for changes and new information regarding dose and contraindications before administering any drug. Caution is especially urged when using new or infrequently ordered drugs.

Library of Congress Cataloging-in-Publication Data

Durham, Roberta F.
  Maternal-newborn nursing : the critical components of nursing care / Roberta F. Durham, Linda Chapman. — 2nd ed.
    p. ; cm.
  Rev. ed. of: Maternal-newborn nursing / Linda Chapman, Roberta F. Durham. c2010.
  Includes bibliographical references and index.
  ISBN 978-0-8036-3704-7 (hbk. : alk. paper)
  I. Chapman, Linda, 1949- II. Chapman, Linda, 1949- Maternal-newborn nursing. III. Title.
  [DNLM: 1. Maternal-Child Nursing. 2. Perinatal Care. WY 157.3]
  RG951
  618.2'0231—dc23   2013009079

To our mothers, Virginia "Ducky" Durham and June Henderson

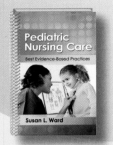
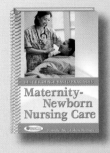
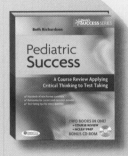
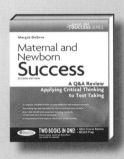
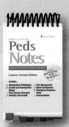
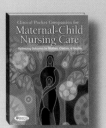
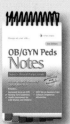
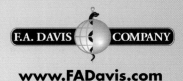

Preface

In this second edition of *Maternal-Newborn Nursing: The Critical Components of Nursing Care* we continue to emphasize the basics of maternity nursing, focusing on evidence-based practice for all levels of nursing programs. Because we realize that today's students lead complex lives and must juggle multiple roles as student, parent, employee, and spouse, we developed this textbook, with its accompanying electronic ancillaries, to present the critical components of maternity nursing in a clear and concise format that lends itself to ease of comprehension while maintaining the integrity of the substantive content. It may be particularly useful for programs designed to present the subject of maternity in an abbreviated or condensed way.

We revised the textbook based on the recommendations of those who have used it—faculty from various states and students in all types of programs—and our own experiences. Revisions include enhanced rationale for nursing actions in all chapters, increased content in pathophysiology in many areas, and expanded high-risk content. We have updated content to keep current in standards in practice, including new guidelines for management of postpartum hemorrhage, management of intrapartal fetal heart rate abnormalities, assessment and care of the late preterm infant, and assessment and care of the newborn with hyperbilirubinemia. We have expanded sections on patient education, patient teaching resources, and complementary and alternative therapies. Professional standards of care for maternity nurses are based on current practice guidelines and research.

ORGANIZATION

This evidence-based text utilizes theory and clinical knowledge of maternity nursing. The conceptual framework is Family Developmental Theory, and substantive theory that forms the foundation for maternity care is presented. The book is organized according to the natural sequence of the perinatal cycle, pregnancy, labor and birth, postpartum, and neonate. We have taken a bio-psycho-social approach dealing with the physiological, psychological adaptation, social, and cultural influences impacting childbearing families, with emphasis on nursing actions and care of women and families. We believe childbirth is a natural, developmental process.

Nursing is an ever-changing science. New research and clinical knowledge expand knowledge and change clinical practice. *Maternal-Newborn Nursing: The Critical Components of Nursing Care* reflects current knowledge, standards, and trends in maternity services, including the trend toward higher levels of intervention in maternity care. These standards and trends are reflected in our inclusion of a chapter on tests during the antepartal period, as well as a chapter devoted to fetal assessment and electronic fetal monitoring. We have devoted a chapter to the care of cesarean birth families; nearly one-third of births in the United States are cesarean.

FEATURES

This textbook presents the critical components of maternity in a pragmatic condensed format by using the following features:

- Information presented in a bulleted format for ease of reading
- Flowcharts, diagrams, tables, clinical pathways, and concept maps to summarize information
- Case studies to assist integration of knowledge

Audio Book

In an effort to help students manage their time more effectively, each book comes with access to downloadable audio files that contain recorded abridged versions of chapters for students to listen to while commuting to and from classes and clinical. Students can use these audio files to reinforce the content in the text, to refresh their reading before class, or to review for an exam. The audio files provide two ways of learning in one product.

Critical Components

This textbook focuses on the critical components of maternity nursing. Critical components are the major areas of knowledge essential for a basic understanding of maternity nursing. The critical components were determined from the authors' combined 50 years of teaching maternity nursing in both traditional and accelerated programs and years of clinical practice in the maternity setting. Current guidelines and standards are integrated and summarized for a pragmatic approach to patient and family-focused care. This focus is especially evident when discussing complications or deviations from the norm.

The focus of the text is on normal pregnancy and childbirth. Chapters on low-risk antenatal, intrapartal, postpartum, and neonate are followed by chapters on high risk and complications in each area. Complications germane to the nursing domain and childbearing population focus on understanding and synthesizing the critical elements for nursing care.

Care of Cesarean Birth Families

Approximately one-third of births are by cesarean section. In response to this increased trend, this book has dedicated a chapter to the intrapartum and postpartum care of the cesarean birth families.

Chapter Format

This textbook clusters physiological changes, nursing assessment, and nursing care content in each chapter. Typically, a chapter is divided into systems in which the physiology; nursing care, including assessment and interventions; expected outcomes; and common deviations of one subsystem are presented. Psychosocial and cultural dimensions of nursing care are highlighted in each chapter.

Flowcharts, Diagrams, Tables, Concept Maps, and Clinical Pathways

Flowcharts, tables, concept maps, and clinical pathways present large amounts of information in a clear and concise format.

Case Studies

Two case studies, one low-risk and one high-risk, are presented in the unit on antepartal care; these are developed further in subsequent chapters. These case studies are presented at the end of each chapter as a strategy to summarize the key elements of the chapter, to assist the students in their development of critical thinking skills, and to help them integrate the content into clinical practice.

The development of the case studies over multiple content areas—antepartum, intrapartum, and postpartum—allows students to analyze the assessment data in relationship to nursing care. This type of teaching/learning activity helps bring content "to life" for students as they synthesize new knowledge.

Review Questions

Review question appear at the end of each chapter to help students review key chapter content.

Teaching Cards

Teaching cards are provided as an electronic resource to help students instruct patients and families. The cards summarize and organize information on key topics related to mother and baby care and discharge teaching and planning. The teaching cards have details regarding newborn care and feeding and postpartum self-care as well as warning signs and guidance about when to call the health-care practitioner.

Special Features

A variety of boxes appears throughout the chapters to highlight information:

- *Critical Component:* Highlights critical information in maternal-newborn nursing
- *Medication:* Highlights the commonly administered medications used during pregnancy, labor and birth, postpartum, and neonatal periods
- *Cultural Awareness:* Stresses the importance of cultural factors in nursing care
- *Evidenced-Based Practice:* Highlights current research and practice guidelines related to nursing care

- *Standards of Care* and *Professional Position Statements:* Highlights key perinatal nursing issues from professional organizations such as Association of Women's Health, Obstetric and Neonatal Nurses (AWHONN)
- Quality and Safety Education in Nursing (QSEN): Highlights QSEN concepts as they apply to the chapter content

Glossary

For ease of looking up definitions, there is a glossary of terms used in the book related to maternal-newborn nursing.

Appendixes

The appendixes include:

- AWHONN guide to breastfeeding
- Common and standard laboratory values for pregnant and nonpregnant women and the neonate
- Temperature equivalents
- Cervical dilation chart
- Newborn weight conversion chart
- Immunization and pregnancy table

IMPORTANT FEATURES FOR INSTRUCTORS

The nursing shortage resulted in the widespread development and expansion of nursing programs. Many nursing programs, which can be as short as 12 months, now teach maternity nursing in a compact or abbreviated format. Faculty are challenged to develop courses with fewer credit units to be taught in 5 or fewer weeks. This requires a critical analysis to identify essential components of the subject area and the appropriate teaching-learning resources. Maternity nursing textbooks are not designed for current approaches to nursing education at the associate, traditional baccalaureate, accelerated baccalaureate, or entry-level masters' nursing programs. This textbook addresses the reality of nursing education today and presents the critical components of maternity in a pragmatic, condensed format with ancillary course materials to facilitate student learning and faculty teaching of maternity nursing.

Current nursing students comprise a diverse group and many are older, more mature learners. They may enter a nursing program with prior degrees and work experience in fields outside of nursing. Most students want materials presented in a clear and concise format that allows them to use their critical thinking skills to integrate the new knowledge into their previous knowledge base and life experiences. Because some nursing students have completed their transition to adulthood, they are believed by education experts to be better poised to master the knowledge they need to arrive at clinical judgments and ethical and moral decisions inherent in nursing practice. Utilization of critical elements, mapping, evidenced-based practice guidelines, and focused activities will satisfy the needs of these specialized learners who are intolerant of "busy work" and extraneous material.

The theme for the new millennium in nursing educations is "We can no longer teach as we were taught." That includes teaching in shorter periods for both theory and clinical and teaching for understanding of critical elements. This book responds to innovations in nursing curricula and the new population of nursing students.

The ancillary products for this text respond to needs and learning styles of current students. For example, some nursing students are already college graduates with academic, life, and work experience contributing to their critical thinking and ability to synthesize complex information and seek evidenced-based solutions to clinical problems. The ancillary resources allow them to utilize a variety of technology-based resources in place of outdated, more traditional approaches used in other maternity textbooks.

Supplemental instructor aids for theory class include:

- An 8-week syllabus guide
- Detailed classroom activities for each content area
- PowerPoint slides
- Image bank
- Fully developed and integrated case studies with critical thinking activities and rationales both for high and low risk.
- Interactive case studies for students to improve critical thinking and priority setting
- Animations to enhance visual learning and application

- Interactive online student exercises
- Exam test bank with over 500 updated questions in ExamViewPro with item descriptors
- Activities using Internet resources

Supplemental instructor materials for clinical include:

- Detailed clinical syllabus for inpatient and community-based perinatal settings
- Clinical integration activities, with critical thinking activities and directions on implementation including:
  - *Family study: format and directions for a community-based postpartum home family study for clinical students*
  - *Topics for clinical integration seminars*
  - *Expectant parent interview activity*
  - *Teaching cards for use with postpartum families*
  - *Medication cards*
  - *Skill laboratory exercises*
  - *Chart review exercises*
  - *Clinical preparation tools*
    - Antepartal data collection worksheet
    - Neonatal intensive care unit (NICU) data collection worksheet
    - Postpartum data collection worksheet
    - Labor and delivery data collection worksheet
    - Newborn assessment worksheet
  - *Nursing care plans for postpartum and labor and delivery*

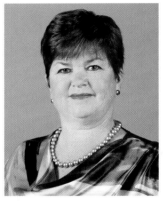

Roberta Durham, RN, PhD, is Professor at California State University, East Bay, in Hayward, California, and a Professor Alumnus at Samuel Merritt University in Oakland, California. She received her bachelor's degree in nursing from the University of Rhode Island and her master's degree in nursing as a perinatal clinical specialist from the University of California, San Francisco. Dr. Durham received her PhD in nursing from the University of California, San Francisco, where she studied grounded theory method with Drs. Anselm Strauss and Leonard Schatzman. Her program of research has been on the management of premature labor and the prevention of premature birth. She has conducted international research and published her substantive and methodological work widely. She was previously a Visiting Professor at the University of Glasgow and is currently involved in international research in Central America to improve perinatal outcomes. She has worked for over 25 years in labor and delivery units in the San Francisco Bay area.

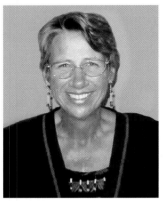

Linda Chapman, RN, PhD, has recently retired from University of Arizona College of Nursing and is a Professor Emeritus at Samuel Merritt University in Oakland, California. She received her diploma in nursing from Samuel Merritt Hospital School of Nursing, her bachelor's degree in nursing from University of Utah, and her master's degree in nursing from the University of California, San Francisco. Dr. Chapman received her PhD from the University of California, San Francisco, where she studied with Drs. Ramona Mercer and Katharyn May. Her program of research has been on the experience of men during the perinatal period. She has conducted research and published her substantive work in practice and research journals. She worked for 25 years in nursery, postpartum, and labor and birthing units at Samuel Merritt Hospital/Summit Medical Center in the San Francisco Bay area.

Contributors

Jessica Bence

Research Assistant
Undergraduate Nursing Student
California State University, East Bay
Hayward, California

Hazel Cortes, RN, BSN

New Graduate
California State University, East Bay
Hayward, California

Sylvia Fischer, MSN, RN, CNM

Clinical Instructor
University of Arizona College of Nursing
Tucson, Arizona

Jill George, RN, BSN

New Graduate
California State University, East Bay
Hayward, California

Melissa Goldsmith, PhD, RNC

Clinical Associate Professor
University of Arizona College of Nursing
Tucson, Arizona

Sarah Hampson, RN, MS

Assistant Professor
Samuel Merritt University
Oakland, California

Megan E. Levy, RN, BSN, PHN

Staff Nurse
Highland Medical Center
Oakland, California

Connie Miller, MSN, RNC

Clinical Assistant Professor
University of Arizona College of Nursing
Tucson, Arizona

Jessica Perez, RN, BSN

Research Assistant
Stanford Medical Center
Palo Alto, California

Kathleen Rehak

Technical Writer and Editor
Richmond, California

Janice Stinson, RN, PhD

Adjunct Assistant Professor/Staff Nurse
University of California, San Francisco
Alta Bates Summit Medical Center
San Francisco, California

Darice Taylor, MSN, RNC

Clinical Instructor
University of Arizona College of Nursing
Staff Nurse and Flight Nurse
Level III Neonatal Intensive Care Unit
Tucson Medical Center
Tucson, Arizona

Contributors to the First Edition

Susan M. Cantrell, MSN, RNC

Assistant Professor
Samuel Merritt University
Oakland, California
Chapter 7

Mabel Choy-Bland, RN, BS

Emergency Department
Kaiser Permanente Hospital
Hayward, California
Research Assistant on chapter development

Deanna Luz Reyes Delgado, RN, BS

Neonatal Intensive Care Unit
Children's Hospital and Research Center Oakland
Oakland, California
*Research Assistant on chapter development and NCLEX
    questions*

Sylvia Fischer, RN, MSN, CNM

Clinical Assistant Professor
University of Arizona College of Nursing
Tucson, Arizona
Chapter 13

Melissa M. Goldsmith, PhD, RNC

Clinical Associate Professor
University of Arizona College of Nursing
Tucson, Arizona
Chapter 17

Stefanie Hahn, RN, BS

Perinatal Staff Nurse
Alta Bates Medical Center
Berkeley, California
Research Assistant on Interactive Computer Exercises

Sarah Hampson, RN, MS

Assistant Professor
Samuel Merritt University
Oakland, California
Chapter 5

Vivian Chioma Nwagwu, RN, MSN

Health Facilities Evaluator
State of California Department of Public Health
Licensing & Certification Program
San Jose, California
Research Assistant on PowerPoint development

Corrine Marie Smith, RN, MS, ANP-c

Nurse Practitioner
Olivetan Benedictine Sisters
Holy Angels Convent
Jonesboro, Arkansas
Chapter 8

Nora Webster, CNM, MSN

Course Faculty
Frontier School of Midwifery and Family Practice
Tuscon, Arizona
Chapter 4

Reviewers

Rebecca L. Allen, RN, MSN
Assistant Professor
Clarkson College
Omaha, Nebraska

Betty Bowles, PhD, RNC
Assistant Professor
Midwestern State University
Wichita Falls, Texas

Tammy Buchholz, RN, MSN
Assistant Professor of Nursing
Sanford College of Nursing
Bismarck, North Dakota

Joan M. Carlson, RN, MSN, CNE
Professor
Harper College
Palatine, Illinois

Cathryn Collings, RN, BSN, MSN
Assistant Professor
Denver School of Nursing
Denver, Colorado

Anita Crawford, RNC-OB, BSN, MSN
Nursing Instructor
Florence-Darlington Technical College
Florence, South Carolina

Carla Crider, MSN, RNC
Instructor
Weatherford College
Weatherford, Texas

Elisabeth Donohoe Culver, PhD, RN, CNM
Assistant Professor/Staff Nurse-Midwife
Bloomsburg University of Pennsylvania/Geisinger
   Medical Center
Bloomsburg/Danville, Pennsylvania

Rachel Derr, RNC-LRN, MSN, DNP
Assistant Professor
Holy Family University
Philadelphia, Pennsylvania

Patricia A. Duclos-Miller, RN, MS, NE-BC
Professor
Capital Community College
Hartford, Connecticut

Laura Dulski, RNC-HROB, CNE, MSN
Assistant Professor
Resurrection University
Oak Park, Illinois

Lisa Everhart, RN, MSN, WHNP-BC
Assistant Professor of Nursing
Columbia State Community College
Franklin, Tennessee

Kara Flowers, RN, MSN, LC, IBCLC
Clinical Assistant Professor
University of Missouri Kansas City School of Nursing
Kansas City, Missouri

Susan Hall, EdD, MSN, RNC, CCE
Instructor/Maternity Coordinator
Winston-Salem State University
Winston-Salem, North Carolina

Stephen Hammer, BSeD, BSN, MA-CS, RN, CCE
Assistant Clinical Nursing Professor
Angelo State University
San Angelo, Texas

Sara Harkness, RN, MS, NP
Clinical Instructor
California State University, East Bay
Hayward, California
Labor and Delivery Staff Nurse
Alta Bates Medical Center
Berkeley, California

Betty J. Hennington, MSN, CNE
Nursing Instructor
Meridian Community College
Meridian, Mississippi

Teresa L. Howell, DNP, RN, CNE
Associate Professor of Nursing
Morehead State University
Morehead, Kentucky

Kerrie Jennings, RN, BSN
Labor and Delivery Staff Nurse
Alta Bates Medical Center
Berkeley, California

Kathryn M. L. Konrad, MS, RNC-OB, LCCE, FACCE
Instructor
The University of Oklahoma College of Nursing
Oklahoma City, Oklahoma

Peggy Korman, MA, CNM, BSN, RN
Assistant Professor
Denver School of Nursing
Denver, Colorado

Kathleen N. Krov, PhD, CNM, RN, CNE
Associate Professor
Raritan Valley Community College
Somerville, New Jersey

Dottie Lay, RN, MSN, MBA, DNP
Professor of Nursing
Norwalk Community College, University of Connecticut
    Adjunct Faculty
Norwalk, Connecticut

Janet G. Marshall, PhD, MSN, RN
Associate Professor
Florida A&M University
Tallahassee, Florida

Margaret McManus, RN, BA
Labor and Delivery/Neonatal Intensive Care Unit Staff
    Nurse II
Alta Bates Medical Center
Berkeley, California

Jacqui McMillian-Bohler, BSN, MSN, CNM
BSN Program Director
Spalding University
Louisville, Kentucky

Cynthia A. Morris, RN, MSN, IBCLC, RLC
Nursing Instructor
Citizens School of Nursing
New Kensington, Pennsylvania

Zula Price, MSN, PhD student
Assistant Clinical Professor
North Carolina A&T State University
Greensboro, North Carolina

Martha C. Ruder, RN, MSN
Coordinator, Associate Degree Nursing
Gulf Coast State College
Panama City, Florida

Benita Kay Ryne, MSN, RNC
Maternal-Newborn Faculty
College of Southern Nevada
Childbirth Education Coordinator
Labor and Delivery Staff Nurse at MountainView Hospital
Las Vegas, Nevada

Cynthia Scaringe, RN, MSN
Nursing Instructor
Skagit Valley College
Mount Vernon, Washington

Carol Thomas, MSN-ED, MSA, RN
Assistant Professor
New York City College of Technology
Brooklyn, New York

Jeanne Tucker, PhD, RN, MSN, HSAD, CHES
Assistant Professor of Nursing
Patty Hanks Shelton School of Nursing
Abilene, Texas

Paulina Van, RN, PhD, CNE
Professor and Chair
Department of Nursing and Health Sciences
California State University, East Bay
Hayward, California

Marcie Weissner, MSN, RNC-OB
Assistant Professor
University of Saint Francis
Fort Wayne, Indiana

Nanette Wong, RNC, BSN
Labor and Delivery Staff Nurse IV
Alta Bates Medical Center
Berkeley, California

Acknowledgments

We are grateful to the following people, who helped us turn an idea into reality:

- Our husbands, Douglas Fredebaugh and Chuck Chapman, for their ongoing support and love
- Our colleagues at Samuel Merritt University who helped us develop from novice to expert teachers
- Our current and past colleagues at the California State University, East Bay, and University of Arizona College of Nursing for their suggestions and support
- Our teachers and mentors Katharyn A. May, RN, DNSc, FAAN, and Ramona T. Mercer, RN, PhD, FAAN
- Our F. A. Davis team, Lisa Houck, Christina Snyder, and Sarah M. Granlund, for their guidance
- Kathleen Rehak for technical document support at key intervals
- Our contributors for sharing their expertise

Contents in Brief

Contents

Unit 3

The Intrapartal Period 185

Unit 4

Postpartal Period 309

Unit 5

Neonatal Period 375

Maternity Nursing Overview

Trends and Issues

EXPECTED STUDENT OUTCOMES

Upon completion of this chapter, the student will be able to:

- ☐ Define key terms.
- ☐ Discuss current trends in the management of labor and birth.
- ☐ Discuss the current trends in maternal and infant health outcomes.
- ☐ Identify leading causes of infant deaths.
- ☐ Discuss current maternal and infant health issues.
- ☐ Identify the primary maternal and infant goals stated in *Healthy People 2020*.

TRENDS

During the past 100 years, maternity nursing has undergone numerous changes in response to advances in technology, medicine, and nursing and to the individual desires of child-bearing couples (**Table 1-1**).

The present trend in an increase in both cesarean births and induction of labor is a significant change in the approach to labor and birth. Management of labor and birth has moved from the low use of obstetrical interventions in the natural childbirth era that began in the 1960s to high use of obstetrical interventions and to a more controlled event. The impetus for this shift has been a childbearing generation whose members embrace technology and who have a desire to control when and how their children are born. The scheduling and method of childbirth are also influenced by physicians' preferences.

Changes have also occurred in fertility and birthrates, preterm rates, neonatal birth weight rates, infant mortality rates, and maternal death and mortality rates.

Fertility and Birthrates

Fertility rate is "the total number of live births, regardless of age of mother, per 1,000 women of reproductive age, 15–44 years" (Centers for Disease Control and Prevention [CDC], 2007).

Birthrate is the number of live births per 1,000 people (CDC, 2007). It is estimated that in 2011 the U.S. birthrate was ranked number 148 out of 221 countries with a birthrate of 13.83 (CIA, 2011). The following is a sample ranking of other countries:

- ■ Niger is ranked 1 with a rate of 50.54.
- ■ Egypt is ranked 64 with rate of 24.63.
- ■ Mexico is ranked 102 with a rate of 19.13.
- ■ Australia is ranked 158 with a rate of 12.33.
- ■ The United Kingdom is ranked 161 with a rate of 12.29.
- ■ Canada is ranked 186 with a rate of 10.28.
- ■ Japan is ranked 220 with a rate of 7.31.
- ■ Monaco is ranked 221 with a rate of 6.94 (CIA, 2011).

In the United States, there was a 49% decrease in the fertility rate and a 57% decrease in the birthrate between 1910 and 2010 (**Table 1-2**). During this period, the fertility rate decreased from 126.8 to 64.1 live births per 1,000 women between the ages of 15 and 44. The birthrate during this same period decreased from 30.1 to 13.0 live births per 1,000.

The decline in fertility rates and birthrates from 1910 to 2010 may be attributed to:

- ■ Availability of a variety of contraceptive methods with a high effectiveness rate
- ■ Increased numbers of women delaying and/or limiting pregnancy/children to focus on careers

Don't have time to read this chapter? Want to reinforce your reading? Need to review for a test?
Listen to this chapter on DavisPlus.

TABLE 1–1   PAST AND PRESENT TRENDS

PAST TRENDS	PRESENT TRENDS
Nursing: Focus on physiological changes and needs of the mother and infant	Family-Centered Maternity Nursing: Focus on both the physiological and psychosocial changes and needs of the childbearing family
Primarily home births	Primarily hospital births
Women labored in one room and delivered in another room	Women labor, deliver, and recover in the same room
Delivery rooms "cold and sterile"	Birthing rooms "warm and homelike"
Expectant fathers and family excluded from the labor and birth experience	Expectant fathers and family/friends involved in the labor and birth experience
Expectant fathers excluded from cesarean births	Expectant fathers or family members in the operating room during cesarean births
Labor pain management: Amnesia or "twilight sleep" to natural childbirth	Labor pain management: analgesics and epidurals.
Hospital postpartum stay of 10 days	Hospital postpartum stay of 48 hours
Infant mortality rate of 58.1 per 1,000 live births in 1933 (Kochanek & Martin, 2004)	Infant mortality rate of 6.1 per 1,000 live births in 2011 (CIA, 2011)
Maternal mortality rate of 619.1 per 100,000 live births in 1933 (Hoyert, 2007)	Maternal mortality rate of 24 per 100,000 live births in 2008 (WHO, 2010)
Induction of labor rate of 9.5% in 1990 (Martin et al., 2006)	Induction of labor rate of 23.2% in 2009 (Martin et al., 2011)
Cesarean section rate of 20.7% in 1996 (Martin et al., 2006)	Cesarean section rate of 32.8% in 2010 (Hamilton et al., 2011)
Low probability of infants surviving who were born at or before 28 weeks of gestation	Increased survival rates of infants born between 24 weeks and 28 weeks of gestation

TABLE 1–2   BIRTH RATES AND FERTILITY RATES 1910–2010 (RATES PER 1,000 LIVE BIRTHS)

YEAR	1910	1930	1950	1970	1980	1990	2000	2010
BIRTHRATE	30.1	21.3	24.1	18.4	15.9	16.7	14.4	13
FERTILITY RATE	126.8	89.2	106.2	87.9	68.4	70.9	65.9	64.1

Hamilton et al. (2006, 2007, 2009, 2011)

■ Legalization and availability of elective abortions
■ Couples limiting number of children due to rising cost of raising children

An interesting trend is noted for the 20-year period from 1990 to 2010 (**Table 1-3**). The birthrates decreased for women age 15–29 but increased for women age 30–45 and older. The greatest increase was seen in women ages 40 years and older. The greatest decrease was in women ages 15–19 years.

In the United States in 2010, there were a total 4,000,279 births; a birthrate of 13.0. The percentages of these births by race are:

■ American Indian or Alaska Native: 1%
■ Asian or Pacific Islanders: 6%
■ Hispanic: 24%
■ Non-Hispanic black: 15%
■ Non-Hispanic white: 54% (Hamilton et al., 2011).

These percentages reflect the multicultural population of the United States and present an exciting challenge to health care workers to adapt their care to reflect an understanding of the health care beliefs and cultural practices of a wide variety of childbearing families.

Preterm Births

■ **Very premature:** Neonates born at less than 32 weeks of gestation
■ **Moderately premature:** Neonates born between 32 and 33 weeks of gestation
■ **Late premature:** Neonates born between 34 and 37 weeks of gestation (Hamilton et al., 2006).

TABLE 1–3 BIRTH RATES BY AGE OF MOTHER (PER 1,000)							
AGE OF MOTHER	15–19	20–24	25–29	30–34	35–39	40–44	45 +
1990	59.9	116.5	120.2	80.8	31.7	5.5	0.2
2000	47.7	109.7	113.5	91.2	39.7	8.0	0.5
2005	40.5	102.2	115.5	95.8	46.3	9.1	0.6
2010	34.1	90.0	108.3	96.6	45.9	10.2	0.7
CHANGE FROM 1990 TO 2010	↓43%	↓23%	↓1%	↑20%	↑45%	↑85%	↑250%

Child Trends Data Bank (2012)

Despite widespread advances in perinatal care, the preterm birthrate continues to rise. The number of premature births rose from 10.61% of live births in 1990 to 11.99% in 2010, reflecting a 13% increase (Hamilton et al., 2011) (**Table 1-4**).

The 2010 percentages of premature births based on race of mother are:

■ American Indian or Alaska Native: 13.6
■ Asian or Pacific Islander: 10.69
■ Hispanic: 11.79
■ Non-Hispanic black: 17.15
■ Non-Hispanic white: 10.78 (Hamilton et al., 2011).

These percentages of preterm birth by race substantially contribute to disparities in health outcomes for infant. Disparities will be discussed later in this chapter.

The increase in preterm birthrate is alarming in that it has an impact on:

■ The emotional well-being of parents
■ The length and quality of life for the preterm infant:
   ■ *A shorter gestational period increases the risk of complications related to immature body organs and systems that can have lifelong negative effects.*
   ■ *68.6% of all infant deaths occur in preterm infants (MacDorman & Mathews, 2008).*
■ The increased cost related to health care of preterm infants.

TABLE 1–4 PERCENTAGES OF PRETERM BIRTHS			
	1990	2005	2010
VERY PRETERM	1.92	2.03	1.97
MODERATELY PRETERM	1.4	1.6	1.53
LATE PRETERM	7.3	9.09	8.49
TOTAL PRETERM	10.61	12.73	11.99

Hamilton et al. (2011)

The increase in preterm birthrate may have a relationship to the increase of birthrates in women 35 years and older. As women age, they are at greater risk for complications during pregnancy such as gestational diabetes and hypertensive disorders. These complications can have an impact on the length of the pregnancy and the overall well-being of the developing fetus.

Neonatal Birth Weight Rates

Neonatal birth weight rates are reported by the CDC in three major categories of low, normal, and high. Normal birth weight is between 2,500 and 3,999 grams; high birth weight is 4,000 grams or greater; low birth weight is below 2,500 grams. Low birth weight is divided into two categories:

■ **Low birth weight (LBW)** is defined as birth weight that is less than 2,500 grams but greater than 1,500 grams.
■ **Very low birth weight (VLBW)** is defined as a birth weight that is less than 1,500 grams.

The National Vital Statistics Reports for 2010 birth data states that:

■ The percentage of LBW neonates has increased from 7.0 in 1990 to 8.15 in 2010.
■ The percentage of VLBW neonates has increased from 1.27 in 1990 to 1.45 in 2010 (Hamilton et al., 2011).

The weight of neonates at birth is an important predictor of future morbidity and mortality rates (Martin et al., 2011).

■ Neonates with birth weights between 4,000 and 4,999 grams have the lowest mortality rate during the first year of life.
■ VLBW neonates are 100 times more likely to die during the first year of life than are neonates with birth weights greater than 2,500 grams.
■ VLBW neonates account for 1.45% of all births but account for 54% of all infant deaths (Martin et al., 2011).

Infant Mortality Rates

Infant mortality is defined as a death before the first birthday. Infant mortality rates in the United States have significantly decreased from 47.0 per 1,000 live births in 1940 to 6.1 in 2011 (**Table 1-5**). This decrease is related to:

■ Improvement and advances in the knowledge and care of high-risk neonates
  ■ *Advances in medical technology such as extracorporeal membrane oxygenation therapy (ECMO) that is used for respiratory distress in preterm infants (see Chapter 17)*
  ■ *Advances in medical treatments such as exogenous pulmonary surfactant (see Chapter 17)*

Although this is a significant decrease, the infant mortality rate remains too high for a nation with the amount of available wealth and health care resources.

■ The 10 major causes of infant deaths are listed in **Table 1-6**.
  ■ *Between 1995 and 2010, there was a significant decrease in infant deaths related to sudden infant death syndrome (SIDS) and respiratory distress syndrome (RDS) of newborns.*
    ■ The decrease in SIDS can be attributed to instructing parents to place their infants on their backs to sleep versus on their stomachs.
    ■ The decrease in deaths related to RDS reflects advances in medical and nursing care of preterm infants.
■ The CDC, and the Health Resources and Service Administration in *Healthy People 2020*, have set a goal to decrease infant mortality rate to 6.0 per 1,000 live births by 2020.

CRITICAL COMPONENT

Infant Mortality

The infant mortality rate is highest for:

■ Mothers 16 years and younger related to socioeconomic status and being biologically immature.
■ Mothers older than 44 years of age related to an increased risk of complications due to age, such as gestational diabetes and hypertensive disorders.

Maternal Death and Mortality Rates

The Department of Health and Human Services classifies maternal deaths as follows:

■ **Maternal death** is defined by the World Health Organization (WHO) as the death of a woman during pregnancy or within 42 days of termination of pregnancy.

The death is related to the pregnancy or aggravated by pregnancy or management of the pregnancy. It excludes death from accidents or injuries.
■ **Direct obstetric death** is a death resulting from complications during pregnancy, labor/birth, and/or postpartum, and from interventions, omission of interventions, or incorrect treatment.
■ **Indirect obstetric death** is defined as a death that is due to a preexisting disease or a disease that develops during pregnancy that does not have a direct obstetrical cause, but its likelihood is aggravated by the changes of pregnancy.
■ **Late maternal death** is defined as a death that occurs more than 42 days after termination of pregnancy from a direct or indirect obstetrical cause.
■ **Pregnancy-related cause** is defined as maternal death during pregnancy or within 42 days of termination of pregnancy regardless of cause of death (Hoyert, 2007).

Maternal mortality rates have significantly decreased from 607.9 per 100,000 live births in 1915 to 7.1 in 1998 (Hoyert, 2007). In 1999, there was a change in the International Classification of Diseases (ICD) that added late maternal death and pregnancy-related causes to the ICD-10. Since the addition of these two classifications, the reported maternal mortality rate has increased from 9.9 per 100,000 in 1999 to 24.0 per 100,000 in 2009 (**Table 1-7**).

■ Worldwide there were an estimated 287,000 maternal deaths in 2010.
  ■ *99% of these deaths occur in developing countries.*
  ■ *Three-fifths of the deaths occur in the sub-Saharan Africa region.*
  ■ *47% decrease in maternal deaths from 1990 to 2010.*
    ■ This decrease of maternal deaths in developing countries is attributed to increased female education, increased use of contraception, improved antenatal care, and increased number of births attended by skilled health personnel (WHO, 2012).
■ Primary causes of maternal deaths worldwide are:
  ■ *Severe hemorrhage*
  ■ *Infections*
  ■ *Eclampsia*
  ■ *Obstructed labor*
  ■ *Complications of abortions*
  ■ *Other causes, such as anemia, HIV/AIDS, and cardiovascular disease (WHO, 2007)*

TABLE 1–5 INFANT MORTALITY RATES (RATES PER 1,000 LIVE BIRTHS)									
	1940	1950	1960	1970	1980	1990	2000	2005	2011
RATE	47.0	29.2	26.0	20.0	12.6	9.2	6.9	6.9	6.1
CIA (2011) and Murphy et al. (2012)									

TABLE 1–6 LEADING CAUSES OF INFANT DEATHS AND MORTALITY RATES (RATES PER 100,000 LIVE BIRTHS)

CAUSE OF DEATH	1995 RATE	CAUSE OF DEATH	2010 RATE
Congenital malformations and chromosomal abnormalities	168.1	Congenital malformations and chromosomal abnormalities	126.9
Disorders related to short gestation and low birth weight	100.9	Disorders related to short gestation and low birth weight	103.2
Sudden infant death syndrome	87.1	Sudden infant death syndrome	47.2
Respiratory distress of newborns	37.3	Newborn affected by maternal complications of pregnancy	38.9
Newborns affected by maternal complications of pregnancy	33.6	Accidents	26.1
Newborns affected by complications of placenta, cord, and membranes	24.7	Newborns affected by complications of placenta, cord, and membranes	25.7
Infections specific to the perinatal period	20.2	Bacteria sepsis of the newborn	14.2
Accidents	20.2	Disease of the circulatory system	12.5
Pneumonia and influenza	12.6	Respiratory distress of newborns	12.4
Intrauterine hypoxia and birth asphyxia	12.2	Necrotizing enterocolotits	11.7

Anderson et al. (1997) and Murphy et al. (2012)

TABLE 1–7 MATERNAL MORTALITY RATIOS 1990 TO 2009 (NUMBER OF MATERNAL DEATHS PER 100,000 LIVE BIRTHS)

DATE	1990	1995	2000	2005	2009
RATE	12	11	14	24	24

WHO (2010) and Martin et al. (2010)

TABLE 1–8 BIRTHRATES FOR TEENAGE WOMEN (RATES PER 1,000 LIVE BIRTHS)

AGE	1990	2005	2010	PERCENTAGE OF CHANGE
10–14	1.4	0.7	0.4	↓71%
15–17	37.5	21.4	17.3	↓54%
18–19	88.6	69.9	58.3	↓34%

Hamilton et al. (2011) and Martin et al. (2011)

ISSUES

Primary issues affecting the health of mothers and infants are birthrates for teenagers, tobacco use during pregnancy, substance abuse during pregnancy, obesity, and health disparities.

Birthrate for Teenagers

The birthrate for women age 10–19 in the United States:

■ Has decreased by 43% from 1990 to 2010 (Hamilton et al., 2011).
  ■ *The greatest percentage of decrease occurred in ages 10–14 (**Table 1-8**).*
■ Is higher than in other developed countries, with birthrate of 34.3 compared to Switzerland's rate of 3.9 (**Table 1-9**).

The U.S. birthrates for women 15–19 years of age by race are:

■ Hispanic—55.7
■ Non-Hispanic black—51.5
■ American Indian/Alaska Native—38.7
■ Non-Hispanic white—23.5
■ Asian/Pacific Islander—10.9 (Hamilton et al., 2011).

Teen births not only affect teen mothers but also have a long-term effect on their children and present a variety of issues for both the teen parents and society.

■ Poverty and income disparities
  ■ *75% of teen mothers begin receiving welfare within 5 years of the birth of their first child (The National Campaign to Prevent Teen Pregnancy, 2012).*

TABLE 1–9		2010 INTERNATIONAL FERTILITY RATE (BIRTHRATE PER 1,000 WOMEN AGES 15–19)	
NATION	RATE	NATION	RATE
Switzerland	3.9	Turkey	30.5
Italy	4.0	Egypt	40.6
Denmark	5.1	Botswana	43.8
France	6.0	Philippines	46.5
Japan	6.0	South Africa	50.4
Iceland	11.6	Argentina	54.2
Canada	11.3	Costa Rica	61.9
Australia	12.5	Mexico	65.5
Saudi Arabia	22.1	India	74.7
Russian Federation	23.2	Brazil	76.0
Unites States of America	27.4	Iraq	85.9
United Kingdom	29.7	Democratic Republic of the Congo	170.6
United Nations Statistics Division (2011)			

- *25% of teen mothers will have a second child within 24 months, which further decreases their ability to complete school and qualify for a well-paying job (The National Campaign to Prevent Teen Pregnancy, 2012).*
- *64% of children of teen mothers live in poverty (March of Dimes, 2009).*
- Health issues for teen mothers
  - *Teen mothers are at higher risk for sexually transmitted illnesses and HIV.*
    - Chlamydia – increased risk of newborn eye infection and pneumonia
    - Syphilis – neonatal blindness and increased risk of maternal and neonatal death
  - *Teen mothers are at higher risk for hypertensive problems during pregnancy.*
- Health issues of infants born to teen mothers
  - *Infants born to teen mothers are at greater risk for health problems that include prematurity and/or low birth weight.*
  - *Prematurity and/or low birth weight places the infant at higher risk for infant death, respiratory distress syndrome, intraventricular bleeding, vision problems, and intestinal problems.*
    - Infant mortality rate is higher: 16.4 for infants of women under 15 years of age compared to 6.8 for infants of women of all ages (National Campaign to Prevent Teen Pregnancy, 2012).

CRITICAL COMPONENT

Teen Pregnancies

- The average related cost for teen pregnancies to federal, state, and/or local government has increased from $9.1 billion in 2004 to $10.9 billion in 2008.
- The majority of the cost is related to consequences to the children of teen women, such as:
  - Increased health issues
  - Reduced educational achievement
  - Increased interactions with child welfare and criminal justice system. *(The National Campaign to Prevent Teen Pregnancy, 2012)*

- Educational issues
  - *Only 40% of teen mothers graduate from high school (The National Campaign to Prevent Teen Pregnancy, 2007).*
  - *Children of teen mothers are at higher risk for not completing high school and they have lower scores on standardized tests.*
- Teen fathers
  - *Teenage males without an involved father are at a higher risk for dropping out of school, abusing alcohol and/or drugs, and being incarcerated (The National Campaign to Prevent Teen Pregnancy, 2007).*
  - *Unmarried teen fathers pay less than $800 a year in child support (The National Campaign to Prevent Teen Pregnancy, 2007).*

Tobacco Use During Pregnancy

Tobacco use during pregnancy is associated with an increased risk of LBW, intrauterine growth restriction, miscarriage, abruptio placenta, premature birth, SIDS, and respiratory problems in the newborn.

- Cigarette smoking during pregnancy declined from 19.5% in 1989 to 13% in 2008 (Tong et al., 2009).
- Women who smoke during pregnancy are less likely to breastfeed their infants.
- 45% of women who smoked prior to pregnancy quit during pregnancy (Tong et al., 2009).
- 17% of women ages 18–24 and 19.8% of women ages 25–44 smoke cigarettes (MMWR, 2011).
- Based on race, the highest percentage of female smokers are American Indian and Alaskan Native (**Table 1-10**).
- Based on educational level, the highest percentage of female smokers are women with a GED (MMWR, 2011).

Substance Abuse During Pregnancy

The use of alcohol and illicit drugs during pregnancy can have a profound effect on the developing fetus and the health of the neonate.

- Exposure to alcohol during pregnancy places the developing fetus at higher risk for fetal death, low birth weight,

TABLE 1–10	PERCENTAGES OF WOMEN WHO ARE CIGARETTE SMOKERS	
RACE	PERCENTAGE
American Indian and Alaskan Native	36.0
Non-Hispanic white	19.6
Non-Hispanic black	17.1
Hispanic	9
Asian or Pacific Islander	4.3
MMWR, 2011	

intrauterine growth retardation, mental retardation, and fetal alcohol syndrome.

■ Exposure to illicit drugs during pregnancy is associated with incidences of preterm birth, abruptio placenta, drug withdrawal for the neonate, and a variety of congenital defects.

Obesity

Obesity is defined as a body mass index (BMI) greater than or equal to 30. In the United States, 35.7% of adults and 16.9% of children are obese (Ogden et al., 2012).

■ 31.9% of women 20–39 years are obese.
■ 17.1% of girls 12–19 years are obese (Ogden et al., 2012).

Obesity in childbearing women has adverse effects on both the woman and her child. Obese pregnant women are at higher risk for:

■ Gestational hypertension
■ Preeclampsia
■ Gestational diabetes
■ Thromboembolism
■ Cesarean birth
■ Wound infections
■ Shoulder dystocia related to macrosomia (birth weight of ≥ 4,000 grams)
■ Sleep apnea
■ Anesthesia complications (Nodine et al., 2012)

The fetuses and/or infants of obese pregnant women are at higher risk for:

■ Fetal abnormalities
  ■ *Spina bifida*
  ■ *Heart defects*
  ■ *Anorectal atresia*
  ■ *Hypospadias*
■ Intrauterine fetal death
■ Birth injuries related to macrosomia
■ Childhood obesity and diabetes (March of Dimes, 2012)

Health Disparities

The topic of health disparities addresses the differences in access, use of health care services, and health outcomes for various factors such as age, race, ethnicity, socioeconomic status, and geographic groups and health status of these populations.

The Agency for Healthcare Research and Quality (AHRQ) evaluates the quality of health care based on six core measures:

■ Effectiveness
■ Patient safety
■ Timeliness
■ Patient centeredness
■ Efficiency
■ Access to care (AHRQ, 2011)

In the AHRQ 2010 National Healthcare Disparities Report, it was reported that:

■ Based on race, Hispanics experienced the worst health care
■ Based on income, poor experienced the worst health care (AHRQ, 2011)

CRITICAL COMPONENT

Prenatal Care

Low-income women are less likely to seek early and continuous prenatal care. These health care behaviors place both the woman and her unborn child at higher risk for complications during pregnancy, labor, and birth, and postpartum.

■ The percentages of women who begin prenatal care late in the pregnancy or receive no prenatal care based on race are listed in **Table 1-11**.
■ Women under 15 years of age are the highest percentage of women of all ages who begin prenatal care late or receive no prenatal care (Martin et al., 2006).
■ Disparities exist in birth outcomes as measured by percentages of premature births and low birth weight (**Table 1-12**).
■ Disparities exist in infant mortality rates based on race (**Table 1-13**).

These disparities can partially be attributed to barriers to access to health care for low-income families. Examples of barriers to access to health care are limited finances, lack of transportation, difficulty with dominant language, and attitudes of the health care team.

POSITION STATEMENT

Access to Health Care
"AWHONN (Association of Women Health, Obstetric and Neonatal Nurses) considers access to affordable and acceptable health care services as a basic human right. Therefore, AWHONN strongly supports policy initiatives that guarantee access to such health care services for all people" (AWHOON, 2008).

TABLE 1–11   PERCENTAGES OF WOMEN RECEIVING LATE OR NO PRENATAL CARE BY RACE AND HISPANIC ORIGIN, 2006

AMERICAN INDIAN OR ALASKA NATIVE	ASIAN OR PACIFIC ISLANDER	HISPANIC	NON-HISPANIC BLACK	NON-HISPANIC WHITE
8.1	3.1	5.0	5.7	2.3

Child Trends (2010a)

TABLE 1–12   2004 REPORTED PERCENTAGES OF PRETERM BIRTH AND LOW BIRTH WEIGHT BY RACE

	PRETERM (BORN PRIOR TO 37 WEEKS)	VERY LOW BIRTH WEIGHT (>1,500 GRAMS)	LOW BIRTH WEIGHT (>2,500 GRAMS)
ALL	12.2	1.5	8.5
AMERICAN INDIAN/ ALASKA NATIVE	13.5	1.3	7.3
ASIAN/PACIFIC ISLANDER	10.8	1.1	8.3
HISPANIC	12.0	1.2	6.9
NON-HISPANIC BLACK	17.2	3.0	13.3
NON-HISPANIC WHITE	11.2	1.5	7.1

Martin et al. (2010)

TABLE 1–13   DEATH RATES OF INFANTS BY RACE AND HISPANIC ORIGIN, 2007 (DEATHS PER 100,000)

AMERICAN INDIAN OR ALASKAN NATIVE	ASIAN OR PACIFIC ISLANDER	HISPANIC	NON-HISPANIC BLACK	NON-HISPANIC WHITE
922	442	587	1,250	560

Child Trends (2010b)

MATERNAL AND CHILD HEALTH GOALS

The health of a nation is reflected in the health of expectant women and their infants (CDC and Health Resources and Service Administration, 2000). Diseases and illness related to complications during pregnancy and the neonatal period can have a lifelong impact on the health of that individual.

Low birth weight and premature neonates are at higher risk for chronic respiratory diseases and abnormalities in neurological development. The CDC and Health Resources and Services have set national health goals that are published in *Healthy People 2020* (**Table 1-14**). Improving the health of women before and during pregnancy and the health of infants will have lifelong effects on the health of the nation.

TABLE 1–14 *HEALTHY PEOPLE 2020* MATERNAL AND INFANT HEALTH GOALS

OBJECTIVES	BASELINE	2010 TARGET
Reduction in fetal and infant deaths.		
• Fetal deaths at 20 or more weeks of gestation	6.2 per 1,000 live births and fetal deaths	5.6 per 1,000 live births and fetal deaths
• Fetal and infant deaths during the perinatal period (28 weeks of gestation to 7 days after birth)	6.6 per 1,000 live births and fetal deaths	5.9 per 1,000 live births and fetal deaths
• All infant deaths	6.7 per 1,000 live births	6.0 per 1,000 live births
• Neonatal deaths	4.5 per 1,000 live births	4.1 per 1,000 live births
• Postnatal	2.2 per 1,000 live births	2.0 per 1,000 live births
• Infant deaths related to birth defects (all birth defects)	1.4 per 1,000 live birth	1.3 per 1,000 live births
• Infant deaths related to congenital heart defects	0.38 per 1,000 live births	0.34 per 1,000 live births
• Infant deaths from sudden infant death syndrome (SIDS)	0.55 per 1,000 live births	0.50 per 1,000 live births
• Infant deaths from sudden unexpected infant deaths (includes SIDS, unknown causes, accidental suffocation, and strangulation in bed)	0.93 per 1,000 live births	0.84 per 1,000 live births
Reduction of 1-year mortality rate for infants with Down syndrome.	48.6 per 1,000 infants diagnosed with Down's syndrome	43.7 per 1,000 infants diagnosed with Down's syndrome
Reduce the rate of maternal mortality.	12.7 maternal deaths per 100,000 live births	11.4 maternal deaths per 100,000 live births
Reduce maternal illness and complications due to pregnancy (complications during hospitalized labor and delivery).	31.1%	28.0%
Reduce cesarean births among low-risk (full-term, singleton, vertex presentation) women.		
• Women giving birth for first time	26.5%	23.9%
• Prior cesarean section	90.8% of low-risk women giving birth with prior cesarean section	81.7%
Reduce low birth weight (LBW) and very low birth weight (VLBW).		
• Low birth weight (LBW)	8.2 % of live births	7.8%
• Very low birth weight (VLBW)	1.5% of live births	1.4%
Reduce preterm births.		
• Total preterm births	12.7% of live births	11.4%
• Live births at 34 to 36 weeks of gestation	9.0%	8.1%
• Live births at 32 to 33 weeks of gestation	1.6%	1.4%
• Live births at less than 32 weeks gestation	2.0%	1.8%
Increase proportion of pregnant women who receive early and adequate prenatal care.		
• Prenatal care beginning in first trimester	70.8% women delivering live births	77.9%
• Early and adequate prenatal care	70.5% of pregnant females	77.6%
Increase abstinence from alcohol, cigarettes, and illicit drugs among pregnant women.		
• Alcohol	89.4% of pregnant females abstained from alcohol	98.3%
• Binge drinking	95% abstained from binge drinking	100%

Continued

TABLE 1–14 *HEALTHY PEOPLE 2020* MATERNAL AND INFANT HEALTH GOALS—cont'd		
OBJECTIVES	BASELINE	2010 TARGET
• Cigarette smoking	89.6% of pregnant females abstained from smoking	98.6
• Illicit drugs	94.9% abstained from illicit drugs	100%
Increase the proportion of women of childbearing potential with intake of at least 400 µg of folic acid from fortified foods or dietary supplements.	23.8% of non-pregnant women aged 15 to 44 years	26.2%
Reduce the proportion of women of childbearing potential who have low red blood cell folate concentrations.	24.5% of non-pregnant females aged 15 to 44 years	22.1%
Increase the proportion of women delivering a live birth who received preconception care services and practiced key recommended preconception health behaviors.		
• Took multivitamins/folic acid prior to pregnancy	30.1%	33.1%
• Did not smoke prior to pregnancy	77.6%	85.4%
• Did not drink alcohol prior to pregnancy (at least 3 months prior to pregnancy)	51%	56.4%
• Had a healthy weight prior to pregnancy	48.5%	53.4%
Increase the proportion of infants who are put to sleep on their backs.	69%	75.9%
Increase the proportion of infants who are breastfed.		
• Ever	74%	81.9%
• At 6 months	43.5%	60.6%
• At 1 year	22.7%	34.1%
• Exclusively through 3 months	33.6%	46.2%
• Exclusively through 6 months	14.1%	25.5%
Increase the proportion of employers that have worksite lactation support programs.	25%	38%
Reduce the proportion of breastfed newborns who receive formula supplementation within the first 2 days of life.	24.2%	14.2%
Increase the proportion of live births that occur in facilities that provide recommended care for lactating mothers and their babies.	2.9%	8.1%
Healthy People 2020 (2011)		

■ ■ ■ **Review Questions** ■ ■ ■

1. The population with the lowest birthrate but highest premature birthrate is:
   A. Non-Hispanic white
   B. Non-Hispanic black
   C. American Indian or Alaska Native
   D. Asian or Pacific Islanders
   E. Hispanic

2. Moderately premature neonates are neonates born:
   A. At less than 28 weeks of gestation
   B. Between 28 weeks and 30 weeks of gestation
   C. Between 30 and 32 weeks of gestation
   D. Between 32 and 34 weeks of gestation
   E. Between 34 and 36 weeks of gestation

3. The two most important predictors of an infant's health and survival after birth are:
   A. Gestational age and birth weight
   B. Gestational age and early prenatal care
   C. Gestational age and complication during labor and birth
   D. Gestational age and Apgar score

4. The greatest increase in birthrate is in women _____.
   A. 15–19 years of age
   B. 25–29 years of age
   C. 30–34 years of age
   D. 40–45+ years of age

5. A maternal and infant goal stated in *Healthy People 2020* is:
   A. Increase abstinence from smoking during pregnancy to 100%.
   B. Reduce cesarean birth for first-time mothers to 23.9%.
   C. Increase the proportion of infants who are breastfed at 6 months to 50%.
   D. Reduce the rate of maternal mortality to 5%.

6. The leading cause of infant death in 2010 was _____.
   A. Sudden infant death syndrome (SIDS)
   B. Congenital malformations
   C. Respiratory distress syndrome of newborns
   D. Accidents

7. The highest percentage of women who smoke during pregnancy are _____.
   A. American Indian and/or Alaskan Native
   B. Asian and/or Pacific Islander
   C. Hispanic
   D. Non-Hispanic black
   E. Non-Hispanic white

8. Infant mortality is defined as a death before _____.
   A. 28 days of age
   B. 6 months of age
   C. 1 year of age
   D. 18 months of age

9. Very low birth weight (VLBW) is defined as a birth weight less than _____.
   A. 500 grams
   B. 1,000 grams
   C. 1,500 grams
   D. 2,000 grams

10. True or False: Very low birth weight (VLBW) neonates account for 1.45% of births but account for 45% of all infant deaths.
    A. True
    B. False

References

Agency for Healthcare Research and Quality. (2011). *National Healthcare Disparities Report 2010.* Retrieved from www.ahrq.gov/qual/nhdr10/nhdr10.pdf

Anderson, R., Kockanek, K., & Murphy, S. (1997). Report of final mortality statistic, 1995. *Monthly vital statistics report, 45,* 11, sup 2. Hyattsville, MD: National Center for Health Statistics. Retrieved from www.cdc.gov/nchs/data/mvsr/supp/mv45

Centers for Disease Control and Prevention (CDC). (2007). *NCHS Definitions* [online]. Retrieved from www.cdc/gov/data/series/sr_21_008acc.pdf

Centers for Disease Control and Prevention, and Health Resources and Service Administration. (2000). *Healthy People 2010* [online]. Retrieved from www.healthypeople.gov/Document/HTML/Volume2/16MICH.htm

Central Intelligence Agency (CIA). (2011). *Rank Order—Infant Mortality Rates.* Retrieved from www.CIA.gov/library/publications/the-world-factbook/rankorder/2011rank.html

Child Trends Data Bank. (2010b). *Infant, child, and youth death rates.* Retrieved from www.childtrendsdatabank.org/?q=node/74

Child Trends Data Bank. (2010a). *Late or no prenatal care.* Retrieved from www.childtrendsdatabank.org/?q=node/243

Child Trends Data Bank. (2012). Birth and fertility rates. Retrieved from www.childtrendsdatabank.org

Hamilton, B., Martin, J., & Ventura, S. (2006). *Births: Preliminary data for 2005. Health E-Stats.* Retrieved from www.cdc/gov/nchs/products/pubs/pubd/hestats/prelimbirths05/prelimbirths05.htm

Hamilton, B., Martin, J., & Ventura, S. (2007). Preliminary data for 2006. *National Vital Statistics Reports, 56,* 1–28 [online]. Hyattsville, MD: National Center for Health Statistics. Retrieved from www.cdc.gov/nchs/data/nvsr/nvsr56/nvsr56_07.pdf

Hamilton, B., Martin, J., & Ventura, S. (2009). Preliminary data for 2007. *National Vital Statistics Reports, 57,* 1–23. Hyattsville, MD: National Center for Health Statistics.

Hamilton, B., Martin, J., & Ventura, S. (2011). Preliminary data for 2010. *National Vital Statistics Reports, 60,* 1–25. Hyattsville, MD: National Center for Health Statistics. Retrieved from www.cdc.gov/nchs/data/nvsr/nvsr60/nvsr60_02.pdf

Healthy People 2020. (2011). *Maternal, infant and child health.* Retrieved from www.healthypeople.gov/2020/topicsobjectives2020/overview.aspx?topics=26

Hoyert, D. (2007). Maternal mortality and related concepts. *National Center for Human Statistics. Vital Health Stats, 3,* 1–13.

MacDorman, M., & Mathews, T. (2008). *Recent trends in infant mortality in the United States.* NCHS data brief no. 9. Hyattsville, MD: National Center for Health Statistics. Retrieved from www.cdc.gov/nchs/data/databriefs/db09.htm

March of Dimes. (2009). Teen pregnancy. Retrieved from www.marchofdimes.com/printableArticles/medicalresources_teenpregnancy.html

March of Dimes. (2012). *Overweight and obesity during pregnancy.* Retrieved from www.marchofdimes.com/pregnancy/complications_obesity.html

Martin, J., Hamilton, B., Sutton, P., Ventura, S., Menacker, F., & Kirmeyer, S. (2006). *Final data for 2004. National vital statistics reports, 55,* 1–20. Retrieved from www.cdc.gov/nchs/data/nvsr/nvsr55/nvsr545_11.pdf

Martin, J., Hamilton, B., Ventura, S., Osterman, M., Kirmeyer, S., Mathews, T., & Wilson, E. (2011). Birth: Final data for 2009. *National Vital Statistic Reports, 57,* 1. Hyattsville, MD: National Center for Health Statistics.

MMWR (2011). Vital signs: Current cigarette smoking among young adults age ≥18 year. Retrieved from www.cdc.gov/tobacco/data_statistics/tables/trends/cig_smoking/index.htnm

Murphy, S., Xu, J., & Kochanek, K. (2012). Deaths: Preliminary data for 2010. *National vital statistics report, 60,* 4. Hyattsville, MD: National Center for Health Science.

The National Campaign to Prevent Teen Pregnancy. (2012). *Counting it up: The public costs of teen childbearing.* Retrieved from www.thenationalcampaign.org

The National Campaign to Prevent Teen Pregnancy. (2007). Why it matters. Retrieved from www.thenationalcampaign.org

Nodine, P., & Hstings-Tolsma, M. (2012). Maternal obesity: Improving pregnancy outcomes. *MCN, 37,* 110–115.

Ogden, C., Carroll, M., Kit, B., & Flegal, K. (2012). Prevalence of obesity in the United States, 2009–2010. *NCHS data brief, no. 82.* Retrieved from www.cdc.gov/nchs/data/databriefs/db82.pdf

Tong, V., Jones, J., Dietz, P., D'Angelo, D., & Bombard, J. (2009). Trends in smoking before, during and after pregnancy—Pregnancy risk monitoring system, United States, 31 sites, 2000–2005. Retrieved from www.cdc.gov/mmwr/preview/mmwrhtml/ss5804a1.htm

United Nations Statistics Division. (2011). Indicators on childbearing. Retrieved from www.unstats.un.org/unsd/demographic/products/socind/childbearing.htm

World Health Organization (WHO). (2007). *Maternal mortality in 2005.* Retrieved from www.who.int/reproductive-health/publications/maternal_mortality_2005/mme_2005.pdf

World Health Organization (WHO). (2012). *Maternal mortality.* Retrieved from www.who.int/mediacentre/factsheet/fs348/en/

Ethics and Standards of Practice Issues

2

EXPECTED STUDENT OUTCOMES

Upon completion of this chapter, the student will be able to:
- ☐ Define key terms.
- ☐ Debate ethical issues in maternity nursing.
- ☐ Explain standards of practice in maternity nursing.
- ☐ Describe legal issues in maternity nursing.
- ☐ Examine concepts in evidence-based practice.

INTRODUCTION

Maternity nursing is an exciting and dynamic area of nursing practice. With that excitement come issues related to ethical challenges, high rates of litigation in obstetrics, and the challenge of practicing safe and evidence-based nursing care that is responsive to the needs of women and families. This chapter presents the foundational principles set forth by the American Nurses Association (ANA) Code of Ethics and specialty practice standards from the Association for Women's Health, Obstetric and Neonatal Nurses (AWHONN) that outline duties and obligations of obstetric and neonatal nurses. Ethical principles are reviewed within the context of perinatal dilemmas and ethical decision making. Common issues in litigation in maternity nursing are presented. Evidence-based practice and challenges in research utilization in the perinatal setting are explored.

ETHICS IN NURSING PRACTICE

The study of ethics is based in philosophical discussions of ancient Greek scholars about the nature of good and evil or right and wrong. Ethics is an integral part of nursing practice and represents the ideal of social order. The ethical tradition of nursing is self-reflective, enduring, and distinctive. Nurses' moral and ethical responsibility to do the right thing is discussed in the ANA Code of Ethics for Nurses (2001).

ANA Code of Ethics

The ANA Code of Ethics makes explicit the primary goals, values, and obligations of the profession of nursing (ANA, 2001). The code of ethics for nursing serves as:

- ■ A statement of the ethical obligations and duties of every nurse

- ■ The profession's non-negotiable ethical standard
- ■ An expression of nursing's own understanding of its commitment to society

The ANA Code of Ethics for Nurses describes the most fundamental values and commitments of the nurse, boundaries of duty and loyalty, and aspects of duties beyond individual patient encounter (**Table 2-1**).

Ethical Principles

Ethical and social issues affecting the health of pregnant women and their fetus are increasingly complex. Some of the complexity arises from technological advances in reproductive technology, maternity care, and neonatal care (McCrink, 2010). Nurses are autonomous professionals who are required to provide ethically competent care. Some ethical principles related to patient care include (Lagana & Duderstadt, 2004):

- ■ **Autonomy:** The right to self-determination
- ■ **Respect for others:** Principle that all persons are equally valued
- ■ **Beneficence:** Obligation to do good
- ■ **Nonmaleficence:** Obligation to do no harm
- ■ **Justice:** Principle of equal treatment of others or that others be treated fairly
- ■ **Fidelity:** Faithfulness or obligation to keep promises
- ■ **Veracity:** Obligation to tell the truth
- ■ **Utility:** The greatest good for the individual or an action that is valued

Ethical Approaches

Clinical situations arise where ethical principles conflict with each other. For example, the patient's right to self-determination, autonomy, includes the right to refuse treatment that may be beneficial to the pregnancy outcome for the

TABLE 2–1	AMERICAN NURSES ASSOCIATION CODE OF ETHICS
PROVISION 1	The nurse, in all professional relationships, practices with compassion and respect for the inherent dignity, worth, and uniqueness of every individual unrestricted by consideration of social or economic status, personal attributes, or nature of the health problems.
PROVISION 2	The nurse's primary commitment is to the patient, whether an individual, family, group, or community.
PROVISION 3	The nurse promotes, advocates for, and strives to protect the health, safety, and rights of the patient.
PROVISION 4	The nurse is responsible and accountable for individual nursing practice and determines the appropriate delegation of tasks consistent with the nurse's obligation to provide optimum care.
PROVISION 5	The nurse owes the same duties to self as to others, including the responsibility to preserve integrity and safety, to maintain competence, and to continue personal and professional growth.
PROVISION 6	The nurse participates in establishing and maintaining health care environments and conditions of employment conducive to the provision of quality health care and consistent with the values of the profession through individual and collective action.
PROVISION 7	The nurse participates in the advancement of the profession through contributions to practice, education, administration, and knowledge development.
PROVISION 8	The nurse collaborates with other health professionals and the public in promoting community, national, and international efforts to meet health needs.
PROVISION 9	The profession of nursing, as represented by associations and their members, is responsible for articulating nursing values, for maintaining the integrity of the profession and its practice, and for shaping social policy.

American Nurses Association. (2001). *Code of ethics for nurses with interpretive statements.* Silver Spring, MD: American Nurses Publishing. Retrieved from http://www.nursingworld.org

fetus. Consideration of ethical approaches can help nurses as they encounter ethical dilemmas. There are a variety of ethical approaches. Two key approaches are:

■ The Rights Approach: The focus is on the individual's right to choose, and the rights include the right to privacy, to know the truth, and to be free from injury or harm.

■ The Utilitarian Approach: This approach posits that ethical actions are those that provide the greatest balance of good over evil and provide for the greatest good for the greatest number.

One can see how these two approaches could result in ethical dilemmas when decisions are made in clinical situations where the individual's right to choose may be in conflict with the greatest good for society.

Ethical Dilemmas

An **ethical dilemma** is a choice that has the potential to violate ethical principles (Lagana & Duderstadt, 2004). In nursing it is often based on the nurse's commitment to advocacy. Action taken in response to our ethical responsibility to intervene on behalf of those in our care is patient **advocacy**. Advocacy also involves accountability for nurses' responses to patients' needs (Lagana, 2000). A unique aspect of maternity nursing is that the nurse advocates for two patients, the woman and the fetus. The maternity nurse's advocacy role is more clearly assigned for the pregnant woman than for the fetus, yet the needs of the mother and fetus are interdependent (Lagana & Duderstadt, 2004). In order to be effective advocates, nurses need to recognize themselves as equal partners in

the health care team (Simmonds, 2008). Examples of ethical dilemmas in clinical practice are presented in **Box 2-1**.

Ethics in Neonatal Care

Ethics involves determining what is good, right, and fair (Pierce, 1998). The role of nurses in the neonatal intensive care unit (NICU) requires a dual role for nurses to protect the well-being of vulnerable infants as well as supporting and respecting parental decisions. According to the ANA Code of Ethics (2001), nurses have an obligation to safeguard the well-being of patients, but they also have the obligation to avoid inflicting harm. One example of a situation in which ethical decision making conflicts can arise is in the care of infants with extreme prematurity. Pierce (1998) suggests three categories for neonates in the NICU:

■ Infants in whom aggressive care would probably be futile, where prognosis for a meaningful life is extremely poor or hopeless

■ Infants in whom aggressive care would probably result in clear benefit to overall well-being, where prevailing knowledge and evidence indicate excellent chances for beneficial outcomes and meaningful interactions

■ Infants in whom the effect of aggressive care is mostly uncertain (**Fig. 2-1**).

Caring for infants in the face of prognostic uncertainty can present ethical dilemmas for nurses as they balance the needs of the infant's well-being with the parents' rights to make decisions. Nurses must continually involve parents in ongoing assessment of the infant's overall well-being. This

BOX 2–1 CLINICAL EXAMPLES OF PERINATAL ETHICAL DILEMMAS

- Court-ordered treatment
- Withdrawal of life support
- Harvesting of fetal organs or tissue
- In vitro fertilization and decisions for disposal of remaining fertilized ova
- Allocation of resources in pregnancy care during the previable period
- Fetal surgery
- Treatment of genetic disorders or fetal abnormalities found on prenatal screening
- Equal access to prenatal care
- Maternal rights versus fetal rights
- Extraordinary medical treatment for pregnancy complications
- Using organs from an anencephalic infant
- Genetic engineering
- Cloning
- Surrogacy
- Drug testing in pregnancy
- Sanctity of life versus quality of life for extremely premature or severely disabled infants
- Substance abuse in pregnancy
- Borderline viability: to resuscitate or not
- Fetal reduction
- Preconception gender selection

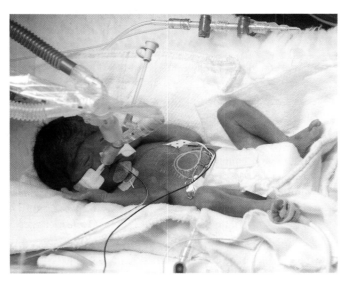

Figure 2-1   Extremely premature baby in NICU.

may be challenging as parents deal with the loss of a "dream" child, the shock of a critically ill neonate, or an unexpected pregnancy outcome. Nurses must report data and perceptions clearly to parents and actively listen to their concerns and understanding of current clinical reality and long-term prognosis. Team conferences with physicians, nurses, parents, and social workers can be crucial to developing plans of care. Lack of consensus about a plan of care can result in profound harm for the infants, families, the health care team, and society (Penticuff, 1998) and can include needless

suffering of the infant, psychological distress and conflict between the family and providers, and inappropriate expenditure of societal resources. Penticuff (1998) proposes that moral responsibility for the good and harm that comes to an infant in the NICU is not borne exclusively by either the parents or the health care team. Nurses and all health care providers are obligated to both respect parental wishes and uphold ethical standards. Legal and ethical precedent suggests that parents ought to be the chief decision makers (Nurse's Legal Handbook, 2004). However, parents often lack the expertise required to make decisions yet are ultimately required to care for the long-term needs of the child.

Collaboration among parents and professionals is essential to work for the infant's good when making treatment decisions for infants in the NICU. Collaborative working relationships encompass working together with mutual respect for the accountabilities of each profession to the shared goal of quality patient outcomes (Asokar, 1998). **Paternalism** is a system under which an authority makes decisions for others and should be avoided in decision making in health care.

Society holds the sanctity of life in high regard, as without life other values are irrelevant (Nurse's Legal Handbook, 2004). Questions emerge about the quality of life when caring for critically ill neonates. Nurses must first be clear about their moral and ethical perspective to be effective as part of the collaborative health care team. Nurses spend more time at the bedside providing care for neonates and interacting with parents than any other health professional. Central concepts in nursing are advocacy and caring. Nurses assume a key role in ethical decision making because of their unique position in all perinatal settings. Ethical sensitivity in professional practice develops in contexts of uncertainty; client suffering and vulnerability; and through relationships characterized by receptivity, responsiveness, and courage on the part of professionals. A little dose of practical wisdom goes a long way.

Ethics and Practice: Nurses' Rights and Responsibilities

AWHONN supports the protection of an individual nurse's right to choose to participate in any reproductive health care service or research activity. Nurses have the right under federal law to refuse to assist in the performance of any health care procedure, in keeping with their personal moral, ethical, or religious beliefs (AWHONN, 2009).

AWHONN considers access to affordable and acceptable health care services a basic human right. AWHONN advocates that nurses adhere to the following principles:

1. Nurses have the professional responsibility to provide nonjudgmental nursing care to all patients.
2. Nurses have the professional responsibility to provide high-quality, impartial nursing care to all patients in emergency situations, regardless of nurses' personal beliefs.
3. Nurses have a professional obligation to inform their employers of any attitudes and beliefs that may interfere with essential job functions.

STANDARDS OF PRACTICE

In addition to a Code of Ethics from the ANA (2001), practice standards help to guide professional nursing practice. AWHONN, the professional organization for maternity nurses, has developed practice standards.

AWHONN (2009) practice standards use ANA (2004) scope and standards of practice as its foundation. The standards summarize what AWHONN (2009) believes is the nursing profession's best judgment and optimal practice based on current research and clinical practice (**Table 2-2**). AWHONN believes that these standards are helpful for all nurses engaged in the functions described. As with most or

TABLE 2–2   STANDARDS FOR PROFESSIONAL NURSING PRACTICE IN THE CARE OF WOMEN AND NEWBORNS
STANDARDS OF CARE
STANDARD I. ASSESSMENT
The nurse gathers health data about women and newborns in the context of woman-centered and family-centered care.
STANDARD II. DIAGNOSIS
The nurse generates nursing diagnosis by analyzing assessment data to identify and differentiate normal physiologic and developmental transitions form pathophysiologic variations and other clinical issues in the context of woman-centered and family-centered care.
STANDARD III. OUTCOME IDENTIFICATION
The nurse individualizes expected outcomes for the women and newborns in the context of woman-centered and family-centered care.
STANDARD IV. PLANNING
The nurse generates a plan of care that includes interventions to attain expected outcomes for women and newborns in the context of woman-centered and family-centered care.
STANDARD V. IMPLEMENTATION
The nurse implements the interventions identified in the woman's or newborn's plan of care in the context of woman-centered and family-centered care.
STANDARD V (a). COORDINATION OF CARE
The nurse coordinates care to women and newborns in the context of woman-centered and family-centered care and within her/his scope of practice.
STANDARD V (b). HEALTH TEACHING AND HEALTH PROMOTION
The nurse uses teaching strategies that promote, maintain, or restore health in the context of woman-centered and family-centered care.
STANDARD VI. EVALUATION
The nurse evaluates the progress of women and newborns toward attainment of expected outcomes in the context of woman-centered and family-centered care.
STANDARDS OF PROFESSIONAL PERFORMANCE
STANDARD VII. QUALITY OF PRACTICE
The nurse evaluates and implements measures to improve quality, safety, and effectiveness of nursing for women and newborns.
STANDARD VIII. EDUCATION
The nurse acquires and maintains knowledge and competencies that utilize current evidence-based nursing practice for women and newborns.
STANDARD IX. PROFESSIONAL PRACTICE EVALUATION
The nurse evaluates her or his own nursing practice in relation to current evidence-based patient care information, professional practice standards and guidelines, statutes, and regulations.
STANDARD X. ETHICS
The nurse's decisions and actions on behalf of women, fetuses, and newborns are determined in an ethical manner and guided by a framework for an ethical decision making process.
STANDARD XI. COLLEGIALITY
The nurse interacts with and contributes to the professional development of other health care providers.

TABLE 2–2 STANDARDS FOR PROFESSIONAL NURSING PRACTICE IN THE CARE OF WOMEN AND NEWBORNS—cont'd

STANDARDS OF PROFESSIONAL PERFORMANCE

STANDARD XII. COLLABORATION AND COMMUNICATION

The nurse collaborates and communicates with women, families, health care providers, and the community in providing safe and holistic care.

STANDARD XII. RESEARCH

The nurse generates and/or uses evidence to identify, examine, validate, and evaluate interprofessional knowledge, theories, and varied approaches in providing care to women and newborns.

STANDARD XIV. RESOURCES AND TECHNOLOGY

The nurse considers factors related to safety, effectiveness, technology, and cost in planning and delivering care to women and newborns.

STANDARD XV. LEADERSHIP

Within appropriate roles in the setting in which the nurse functions, she or he should seek to serve as a role model, change agent, consultant, and mentor to women, families, and other health care professionals.

Association for Women's Health, Obstetric and Neonatal Nurses (AWHONN). (2009). *Standards for professional nursing practice in the care of women and newborns* (7th ed.). Washington, DC: Author.

all such standards, certain qualifications should be borne in mind.

- These standards articulate general guidelines; additional considerations or procedures may be warranted for particular patients or settings. The best interest of an individual patient is always the touchstone of practice.
- These standards are but one source of guidance. Nurses also must act in accordance with applicable law, institutional rules and procedures, and established interprofessional arrangements concerning the division of duties.
- These standards represent optimal practice. Full compliance may not be possible at all times with all patients in all settings.
- These standards serve as a guide for optimal practice. They are not designed to define standards of practice for employment, licensure, discipline, reimbursement, or legal or other purposes.
- These standards may change in response to changes in research and practice.
- The standards define the nurse's responsibility to the patient and the roles and behaviors to which the nurse is accountable. The definition of terms delimits the scope of the standards (**Table 2-3**).

The Standards of Practice set forth in this seventh edition are intended to define the roles, functions, and competencies of the nurse who strives to provide high-quality services to patients. The Standards of Professional Performance delineate the various roles and behaviors for which the professional nurse is accountable. The standards are enduring and should remain largely stable over time because they reflect the philosophical values of the profession (ANA, 2004).

LEGAL ISSUES IN DELIVERY OF CARE

Maternity nursing is the most litigious of all the areas of nursing. Contributing to this is the complexity of caring for two patients, the mother and the fetus. There are five clinical situations that account for a majority of fetal and neonatal injuries and litigation in obstetrics (Feinstein, Torgersen, & Atterbury, 2003):

- Inability to recognize and/or inability to appropriately respond to intrapartum fetal compromise
- Inability to effect a timely cesarean birth (30 minutes from decision to incision) when indicated by fetal or maternal condition
- Inability to appropriately initiate resuscitation of a depressed neonate
- Inappropriate use of oxytocin or misoprostol leading to uterine hyperstimulation, uterine rupture, and fetal intolerance of labor and/or fetal death
- Inappropriate use of forceps/vacuum and/or preventable shoulder dystocia

The number of obstetric malpractice claims represents only about 5% of all malpractice claims, but the dollar amount for the claims represents up to 35% of the total financial liability of a hospital or health care system (Simpson & Creehan, 2008). The literature indicates that patients who are more dissatisfied with the interpersonal interaction with health care providers are more likely to pursue litigation (Lagana, 2000). It has also been suggested that increased use of technology may interfere with a nurse's ability to engage with women and families in a therapeutic and caring interaction.

TABLE 2-3   TERMS RELATED TO STANDARDS

TERM	DEFINITION
ASSESSMENT	A systematic, dynamic process by which the nurse, through interaction with women, newborns and families, significant others, and health care providers, collects, monitors, and analyzes data. Data may include the following dimensions: psychological, biotechnological, physical, sociocultural, spiritual, cognitive, developmental, and economic, as well as functional abilities and lifestyle.
CULTURAL CONSCIOUSNESS	The acceptance of and respect for the attributes of diversity and includes the acknowledgement of both similarities and differences. Culturally competent care includes recognition and awareness of the cultural perspective of those who are served. Within the scope of law and institutional policies, providers should consider how best to adapt their treatment approach in light of the values and cultural preferences of the client.
CHILDBEARING AND NEWBORN HEALTH CARE	A model of care addressing the health promotion, maintenance, and restoration needs of women from the preconception through the postpartum period; and low-risk, high-risk, and critically ill newborns from birth through discharge and follow-up, within the social, political, economic and environmental context of the mother's, her newborn's, and the family's lives.
DIAGNOSIS	A clinical judgment about the patient's response to actual or potential health conditions or needs. Diagnoses provide the basis for determination of a plan of nursing care to achieve expected outcomes.
DIVERSITY	A quality that encompasses acceptance and respect related to but not limited to age, class, culture, people with special health care needs, education level, ethnicity, family structure, gender, ideologies, political beliefs, race, religion, sexual orientation, style, and values.
EVALUATION	The process of determining the patient's progress toward attainment of expected outcomes and the effectiveness of nursing care.
EXPECTED OUTCOMES	Response to nursing interventions that is measurable, desirable, and observable.
FAMILY-CENTERED MATERNITY CARE	A model of care based on the philosophy that the physical, sociocultural, psychological, spiritual, and economic needs of the woman and her family, however the family may be defined, should be integrated and considered collectively. Provisions of FCC require mutual trust and collaboration between the woman, her family, and health care professionals.
GUIDELINE	A framework developed through experts' consensus and review of the literature, which guides patient-focused activities that affect the provisions of care.
IMPLEMENTATION	The process of taking action by intervening, delegating, and/or coordinating. Women, newborns, families, significant others, or health care providers may direct the implementation of interventions within the plan of care.
OUTCOME	A measurable individual, family, or community state, behavior, or perception that is responsive to nursing interventions.
STANDARD	Authoritative statement defined and promoted by the profession and by which the quality of practice, service, or education can be evaluated.
STANDARDS OF PRACTICE	Authoritative statements that describe competent clinical nursing practice for women and newborns demonstrated through assessment, diagnosis, outcome identification, planning, implementation, and evaluation.
STANDARDS OF PROFESSIONAL PERFORMANCE	Authoritative statements that describe competent behavior in the professional role, including activities related to quality of practice, education, professional practice evaluation, ethics, collegiality, collaboration, communication, research, resources and technology, and leadership.
STANDARDS OF PROFESSIONAL PERFORMANCE	Authoritative statements that describe competent behavior in the professional role, including activities related to quality of care, performance appraisal, resource utilization, education, collegiality, ethics, collaboration, research, and research utilization.
WOMEN'S HEALTH CARE	A model of care addressing women's health promotion, maintenance, and restoration needs occurring across the lifespan and relating to one or more life strategies: adolescence, young adulthood, middle years, and older within the social, political, economic, and environmental context of their lives (AWHONN, 1999).

Association for Women's Health, Obstetric and Neonatal Nurses (AWHONN). (2009). *Standards for professional nursing practice in the care of women and newborns* (7th ed.). Washington, DC: Author.

Fetal Monitoring

One clinical issue that is often a key element of litigation is related to interpretation of fetal heart rate (FHR) monitoring and is related to the nurse's ability to recognize and appropriately respond to intrapartal fetal compromise. For that reason, this is the focus of this section and serves as an example of how nursing standards, guidelines, and policies should be the foundation of safe practice. Common allegations related to fetal monitoring are:

■ Failure to accurately assess maternal and fetal status
■ Failure to appreciate a deteriorating fetal status
■ Failure to treat an abnormal or indeterminate FHR
■ Failure to reduce or discontinue oxytocin with an abnormal or indeterminate FHR
■ Failure to correctly communicate maternal/fetal status to the care provider
■ Failure to institute the chain of command when there is a clinical disagreement

Nurses are accountable for safe and effective FHR assessment, and failure to do so contributes to claims of nursing negligence (Gilbert, 2007; Mahlmeister, 2000; Pearson, 2011). AWHONN (2000) provides a position statement on fetal assessment that states:

■ AWHONN strongly advises that nurses should complete a course of study that includes physiological interpretation of electronic fetal monitoring (EFM) and its implications for care in labor.
■ Each facility should develop a policy that defines when to use EFM and auscultation of FHR and that specifies frequency and documentation based on best available evidence, professional association guidelines, and expert consensus.

Timely communication and collaboration with care providers is essential to ensure Category II (indeterminate) or Category III (abnormal) FHR patterns are managed appropriately. Organizational resources and systems should be in place to support timely interventions when FHR is indeterminate or abnormal (Simpson & Knox, 2003). Uniform FHR terminology and interpretation are necessary to facilitate appropriate communication and legally defensible documentation (Lyndon & Ali, 2009).

Interpretation of FHR data can sometimes result in conflict. There may be agreement about ominous patterns and normal patterns, but often care providers encounter patterns that fall between these extremes (Freeman, 2002). Some issues of conflict in the clinical setting cannot be resolved between the caregivers immediately involved, yet need to be resolved quickly.

1. The nurse must initiate the course of action when the clinical situation is a matter of maternal or fetal well-being.
2. In a case of a primary care provider not responding to an abnormal FHR or a deteriorating clinical situation, the nurse should use the chain of command to resolve the situation, advocate for the patient's safety, and seek necessary interventions to avoid a potentially adverse outcome.
3. At the first level, notify the immediate supervisor to provide assistance. Further steps are defined by the structure of the institution, and a policy outlining communication for the chain of command should be present (**Fig. 2-2**).

Risk Management

Risk management is a systems approach to the prevention of litigation. It involves the identification of systems problems, analysis, and treatment of risks before a suit is brought (Gilbert, 2007). There are two key components of a successful risk management program:

■ Avoiding preventable adverse outcomes to the fetus during labor requires competent care providers who use consistent and current FHR monitoring language and who are in practice environments with systems in place that permit timely clinical intervention.
■ Decreasing risk of liability exposure includes methods to demonstrate evidence that appropriate timely care was provided that accurately reflects maternal fetal status before, during, and after interventions occurred.

Not all adverse or unexpected outcomes are preventable or are the result of poor care. Authors suggest (Simpson & Creehan, 2008; Simpson & Knox, 2003) the risk of liability can be reduced and injuries to mothers and neonates can be reduced when all members of the perinatal team follow two basic tenets:

■ Use applicable evidence and/or published standards and guidelines as the foundation of care.
■ Make patient safety a priority over convenience, productivity, and costs.

All nurses need to bear in mind that the most and sometimes the only defensible nursing actions are those that have

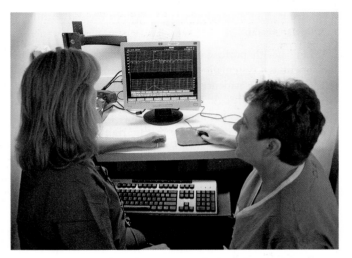

Figure 2–2 Together the nurse and physician review an EFM strip.

as their sole focus the health and well-being of the patient (Greenwald & Monder, 2003).

EVIDENCE-BASED PRACTICE

Health care professions are moving toward thinking that practice decisions ought to be made with the best available knowledge or evidence. Evidence-based practice (EBP) and terms such as evidence-based medicine (EBM) and evidence-based nursing (EBN) reflect a very important global paradigm shift in how to view health care outcomes, how the discipline is taught, how practice is conducted, and how health care practices are evaluated for quality (Milton, 2007).

In the early 1990s in the United States, the Agency for Health Care Policy and Research (AHCPR) was established with interdisciplinary teams to gather and assess available research literature and develop evidence-based clinical guidelines. Nurses were prominent members of the interdisciplinary teams who performed this early work. In the mid-1990s, AHCPR was changed to the Agency for Healthcare Research and Quality (AHRQ), and it now has a clearinghouse for clinical guidelines (http://www.guidelines.gov).

The National Guideline Clearinghouse is a publicly available database of evidence-based clinical practice guidelines (CPGs). The database is regularly updated and is therefore an important resource for clinicians. We recommend the National Guideline Clearinghouse as the first place clinicians go to assess whether an established guideline is available. For CPG to be considered by the National Guideline Clearinghouse it must meet four rigorous criteria (AHRQ, 2000):

1. Contains systematically developed recommendations, strategies, or other information to assist health care decision making in specific clinical circumstances.
2. Produced under the auspices of a relevant professional organization.
3. Development process included a verifiable, systematic literature search and review of the existing literature published in peer-reviews journals.
4. Current, that is developed, reviewed, or revised within the last 5 years.

Many health professionals have chosen to view the EBP movement as a systematic approach to determine the most current and relevant evidence upon which to base decisions about patient care (Melnyk & Fineout-Overholt, 2005). Rigorously conducted research that reports findings that are "good evidence" may not always translate to the "right" decisions for an individual patient. Most authors and clinicians have extended the definition of **evidence-based practice (EBP)** to include the integration of best *research evidence, clinical expertise,* and *patient values* in making decisions about the care of patients (Reilly, 2004). Clinical expertise comes from knowledge and experience over time. Patient values are the unique circumstances of each patient and should include patient preferences. Characteristics of best research evidence are quantitative evidence such as clinical trials and laboratory experiments, evidence from qualitative research, and evidence from experts in practice.

Quality and Safety Education for Nurses (QSEN) Evidence-Based Practice

QSEN EBP definition: Integrate best current evidence with clinical expertise and patient/family preferences and values for delivery of optimal health care.

Nurses are in a unique position to explore a woman's preferences, and advocate for the use of best current evidence and clinical expertise for delivery of optimal health care. Some suggestions to foster EBP in clinical settings include:

■ Describe and be able to locate reliable sources for locating evidence reports and clinical practice guidelines
■ Question rationale for routine approaches to care that result in less-than-desired outcomes or adverse events
■ Base individualized care plan on patient values, clinical expertise, and evidence

---

Evidence-Based Practice Research: Cochrane Reviews

An important resource for evidence-based practice is systematic reviews. One such source is Cochrane Reviews (http://www.cochrane.org). The Cochrane Review is an international consortium of experts who perform systematic reviews and meta-analysis on all available data, evaluating the body of evidence on a particular clinical topic for quality of study design and study results. These reviews look at randomized clinical trials of interventions related to a specific clinical problem and, after assessing the findings from rigorous studies, make recommendations for clinical practice. They consider the randomized controlled trial (RCT) as the gold standard of research evidence.

Although not absolute, a hierarchy of evidence can be helpful when evaluating research evidence. When considering potential interventions, nurses should look for the highest level of available evidence relevant to the clinical problem. A hierarchy of strength of evidence for treatment decisions is presented in **Box 2-2**, indicating unsystematic clinical observations as the lowest level and systematic reviews of RCTs as the highest level of evidence.

Evidence-Based Nursing

Evidence-based nursing (EBN) has become an internationally recognized although sometimes contested part of nursing practice (Flemming, 2007). EBN is central to the knowledge base for nursing practice. Critics of EBN dislike the central role that randomized controlled trials (RCTs) take in providing evidence for nursing, claiming that the context and experience of nursing care are removed from evaluation of evidence. One of the principles of evidence-based health care has been driven by requirements to deliver quality care within economically constrained conditions (Critical Component: Evidence-Based Nursing).

Some nurses have adopted a predominantly medical model of evidence, with RCTs as the central, methodological approach to define good evidence. EBN has been criticized for this stance, focusing on the lack of relevance of RCTs for nursing practice. Criticisms stem from the fact that RCTs are

CRITICAL COMPONENT

Evidence-Based Nursing

To practice EBN, a nurse is expected to combine the best research evidence with clinical expertise while taking into account the patients' preferences and their situation in the context of the available resources. Evidence-based decision making should include consideration of the patients' clinical state, clinical setting, and clinical circumstances (DiCenso, Ciliska, & Guyatt, 2005).

BOX 2–2 HIERARCHY OF STRENGTH OF EVIDENCE FOR TREATMENT DECISIONS

Systematic reviews of randomized clinical trials (i.e., Cochrane Reviews)

↑

Single randomized trial (individual RCT research)

↑

Systematic review of observational studies addressing patient important outcomes

↑

Single observational studies addressing patient important outcomes

↑

Physiological studies (i.e., studies of indicators such as blood pressure)

↑

Unsystematic clinical observations (clinical observations made by practitioners over time)

DiCenso, A., Guyatt, G., & Ciliska, D. (Eds.) (2005) , *Evidence-based nursing: A guide to clinical practice*. St. Louis, MO: Elsevier Mosby.; DiCenso, A., Bayley, L., & Haynes, R. (2009). Accessing preappraised evidence: fine-tuning the 5S model into a 6S model (Editorial). ACP Journal Club, 151(3), 1.

given an illusionary stance of credibility, when there may not be credible evidence relevant to nursing practice.

Utilization of Research in Clinical Practice

To enhance EBP and support the choices of childbearing women and families, we must utilize qualitative research findings in practice (Durham, 2002). Although nursing has developed models for assisting a practitioner in applying research findings in practice (Cronenwett, 1995; Stetler, 1994; Titler & Goode, 1995), these models only assist in applying quantitative research.

Qualitative research is increasingly recognized as an integral part of the evidence that imforms evidence-based practice. Qualitative researchers investigate naturally occurring phenomena and describe, analyze, and sometimes develop a theory on the phenomena. They also describe the context and relationships of key factors related to the phenomena. This kind of work is conducted in the "real world," not in a controlled situation, and yields important findings for practice. Practitioners may not be aware of qualitative research findings, or, if they are, they may not be able to apply the findings. Reports of qualitative research

should be more readily understood by persons in practice as they are conveyed in language that is more understandable to the practitioner. Story lines from qualitative research are often a more compelling and culturally resonant way to communicate research findings, particularly to staff, affected groups, and policy makers (Sandelowski, 1996). Despite the fact that qualitative research is conducted in the "real world" and is more understandable to many practitioners, as with quantitative research utilization, a gap sometimes exists between the world of qualitative research and the world of practice. A creative bridge between these worlds is needed. Some guidelines for bridging that gap are outlined by Swanson, Durham, and Albright (1997) and include evaluating the findings or proposed theory for its context, generalizability, and fit with one's own practice; evaluating the concepts, conditions, and variation explained in the findings; and evaluating findings for enhancing and informing one's practice.

In the current era of cost containment, nurses must know what is going on in the real world of their patients because practitioners are limited to interacting with clients within an ever-smaller window of time and space. Qualitative research can assist in bringing practitioners an awareness of that larger world and its implications for their scope of practice (Swanson, Durham, & Albright, 1997). Qualitative research describes and analyzes our patients' realities. The research findings have the capacity to influence conceptual thinking and cause practitioners to question assumptions about a phenomenon in practice (Cronenwett, 1995). Incorporating qualitative research as evidence to support research-based practice has the capacity not only to enhance nursing practice but also to resolve some of the tensions between art and science with which nurses sometimes find themselves struggling (Durham, 2002).

Research Utilization Challenges

Health care often falls short in translating research into practice and improvement of care. While adopting EBP has resulted in improvements in patient outcome, large gaps remain between what we know and what we do (Scott, 2010). Failing to use the latest health care research is costly, harmful, and can lead to use of ineffective care.

Many innovations have become common practice in perinatal nursing:

■ Fetal monitoring
■ Mother/baby care
■ Early postpartum discharge

These changes in care were influenced by:

■ Medical and technological innovations
■ Social context of the time and families' preferences
■ Health care costs

How nurses respond to the increasing use of technology during birth, threats of litigation, and providing the best care under time and cost constraints are the realities facing current perinatal nursing care today (Martell, 2006; Lothian, 2009).

Continuous electronic fetal monitoring (EFM) in labor is one of the most common interventions during labor. However, there is little evidence to support the use of continuous electronic fetal monitoring, in particular with low-risk patients. Two Cochrane Reviews compared the efficacy and safety of routine continuous EFM of labor with intermittent auscultation (Alfirevic, Devane, & Gyte, 2008; Thacker, Stroup, & Chang, 2006). The reviewers concluded that use of routine EFM has no measurable impact on infant morbidity and mortality. In the latest review the authors concluded continuous EFM during labor is associated with a reduction in neonatal seizures but no significant differences in cerebral palsy, infant mortality, or other standard measures of neonatal well-being. However, continuous EFM was associated with an increase in caesarean births and operative vaginal births. They noted the real challenge is how best to convey this uncertainty to women to enable them to make an informed choice without compromising the normality of labor.

Although EBP is the goal of nursing care and has become the standard of care in the United States, the evidence about EFM has not been used in practice (Wood, 2003). Research evidence does not support the use of continuous EFM. Despite this, many reasons contribute to its continued use, such as habit, convenience, liability, staffing, and economics (Woods, 2003). It is no longer acceptable for nurses to continue doing things the way they have always been done, by tradition without questioning whether or not it is the best approach. One way nurses can ensure EBP in their setting is by participating in multidisciplinary teams that generate research-based practice guidelines.

■ ■ ■ **Review Questions** ■ ■ ■

1. The organization that publishes standards and guidelines for maternity nursing is the:
   A. National Perinatal Association
   B. American Nurses Association
   C. American Academy of Pediatrics
   D. Association of Women's Health, Obstetrics and Neonatal Nursing

2. Autonomy is defined as the right to:
   A. Do good
   B. Equal treatment
   C. Self-determination
   D. Be valued

3. An ethical dilemma is:
   A. A violation of patient autonomy
   B. A choice that violates ethical principles
   C. A conflict between advocacy and respect
   D. A conflict between what is just and good

4. Evidence-based decision making should include consideration of:
   A. Best research evidence, patient's clinical state, and clinical setting
   B. Best research evidence, patient's acuity, and financial considerations
   C. Best research evidence, clinical expertise, and patient values
   D. Best research evidence, clinical resources, and patient values

5. Risk management is an approach to the prevention of:
   A. Morbidity and mortality
   B. Litigation
   C. Staff conflicts
   D. Poor care

6. A response to nursing interventions that are measurable and observable are:
   A. Variables
   B. Guidelines
   C. Health dimensions
   D. Expected outcomes

7. A _____ is a framework developed through expert consensus and review of the literature.
   A. Guideline
   B. Outcome
   C. Standard
   D. Evaluation

8. Failing to use the latest health care research is
   A. Unsafe
   B. Costly and harmful
   C. Costly, harmful, and can lead to use of ineffective care
   D. Risky

9. Nurses have the professional responsibility to provide high-quality, impartial nursing care to all patients in _____, regardless of the nurses' personal beliefs.
   A. Emergency situations
   B. Urgent situations
   C. Safe situations
   D. Every situation

10. To be effective advocates for patients and their families, the nurse needs to:
    A. Talk to patients about their concerns
    B. Recognize themselves as equal partners in the health care team
    C. Assume the patients' needs
    D. Ask family members about key health care decisions

References

Alfirevic, Z. D., Devane, D., & Gyte G. M. (2008). Continuous cardiotocography (CTG) as a form of electronic fetal monitoring (EFM) for fetal assessment during labour. *Cochrane Database of Systematic Reviews* 2006, Issue 3. Art. No.: CD006066. doi:10.1002/14651858.CD006066.

American Nurses Association. (2004). Nursing: Scope and standards of practice. Washington, DC: Author.

American Nurses Association (ANA). (2001). *Code of ethics for nurses with interpretive statements*. Silver Spring, MD: American Nurses Publishing. Retrieved from http://www.nursingworld.org/ethics/ecode.htm

Aroskar, M. (1998). Ethical working relationships in patient care: Challenges and possibilities. *Nursing Clinics of North America, 33*(2), 287–293.

Association for Women's Health, Obstetric ad Neonatal Nurses (AWHONN). (2009). Ethical Decision Making in the Clinical Setting: Nurses' Rights and Responsibilities. *Journal of Obstetrics/Gynecology and Neonatal Nursing, 741,* 38.

Association for Women's Health, Obstetric and Neonatal Nurses (AWHONN). (2000). *Fetal Assessment Clinical Position Statement.* Washington, DC: Author.

Association for Women's Health, Obstetric and Neonatal Nurses (AWHONN). (2009). *Standards for professional nursing practice in the care of women and newborns* (7th ed.). Washington, DC: Author.

Cronenwett, L. (1995). Effective methods for disseminating research findings to nurses in practice. *Nursing Clinics of North America, 30*(3), 429–438.

DiCenso, A., Bayley, L., & Haynes, R. (2009). Accessing preappraised evidence: fine-tuning the 5S model into a 6S model (Editorial). ACP Journal Club, *151*(3), 1.

DiCenso, A., Ciliska, D., & Guyatt, G. (2005). Introduction to evidence-based nursing. In: A. DiCenso, G. Guyatt, & D. Ciliska (Eds.), *Evidence-based nursing: A guide to clinical practice* (pp. 3–19). St. Louis: Elsevier Mosby.

Durham, R. (2002). Women, work and midwifery. In R. Mander & V. Flemming (Eds.), *Failure to progress* (pp. 122–132). London: Routledge.

Flemming, K. (2007). The knowledge base for evidence-based nursing: A role for mixed methods research? *Advances in Nursing Science, 30*(1), 41–51.

Freeman, R. (2002). Problems with intrapartal fetal heart rate monitoring interpretation and patient management. *American Journal of Obstetrics and Gynecology, 100*(4), 813–816.

Gilbert, E. (2007). *Manual of high risk pregnancy and delivery.* St. Louis: C. V. Mosby.

Greenwald, L., & Mondor, M. (2003). Malpractice and the Perinatal Nurse. *Journal of Perinatal & Neonatal Nursing, 17*(2), pp. 101–109.

Lagana, K. (2000). The "right" to a caring relationship: The law and ethic of care. *Journal of Perinatal & Neonatal Nursing, 14*(2), 12–24.

Lagana, K., & Duderstadt, K. (2004). *Perinatal and neonatal ethics: Facing contemporary challenges.* White Plains, NY: March of Dimes.

Lothian, J. (2009). Ethics and Maternity Care: From Principles to Practice. *Journal of Perinatal Education, 18*(1), 1–3.

Lyndon, A., & Ali, L. (Eds.). (2009). *AWHONN's Fetal Heart Monitoring Principles and Practices* (4th ed.). Washington, DC: Association of Women's Health, Obstetric and Neonatal Nurses.

Mahlmeister, L. (2000). Legal implications of fetal heart rate assessment. *JOGNN, 29*, 517–526.

Martell, L. (2006). From innovation to common practice: Perinatal nursing pre 1970 to 2005. *Journal of Perinatal & Neonatal Nursing, 20*(1), 8–16.

McCrink, A. (2010). Ethical Nursing Practice. *Nursing for Women's Health, 14*(6), 443–446.

Melnyk, B. M., & Fineout-Overholt, E. (2005). *Evidence-based practice in nursing and healthcare: A guide to best practice.* Philadelphia: Lippincott Williams & Wilkins.

Milton, C. L. (2007). Evidence-based practice: Ethical questions for nursing. *Nursing Science Quarterly, 20*(2), 123–126.

Nurse's Legal Handbook (5th ed.) (2004). Philadelphia: Lippincott Williams & Wilkins.

Pearson, N. (2011). Oxytocin Safety. *Nursing for Women's Health, 15*(2), 110–117.

Penticuff, J. (1998). Defining futility in neonatal intensive care. *Nursing Clinics of North America, 33*(2), 339–352.

Pierce, S. F. (1998). Neonatal intensive care: Decision making in the face of prognostic uncertainty. *Nursing Clinics of North America, 33*(2), 287–293.

Reilly, B. (2004). The essence of EBM. *British Medical Journal, 329*, 991–992.

Sandelowski, M. (1996). Using qualitative methods in intervention studies. *Research in Nursing and Health, 19*, 359–364.

Scott, S. D. (2010). Achieving Consistent Quality Care. Using Research to Guide Clinical Practice. Second Ed. Association of Women's Health, Obstetrics and Neonatal Nursing (AWHONN).

Simmonds, A. H. (2008). Autonomy and Advocacy in Perinatal Nursing Practice. *Nursing Ethics, 15*(3), 360–370.

Simpson, K., Creehan, P., & Association of Women's Health, Obstetrics and Neonatal Nursing. (2008). *Perinatal nursing* (3rd ed.). Philadelphia: Lippincott Williams & Wilkins.

Simpson, K., & Knox, E. (2003). Common area of litigation related to care during labor and birth: Recommendations to promote patient safety and decrease risk exposure. *Journal of Perinatal and Neonatal Nursing, 17*(2), 110–125.

Stetler, C. (1994). Refinement of the Stetler/Marram model for application of research findings to practice. *Nursing Outlook, 42*, 15–25.

Swanson, J., Durham, R., & Albright, J. (1997). Clinical utilization/application of qualitative research. In J. Morse (Ed.), *Completing a qualitative project: Details and dialogue* (pp. 253–282). Thousand Oaks, CA: Sage.

Thacker, S., Stroup, D., & Chang, M. (2006). *Continuous electronic heart rate monitoring for fetal assessment during labor.* (Cochrane Review). In: The Cochrane Library Issue 3, 2006. Art No: CD000063. DO1:10, 1002/14651858 CD000063. pub.2.

Titler, M., & Goode, C. (1995). Research utilization. *Nursing Clinics of North America, 30*(3), xv.

Woods, S. (2003). Should women be given a choice about fetal assessment in labor? *The American Journal of Maternal/Child Nursing, 28*(5), 292–298.

Genetics, Conception, Fetal Development, and Reproductive Technology

EXPECTED STUDENT OUTCOMES

Upon completion of this chapter, the student will be able to:

☐ Define key terms.
☐ Discuss the relevance of genetics within the context of the care of the childbearing family.
☐ Identify critical components of conception, embryonic development, and fetal development.
☐ Describe the development and function of the placenta and amniotic fluid.
☐ List the common causes of infertility.
☐ Describe the common diagnostic tests used in diagnosing causes of infertility.
☐ Describe the most common methods used in assisted fertility.
☐ Discuss the ethical and emotional implications of assisted reproductive therapies.

GENETICS AND THE CHILDBEARING FAMILY

Advances in **genetics,** the study of heredity, and **genomics,** the study of genes and their function and related technology, are providing better methods for:

- preventing diseases and abnormalities,
- diagnosing diseases,
- predicting health risks, and
- personalizing treatment plans.

CRITICAL COMPONENT

Genetics and Genomics

"The main difference between genomics and genetics is that genetics scrutinizes the functioning and composition of the single gene whereas genomics addresses all genes and their interrelationships in order to identify their combined influence on the growth and development of the organism."

WHO, 2012

Genes

- Genes are composed of DNA (hereditary material) and protein.
- They are the basic functional and physical units of heredity.
- There are approximately 30,000 genes in the human genome.
  - *The **genome** is an organism's complete set of DNA.*
- Numerous genes are located on each human chromosome.
  - *Each human cell contains 46 chromosomes.*
  - *There are 22 homologous pairs of chromosomes and one pair of sex chromosomes (XX or XY).*
- **Genotype** refers to a person's genetic makeup.
- **Phenotype** refers to how the genes are outwardly expressed (i.e., eye color, hair color, height).

Dominant and Recessive Inheritance

- Genes are either dominant or recessive. When there is both a dominant and a recessive gene in the pair, the traits of the dominant gene are present.
- The traits of the recessive gene are present when both genes of the pair are recessive.

Don't have time to read this chapter? Want to reinforce your reading? Need to review for a test?
Listen to this chapter on Davis*Plus*.

■ Genetic diseases or disorders are usually related to a defective recessive gene and present in the developing human when both pairs of the gene have the same defect.
  ■ *Examples of common recessive genetic disorders are cystic fibrosis, sickle cell anemia, thalassemia, and Tay-Sachs disease (**Table 3-1**).*
  ■ *A person who has only one recessive gene for a disorder is known as a carrier and does not present with the disorder.*
■ Genetic disorders related to a dominant gene are rare.

Sex-Linked Inheritance

■ Also referred to as X-linked inheritance or traits (see Table 3-1)
■ These are genes or traits that are located only on the X chromosome. These genes can be either recessive or dominant. The Y chromosome does not have the corresponding genes for some of the X chromosome's genes.
■ A male child who receives an X chromosome with a disorder of one or more of its genes presents with the disorder when the Y chromosome does not carry that gene; the gene, even though it may be recessive, becomes dominant.
■ Female children who have one X chromosome with a sex-linked trait disorder do not present with the trait, but are carriers of the trait.

Relevance of Genetics in the Care of the Childbearing Family

■ The scientific knowledge of genetics is rapidly increasing with the desire that gene therapy will be used to correct genetic disorders such as heart disease, diabetes, and Down syndrome.

■ The Human Genome Project, a 13-year international, collaborative research program that was completed in 2003, has provided the scientific community with valuable information that is being used in the diagnosis, treatment, and prevention of genetically linked disorders.
■ 10% of all abnormalities of the developing human are due to genetic factors (Sadler, 2004).

Genetic Testing

■ There are several genetic tests that are selectively used in the care of the childbearing families. These include:
  ■ *Carrier testing*
    ■ Used to identify individuals who carry one copy of a gene mutation that, when present in two copies, causes a genetic disorder.
    ■ Used when there is a family history of a genetic disorder.
      ■ *When both prospective parents are tested, the test can provide information about their risk of having a child with a genetic condition.*
  ■ *Preimplantation testing, also known as preimplantation genetic diagnosis (PGD)*
    ■ Used to detect genetic changes in embryos that are created using assisted reproductive techniques.
  ■ *Prenatal testing*
    ■ Allows for the early detection of genetic disorders, such as trisomy 21, hemophilia, and Tay-Sachs disease.
  ■ *Newborn screening*
    ■ Used to detect genetic disorders that can be treated early in life.

TABLE 3–1   GENETIC DISEASES

DISEASE (PATTERN OF INHERITANCE)	DESCRIPTION
SICKLE-CELL ANEMIA (R)	The most common genetic disease among people of African ancestry. Sickle-cell hemoglobin forms rigid crystals that distort and disrupt red blood cells (RBCs); oxygen-carrying capacity of the blood is diminished.
CYSTIC FIBROSIS (R)	The most common genetic disease among people of European ancestry. Production of thick mucus clogs in the bronchial tree and pancreatic ducts. Most severe effects are chronic respiratory infections and pulmonary failure.
TAY-SACHS DISEASE (R)	The most common genetic disease among people of Jewish ancestry. Degeneration of neurons and the nervous system results in death by the age of 2 years.
PHENYLKETONURIA OR PKU (R)	Lack of an enzyme to metabolize the amino acid phenylalanine leads to severe mental and physical retardation. These effects may be prevented by the use of a diet (beginning at birth) that limits phenylalanine.
HUNTINGTON'S DISEASE (D)	Uncontrollable muscle contractions between the ages of 30 and 50 years, followed by loss of memory and personality. There is no treatment that can delay mental deterioration.
HEMOPHILIA (X-LINKED)	Lack of factor VIII impairs chemical clotting; may be controlled with factor VIII from donated blood.
DUCHENNE'S MUSCULAR DYSTROPHY (X-LINKED)	Replacement of muscle by adipose or scar tissue, with progressive loss of muscle function; often fatal before age 20 years due to involvement of cardiac muscle.

R = recessive; D = dominant.
Scanlon & Sanders (2007).

■ Couples who have a higher risk for conceiving a child with a genetic disorder include:
  ■ *Maternal age older than 35*
  ■ *History of previous pregnancy resulting in a genetic disorder or newborn abnormalities*
  ■ *Man and/or woman who has a genetic disorder*
  ■ *Family history of a genetic disorder*
■ Diagnosis of genetic disorders during pregnancy provides parents with options to:
  ■ *Continue or terminate the pregnancy*
  ■ *Prepare for a child with this genetic disorder*
  ■ *Use gene therapy when available*
■ Nursing Actions
  ■ *Nursing actions for couples who elect to terminate the pregnancy based on information from genetic testing are:*
    ■ Explain the stages of grief they will experience.
    ■ Inform the couple that grief is a normal process.
    ■ Encourage the couple to communicate with each other and share their emotions.
    ■ Refer the couple to a support group if available in their community.
  ■ *Nursing actions for couples who elect to continue the pregnancy based on information from genetic testing are:*
    ■ Provide them additional information about the genetic disorder.
    ■ Refer them to support groups for parents who have children with the same genetic disorder.
    ■ Provide a list of Web sites that contain accurate information about the disorder.
    ■ Explain that they will experience grief over the loss of the "dream child" and this is normal.
    ■ Encourage them to talk openly to each other about their feelings and concerns.
  ■ *A general understanding of genetics and the possible effects on the developing human are necessary for nurses, especially those practicing in the obstetrical or pediatric areas. Nurses may need to:*
    ■ *Explain/clarify diagnostic procedures used in genetic testing (i.e., purpose, findings, and possible side effects).*
    ■ *Clarify or reinforce information the couple received from their health care provider or genetic counselor.*
  ■ *Maternal–child nurses need to have knowledge and information regarding:*
    ■ *Genetic counseling services available in the parents' community*
    ■ *Access to genetic services*
    ■ *Procedure for referral to the different services*
    ■ *The information or services these agencies provide*

TERATOGENS

■ **Teratogens** are defined as any drugs, viruses, infections, or other exposures that can cause embryonic/fetal developmental abnormality (**Table 3-2**).
■ Birth defects can occur from genetic disorders or be the result of teratogen exposure.
■ The degree or types of malformation vary based on length of exposure, amount of exposure, and when it occurs during human development.

TABLE 3–2 TERATOGENIC AGENTS

AGENT	EFFECT
DRUGS AND CHEMICALS ALCOHOL	Increased risk of fetal alcohol syndrome occurring when the pregnant woman ingests six or more alcoholic drinks a day. No amount of alcohol is considered safe during pregnancy. Newborn characteristics of fetal alcohol syndrome include: • Low birth weight • Microcephaly • Mental retardation • Unusual facial features due to midfacial hypoplasia • Cardiac defects
ANGIOTENSIN-CONVERTING ENZYME (ACE) INHIBITORS	Increased risk for: • Renal tubular dysplasia that can lead to renal failure and fetal or neonatal death • Intrauterine growth restriction
CARBAMAZEPINE (ANTICONVULSANTS)	Increased risk for: • Neural tubal defects • Craniofacial defects, including cleft lip and palate • Intrauterine growth restriction
COCAINE	Increased risk for: • Heart, limbs, face, gastrointestinal tract, and genitourinary tract defects • Cerebral infarctions • Placental abnormalities
WARFARIN (COUMADIN)	Increased risk for: • Spontaneous abortion • Fetal demise • Fetal or newborn hemorrhage • Central nervous system abnormalities
INFECTIONS/VIRUSES CYTOMEGALOVIRUS	Increased risk for: • Hydrocephaly • Microcephaly • Cerebral calcification • Mental retardation • Hearing loss
HERPES VARICELLA (CHICKEN POX)	Increased risk for: • Hypoplasia of hands and feet • Blindness/cataracts • Mental retardation

Continued

TABLE 3–2 TERATOGENIC AGENTS—cont'd	
AGENT	**EFFECT**
RUBELLA	Increased risk for: • Heart defects • Deafness and/or blindness • Mental retardation • Fetal demise
SYPHILIS	Increased risk for: • Skin, bone and/or teeth defects • Fetal demise
TOXOPLASMOSIS	Increased risk for: • Fetal demise • Blindness • Mental retardation

Sources: American College of Obstetricians and Gynecologists (ACOG; 1997); Scanlon & Sanders (2007).

CRITICAL COMPONENT

Teratogens

The developing human is most vulnerable to the effects of teratogens during the period of organogenesis, the first 8 weeks of gestation.

CRITICAL COMPONENT

Toxoplasmosis

- Can cause fetal demise, mental retardation, and blindness when the embryo is exposed to *Toxoplasma* during pregnancy (see Table 3-2).
- *Toxoplasma* is a protozoan parasite found in cat feces and uncooked or rare beef and lamb.
- Pregnant women or women who are attempting pregnancy need to avoid contact with cat feces (i.e., changing a litter box).
- Pregnant women or women who are attempting pregnancy should avoid eating rare beef or lamb.

■ The developing human is most vulnerable to the effects of teratogens during organogenesis, which occurs during the first 8 weeks of gestation. Exposure during this time can cause gross structural defects (American College of Obstetricians and Gynecologists [ACOG], 1997).

■ Exposure to teratogens after 13 weeks of gestation may cause fetal growth restriction or reduction of organ size (ACOG, 1997).

ANATOMY AND PHYSIOLOGY REVIEW

Female

The major structures and functions of the female reproductive system are (**Figs. 3-1** and **3-2**):

■ Ovaries
  ■ *There are two oval shaped ovaries; one on each side of uterus.*
  ■ *The ovarian ligament and broad ligament help keep the ovaries in place.*

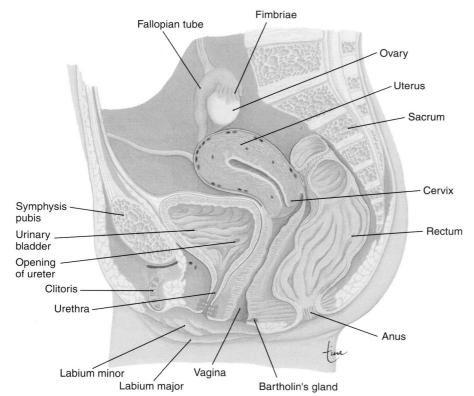

Figure 3–1   Female reproductive system shown in a midsagittal section through the pelvic cavity.

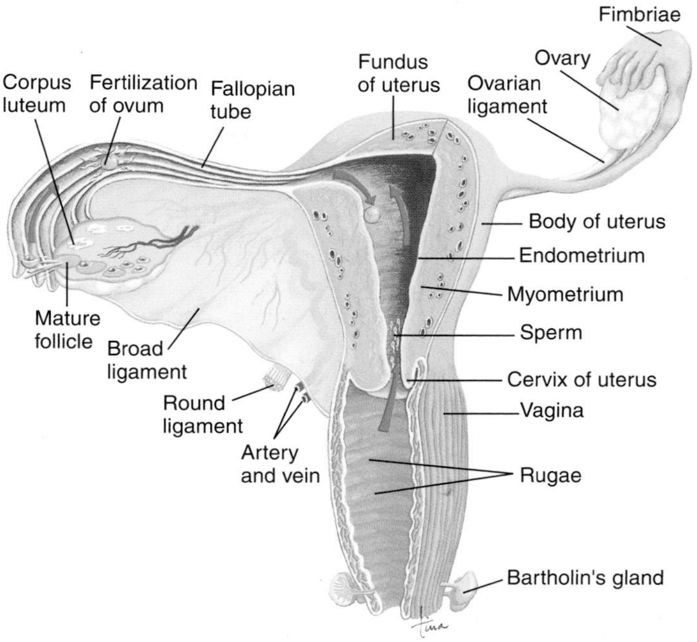

Figure 3–2 Female reproductive system shown in anterior view. The ovary left of the illustration has been sectioned to show the developing follicles. The fallopian tube at the left of the illustration has been sectioned to show fertilization. The uterus and vagina have been sectioned to show internal structures. Arrows indicate the movement of the ovum toward the uterus and the movement of sperm from the vagina toward the fallopian tube.

- *Primary follicles are present in the ovaries.*
  - Several thousand follicles are present at birth.
  - Each follicle contains an oocyte.
  - The follicle cells secrete estrogen.
  - Graafian follicle is a mature follicle.
- Fallopian tubes
  - *There are two fallopian tubes (also referred to as oviducts).*
  - *The lateral end partially surrounds the ovary.*
    - Fimbriae (fringelike projections) from the lateral end create a current within the fluid to pull the ovum into the fallopian tube (Scanlon & Sanders, 2007).
    - Peristaltic waves created by the smooth muscle contractions of the fallopian tubes move the ovum through the tube and into the uterus (Scanlon & Sanders, 2007).
  - *The medial end opens into the uterus.*
  - *Fertilization occurs within the fallopian tube.*
- Uterus
  - *It is shaped like an upside-down pear.*
  - *It is approximately 3 inches long; 2 inches wide; 1 inch deep.*
  - *The **fundus** is the upper portion of the uterus.*
  - *The body of the uterus is the large central portion.*
  - *The cervix of the uterus is the narrow, lower end that opens to the vagina.*
  - *The inner lining of the uterus is the endometrium.*
    - The endometrium consists of the basilar layer (a permanent layer) and the functional layer (a regenerative layer).
    - Estrogen and progesterone stimulate the functional layer of the endometrium to thicken in preparation for implantation.
    - The endometrium continues to thicken when implantation occurs.
    - The functional layer is lost during the menstrual cycle when implantation does not occur.

- *Implantation normally occurs in the uterus.*
- *The uterus expands during pregnancy to accommodate the developing embryo/fetus and placenta.*
- Vagina
  - *A muscular tube approximately 4 inches in length that extends from the cervix to the perineum.*
  - *Functions*
    - Receive sperm during sexual intercourse
    - Provide exit for menstrual blood flow
    - Birth canal during second stage of labor
- External genital structure, also known as the vulva
  - *Clitoris*
    - A small mass of erectile tissue anterior to the urethral orifice
    - Responds to sexual stimulation.
  - *Labia majora and minora*
    - Paired folds of skin that cover the openings to the urethra and vagina and prevent drying of their mucous membranes.
  - *Bartholin's glands*
    - They are located in the floor of the vestibule.
    - The ducts of the gland open onto the mucus of the vaginal orifice.
    - Their secretions keep the mucsa moist and lubricate the vagina during sexual intercourse.

Male

The major structures and functions of the male reproductive system are (**Figs. 3-3** and **3-4**):

- Scrotum
  - *A loose bag of skin and connective tissue which holds the testes suspended within it.*
  - *Temperature inside the scrotum is approximately 96˚F, which is lower than the body temperature and necessary for the production of viable sperm (Scanlon & Sanders, 2007).*

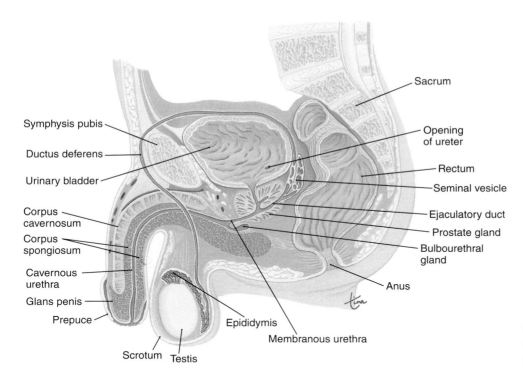

Figure 3–3 Male reproductive system shown in a midsagittal section through the pelvic cavity.

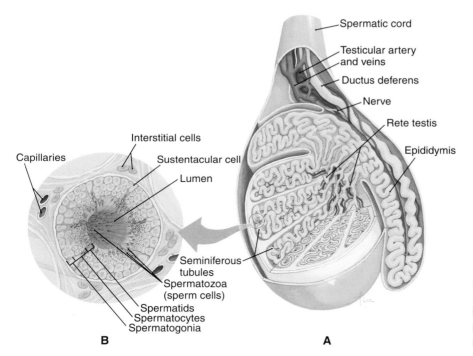

Figure 3–4 (A) Midsagittal section of portion of the testis; the epididymis is on the posterior side of the testis. (B) Cross section through a somniferous tubule showing development of the sperm.

■ Testes
  ■ *A pair of testis lies suspended in the scrotum.*
  ■ *Testes develop in the fetus near the kidney and normally descend into the scrotum prior to birth.*
  ■ *Each testis is divided into lobes which contain several seminiferous tubules.*
    ▨ Spermatogenesis takes place in the seminiferous tubules.
    ▨ Sustentacular (Sertoli) cells within the tubules produce the inhibin hormone when stimulated by testosterone.

▨ Inhibin hormone decreases the secretion of follicle-stimulating hormone (FSH); decreased levels of FSH causes a decrease testosterone levels.
■ *Sperm travel from the seminiferous tubules though the testis (a tubular network) and enter the epididymis.*
■ Epididymis
  ■ *A coiled tube-like structure on the posterior surface of each testis*
  ■ *Sperm complete their maturation within the epididymis.*

- Ductus deferens, also referred to as vas deferens
  - *It extends from the epididymis into the abdominal cavity. In the abdominal cavity, it extends over the urinary bladder and down the posterior side of the bladder and joins with the ejaculatory duct.*
- Ejaculatory ducts
  - *There are two ejaculatory ducts.*
  - *They receive sperm from the ductus deferens and secretions from the seminal vesicles.*
  - *They empty into the urethra.*
- Seminal vesicles
  - *They are located posterior to the urinary bladder.*
  - *They produce secretions that contain fructose, which is an energy source for sperm.*
  - *The secretions are alkaline, which enhances sperm motility.*
- Prostate gland
  - *It is a muscular gland located below the urinary bladder.*
  - *It surrounds the first inch of the urethra as the urethra extends from the bladder.*
  - *It secretes an alkaline fluid that enhances sperm mobility.*
- Bulbourethral glands, also referred to as Cowper's glands
  - *They are located below the prostate gland.*
  - *They secrete an alkaline solution that coats the interior of the urethra to neutralize the acidic urine that is present.*

- Urethra
  - *It is located within the penis.*
  - *It is the final duct that the semen passes through as it exits the body.*
- Penis
  - *It is the external male genital organ.*
  - *It consists of smooth muscle, connective tissue, and blood sinuses.*
  - *The penis is flaccid when blood flow to the area is minimal.*
  - *The penis is erect when the arteries of the penis dilate and the sinuses fill with blood.*

Menstrual Cycle

A woman's menstrual cycle is influenced by the ovarian cycle and endometrial cycle (**Fig. 3-5**).

Ovarian Cycle

The **ovarian cycle** pertains to the maturation of ova and consists of three phases:

- The **follicular phase** begins the first day of menstruation and last 12–14 days. During this phase, the graafian follicle is maturing under the influence of two pituitary hormones: luteinizing hormone (LH) and follicle-stimulating hormone (FSH). The maturing graafian follicle produces estrogen.

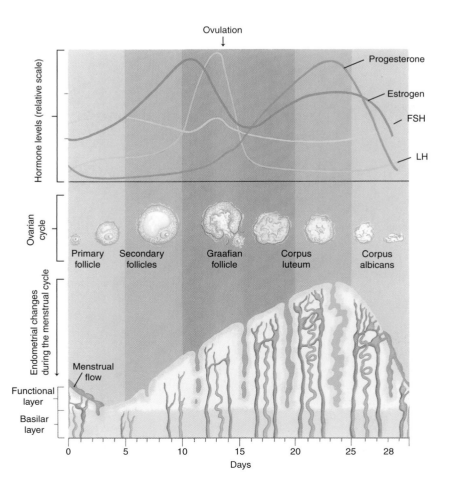

Figure 3-5 The menstrual cycle. The levels of the major hormones are shown in relationship to one another throughout the cycle. Changes in the ovarian follicle are depicted. The relative thickness of the endometrium is also shown.

■ The **ovulatory phase** begins when estrogen levels peak and ends with the release of the oocyte (egg) from the mature graafian follicle. The release of the oocyte is referred to as ovulation.
  ■ *There is a surge in LH levels 12–36 hours before ovulation.*
  ■ *There is a decrease in estrogen levels and an increase in progesterone levels before the LH surge.*
■ The **luteal phase** begins after ovulation and lasts approximately 14 days. During this phase, the cells of the empty follicle undergo changes and form into the corpus luteum.
  ■ *The corpus luteum produces high levels of progesterone along with low levels of estrogen.*
  ■ *If pregnancy occurs, the corpus luteum continues to release progesterone and estrogen until the placenta matures and assumes this function.*
  ■ *If pregnancy does not occur, the corpus luteum degenerates and results in a decrease in progesterone and the beginning of menstruation.*

Endometrial Cycle

The **endometrial cycle** pertains to the changes in the endometrium of the uterus in responses to the hormonal changes that occur during the ovarian cycle. This cycle consists of three phases:

■ The **proliferative phase** occurs following menstruation and ends with ovulation. During this phase, the endometrium is preparing for implantation by becoming thicker and more vascular. These changes are in response to the increasing levels of estrogen produced by the graafian follicle.
■ The **secretory phase** begins after ovulation and ends with the onset of menstruation. During this phase, the endometrium continues to thicken. The primary hormone during this phase is progesterone, which is secreted from the corpus luteum.
  ■ *If pregnancy occurs, the endometrium continues to develop and begins to secrete glycogen.*
  ■ *If pregnancy does not occur, the corpus luteum begins to degenerate and the endometrial tissue degenerates.*
■ The **menstrual phase** occurs in response to hormonal changes and results in the sloughing off of the endometrial tissue.

OOGENESIS

Oogenesis is the formation of a mature ovum (egg).

■ Oogenesis is regulated by two primary hormones.
  ■ *Follicle-stimulating hormone (FSH) secreted from the anterior pituitary gland stimulates growth of the ovarian follicles and stimulates the follicles to secrete estrogen.*
  ■ *Estrogen secreted from the follicle cells promotes the maturation of the ovum.*
■ Process of oogenesis (**Fig. 3-6**)
  ■ *FSH stimulates the growth of ovarian follicle which contains an oogonium (stem cell).*

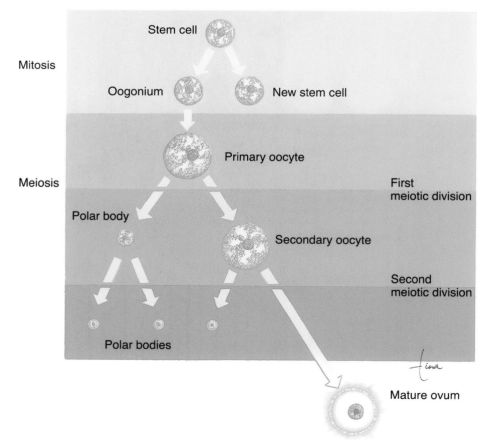

Figure 3-6 Oogenesis. The process of mitosis and meiosis are shown. For each primary oocyte that undergoes meiosis, only one functional ovum is formed.

■ *Through the process of mitosis, the oogonium within the ovary forms into two daughter cells: the primary oocyte and a new stem cell.*
  ■ **Mitosis** is the process by which a cell divides and forms two genetically identical cells (daughter cells) each containing the diploid number of chromosomes.
■ *Through the process of meiosis, the primary oocyte forms into the secondary oocyte and a polar body. The polar body forms into two polar bodies. The secondary oocyte forms into a polar body and a mature ovum.*
  ■ **Meiosis** is a process of two successive cell divisions that produces cells that contain half the number of chromosomes (haploid).

SPERMATOGENESIS

Spermatogenesis is the formation of mature spermatozoa (sperm).

■ Spermatogenesis is regulated by three primary hormones.
  ■ *Follicle-stimulating hormone (FSH) secreted from the anterior pituitary gland stimulates sperm production.*

■ *Luteinizing hormone (LH) secreted from the anterior pituitary gland stimulates testosterone production.*
■ *Testosterone secreted by the testes promotes the maturation of the sperm.*
■ Process of spermatogenesis (**Fig. 3-7**):
  ■ *Through the process of mitosis, the spermatogonium (stem cell) within the seminiferous tubules of the testis forms into two daughter cells: a new spermatogonia and a spermatogonium.*
  ■ *The spermatogonium differentiates and is referred to as the primary spermatocyte.*
  ■ *Through the process of meiosis, the primary spermatocyte forms into two secondary spermatocytes and each secondary spermatocyte forms into two spermatids and contain the haploid number of chromosomes.*
  ■ *Spermatids mature and are referred to as spermatozoa.*

CONCEPTION

Conception, also known as fertilization, occurs when a sperm nucleus enters the nucleus of the oocyte (**Fig. 3-8**).

■ Fertilization normally occurs in the outer third of the fallopian tube.

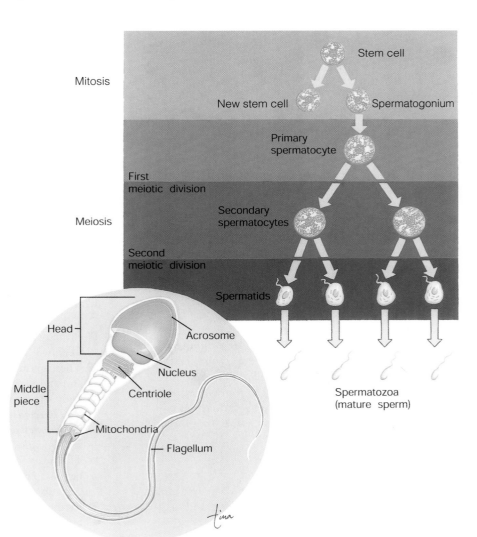

Figure 3–7   Spermatogenesis. The process of mitosis and meiosis are shown. For each primary spermatocyte that undergoes meiosis, four functional sperm cells are formed. The structure of the sperm cell is also shown.

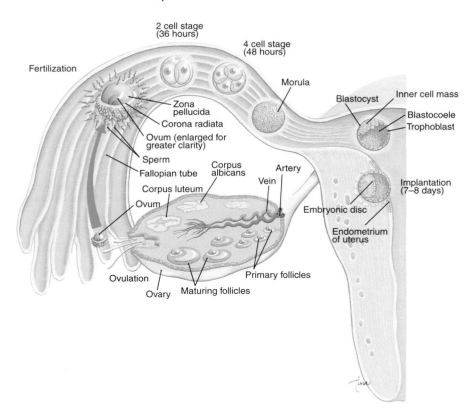

Figure 3–8   Ovulation, fertilization, and early embryonic development. Fertilization takes place in the fallopian tube, and the embryo has reached the blastocyst stage when it becomes implanted in the endometrium of the uterus.

■ The fertilized oocyte is called a **zygote** and contains the diploid number of chromosomes (46).

Cell Division

■ The single-cell zygote undergoes mitotic cell division known as **cleavage.**

■ Three days after fertilization, the zygote forms into a 16-cell, solid sphere that is called a **morula.**

■ Mitosis continues, and around day 5 the developing human is known as the blastocyst and enters the uterus.

■ The **blastocyst** is composed of an inner cell mass known as the **embryoblast,** which will develop into the embryo, and an outer cell mass known as the **trophoblast,** which will assist in implantation and become part of the placenta.

■ **Multiple gestation** refers to more than one developing embryo such as twins and triplets.

  ■ *Twins can be either monozygotic or dizygotic.*

  ■ *Monozygotic twins, also referred to as identical twins, are the result of one fertilized ovum splitting during the early stages of cell division and forming two identical embryos. These developing fetuses are genetically the same.*

  ■ *Dizygotic twins, also referred to as fraternal twins, are the result of two separate ova being fertilized by two separate sperm. These developing fetuses are not genetically the same.*

Implantation

■ **Implantation,** the embedding of the blastocyst into the endometrium of the uterus, begins around day 5 or 6.

■ Progesterone stimulates the endometrium of the uterus, which becomes thicker and more vascular in preparation for implantation.

■ Enzymes secreted by the trophoblast, now referred to as the chorion, digest the surface of the endometrium in preparation for implantation of the blastocyst.

■ Implantation normally occurs in the upper part of the posterior wall of the uterus.

EMBRYO AND FETAL DEVELOPMENT

Embryo

The developing human is referred to as an **embryo** from the time of implantation through 8 weeks of gestation. **Organogenesis,** the formation and development of body organs, occurs during this critical time of human development.

■ Primary germ layers begin to develop around day 14 (**Table 3-3**).

■ These germ layers, known as the ectoderm, mesoderm, and endoderm, form the different organs, tissues, and body structure of the developing human.

  ■ *The **ectoderm** is the outer germ layer.*

  ■ *The **mesoderm** is the middle germ layer.*

  ■ *The **endoderm** is the inner germ layer.*

■ The heart forms during the 3rd gestational week and begins to beat and circulate blood during the 4th gestational week.

■ By the end of the 8th gestational week the developing human has transformed from the primary germ layers to

TABLE 3–3 STRUCTURES DERIVED FROM THE PRIMARY GERM LAYERS

LAYER	STRUCTURES DERIVED*
ECTODERM	Epidermis; hair and nail follicles; sweat glands
	Nervous system; pituitary gland; adrenal medulla
	Lens and cornea; internal ear
	Mucosa of oral and nasal cavities; salivary glands
MESODERM	Dermis; bone and cartilage
	Skeletal muscles; cardiac muscles; most smooth muscles
	Kidneys; adrenal cortex
	Bone marrow and blood; lymphatic tissue; lining of blood vessels
ENDODERM	Mucosa of esophagus, stomach, and intestines
	Epithelium of respiratory tract, including lungs
	Liver and mucosa of gallbladder
	Thyroid gland; pancreas

*These are representative lists, not all-inclusive ones. Most organs are combinations of tissues from each of the three germ layers. Scanlon & Sanders (2007).

a clearly defined human that is 3 cm in length with all organ systems formed (**Fig. 3-9**).

Fetus

The developing human is referred to as a **fetus** from week 9 to birth. During this stage of development, organ systems are growing and maturing (**Table 3-4**).

Fetal Circulation

- The cardiovascular system begins to develop within the first few weeks of gestation.
- The heart begins to beat during the 4th gestational week.
- Unique features of fetal circulation are (**Fig. 3-10**):
  - *High levels of oxygenated blood enter the fetal circulatory system from the placenta via the umbilical vein.*
  - *The **ductus venosus** connects the umbilical vein to the inferior vena cava. This allows the majority of the high levels of oxygenated blood to enter the right atrium.*
  - *The **foramen ovale** is an opening between the right and left atria. Blood high in oxygen is shunted to the left atrium via the foramen ovale. After delivery, the foramen ovale closes in response to increased blood returning to the left atrium. It may take up to 3 months for full closure.*

- *The **ductus arteriosus** connects the pulmonary artery with the descending aorta. The majority of the oxygenated blood is shunted to the aorta via the ductus arteriosus with smaller amounts going to the lungs. After delivery, the ductus arteriosus constricts in response to the higher blood oxygen levels and prostaglandins.*

PLACENTA, MEMBRANES, AMNIOTIC FLUID, AND UMBILICAL CORD

Placenta

- The placenta is formed from both fetal and maternal tissue (**Fig. 3-11**).
  - *The chorionic membrane that develops from the trophoblast along with the chorionic villi form the fetal side of the placenta. The **chorionic villi** are projections from the chorion that embed into the decidua basalis and later form the fetal blood vessels of the placenta.*
  - *The endometrium is referred to as the decidua and consists of three layers: decidua basalis, decidua capsularis, and decidua vera. The **decidua basalis**, the portion directly beneath the blastocyst, forms the maternal portion of the placenta.*
- The maternal side of the placenta is divided into compartments or lobes known as **cotyledons.**
- The placental membrane separates the maternal and fetal blood and prevents fetal blood mixing with maternal blood, but allows for the exchange of gases, nutrients, and electrolytes.

Function of the Placenta

- Metabolic and gas exchange: In the placenta, fetal waste products and CO_2 are transferred from the fetal blood into the maternal blood sinuses by diffusion. Nutrients, such as glucose and amino acids, and O_2 are transferred from the maternal blood sinuses to the fetal blood through the mechanisms of diffuse and active transport.
- Hormone production: The major hormones the placenta produces are progesterone, estrogen, human chorionic gonadotropin (hCG), and human placental lactogen (hPL), also known as human chorionic somatomammotropin.
  - *Progesterone facilitates implantation and decreases uterine contractility.*
  - *Estrogen stimulates the enlargement of the breasts and uterus.*
  - *hCG stimulates the corpus luteum so that it will continue to secrete estrogen and progesterone until the placenta is mature enough to secrete these hormones. This is the hormone assessed in pregnancy tests. hCG rises rapidly during the first trimester and then has a rapid decline.*
  - *hPL:*
    - Promotes fetal growth by regulating glucose available to the developing human.
    - Stimulates breast development in preparation for lactation.

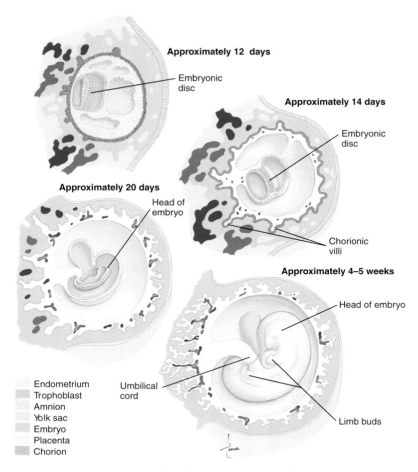

Figure 3-9 Embryonic development at 12 days (after fertilization), 14 days, 20 days, and 4-5 weeks. By 5 weeks, the embryo has distinct parts but does not yet look definitely human.

TABLE 3–4 SUMMARY OF FETAL DEVELOPMENT		
GESTATIONAL WEEK	**LENGTH* AND WEIGHT**	**FETAL DEVELOPMENT/CHARACTERISTICS**
12	8 cm 45 grams	Red blood cells are produced in the liver. Fusion of the palate is completed. External genitalia are developed to the point that sex of fetus can be noted with ultrasound. Eyelids are closed. Fetal heart tone can be heard by Doppler device.
16	14 cm 200 grams	Lanugo is present on head. Meconium is formed in the intestines. Teeth begin to form. Sucking motions are made with the mouth. Skin is transparent.
20	19 cm 450 grams	Lanugo covers the entire body. Vernix caseosa covers the body. Nails are formed. Brown fat begins to develop.

TABLE 3-4   SUMMARY OF FETAL DEVELOPMENT—cont'd

GESTATIONAL WEEK	LENGTH* AND WEIGHT	FETAL DEVELOPMENT/CHARACTERISTICS
24	23 cm 820 grams	Eyes are developed. Alveoli form in the lungs and begin to produce surfactant. Footprints and fingerprints are forming. Respiratory movement can be detected.
28	27 cm 1,300 grams	Eyelids are open. Adipose tissue develops rapidly. The respiratory system has developed to a point that gas exchange is possible, but lungs are not fully mature.
32	30 cm 2,100 grams	Bones are fully developed. Lungs are maturing. Increased amounts of adipose tissue are present.
36	34 cm 2,900 grams	Lanugo begins to disappear. Labia majora and minora are equally prominent. Testes in upper portion of scrotum
40	36 cm 3,400 grams	Fetus is considered full term at 38 weeks. All organs/systems are fully developed.

*Length is measured from the crown (top of head) to the rump (buttock). This is referred to as the CRL.
Sources: Sadler (2004); Scanlon & Sanders (2007).

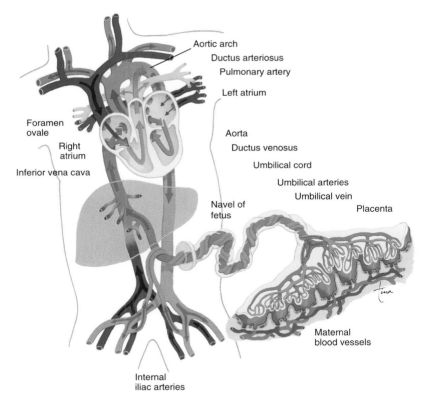

Figure 3-10   Fetal circulation. Fetal heart and blood vessels are shown on the left. Arrows depict direction of blood flow. The placenta and umbilical vessels are shown on the right.

- Viruses, such as rubella and cytomegalovirus, can cross the placental membrane and enter the fetal system and cause fetal death or defects.
- Drugs can cross the placental membrane. Women should consult with their health care provider before taking any medication/drugs. Drugs with an FDA pregnancy category C, D, or X should be avoided during pregnancy or when attempting pregnancy.
- The placenta becomes fully functional between the 8th and 10th weeks of gestation.
- By the 9th month, the placenta is between 15 and 25 cm in diameter, 3 cm thick, and weighs approximately 600 grams.

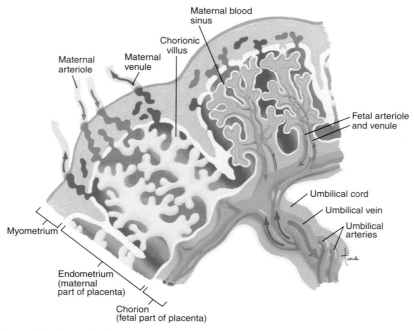

Figure 3–11   Placenta and umbilical cord. The fetal capillaries in the chorionic villi are within the maternal blood sinuses. Arrows indicate the direction of blood flow in the maternal and fetal vessels.

CRITICAL COMPONENT

Medications

Women who are pregnant or attempting pregnancy should consult with their health care provider before taking any prescribed or over-the-counter medications, as medications can cross the placental membrane.

Embryonic Membranes

■ Two membranes (amnion and chorion) form the amniotic sac (also referred to as the bag of waters).
■ The chorionic membrane (outer membrane) develops from the trophoblast.
■ The amniotic membrane (inner membrane) develops from the embryoblast.
■ The embryo and amniotic fluid are contained within the amniotic sac.
■ The membranes stretch to accommodate the growth of the developing fetus and the increase of amniotic fluid.

Amniotic Fluid

■ Amniotic fluid is the fluid contained within the amniotic sac (**Fig. 3-12**).
■ Amniotic fluid is clear and is mainly composed of water. It also contains proteins, carbohydrates, lipids, electrolytes, fetal cells, lanugo, and vernix caseosa.
■ Amniotic fluid during the first trimester is produced from the amniotic membrane. During the second and

third trimesters, the fluid is produced by the fetal kidneys.
■ Amniotic fluid increases during pregnancy and peaks around 34 weeks at 800–1,000 mL and then decreases to 500–600 mL at term.

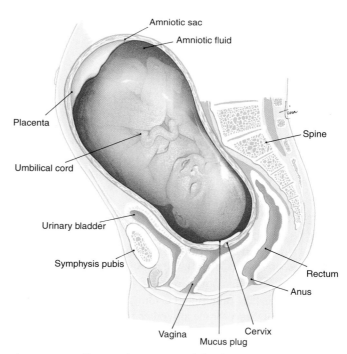

Figure 3-12   Fetus, placenta, umbilical cord, and amniotic fluid.

Function of Amniotic Fluid

■ Acts as a cushion for the fetus when there are sudden maternal movements
■ Prevents adherence of the developing human to the amniotic membranes
■ Allows freedom of fetal movement, which aids in symmetrical musculoskeletal development
■ Provides a consistent thermal environment

Abnormalities

■ **Polyhydramnios** or hydramnios refers to excess amount of amniotic fluid (1,500–2,000 mL). Newborns of mothers who experienced polyhydramnios have an increased incidence of chromosomal disorders and gastrointestinal, cardiac, and/or neural tube disorders.
■ **Oligohydramnios** refers to a decreased amount of amniotic fluid (<500 mL at term or 50% reduction of normal amount), which is generally related to a decrease in placental function. Newborns of mothers who experienced oligohydramnios have an increased incidence of congenital renal problems.

Umbilical Cord

■ Connects the fetus to the placenta
■ Consist of two umbilical arteries and one umbilical vein
  ■ *Arteries carry deoxygenated blood.*
  ■ *The vein carries oxygenated blood.*
■ The vessels are surrounded by **Wharton's jelly,** a collagenous substance, which protects the vessels from compression.
■ Usually inserted in the center of the placenta.
■ Average length of the cord is 55 cm.

CRITICAL COMPONENT

Umbilical Vessels

■ After delivery of the newborn, assess the number of vessels in the cord.
■ Newborns with two vessels (one artery and one vein) have a 20% chance of having a cardiac or other vascular defect.
■ Document the number of vessels present in the newborn. Record and report abnormalities to the pediatrician or pediatric nurse practitioner.

INFERTILITY AND REPRODUCTIVE TECHNOLOGY

Infertility is defined as the inability to conceive and maintain a pregnancy after 12 months (6 months for woman older than 35 years old age) of unprotected sexual intercourse. More than 5 million couples experience difficulties in conceiving (Storment, 2006). In approximately 80% of these couples, a cause can be identified. Infertility affects the physical, social, psychological, sexual, and economic dimensions of the couple's lives.

Causes

One third of the causes are related to female factors alone, one third to male factors alone, and one third to a combination of male and female factors (Frey & Patel, 2004).

■ Male causative factors are classified into five categories: endocrine, spermatogenesis, sperm antibodies, sperm transport, and disorders of intercourse (Porche, 2006).
  ■ *Endocrine: Pituitary diseases, pituitary tumors, and hypothalamic diseases may interfere with male fertility. Low levels of luteinizing hormone (LH), follicle-stimulating hormone (FSH), or testosterone can also decrease sperm production.*
  ■ *Spermatogenesis is the process in which mature functional sperm are formed. Several factors can affect the development of mature sperm. These factors are referred to as gonadotoxins and include:*
    ■ Drugs (e.g., chemotherapeutics, calcium channel blockers, heroin, alcohol, and nicotine)
    ■ Infections (e.g., prostatitis, sexually transmitted illnesses, and contracting mumps after puberty)
    ■ Systemic illness
    ■ Heat exposure: Prolonged heat exposure to the testicles (e.g., use of hot tubs, wearing tight underwear, and frequent bicycle riding)
    ■ Pesticides
    ■ Radiation to the pelvic region
    ■ **Sperm antibodies** are an immunological reaction against the sperm that causes a decrease in sperm motility. This is seen mainly in men who have had either a vasectomy reversal or experienced testicular trauma.
    ■ Sperm transport factor addresses the structures related to the male reproductive anatomy that might be missing or blocked, thus interfering with the transportation of sperm. These causes can include vasectomy, prostatectomy, inguinal hernia, and congenital absence of the vas deferens.
    ■ Disorders of intercourse include erectile dysfunction (inability to achieve and/or maintain an erection), ejaculatory dysfunctions (retrograde ejaculation), anatomical abnormalities (hypospadias), and psychosocial factors that can interfere with fertility.
■ Female causative factors are classified into three major categories: ovulatory dysfunction, tubal and pelvic pathology, and cervical mucus factor (Frey & Patel, 2004).
  ■ *Ovulatory dysfunction includes anovulation or inconsistent ovulation. These factors affect 15%–25% of couples experiencing infertility and have a very high success rate with appropriate treatment (Storment, 2006).*
  ■ *Tubal and pelvic pathology include (1) damage to the fallopian tubes most commonly related to previous pelvic inflammatory disease or endometriosis and (2) uterine fibroids, benign growths of the muscular wall of the uterus, which can cause a narrowing of the uterine cavity and interfere with embryonic and fetal development, causing a spontaneous abortion.*
  ■ *Cervical mucus factors include (1) cervical surgeries such as cryotherapy, a medical intervention used to treat cervical dysplasia, and (2) infection. These may interfere with the ability of sperm to survive or enter the uterus.*

CRITICAL COMPONENT

Risk Factors for Infertility

Women:

Autoimmune disorders
Diabetes
Eating disorders or poor nutrition
Excessive alcohol drinking
Excessive exercising
Obesity
Older age
Sexually transmitted infections

Men:

Environmental pollutants
Heavy use of alcohol, marijuana, or cocaine
Impotence
Older age
Sexually transmitted infections
Smoking

PubMed Health, 2011

Diagnosis of Infertility

When a couple is experiencing difficulty in conceiving, both the man and the woman need to be evaluated. Initial screening for the female partner can be provided by her gynecologist (history, physical examination, and pelvic examination) (**Table 3-5**). Initial screening for the male partner should be performed by a urologist and includes history and physical (**Table 3-6**). The couple may be referred to a reproductive specialist after this initial screening.

Common Diagnostic Tests

■ Screening for sexually transmitted illnesses (STIs)
■ Laboratory test to assess hormonal levels (TSH, FSH, LH, and testosterone)
■ Semen analysis
   ■ *The male partner abstains for 2–3 days before providing a masturbated sample of his semen.*
   ■ *Specimens are either collected at the site of testing or brought to the site within an hour of collection.*
   ■ *The semen analysis includes volume, sperm concentration, motility, morphology, white blood cell count, immunobead, and mixed agglutination reaction test.*
   ■ *Several semen analyses may be required because sperm production normally fluctuates.*
■ Assessing for ovulatory dysfunction
   ■ *Basal body temperature (BBT): The female partner takes her temperature each morning before rising using a basal thermometer and records her daily temperature. Ovulation has occurred if there is a rise in the temperature by 0.4°F for 3 consecutive days.*
   ■ *Ovarian reserve testing: On day 3 of the menstrual cycle a serum FSH and estradiol test is performed. Further evaluation is needed by a reproductive specialist when the FSH is greater than 10 IU/L (Frey & Patel, 2004).*

TABLE 3–5   AREAS OF FOCUS FOR THE MEDICAL HISTORY OF THE FEMALE PARTNER

HISTORY COMPONENTS	FOCUS OF ASSESSMENT
MEDICAL HISTORY AND REVIEW OF SYSTEMS	Abnormal hair growth
	Weight gain
	Breast discharge
	Hypothyroid or hyperthyroid symptoms
	History of diabetes mellitus or current symptoms of DM
	Current medical problems and medications
	Vaccination history
	Allergies
SURGICAL HISTORY	Fallopian tube surgery
	Ectopic pregnancy
	Appendectomy
	Other pelvic surgeries
MENSTRUAL CYCLE AND DEVELOPMENTAL HISTORY	Age of menarche
	Breast development
	Dysmenorrhea
	History of sexually transmitted illnesses
	Use of prior contraception
	History of diethylstilbestrol (DES) exposure
	History of abnormal results from Papanicolaou smear and subsequent treatment
SEXUAL HISTORY	Frequency of sexual intercourse
	Timing of intercourse with basal body temperature charting or ovulation predictor kits
	Dyspareunia (painful intercourse)
	Use of lubrications
	Previous births
INFERTILITY HISTORY	History of infertility treatment in pregnancy
	Duration of current infertility
SOCIAL HISTORY	Use of alcohol, tobacco, caffeine, recreational drugs
	Exposure to chemotherapy or radiation
	Excessive stress
FAMILY HISTORY OF GENETIC DISEASES	Ancestry-based genetic diseases, i.e., cystic fibrosis, sickle cell disease, and thalassemia

Frey & Patel (2004).

TABLE 3–6 AREAS OF FOCUS FOR THE MEDICAL HISTORY OF THE MALE PARTNER

HISTORY COMPONENTS	FOCUS OF ASSESSMENT
MEDICAL HISTORY AND REVIEW OF SYSTEMS	General health
	Erectile function
	Degree of virilization
	History of sexually transmitted illnesses
	Testicular infections (mumps), genital trauma, or undescended testicle
	Pubertal development
	History of exposure to high temperatures (hot tubs) or recent fever
	Current medical problems and medications such as calcium channel blockers
	Vaccination history
	Allergies
SURGICAL HISTORY	History of hernia or testicular or varicocele surgery
SEXUAL HISTORY	Previously fathered a pregnancy
	History of contraception use
	History of infertility in a previous relationship
	Excessive use of lubricants
FAMILY HISTORY OF GENETIC DISEASES	Ancestry-based genetic diseases, i.e., cystic fibrosis, sickle cell disease, and thalassemia
	Family history of male infertility

Frey & Patel (2004).

■ *Detecting LH surge:* There is a rapid increase in LH 36 hours before ovulation that is referred to as the LH surge and can be tested with urine or serum. The urine test can be performed at home and be used to assist in identifying the ideal time for intercourse when pregnancy is desired.

■ **Endometrial biopsy** is performed to assess the response of the uterus to hormonal signals that occur during the cycle. The biopsy is performed at the end of the menstrual cycle. The procedure is performed in the clinical or medical office.

■ **Hysterosalpingogram** is a radiological examination that provides information about the endocervical canal, uterine cavity, and the fallopian tubes. Under fluoroscopic observation, dye is slowly injected through the cervical canal into the uterus. This examination can detect tubal problems such as adhesions or occlusions; and uterine abnormalities such as fibroids, bicornate uterus, and uterine fistulas.

■ Laparoscopy is performed with a laparoscope that is used to visualize and inspect the ovaries, fallopian tubes, and the uterus for abnormalities such as endometriosis and scarring.

Treatment

■ Treatment for the male partner ranges from lifestyle changes to surgery.
  ■ *Treatment for endocrine factors may include hormonal therapy.*
  ■ *Treatment for abnormal sperm count may focus on lifestyle changes such as stress reduction, improved nutrition, elimination of tobacco, and elimination of drugs known to have an adverse effect on fertility.*
  ■ *Treatment for sperm antibodies is corticosteroids to decrease the production of antibodies.*
  ■ *Treatment for infections of the genitourinary tract may include antibiotics.*
  ■ *Treatment for sperm transport factor may include repair of varicocele or inguinal hernia.*
  ■ *Treatment for disorders related to intercourse may include surgery such as transurethral resection of ejaculatory ducts.*
■ Treatment for the female partner also ranges from lifestyle changes to surgery.
  ■ *Treatment for anovulation can focus on lifestyle changes such as stress reduction, improved nutrition, elimination of tobacco, and elimination of drugs known to have an adverse effect on fertility. Treatment also includes the use of a variety of medications that stimulate egg production. The most common medication used is clomiphene citrate.*
  ■ *Treatment for tubal abnormalities may include surgery to open the tubes.*
  ■ *Treatment for uterine fibroids may include surgical removal of the fibroids known as a* **myomectomy.**
  ■ *Treatment for cervical factor related to infection is antibiotics.*

Medication

Clomiphene Citrate

■ Indication: Anovulatory infertility
■ Action: Stimulates release of FSH and LH, which stimulates ovulation
■ Common side effects: Hot flashes, breast discomfort, headaches, insomnia
■ Route and dose: PO; 50–200 mg/day from cycle day 3–7.
(Data from Vallerand & Sanoski, 2013)

Common Methods of Assisted Fertility

When the previously mentioned treatments are not successful, the couple is usually referred to an infertility expert. This is an obstetrician who has specialized in infertility. Additional testing is done, and based on the outcome there are a variety of procedures that can be used to assist in fertility (**Table 3-7**).

TABLE 3–7 COMMON ASSISTED FERTILITY TECHNOLOGIES

TECHNOLOGY	PROCEDURE
ARTIFICIAL INSEMINATION (AI): Intracervical Intrauterine Partner's sperm Donor sperm	Sperm that has been removed from semen is deposited directly into the cervix or uterus using a plastic catheter. The sample is collected by masturbation and the sperm is separated from the semen and prepared for insemination. Sperm can be from the partner or from a donor when the male partner does not produce sperm. Examples of fertility conditions where this procedure is used include (1) poor cervical mucus production as a result of previous surgery of the cervix, (2) anti-sperm antibodies, (3) diminished amount of sperm, and (4) diminished sperm motility.
TESTICULAR SPERM ASPIRATION	Sperm are aspirated or extracted directly from the testicles. Sperm are then microinjected into the harvested eggs of the female partner. Examples of fertility conditions where this procedure is used is with men who (1) had an unsuccessful vasectomy reversal, (2) have an absence of vas deferens, and (3) have an extremely low sperm count or no sperm in their ejaculated semen.
IN VITRO FERTILIZATION (IVF)	IVF is a procedure in which oocytes are harvested and fertilization occurs outside the female body in a laboratory.
ZYGOTE INTRAFALLOPIAN TRANSFER (ZIFT)	In ZIFT, a zygote is placed into the fallopian tube via laparoscopy 1 day after the oocyte is retrieved from the woman and IVF is used.
GAMETE INTRAFALLOPIAN TRANSFER (GIFT)	In GIFT, sperm and oocytes are mixed outside of the woman's body and then placed into the fallopian tube via laparoscopy. Fertilization takes place inside the fallopian tube. Examples of fertility conditions in which these procedures are used are (1) a history of failed infertility treatment for anovulation, (2) unexplained infertility, and (3) low sperm count.
EMBRYO TRANSFER (ET)	ET is when through IVF an embryo is placed in the uterine cavity via a catheter. Example of fertility condition in which this procedure is used is when the fallopian tubes are blocked.

Emotional Implications

■ Couples experience a "roller coaster" effect during diagnosis and treatment. Each month they become excited and hopeful that they will conceive, and then the woman has a period and their excitement and hopes turn to sadness and possibly depression.

■ Infertility can be seen as a crisis in the couple's lives and relationship (Sherrod, 2004).

■ Diagnosis and treatment of infertility can cause:
  ■ *Stress, anxiety, and depression for both the female and/or male partner*
    ■ *One or both partners may experience guilt and blame him- or herself or the partner for the inability to conceive.*
  ■ *Strain between the partners*
    ■ *Sexual activity becomes prescribed due to the type of testing required and the method of treatment, causing sexual dysfunction (Read, 2004).*
  ■ *Strain within the extended family*
    ■ *The couple may avoid family gatherings, especially those that involve children because they remind them of their infertility problems.*
  ■ *Social isolation*
    ■ *Some couples withdraw from social interaction because it is too painful to be around other couples who have children.*

■ *Some couples do not share with others that they are experiencing problems with fertility; thus, they do not have people who can be supportive during diagnosis and treatment.*
■ *Self-esteem issues*
  ■ *The individual's self-esteem can be affected by infertility.*
  ■ *The woman may feel less like a woman because she cannot conceive, or the man may feel less like a man when he cannot impregnate his partner.*
  ■ *The man or woman may feel like he or she has a defective body and is ashamed of it.*

■ Counseling
  ■ *Most couples can benefit from counseling during the time of diagnosis and treatment and after treatment has stopped.*
  ■ *Ideally, counseling should start before treatment begins. Couples may have too high expectations regarding reproductive technology and may not want to recognize that treatment may not be successful.*
  ■ *Counseling includes:*
    ■ Discussion on how treatment may have an effect on them as a couple, as an individual, and as a family
    ■ Discussion on the different treatment methods and any ethical dilemmas that might be related to these treatments
    ■ Discussion on the effects, consequences, and resolution of treatment
    ■ Discussion on when to stop treatment
    ■ Discussion on adoption

Olshanky, E. (2003). A theoretical explanation for previously infertile mothers' vulnerability to depression. *Journal of Nursing Scholarship, 35*, 263-268.

Evidence-Based Practice Research

Since the 1980s, the focus of the research of Ellen Olshanky, DNSc, RNC, has been on the psychosocial effects of infertility. In this article, Dr. Olshanky synthesized the results of several grounded theory studies on the experience of infertility and summarized her theory of identity as infertility. According to her theory:

■ Women who are distressed by their infertility become consumed with concerns about the infertility and often neglect their relationships with friends, spouse, or family members. This can lead to social isolation.
■ Infertility becomes the focus of the marriage or couple relationship, and other aspects of the relationship are often ignored. This can lead to a dysfunctional marriage or couple relationship.
■ Career women may experience a sense of loss of self due to the shift of focus from career to infertility. This also contributes to social isolation.
■ Once pregnancy has been achieved, women often have difficulty perceiving themselves as pregnant women.

Ethical Implications

Assisted reproductive technologies (ART) are treatments that involve the surgical removal of the oocytes and combining them with sperm in a laboratory setting. These treatments include IVF, ZIFT, GIFT, and ET. ART has created numerous ethical dilemmas. The primary one is what to do with the "surplus" embryos. This refers to the embryos produced from hyperstimulation of the ovaries that occurs when IVF technologies are being used. Several eggs from the woman may be harvested and fertilized using IVF, but only two or three are returned to the woman's body. The "surplus" embryos are either frozen for future use or allowed to perish. This has raised the question of when life begins and the rights of the embryo. Other ethical questions that arise are:

■ Who owns the embryos—the woman or the man?
■ Who decides what will happen with the "surplus" embryos?
■ Who has access to ART, as health insurance providers may not pay for the costs of ART?
■ At what point should the health care provider tell the couple to stop using ART?
■ When artificial insemination with donor sperm is used, do you tell the child and if so, when?
■ Does the sperm donor have any rights or responsibilities regarding the child produced from his donation?

The Nurse's Role

■ The role of the nurse varies based on where he or she interfaces with the couple who is experiencing infertility.
■ Nurses who work in an infertility clinic take on a variety of roles (e.g., counseling, teaching, supporting, and assisting in the procedures).

■ Nurses, whether they work in acute care settings or in clinics, need to be aware of the emotional impact infertility has on the individual as well as on the couple. Couples become frustrated when they work with health care professionals who do not understand the effect infertility has on their lives (Sherrod, 2004).

CRITICAL COMPONENT

Infertility

■ The experience of infertility has an effect on the individual's as well as the couple's emotional well-being.
■ Nurses' awareness of how infertility affects all aspects of the individual's and of the couple's relationship will enhance the effectiveness of the nursing care provided to these couples or individuals.

■ ■ ■ Review Questions ■ ■ ■

1. Your patient delivered a full-term baby 12 hours ago. The woman and her husband, who are in their early 20s, have just been informed by their pediatrician that their baby has trisomy 21 (Down syndrome). This is their first child and they did not have prenatal genetic testing. Your nursing care will include (select all of the correct nursing actions):
   A. Explaining that they will go through a grieving process over the loss of their "dream" child.
   B. Explaining the importance of talking openly to each other about their feelings and concerns regarding their child.
   C. Explaining they will benefit from seeing a genetic counselor.
   D. Explaining that they should direct questions regarding the baby's diagnosis to their pediatrician.

2. The developing human is most vulnerable to teratogens during
   A. The first 4 weeks of gestation
   B. The first 8 weeks of gestation
   C. The first 12 weeks of gestation
   D. The first 16 weeks of gestation

3. Fertilization takes place in the _____.
   A. Ovaries
   B. Fallopian tube
   C. Uterus

4. You are a nurse working in a prenatal clinic. Your patient, an 18-year-old woman, is in her 10th gestational week. She wants to know when her baby's heart will start to beat. You inform her that it usually begins to beat around:
   A. The 2nd week of gestation
   B. The 3rd week of gestation
   C. The 4th week of gestation
   D. The 5th week of gestation

5. Which placental hormone is responsible for regulating glucose availability to the fetus?
   A. Progesterone
   B. Estrogen
   C. hCG
   D. hPL

6. You are a nurse in a family planning clinic. Your patient has been married for 5 years. She used an IUD, which was removed 12 months ago. She informs you that she and her husband have been trying to get pregnant for the past 12 months. Initial screening to determine the cause of infertility includes (select all of the correct answers):
   A. Sperm analysis
   B. Testicular biopsy
   C. Assessing for ovulation
   D. Hysterosalpingogram

7. True or false: Meiosis is a process of two successive cell divisions that produces two haploid cells.
   A. True
   B. False

8. A 25-year-old woman is seeing her gynecologist for a preconception visit. She has been married for 3 years. Her brother has hemophilia. Which of these genetic tests would be recommended for this woman?
   A. Carrier testing
   B. Predictive testing
   C. Preimplantation testing
   D. Prenatal testing

9. Factors that place a man at risk for infertility are: (select all of the correct answers)
   A. Cigarette smoking
   B. Eating disorders
   C. Excessive exercising
   D. Use of marijuana

10. True or False: Genetics is the study of genes and their function and related technology.
    A. True
    B. False

References

American College of Obstetricians and Gynecologists (ACOG). (1997). *Teratology* (educational bulletin no. 236). Washington, DC: Author.

Frey, K., & Patel, K. (2004). Initial evaluation and management of infertility by primary care physician. *Mayo Clinical Proceedings, 79,* 1439–1443.

Olshansky, E. (2003). A theoretical explanation of previously infertile mothers' vulnerability to depression. *Journal of Nursing Scholarship, 35,* 236–268.

Porche, D. (2006). Male infertility: Etiology, history, and physical assessment. *JNP, 2,* 226–228.

PubMed Health (2011). Infertility. Retrieved from www.ncbi.nlm. gov/pubmedhealth/PMH0002173

Read, J. (2004). Sexual problems associated with infertility, pregnancy, and ageing. *BMJ, 329,* 559–561.

Sadler, T. W. (2004). *Langman's medical embryology.* Philadelphia: Lippincott Williams & Wilkins.

Scanlon, S., & Sanders, T. (2007). *Essentials of anatomy and physiology* (5th ed.). Philadelphia: F.A. Davis.

Sherrod, R. (2004). Understanding the emotional aspects of infertility: Implications for nursing practice. *Journal of Psychosocial Nursing and Mental Health Services, 42,* 40–47.

Storment, J. (2006). Infertility and recurrent pregnancy loss. In Curtis, M., Overholt, S., & Hopkins, M., *Glass' office gynecology* (6th ed.). Philadelphia: Lippincott Williams & Wilkins.

Vallerand, A., Sanoski, C. (2013). *Davis's drug guide for nurses (13 ed.).* Philadelphia, PA: F. A. Davis.

WHO (2012). Human Genetics Programme. Retrieved from www.who.int/genomics/geneticsVSgenomics/en

Physiological Aspects of Antepartum Care

4

EXPECTED STUDENT OUTCOMES

On completion of this chapter, the student will be able to:

- ☐ Define key terms.
- ☐ Identify the major components of preconception health care.
- ☐ Describe methods for diagnosis of pregnancy and determination of estimated date of delivery.
- ☐ Identify the progression of anatomical and physiological changes over the course of a pregnancy.
- ☐ Link the anatomical and physiological changes of pregnancy to signs and symptoms and common discomforts of pregnancy.
- ☐ Describe appropriate interventions to relieve common discomforts of pregnancy.
- ☐ Identify the critical elements of assessment and nursing care during initial and subsequent prenatal visits.
- ☐ Describe the elements of patient education and anticipatory guidance appropriate for each trimester of pregnancy.

Nursing Diagnosis

- ▪ Knowledge deficit related to physiological changes of pregnancy
- ▪ Knowledge deficit related to nutritional requirements during pregnancy
- ▪ Altered health maintenance related to knowledge deficit regarding self-care measures during pregnancy
- ▪ Knowledge deficit of warning signs of pregnancy
- ▪ Sleep pattern disturbance related to discomforts of late pregnancy
- ▪ Constipation related to changes in gastrointestinal tract during pregnancy
- ▪ Anxiety related to physiologic changes of pregnancy

Nursing Outcomes

- ▪ The pregnant woman will verbalize an understanding of expected anatomical and physiological changes of pregnancy.
- ▪ The pregnant woman will report eating a diet following food pyramid guidelines with the recommended calorie intake and will achieve the recommended weight gain throughout pregnancy.
- ▪ The pregnant woman will verbalize understanding of self-care needs in pregnancy such as posture/body mechanics, rest and relaxation, personal hygiene, and activity and exercise.
- ▪ The pregnant woman will verbalize an understanding of how to implement measures for relieving discomforts associated with normal physical changes such as: pregnant woman will verbalize an understanding of strategies for constipation management in pregnancy and will resume normal bowel function.
- ▪ The pregnant woman will verbalize understanding of warning signs of pregnancy and when to call provider.
- ▪ The pregnant woman will verbalize understanding of strategies to accommodate sleep disturbance during pregnancy.
- ▪ The pregnant woman will report experiencing a reduction in anxiety.

Don't have time to read this chapter? Want to reinforce your reading? Need to review for a test?
Listen to this chapter on Davis*Plus*.

INTRODUCTION

The scope of this chapter is nursing care and interventions prior to conception and throughout a normal pregnancy based on an understanding of the physiological aspects of pregnancy. Chapter 5 addresses the psychosocial and cultural components of the antepartum period.

The focus of nursing care during the preconception and antepartum period is:

- Prior to pregnancy:
  - *Assessment of the health of the woman and potential risk factors*
  - *Education on health promotion and disease prevention*
- During pregnancy:
  - *Regular assessment of the health of the pregnancy*
  - *Regular assessment and screening of risk factors for potential complications*
  - *Education on health promotion and disease prevention*
  - *Inclusion of significant others/family in care and education to promote pregnancy adaptation*
  - *Implementation of appropriate interventions based on risk status or actual complications*

PRECONCEPTION HEALTH CARE

Preconception care is defined as a set of interventions that aim to identify medical, behavioral, and social risks to a woman's health or pregnancy outcome through prevention and management (Centers for Disease Control and Prevention [CDC], 2006). Preconception care consists of health promotion, risk screening, and implementation of interventions for childbearing-aged women before a pregnancy with the goal of modifying risk factors that could negatively impact a pregnancy (CDC, 2006; **Table 4-1**). This care is critical because several risk behaviors (i.e., smoking) and exposures negatively affect fetal development and pregnancy outcomes (see Critical Component: Preconception Health Care). In addition, because almost half of pregnancies are unintended (i.e., mistimed or unwanted at the time of conception), preconception care optimizes a woman's health for a potential pregnancy (Martin, Hamilton, Menacker, Sutton, & Mathews, 2007).

CRITICAL COMPONENT

Preconception Health Care

Assessing a woman for risk factors and implementing interventions when appropriate can positively impact her current or future health as well as the health of any future pregnancies, resulting in better health outcomes for women and families (CDC, 2006).

Routine Physical Examination and Screening

Two of the primary components of a preconception health care visit are a physical examination and relevant health screening in the form of laboratory or diagnostic testing (see Table 4-1).

- The physical examination includes:
  - *Height and weight measurements to calculate BMI and assess whether at a healthy weight*
  - *Comprehensive physical examination*
  - *Breast examination*
  - *Pelvic examination*

TABLE 4–1	COMPONENTS OF HEALTH HISTORY AND RISK FACTOR ASSESSMENT IN PRECONCEPTION CARE
COMPONENT	**PURPOSE AND ACTIONS**
IDENTIFYING INFORMATION Age, gravida/para, address, race/ethnicity, religion, marital/family status, occupation, education	To determine specific risks based on sociodemographic characteristics • Provide education and anticipatory guidance. • To identify psychosocial resources and available sources of support (See Chapter 5 for detailed information on psychosocial and cultural assessment.) • Refer for social services, counseling services, spiritual support.
HEALTH STATUS Prior and present health status	To determine past and present health status: • Provide education and anticipatory guidance. • Refer for additional testing/procedures. • Refer to physician specialist, counseling services, substance abuse treatment, genetic counseling, dietician, social services as indicated. • Administer rubella and/or hepatitis and flu vaccines as indicated. • Refer to cessation programs as appropriate (e.g., smoking).

TABLE 4–1	COMPONENTS OF HEALTH HISTORY AND RISK FACTOR ASSESSMENT IN PRECONCEPTION CARE—cont'd
COMPONENT	**PURPOSE AND ACTIONS**
DISEASE/COMPLICATIONS History of or current medical conditions/diseases (may include thromboembolytic blood dyscrasias, autoimmume, thyroid disorders) Surgeries (including blood transfusions) History of physical/sexual abuse Medication use (prescription, OTC, complementary) Allergies Immunizations	To identify any components in medical history that may increase risk in the well-woman population • Initiate actions to minimize risks.
FAMILY MEDICAL Current health status Genetic Medical conditions/diseases	To determine both modifiable and non-modifiable risk factors related to family and genetic history • Initiate actions to minimize risks.
REPRODUCTIVE Menstrual Obstetric Gynecological Contraceptive Sexual	To ascertain details about menstrual cycles, past pregnancies and their outcomes, any gynecological disorders including infertility, past or present contraceptive use, history of sexually transmitted infections, sexual orientation, past or present sexuality issues, use of safe sex practices. Asess prior pregnancy losses
SELF-CARE/LIFESTYLE/SAFETY BEHAVIORS	To determine: • Frequency of health maintenance visits (well-woman and dental) • Bowel patterns • Sleep patterns • Stress management • Nutrition, BMI, and exercise history • *Counseling on the importance of achieving a normal BMI prior to conception* To identify tobacco, alcohol, and substance use/abuse, caffeine use To identify use of complementary and alternative medicine (CAM) modalities To identify spiritual or religious practices To determine safety practices such as use of seat belts, sunscreen, smoke alarms and carbon monoxide detectors, gun safety • Initiate actions to minimize risks.
PSYCHOSOCIAL Mental health Social	To ascertain past and present psychological and emotional health To identify social patterns and sources of emotional and social support in family and friends • Refer to mental health providers as needed.
CULTURAL Beliefs/values Practices Primary language	To identify cultural practices and beliefs/values impacting health and pregnancy • Incorporate knowledge of beliefs and practices in care. To determine need for translation • Obtain translation assistance as needed. • Provide educational materials in woman's primary language.

Continued

TABLE 4–1   COMPONENTS OF HEALTH HISTORY AND RISK FACTOR ASSESSMENT IN PRECONCEPTION CARE—cont'd

COMPONENT	PURPOSE AND ACTIONS
ENVIRONMENTAL Home Workplace	To identify past and current exposure to environmental or occupational hazards/toxins • Refer for environmental exposure counseling, genetic counseling when indicated.
FINANCIAL Basic needs related to food and housing Resources Health insurance	To determine adequacy of resources to meet basic ongoing needs • Refer for social services, economic support services as indicated.

■ Laboratory and diagnostic tests include:
  ■ *Papanicolaou smear (Pap smear), a screening test for cervical cancer*
  ■ *Blood type and Rh factor*
  ■ *Complete blood count (CBC)*
  ■ *Serum cholesterol*
  ■ *Serum glucose*
  ■ *Urinalysis*
  ■ *Human immunodeficiency virus (HIV)*
  ■ *Syphilis*
  ■ *Sexually transmitted disease (STD) cultures*
■ Additional testing may be ordered based on history and physical examination findings.

Preconception Anticipatory Guidance and Education

Anticipatory guidance is the provision of information and guidance to women and their families that enables them to be knowledgeable and prepared as the process of pregnancy and childbirth unfolds. Anticipatory guidance and education in the childbearing-aged population spans topics from health maintenance, self-care, and lifestyle choices to contraception and safety behaviors. The nurse is key in providing this aspect of care. It is imperative that a woman's age, sexual orientation, culture, religion, and additional values and beliefs are acknowledged and respected, and that this information is incorporated appropriately into the nurse's teaching plan

Preconception Education

The goal of preconception education is to provide a woman with information she can use to enhance her health before becoming pregnant. When a woman seeks care specifically because she is planning for a future pregnancy, more emphasis is placed on counseling and anticipatory guidance related to preparation and planning for a pregnancy.

Preconception anticipatory guidance and education topics:

■ Nutrition
■ Prenatal vitamins
■ Exercise
■ Self-care
■ Contraception cessation
■ Timing of conception
■ Modifying behaviors to reduce risks

Nutrition

Maintaining a healthy weight is especially important for women planning a pregnancy. The **body mass index (BMI),** a number calculated based on a person's height and weight, represents a measure of body fat. The BMI can be used as an easy method of screening the nutritional status of women and to identify weight categories that may lead to health problems. The Institute of Medicine (IOM) and the Centers for Disease Control and Prevention (CDC) use the following table to interpret the BMI (see **Box 4-1**).

Currently 35.7% of adults in the United States are obese (Ogden, Carroll, Kit, & Flegal, 2012). The number of women in childbearing years who are overweight or obese has grown over the last three decades, and maternal obesity prior to conception has been linked to childhood obesity in their offspring (Whitaker, 2004). Taking into consideration the lifelong health consequences associated with obesity, the IOM published new guidelines in 2009 recommending that women achieve their normal BMI prior to conceiving (see Critical Component: Pre-Pregnancy Weight).

CRITICAL COMPONENT

Pre-Pregnancy Weight

An overweight or obese pre-pregnancy weight increases the risk for poor maternal and neonatal outcomes and may have far-reaching implications for long-term health and development of chronic disease. At the other end of the spectrum, underweight pre-pregnancy weight and/or inadequate weight gain increases the risk for poor fetal growth and low birth weight. Women who are either significantly overweight or underweight should be referred for dietary counseling and planning in order to achieve a healthier weight before conception. (IOM, 2009)

BOX 4-1 BMI SCALE

BMI Classification	BMI (KG/M²)
Underweight	<18.5
Normal range	18.5-24.9
Overweight	25.0-29.9
Obese	≥30.0

World Health Organization (2011).

Obesity increases a woman's risk for infertility, and when pregnant, is associated with increased perinatal morbidity and mortality from a variety of causes such as:

■ Increased risk for antepartum complications such as hypertension, preeclampsia, gestational diabetes, thromboembolism, and urinary tract infections.
■ Complications during childbirth due to large for gestational age (LGA) infants and macrosomia
■ Prolonged labor and difficult delivery
■ Cesarean delivery
■ Postpartum hemorrhage
■ Poor wound healing following a cesarean birth.

Given the detrimental influence of maternal overweight and obesity on reproductive and pregnancy outcomes for the mother and child, it is the position of the American Dietetic Association and the American Society for Nutrition that all overweight and obese women of reproductive age should receive counseling prior to pregnancy, during pregnancy, and in the interconceptional period on the roles of diet and physical activity in reproductive health, in order to ameliorate these adverse outcomes (American Dietetic Association and American Society for Nutrition, 2009).

Poor perinatal outcomes can also result from inadequate maternal weight during pregnancy such as small for gestational age (SGA) infants and preterm birth (Gussler & Arensberg, 2011; Cunningham, Leveno, Bloom, Hauth, Rouse, & Sprong, 2010).

Nutritional education for women of childbearing years:

■ Educate on diet and physical activity and their role in reproductive health.
■ Advise on the importance of achieving and maintaining a healthy weight prior to conception.
■ Encourage nutritious food choices with an emphasis on fresh fruits and vegetables, lean protein sources, low-fat or non-fat dairy foods, whole grains, and small amounts of healthy fats.
■ Help choose appropriate foods and serving sizes (see Fig. 4-8).

Prenatal Vitamins

Many women planning a pregnancy begin taking a prenatal vitamin supplement. Prenatal vitamins contain a wide range of vitamins and minerals important for good health during pregnancy:

■ Folic acid supplementation: Decreases risk of neural tube defects (see Critical Component: Folic Acid Supplements).

■ Calcium, magnesium, and vitamin D: Contribute to bone health and osteoporosis prevention throughout the life span, including during the childbearing years.
■ Iron supplementation is commonly prescribed during pregnancy, although there is some controversy about the benefit of this practice as a routine recommendation.
■ A woman who is anticipating a short time period between pregnancies is at risk for iron-deficiency anemia. Iron supplementation may be prescribed, and she is encouraged to include iron-rich foods in her diet in between pregnancies since she is likely to have reduced iron stores and may also be anemic from the previous recent pregnancy.
■ Megadoses of vitamins and minerals are not recommended, as they may be toxic to the developing fetus.

CRITICAL COMPONENT

Folic Acid Supplements

In 1992, the CDC began recommending daily folic acid supplementation of 0.4 mg daily for childbearing-aged women after folic acid was shown to reduce the incidence of neural tube defects (NTDs) such as spina bifida, with an expected reduction in NTD incidence in the United States of 50%. The beneficial impact of folic acid supplementation is greatest between 1 month before pregnancy and through the first trimester, the period of neural tube development (CDC, 1992)

Exercise

A program of regular exercise positively impacts a woman's health and may generally be continued once she has conceived. It is best to implement such a program several months in advance of conception so that when pregnancy occurs, regular exercise is already comfortable and routine. Women embarking on a new exercise regime may want to confer with their providers.

■ Some form of aerobic activity, including regular weight-bearing exercise such as walking or running, as well as stretching exercises and some type of weight work/muscle strengthening together provide overall body conditioning.
■ The weight-bearing exercise and weight/strengthening work also enhance bone health and help prevent osteoporosis.

Self-Care

Most women are pregnant for at least 1–2 weeks before being aware of their pregnancy. For this reason, it is helpful to counsel the preconception woman to decrease risk behaviors and eliminate exposure to substances that are known or suspected to be harmful during gestation as soon as she stops using contraception or begins trying to become pregnant (**Fig. 4-1**). The woman should avoid:

■ Alcohol
■ Tobacco
■ Secondhand smoke

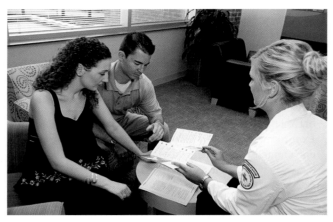

Figure 4–1 Nurse providing anticipatory guidance and education on self-care.

- Excessive use of caffeine
- Illicit drugs
- Medications contraindicated in pregnancy (prescription, over-the-counter, and herbal supplements)
- Environmental toxins

The woman should be encouraged to:

- Use safer sex practices to prevent STIs
- Use seat belts in a car
- Ensure that smoke alarms and carbon monoxide detectors are in working order
- Apply sunscreen when outdoors
- Maintain adequate relaxation and sleep
- Maintain optimal oral health and treat any periodontal disease before pregnancy, as it has been associated with adverse pregnancy outcomes including preterm birth and low birth weight (CDC, 2006).
- Discuss the use of complementary or alternative medicine modalities, such as acupuncture, herbal supplements, homeopathy, and massage, with her primary health care provider. Some of these interventions may need to be discontinued before a pregnancy for safety reasons.

Contraception Cessation

Before conception, it is ideal for a woman to have at least two or three normal menstrual periods. For all women planning a pregnancy, discontinuation of contraception and tracking of menstrual cycles will aid in facilitating conception and subsequently in dating the pregnancy once conception is achieved.

- Women using some form of hormonal contraception need to stop hormonal contraception and begin the use of a barrier method of birth control or fertility awareness family planning techniques for the next few months before conception.
- Women using Depo-Provera for contraception need to be informed that it may take from several months up to more than a year to conceive after discontinuing injections.
- Women using an intrauterine device (IUD) need to have the device removed.

Timing of Conception

Many women are interested in learning more about their menstrual cycles in order to gain more control over their ability to conceive.

- Preconception counseling can include basic information about the menstrual cycle, when in the cycle a woman is able to conceive, signs of ovulation, the life span of ovum and sperm, and how to time sexual intercourse in order to increase the likelihood of conception.
- Women who have used fertility awareness family planning principles are familiar with these concepts and can simply reverse the behaviors they practiced when using the method to avoid conception.

Modifying Behaviors to Reduce Risk

With each topic of conversation in preconception counseling, women gain information allowing them to positively affect their overall health and reduce perinatal risk. Several factors contribute to risk reduction or elimination by modifying risk factors related to preexisting medical conditions, high-risk behaviors, and self-care and safety behavior deficits to improve outcomes of future pregnancies (Evidence-Based Practice: Recommendations to Improve Preconception Health and Health Care in the United States).

Nursing Actions in Preconception Care

- Provide comfort and privacy.
- Use therapeutic communication techniques.
- Obtain the health history.
- Conduct a review of systems.
- Provide teaching about procedures.
- Assist with physical and pelvic exams.
- Assist with obtaining specimens.
- Provide anticipatory guidance and education related to plan of care and appropriate follow-up.
- Assess the patient's understanding.
- Provide education, recommendations, and referrals to help women make appropriate behavioral, lifestyle, or medical changes based on history or physical examination.

Evidence-Based Practice: Recommendations to Improve Preconception Health and Health Care in the United States

The Centers for Disease Control and Prevention (CDC) recommendations emphasize that preconception care is not limited to a single visit to a health professional but is a process of care that is designed to meet the needs of a woman during the different stages of her reproductive life. All women of reproductive age are candidates for preconception care; however, preconception care must be tailored to meet the needs of the individual (CDC, 2006; Jack, Atrash, Coonrod, Moos, O'Donnell, & Johnson, 2008).

See **Table 4-2** for categories of clinical content for preconception care.

Preconception Care for Men

Preconception care for men offers an opportunity, similar to the opportunity it presents for women, for disease prevention and health promotion. In addition, preconception care for men is an important factor in improving family planning and pregnancy outcomes for women, enhancing the reproductive health and health behaviors of men and their partners, and preparing for fatherhood. The CDC recommends that each male planning with his partner to conceive a pregnancy should have a comprehensive medical evaluation for the purposes of preventing and finding disease and providing preconception education. Management should be optimized for any high-risk behaviors or poorly controlled disease states prior to attempting conception (Frey, Navarro, Kotelchuck, & Lu, 2008).

DIAGNOSIS OF PREGNANCY

The diagnostic confirmation of pregnancy is based on a combination of the presumptive, probable, and positive changes/signs of pregnancy. This information is obtained through history, physical and pelvic examinations, and laboratory and diagnostic studies.

Presumptive Signs of Pregnancy

The **presumptive signs** of pregnancy include all subjective signs of pregnancy (i.e., physiological changes perceived by the woman herself):

- **Amenorrhea:** Absence of menstruation
- Nausea and vomiting: Common from week 2–12
- Breast changes: Changes begin to appear at 2 to 3 weeks
  - *Enlargement, tenderness, and tingling of breasts*
  - *Increased vascularity of breasts*

TABLE 4–2   CATEGORIES OF CLNICAL CONTENT FOR PRECONCEPTION CARE

Health Promotion	Personal History	Nutrition
• Family Planning and Reproductive Life Plan	• Family History	• Calcium
• Weight Status	• Known Genetic Conditions	• Dietary Supplements
• Physical Activity	• Prior Cesarean Delivery	• Essential Fatty Acids
• Nutrient Intake	• Prior Miscarriage	• Folic Acid
• Folate	• Prior Preterm Birth	• Iodine
• Substance Use	• Prior Stillbirth	• Iron
• STIs	• Uterine Anomalies	
Immunizations	**Infectious Diseases**	**Medical Conditions**
• Hepatitis B	• Cytomegalovirus	• Asthma
• HPV	• Hepatitis C	• Cardiovascular Disease
• Influenza	• Herpes Simplex Virus	• Diabetes Mellitus
• Measles, Mumps, and Rubella (MMR)	• HIV	• Eating Disorders
• Tetanus, Diphtheria, Pertussis (TDAP)	• Listerosis	• Hypertension
• Varicella	• Malaria	• Lupus
	• Sexually Transmitted Infections	• PKU
	• Syphilis	• Psychiatric Conditions
	• Toxoplasmosis	• Renal Disease
	• Tuberculosis	• Rheumatoid Arthritis
		• Seizure Disorders
		• Thrombophilia
		• Thyroid Disease
Exposures	**Psychosocial Risks**	**Special Populations**
• Alcohol, Tobacco, Illicit Substances	• Access to Care	• Disability
• Environmental	• Inadequate Financial Resources	• Immigrant and Refugee Populations
• Hobbies		• Survivors of Cancer
• Medications		

■ Fatigue: Common during the first trimester
■ Urination frequency: Related to pressure of enlarging uterus on bladder; decreases as uterus moves upward and out of pelvis
■ **Quickening:** A woman's first awareness of fetal movement; occurs around 18–20 weeks' gestation in primigravidas (between 14–16 weeks in multigravidas)

All of these changes could have causes outside of pregnancy and are not considered diagnostic.

Probable Signs of Pregnancy

The **probable signs** of pregnancy are objective signs of pregnancy and include all physiological and anatomical changes that can be perceived by the health care provider:

■ **Chadwick's sign:** Bluish-purple coloration of the vaginal mucosa, cervix, and vulva seen at 6–8 weeks
■ **Goodell's sign:** Softening of the cervix and vagina with increased leukorrheal discharge; palpated at 8 weeks
■ **Hegar's sign:** Softening of the lower uterine segment; palpated at 6 weeks
■ Uterine growth and abdominal growth
■ Skin hyperpigmentation
  ■ *Melasma (chloasma), also referred to as the mask of pregnancy: Brownish pigmentation over the forehead, temples, cheek, and/or upper lip*
  ■ *Linea nigra: Dark line that runs from the umbilicus to the pubis*
  ■ *Nipples and areola: Become darker; more evident in primigravidas and dark-haired women*
■ **Ballottement:** A light tap of the examining finger on the cervix causes fetus to rise in the amniotic fluid and then rebound to its original position; occurs at 16–18 weeks
■ Positive pregnancy test results
  ■ *Laboratory tests are based on detection of the presence of human chorionic gonadatropin (hCG) in maternal urine or blood.*
  ■ *The tests are extremely accurate, but not 100%. There can be both false-positive and false-negative results. Because of this, a positive pregnancy test is considered a probable rather than a positive sign of pregnancy.*
  ■ *A maternal blood pregnancy test can detect hCG levels before a missed period.*
  ■ *A urine pregnancy test is best performed using a first morning urine specimen, which has the highest concentration of hCG, and becomes positive about 4 weeks after conception.*
  ■ *Home pregnancy tests are also accurate (but not 100%) and are simple to perform. These urine tests use enzymes and rely on a color change when agglutination occurs, indicating a pregnancy. The home tests can be performed at the time of a missed menstrual period or as early as 1 week before a missed period. If a negative result occurs, the instructions suggest that the test be repeated in one week if a menstrual period has not begun.*

All of these changes could also have causes other than pregnancy and are not considered diagnostic. The presumptive and probable signs of pregnancy are important components of the assessment in confirming a pregnancy. Early in gestation, before any positive signs of pregnancy, a combination of presumptive and probable signs is used to make a practical diagnosis of pregnancy.

Positive Signs of Pregnancy

The **positive signs** of pregnancy are the objective signs of pregnancy (noted by the examiner) that can only be attributed to the fetus:

■ Auscultation of the fetal heart, by 10–12 weeks' gestation with a Doppler
■ Observation and palpation of fetal movement by the examiner after about 20 weeks' gestation
■ Sonographic visualization of the fetus: Cardiac movement noted at 4–8 weeks

Sonographic Diagnosis of Pregnancy

Ultrasound using a vaginal probe can confirm a pregnancy slightly earlier than with the transabdominal method. With a transvaginal ultrasound the gestational sac is visible by 4.5–5 weeks' gestation and fetal cardiac movement can be observed as early as 4 weeks' gestation. Ultrasound visualization of a pregnancy has increasingly become a routine and expected part of prenatal care. Indications for ultrasound examination of an early pregnancy for purposes of diagnosis include:

■ Pelvic pain or vaginal bleeding in the first trimester
■ History of repeated pregnancy loss or ectopic pregnancy (the implantation of a fertilized ovum outside the uterus)
■ Uncertain menstrual history
■ Discrepancy between actual size and expected size of pregnancy based on history

PREGNANCY

The **antepartum (antepartal) period,** also referred to as the prenatal period, begins with the first day of the **last normal menstrual period** (LMP) and ends with the onset of labor (known as the intrapartal period).

Pregnancy is also counted in terms of trimesters, each roughly 3 months in length:

Trimesters

First trimester:	First day of LMP through 14 completed weeks
Second trimester:	15 weeks through 28 completed weeks
Third trimester:	29 weeks through 40 completed weeks

Calculation of Due Date

An important piece of information to share with a newly pregnant woman and her family is her "due date" or **estimated date of birth (EDB).** It is more commonly known now as **estimated date of delivery (EDD).** This date represents a best estimation as to when a full-term infant will be born.

The original term used for this date was the **estimated date of confinement (EDC).**

Calculation of the EDD is best accomplished with a known and certain last menstrual period date (LMP). Other tools are used to determine the most accurate EDD possible if the LMP is not known and are used throughout the pregnancy to confirm EDD based on an LMP. These tools are:

■ Physical examination to determine uterine size
■ First auscultation of fetal heart rate with a Doppler and/or a fetoscope (stethoscope for auscultation of fetal heart tones)
■ Date of quickening
■ Ultrasound examination
■ History of assisted reproduction

Naegele's Rule

Naegele's rule is the standard formula for determining an EDD based on the LMP. The formula is: First day of LMP – 3 months + 7 days (see **Box 4-2**).

FORMULA FOR NAEGELE'S RULE

LMP	Sept 7
	–3 months
	June 7
	+7 days
EDD	June 14

It is important to remember that the EDD as determined by Naegele's rule is only a best guess of when a baby is likely to be born. Two factors influence the accuracy of Naegele's rule:

■ Regularity of a woman's menstrual cycles
■ Length of a woman's menstrual cycles
  ■ *Results may not be accurate if menstrual cycles are not regular or are greater than 28 days apart.*

Most women give birth within the time period of 3 weeks before to 2 weeks after their EDD. The length of pregnancy is approximately 280 days or 40 weeks from the first day of the LMP. In recent years there has been conflicting or inconsistent information on the definition of a "term" pregnancy. The window for **term gestation** has traditionally been defined as between the 5 weeks from 37 to 42 weeks from the LMP. Statisticians or some experts now define term pregnancy as one that begins after the 37th competed week of pregnancy through the end of the

BOX 4–2 GESTATIONAL AGE

Gestational age refers to the number of completed weeks of fetal development, calculated from the first day of the last normal menstrual period. Embryologists date fetal age and development from the time of conception (known as conceptual or embryological age), which is usually 2 weeks less. Unless otherwise specified, all references to dating or fetal age in this textbook will be gestational ages (based on time since the last menstrual period and not time since conception).

41st week of pregnancy. According to the American Academy of Pediatrics (AAP) and the American College of Obstetricians and Gynecologists (ACOG) (2007), neonates born prior to 37 completed weeks (<37 6/7 weeks or <259 days) of pregnancy are referred to as preterm, and those delivered after 42 weeks (>42 6/7 or >294) are classified as post term (AAP & ACOG, 2007).

Weeks of Gestation

Once an EDD has been determined, a pregnancy is counted in terms of weeks of gestation beginning with the first day of the LMP and ending with 40 completed weeks (the EDD). A useful tool for quickly and easily calculating the EDD is the gestational wheel (**Fig. 4-2**), but it is less reliable than Naegele's rule due to variations of up to a few days between wheels. It is best to calculate a due date initially using Naegele's rule and then employ a gestational wheel to determine a woman's current gestational age.

To use the gestational wheel, place the arrow labeled "first day of last period" from the inner circle on the date of the LMP on the outer circle. The EDD is then read as the date on the outside circle that lines up with the arrow at 40 completed weeks on the inside circle. With the example the LMP is _____ and the EDD is _____.

Prenatal Assessment Terminology

A set of terms is used to describe obstetrical history and to define a woman's obstetrical status. An important shorthand system for explaining a woman's obstetrical history uses the

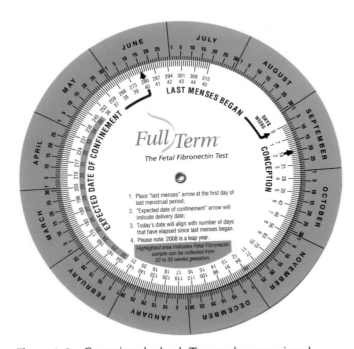

Figure 4–2 Gestational wheel. To use the gestational wheel, place the arrow labeled "first day of last period" from the inner circle on the date of the LMP on the outer circle. The EDD is then read as the date on the outside circle that lines up with the arrow at 40 completed weeks on the inside circle. With the example in Figure 4-2, the LMP is Sept 7 and the EDD is June 14.

terms *gravida* and *para* in describing numbers of pregnancies and births.

- **G/P** is a two-digit system to denote pregnancy and birth history.
  - **Gravida** *refers to the total number of times a woman has been pregnant, without reference to how many fetuses there were with each pregnancy or when the pregnancy ended. It is simply how many times a woman has been pregnant, including the current pregnancy.*
  - **Para** *refers to the number of births after 20 weeks' gestation whether live births or stillbirths. There is no reference to number of fetuses delivered with this system, so twins count as one delivery, just like a singleton birth. A pregnancy that ends before the end of 20 weeks' gestation is considered an abortion, whether it is spontaneous (miscarriage) or induced (elective or therapeutic), and is not counted using the G/P system.*
- **GTPAL** (meaning *gravida, term, para, abortion,* and *living*) is a more comprehensive system that gives information about each infant from prior pregnancies. This system designates numbers of infants as follows:
  - **G** = *total number of times pregnant (same as G/P system above)*
  - **T** = *number of* term *infants born (after 37 completed or 37 6/7 weeks' gestation)*
  - **P** = *number of* preterm *infants born between 20 and 37 completed weeks' gestation or 37 6/7 weeks)*
  - **A** = *number of abortions (either spontaneous or induced) before 20 weeks' gestation (or <500 grams at birth)*
  - **L** = *the number of children currently* living.

- **GTPALM may be used, and the M represents pregnancies with multiple gestations.**
- **Nulligravida** is a woman who has never been pregnant or given birth.
- **Primigravida** is a woman who is pregnant for the first time.
- **Multigravida** is someone who is pregnant for at least the second time.

PHYSIOLOGICAL PROGRESSION OF PREGNANCY

Pregnancy results in maternal physiologic adaptations involving every body system. Every change has either the maintenance of the pregnancy, the development of the fetus, or preparation for the labor and birth as its basis and is protective of the woman and/or the fetus. To both understand a woman's experience of normal pregnancy and be effective in identifying deviations from normal, the nurse must have a basic foundation in the physiology of pregnancy.

This understanding is critical not only for risk assessment and implementation of appropriate nursing interventions to reduce risk but also for providing effective patient education and anticipatory guidance grounded in knowledge of the physiological basis for the normal physical changes in pregnancy and their resulting common, and normal, discomforts. The next sections present the changes that occur in each system, and **Table 4-3** summarizes the major physiological changes and factors that influence these changes.

TABLE 4–3 PHYSIOLOGICAL CHANGES IN PREGNANCY

PHYSIOLOGICAL CHANGES	CLINICAL SIGNS AND SYMPTOMS
REPRODUCTIVE SYSTEM—Breasts Increase of estrogen and progesterone levels: Initially produced by the corpus luteum and then by the placenta Increased blood supply to breasts	Tenderness, feeling of fullness, and tingling sensation Increase in weight of breast by 400 grams Enlargement of breasts, nipples, areola, and Montgomery follicles (small glands on the areola around the nipple) Striae: Due to stretching of skin to accommodate enlarging breast tissue Prominent veins due to a twofold increase in blood flow
Increase of prolactin: Produced by the anterior pituitary	Increased growth of mammary glands Increase in lactiferous ducts and alveolar system Production of colostrum, a yellow secretion rich in antibodies, begins to be produced as early as 16 weeks
REPRODUCTIVE SYSTEM—Uterus, cervix, and vagina Increased levels of estrogen and progesterone	Hypertrophy of uterine wall Softening of vaginal muscle and connective tissue in preparation for expansion of tissue to accommodate passage of fetus through the birth canal Uterus contractibility increases in response to increased estrogen levels, leading to Braxton-Hicks contractions. Hypertrophy of cervical glands leads to formation of mucus plug, which serves as a protective barrier between uterus/fetus and vagina. Increased vascularity and hypertrophy of vaginal and cervical glands leads to increase in leukorrhea. Cessation of menstrual cycle (amenorrhea) and ovulation

TABLE 4–3 PHYSIOLOGICAL CHANGES IN PREGNANCY—cont'd

PHYSIOLOGICAL CHANGES	CLINICAL SIGNS AND SYMPTOMS
Enlargement and stretching of uterus to accommodate developing fetus and placenta	Increase in uterine size to 20 times that of non-pregnant uterus
	Weight of uterus increases from 70 grams to 1,100 grams.
	Capacity increases from 10 ml to 5000 ml; 80% of that to uteroplacental
Expanded circulatory volume leads to increased vascular congestion.	Blood flow to the uterus is 500–600 mL/min at term.
	Goodell's sign: Softening of the cervix
	Hegar's sign: Softening of the lower uterine segment
	Chadwick's sign: Bluish coloration of cervix, vaginal mucosa, and vulva
Acid pH of vagina	Acid environment inhibits growth of bacteria.
	Acid environment allows growth of *Candida albicans*, leading to increased risk of candidiasis (yeast infection).
CARDIOVASCULAR SYSTEM Decrease in peripheral vascular resistance	Decrease in blood pressure
Increase in blood volume by 40%–45%	Hypervolemia of pregnancy
Increase in cardiac output by 40%	Increased heart rate of 15–20 bpm
BMR increased 10%–20% by 3rd trimester	Increased stroke volume of 25%–30%
Increase in peripheral dilation	Systolic murmurs, load and wide S1 split, load S2, obvious S3
	Increase in heart size
Increase in RBC count by 30%	Physiological anemia of pregnancy
Increase in RBC volume by 18%–33%	Hemodilution is caused by the increase in plasma volume being relatively larger than the increase in RBCs, which results in decreased hemoglobin and hematocrit values. (See Appendix B for pregnancy laboratory values.)
Increase in plasma volume by 50%	
Increase in WBC count	Values up to 16,000 mm^3 in the absence of infection
Increased demand for iron in fetal development	Iron-deficiency anemia: Hemoglobin <11 g/dL and hematocrit<33%
Plasma fibrin increase of 40%	Hypercoagulability
Fibrinogen increase of 50%	
Decrease in coagulation inhibiting factors	
Protective of inevitable blood loss during birth	
Increased venous pressure and decreased blood flow to extremities due to compression of iliac veins and inferior vena cava	Edema of lower extremities
	Varicosities in legs and vulva
	Hemorrhoids
In supine position the enlarged uterus compresses the inferior vena cava, causing reduced blood flow back to the right atrium and a drop in cardiac output and blood pressure.	Supine hypotensive syndrome
RESPIRATORY SYSTEM Hormones of pregnancy stimulate the respiratory center and act on lung tissue to increase and enhance respiratory function.	Increase in tidal volume by 35%–50%
	Slight increase in respiratory rate
	Increase in inspiratory capacity
	Decrease in expiratory volume
Increase of oxygen consumption by 15%–20%	Slight hyperventilation
	Slight respiratory alkalosis
Estrogen, progesterone, and prostaglandins cause vascular engorgement and smooth muscle relaxation.	Dyspnea
	Nasal and sinus congestion
	Epistaxis

Continued

TABLE 4–3   PHYSIOLOGICAL CHANGES IN PREGNANCY—cont'd

PHYSIOLOGICAL CHANGES	CLINICAL SIGNS AND SYMPTOMS
Upward displacement of diaphragm by enlarging uterus Estrogen causes a relaxation of the ligaments and joints of the ribs. Slight decrease in lung capacity	Shift from abdominal to thoracic breathing Chest and thorax expand to accommodate thoracic breathing and upward displacement of diaphragm.
RENAL SYSTEM Alterations in cardiovascular system (increased cardiac output and increased blood and plasma volume) lead to increased renal blood flow of 50%–80% in first trimester and then decreases. Increased progesterone levels, which cause a relaxation of smooth muscles	Urinary frequency and incontinence and increased risk of urinary tract infection (UTI)
Dilation of renal pelvis and ureters Ureters become elongated with decreased motility. Decreased bladder tone with increased bladder capacity	Increased risk of UTI
Pressure of enlarging uterus on renal structures Displacement of bladder in third trimester	Urinary frequency and nocturia
Increased glomerular filtration rate	Increased urinary output
Increased renal excretion of glucose and protein	Glucosuria and proteinuria
Decreased renal flow in third trimester	Dependent edema
Increased vascularity	Hyperemia of bladder and urethra
GASTROINTESTINAL SYSTEM Increased levels of hCG and altered carbohydrate metabolism	Nausea and vomiting during early pregnancy
Increased progesterone levels slow stomach emptying and relax the esophageal sphincter.	Reflux of gastric contents into lower esophagus resulting in heartburn
Increased progesterone levels relax smooth muscle to slow the digestive process and movement of stool.	Bloating, flatulence, and constipation
Increased progesterone levels decrease muscle tone of gallbladder and result in prolonged emptying time.	Increased risk of gallstone formation and cholestasis
Changes in senses of taste and smell	Increase or decrease in appetite Nausea Pica: Abnormal; craving for and ingestion of nonfood substances such as clay or starch
Displacement of intestines by uterus	Flatulence, abdominal distension, abdominal cramping, and pelvic heaviness
Increased levels of estrogen lead to increased vascular congestion of mucosa.	Gingivitis, bleeding gums, increase risk of periodontal disease
MUSCULOSKELETAL SYSTEM Increased progesterone and relaxin levels lead to softening of joints and increased joint mobility, resulting in widening and increased mobility of the sacroiliac and symphysis pubis.	Altered gait: "Waddle" gait Facilitates birthing process Low back pain or pelvic discomfort Pelvis tilts forward, leading to shifting of center of gravity that results in change in posture and walking style, increasing lordosis. Increased risk of falls due to shift in center of gravity and change in gait and posture

TABLE 4–3 PHYSIOLOGICAL CHANGES IN PREGNANCY—cont'd

PHYSIOLOGICAL CHANGES	CLINICAL SIGNS AND SYMPTOMS
Distension of abdomen related to expanding uterus, reduced abdominal tone, and increased breast size	Round ligament spasm
Increased estrogen and relaxin levels lead to increased elasticity and relaxation of ligaments.	Increase risk of joint pain and injury
Abdominal muscles stretch due to enlarging uterus.	Diastasis recti
INTEGUMENTARY SYSTEM Estrogen and progesterone levels stimulate increased melanin deposition, causing light brown to dark brown pigmentation.	Linea nigra Melasma (chloasma) Increased pigmentation of nipples, areola, vulva, scars, and moles
Increased blood flow, increased basal metabolic rate, progesterone-induced increase in body temperature, and vasomotor instability	Hot flashes, facial flushing, alternating sensation of hot and cold Increased perspiration
Increased action of adrenocorticosteroids leads to cutaneous elastic tissues becoming fragile.	Striae gravidarum (stretch marks) on abdomen, thighs, breast, and buttocks
Increased estrogen levels lead to color and vascular changes.	Angiomas (spider nevi) Palmarerythema: Pinkish-red mottling over palms of hands and redness of fingers
Increased androgens lead to increase in sebaceous gland secretions.	Increased oiliness of skin and increase of acne
ENDOCRINE SYSTEM Decreased follicle-stimulating hormone	Amenorrhea
Increased progesterone	Maintains pregnancy by relaxation of smooth muscles, leading to decreased uterine activity, which results in decreased risk of spontaneous abortions Decreases gastrointestinal motility and slows digestive processes
Increased estrogen	Facilitates uterine and breast development Facilitates increases in vascularity Facilitates hyperpigmentation Alters metabolic processes and fluid and electrolyte balance
Increased prolactin	Facilitates lactation
Increased oxytocin	Stimulates uterine contractions Stimulates the milk let-down or ejection reflex in response to breastfeeding
Increased human chorionic gonadotropin (hCG)	Maintenance of corpus luteum until placenta becomes fully functional
Human placental lactogen/human chorionic somatomammotropin	Facilitates breast development Alters carbohydrate, protein, and fat metabolism Facilitates fetal growth by altering maternal metabolism; acts as an insulin antagonist
Hyperplasia and increased vascularity of thyroid	Enlargement of thyroid Heat intolerance and fatigue
Increased BMR related to fetal metabolic activity	Depletion of maternal glucose stores leads to increased risk of maternal hypoglycemia.
Increased need for glucose due to developing fetus	Increased production of insulin
Increase in circulating cortisol	Increase in maternal resistance to insulin leads to increased risk of hyperglycemia.
NEUROLOGICAL SYSTEM	Headache Syncope

Blackburn (2007); Cunningham et al. (2010); Kahn & Hoos (2010); Mattson & Smith, 2011; Blackburn (2014).

Reproductive System

Maternal physiologic adaptations to pregnancy are most profound in the reproductive system. The uterus undergoes phenomenal growth, breasts prepare for lactation, and the vagina changes to accommodate the birthing process (**Fig. 4-3**).

Breasts

Breast changes begin early in pregnancy and continue throughout gestation and into the postpartum period. These changes are primarily influenced by increases in hormone levels and occur in preparation for lactation (see Table 4-3).

Uterus

The uterus is described in three parts:

- **Fundus** or upper portion
- **Isthmus** or lower segment
- **Cervix,** the lower narrow part, or neck; the external part of the cervix interfaces with the vagina. The **Cervical Os** is the opening of the cervix that dilates (opens) during labor to allow passage of the fetus through the vagina.

Uterine changes over the course of pregnancy are profound (see Table 4-3).

- Before pregnancy, this elastic, muscular organ is the size and shape of a small pear weighing 40–50 g.

- During pregnancy, the uterine wall progressively thins as the uterus expands to accommodate the developing fetus.
- By mid-pregnancy, the uterine fundus reaches the level of the umbilicus abdominally.
- Toward the end of pregnancy, the enlarged uterus, containing a full-term fetus, fills the abdominal cavity and has altered the placement of the lungs and rib cage in addition to the abdominal organs (**Fig. 4-4**).
- Intermittent, painless, and physiological uterine contractions, referred to as **Braxton-Hicks contractions,** begin in the second trimester but some women do not feel them until the third trimester. These contractions are irregular with no particular pattern. As the uterus enlarges, they are more noticeable.
- At term, the uterus weighs 1100–1200 g.

Vagina

The vagina is an elastic muscular canal. As pregnancy progresses, various changes take place in the vasculature and tone (see Table 4-3).

- An increase of vascularity due to the expanded circulatory needs
- An increase of vaginal discharge (**leukorrhea**), which is in response to the estrogen-induced hypertrophy of the vaginal glands
- Relaxation of the vaginal wall and perineal body, which allows stretching of tissues to accommodate the birthing process.

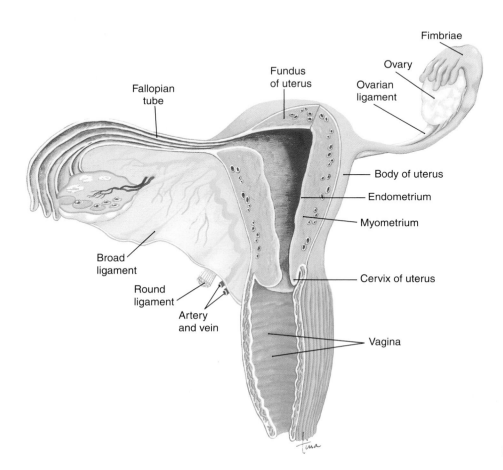

Figure 4–3   Reproductive system.

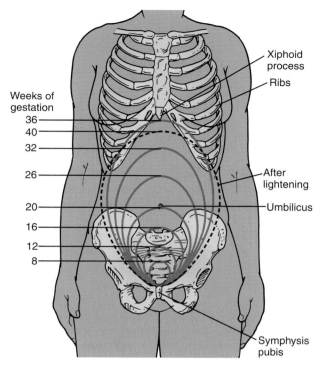

Figure 4-4 Uterine heights by weeks of gestation with anatomical landmarks.

■ Acid pH of the vagina, which inhibits growth of bacteria but allows overgrowth of *Candida albicans.* This places the pregnant woman at risk for candidiasis (yeast infection).

Ovaries

The corpus luteum, which normally degrades after ovulation when the egg is not fertilized, is maintained during the first couple months of pregnancy by high levels of human chorionic gonadatropin (hCG). At the beginning of pregnancy, the corpus luteum produces progesterone in order to maintain the thick lining of the uterus, referred to as the **endometrium,** to allow for implantation and establishment of the pregnancy. There is subsequently no shedding of the endometrium that would result in menstruation. Ovulation ceases as the hormones of pregnancy inhibit follicle maturation and release. By 6–7 weeks' gestation, the placenta begins producing progesterone and the corpus luteum degenerates.

PATIENT EDUCATION

- Discuss reasons for breast changes such as tenderness, enlargement, or heaviness and encourage the woman to wear a properly fitted supportive bra.
- Explain the possibility of breasts to leaking colostrum.
- Educate on Braxton-Hicks contractions and contraction patterns that should be reported to her health care provider.
- Discuss self-care measures to prevent yeast infections.

Cardiovascular System

The cardiovascular system undergoes significant adaptations during pregnancy to support the maintenance and development of the fetus while also meeting maternal physiological needs during both the pregnancy and the postpartum period. The hemodynamic changes are also a protective mechanism for the inevitable maternal blood loss during the intrapartum period (see Table 4-3). Cardiovascular system changes include:

■ Cardiac output (CO) increases 30%–50% and reaches a peak at 25–30 weeks.
■ The heart rate increases 15–20 beats per minute (bpm).
■ Stroke volume increases by 25%–30%.
■ Basal metabolic rate (BMR) increases 10%–20% by the third trimester.
■ The white blood cell (WBC) count increases, with values up to 16,000 mm^3 in the absence of infection.
　■ *The increase is hormonally induced and similar to elevations seen in physiological stress such as exercise.*
■ Plasma volume increases 40%–50% during pregnancy until reaching a peak about 32–34 weeks and remaining there until term.
■ In response to increased oxygen requirements of pregnancy, the red blood cell (RBC) count increases 30% and RBC volume increases up to 33% with iron supplementation (up to 18% without supplementation).
　■ *The increase in plasma volume is relatively larger than the increase in RBCs. This hemodilution is evidenced by decreased hemoglobin and hematocrit values and is known as* **physiological anemia of pregnancy,** *or pseudo anemia of pregnancy. See Appendix B for laboratory values during pregnancy.*
　■ *Cardiac work is eased as the decrease in blood viscosity facilitates placental perfusion.*
■ Iron-deficiency anemia is defined as hemoglobin less than 11.0 g/dL and hematocrit less than 33%.
　■ *Maternal iron stores are insufficient to meet the demands for iron in fetal development.*
■ Blood volume increases by 1,500 mL or by 40%–45% to support uteroplacental demands and maintenance of pregnancy. This is referred to as **hypervolemia of pregnancy.**
■ The heart enlarges slightly as a result of hypervolemia and increased cardiac output.
■ The heart shifts upward and laterally as the growing uterus displaces the diaphragm (**Fig. 4-5**).
■ Hypercoagulation occurs during pregnancy to decrease the risk of postpartum hemorrhage. These changes place the woman at increased risk for thrombosis and coagulopathies.
　■ *Plasma fibrin increase of 40%*
　■ *Fibrinogen increase of 50%*
　■ *Coagulation inhibiting factors decrease*
■ Blood pressure decreases in the first trimester due to a decrease in peripheral vascular resistance. The blood pressure returns to normal by term.
■ **Supine hypotension** can occur when the woman is in the supine position as the enlarging uterus can compress the

(Text continued on page 65)

TABLE 4–4   SELF-CARE/RELIEF MEASURES FOR PHYSICAL CHANGES AND COMMON DISCOMFORTS OF PREGNANCY

BODY SYSTEM	PHYSICAL CHANGES AND COMMON DISCOMFORTS OF PREGNANCY (COMMON TIMING)	NURSING ACTIONS FOR PATIENT EDUCATION FOR SELF-CARE AND RELIEF MEASURES
GENERALIZED OR MULTISYSTEM	Fatigue (first and third trimesters)	Reassure the woman of the normalcy of her response. Encourage the woman to plan for extra rest during the day and at night; focus on "work" of growing a healthy baby. Enlist support and assistance from friends and family. Encourage the woman to eat an optimal diet with adequate caloric intake and iron-rich foods and iron supplementation if anemic.
	Insomnia (throughout pregnancy)	Instruct the woman to implement sleep hygiene measures (regular bedtime, relaxing or low-key activities pre-bedtime). Encourage the woman to create a comfortable sleep environment (body pillow, additional pillows). Teach breathing exercises and relaxation techniques/measures [progressive relaxation, effleurage (a massage technique using a very light touch of the fingers in two repetitive circular patterns over the gravid abdomen), warm bath or warm beverage pre-bedtime]. Evaluate caffeine use.
	Emotional lability (throughout pregnancy)	Reassure the woman of the normalcy of response. Encourage adequate rest and optimal nutrition. Encourage communication with partner/significant support people. Refer to pregnancy support group.
REPRODUCTIVE Breasts	Tenderness, enlargement, upper back pain (throughout pregnancy; tenderness mostly in the first trimester)	Encourage the woman to wear a well-fitting, supportive bra. Instruct woman in correct use of good body mechanics.
	Leaking of colostrum from nipples (starting second trimester onward)	Reassure the woman of the normalcy. Recommend soft cotton breast pads if leaking is troublesome.
Uterus	Braxton-Hicks contractions (mid-pregnancy onward)	Reassure the woman that occasional contractions are normal. Instruct the woman to call her provider if contractions become regular and persist before 37 weeks. Ensure adequate fluid intake. Recommend a maternity girdle for uterus support.
Cervix/vagina	Increased secretions Yeast infections (throughout pregnancy)	Encourage daily bathing. Recommend cotton underwear. Recommend wearing panty liner, changing pad frequently. Instruct the woman to avoid douching or using feminine hygiene sprays. Inform provider if discharge changes in color, or accompanied by foul odor or pruritus.
	Dyspareunia (throughout pregnancy)	Reassure the woman/couple of normalcy of response, provide information. Suggest alternative positions for sexual intercourse and alternative sexual activity to sexual intercourse.

TABLE 4–4	SELF-CARE/RELIEF MEASURES FOR PHYSICAL CHANGES AND COMMON DISCOMFORTS OF PREGNANCY—cont'd	
BODY SYSTEM	**PHYSICAL CHANGES AND COMMON DISCOMFORTS OF PREGNANCY (COMMON TIMING)**	**NURSING ACTIONS FOR PATIENT EDUCATION FOR SELF-CARE AND RELIEF MEASURES**
CARDIOVASCULAR	Supine hypotension (mid-pregnancy onward)	Instruct the woman to avoid supine position from mid-pregnancy onward. Advise her to lie on her side and rise slowly to decrease the risk of a hypotensive event.
	Orthostatic hypotension	Advise woman to keep feet moving when standing and avoid standing for prolonged periods. Instruct to rise slowly from a lying position to sitting or standing to decrease the risk of a hypotensive event.
	Anemia (throughout pregnancy; more common in late second trimester)	Encourage the woman to include iron-rich foods in daily dietary intake and take iron supplementation.
	Dependent edema lower extremities and/or vulva (late pregnancy)	Instruct the woman to: • Wear loose clothing • Use a maternity girdle (abdominal support), which may help reduce venous pressure in pelvis/lower extremities and enhance circulation • Avoid prolonged standing or sitting • Dorsiflex feet periodically when standing or sitting • Elevate legs when sitting • Position on side when lying down
	Varicosities (later pregnancy)	Instruct woman in all measures for dependent edema (see above). Suggest the woman wear support hose (put on before rising in the morning, before legs have been in dependent position). Instruct the woman to lie on her back with legs propped against a wall in an approximately 45-degree angle to spine periodically throughout the day. Instruct the woman to avoid crossing legs when sitting.
RESPIRATORY	Hyperventilation and dyspnea (throughout pregnancy; may worsen in later pregnancy)	Reassure the woman of the normalcy of her response and provide information. Instruct the woman to slow down respiration rate and depth when hyperventilating. Encourage good posture. Instruct the woman to stand and stretch, taking a deep breath, periodically throughout the day; stretch and take a deep breath periodically throughout the night. Suggest sleeping semi-sitting with additional pillows for support.
	Nasal and sinus congestion/ Epistaxis (throughout pregnancy)	Suggest the woman try a cool-air humidifier. Instruct the woman to avoid use of decongestants and nasal sprays and instead to use normal saline drops.

Continued

TABLE 4–4	SELF-CARE/RELIEF MEASURES FOR PHYSICAL CHANGES AND COMMON DISCOMFORTS OF PREGNANCY—cont'd	
BODY SYSTEM	**PHYSICAL CHANGES AND COMMON DISCOMFORTS OF PREGNANCY (COMMON TIMING)**	**NURSING ACTIONS FOR PATIENT EDUCATION FOR SELF-CARE AND RELIEF MEASURES**
RENAL	Frequency and urgency/nocturia (may be throughout pregnancy; most common in first and third trimesters)	Reassure the woman of normalcy of response. Encourage the woman to empty her bladder frequently, always wiping front to back. Stress the importance of maintaining adequate hydration, reducing fluid intake only near bedtime. Instruct her to urinate after intercourse. Teach the woman to notify her provider if there is pain or blood with urination. Encourage Kegel exercises; wear perineal pad if needed.
GASTROINTESTINAL	Nausea and/or vomiting in pregnancy (NVP) (first trimester and sometimes into the second trimester)	Reassure the woman of normalcy and self-limiting nature of response. Avoid strong odors and causative factors (e.g., spicy foods, greasy foods, large meals, stuffy rooms, hot places or loud noises). Encourage women to experiment with alleviating factors: • Eating small, frequent meals as soon as, or before, feeling hungry • Eat a slow pace • Eat crackers or dry toast before rising or whenever nauseous • Drink cold, clear carbonated beverages such as ginger ale, or sour beverages such as lemonade • Avoid fluid intake with meals • Eat ginger-flavored lollipops or peppermint candies • Brush teeth after eating • Wear P6 acupressure wrist bands • Take vitamins at bedtime with a snack (not in the morning) • Suggest vitamin B6, 25 mg by mouth three times daily or ginger, 250 mg by mouth four times daily Oral or rectal medications may be prescribed for management of troublesome symptoms. Identify, acknowledge, and support women with significant NVP to offer additional treatment options.
	Increase or sense of increase in salivation (mostly first trimester if associated with nausea)	Suggest use of gum or hard candy or use astringent mouthwash.
	Bleeding gums (throughout pregnancy)	Encourage the woman to maintain good oral hygiene (brush gently with soft toothbrush, daily flossing). Maintain optimal nutrition.
	Flatulence (throughout pregnancy)	Encourage the woman to: • Maintain regular bowel habits • Engage in regular exercise • Avoid gas-producing foods • Chew food slowly and thoroughly • Use the knee-chest position during periods of discomfort

TABLE 4–4	SELF-CARE/RELIEF MEASURES FOR PHYSICAL CHANGES AND COMMON DISCOMFORTS OF PREGNANCY—cont'd	
BODY SYSTEM	**PHYSICAL CHANGES AND COMMON DISCOMFORTS OF PREGNANCY (COMMON TIMING)**	**NURSING ACTIONS FOR PATIENT EDUCATION FOR SELF-CARE AND RELIEF MEASURES**
	Heartburn (later pregnancy)	Suggest: • Small, frequent meals • Maintain good posture • Maintain adequate fluid intake, but avoid fluid intake with meals • Avoid fatty or fried foods • Remain upright for 30–45 minutes after eating • Refrain from eating at least 3 hours prior to bedtime
	Constipation (throughout pregnancy) (see Concept Map)	Encourage the woman to: • Maintain adequate fluid intake • Engage in regular exercise such as walking • Increase fiber in diet • Maintain regular bowel habits • Maintain good posture and body mechanics
	Hemorrhoids (later pregnancy)	Avoid constipation (see above) Instruct the woman to avoid bearing down with bowel movements. Instruct the woman in comfort measures (e.g., ice packs, warm baths or sitz baths, witch hazel compresses). Elevate the hips and lower extremities during rest periods throughout the day. Gently reinsert into the rectum while doing Kegel exercises.
MUSCULOSKELETAL	Low back pain/joint discomfort/difficulty walking (later pregnancy)	Instruct the woman to: • Utilize proper body mechanics (e.g., stoop using knees vs. bend for lifting) • Maintain good posture • Do pelvic rock/pelvic tilt exercises • Wear supportive shoes with low heels • Apply warmth or ice to painful area • Use of maternity girdle • Use massage • Use relaxation techniques • Sleep on a firm mattress with pillows for additional support of extremities, abdomen, and back
	Diastasis recti (later pregnancy)	Instruct the woman to do gentle abdominal strengthening exercises (e.g., tiny abdominal crunches, may cross arms over abdomen to opposite sides for splinting, no sit-ups). Teach proper technique for sitting up from lying down (i.e., roll to side, lift torso up using arms until in sitting position).

Continued

TABLE 4–4   SELF-CARE/RELIEF MEASURES FOR PHYSICAL CHANGES AND COMMON DISCOMFORTS OF PREGNANCY—cont'd

BODY SYSTEM	PHYSICAL CHANGES AND COMMON DISCOMFORTS OF PREGNANCY (COMMON TIMING)	NURSING ACTIONS FOR PATIENT EDUCATION FOR SELF-CARE AND RELIEF MEASURES
	Round ligament spasm & pain (late second and third trimester)	Instruct the woman to: • Lie on side and flex knees up to abdomen • Bend toward pain • Do pelvic tilt/pelvic rock exercises • Use warm baths or compresses • Use side-lying in exaggerated Sim's position with pillows for additional support of abdomen and in between legs • Use maternity belt
	Leg cramps (throughout pregnancy)	Instruct the woman to: • Dorsiflex foot to stretch calf muscle • Warm baths or compresses to the affected area • Change position slowly • Massage the affected area • Regular exercise and muscle conditioning
INTEGUMENTARY	Striae (stretch marks) (later pregnancy)	Reassure the woman that there is no method to prevent them. Suggest maintaining skin comfort (e.g., lotions, oatmeal baths, non-binding clothing). Encourage good weight control.
	Dry skin or pruritus (itching) (later pregnancy)	Suggestions for maintaining skin comfort use tepid water for baths and showers and rinse with cooler water. Avoid hot water (drying effect and may increase itching). Use moisturizing soaps or body wash. Avoid exfoliating scrubs or deodorant soaps (has drying effect and may increase itching). Use of lotions, oatmeal baths, non-binding clothing may lessen itching.
	Skin hyperpigmentation	Limit sun exposure. Wear sunscreen regularly.
	Acne	Use products developed for the face only (e.g., cleansers, sunscreen), avoid body soaps and facial scrubs (both have drying effects), body lotions/creams (clog pores); use tepid water when washing face and always follow with cold rinse to close pores before applying moisturizers (if needed) or sunscreen.
NEUROLOGICAL	Headaches	Maintain adequate hydration
	Syncope	Rise slowly from sitting to standing Instruct the woman to avoid supine position from mid-pregnancy onward. Advise her to lie on her side and rise slowly to decrease the risk of a hypotensive event.

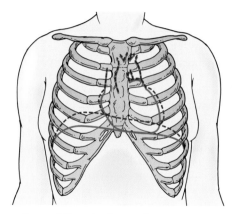

Figure 4–5 Dotted lines indicate displacement of heart and lungs as pregnancy progresses and uterus enlarges.

inferior vena cava (see Critical Component: Supine Hypotensive Syndrome).

- In the majority of women, a systolic heart murmur or a third heart sound (gallop) may be heard by mid-pregnancy.
- Peripheral dilation is increased.
- Varicosities may develop in the legs or vulva as a result of increased venous pressure below the level of the uterus.
- Dependent edema in the lower extremities is caused by increased venous pressure from the enlarging uterus.

PATIENT EDUCATION (SEE TABLE 4-4)

- Educate on the causes of supine and orthostatic hypotension and advice on self-care measures to prevent a hypotensive event.
- Encourage the woman to include iron-rich foods and take iron supplementation to prevent anemia.
- Instruct the woman in prevention and relief measures for dependent edema and varicosities.

Respiratory System

Throughout the course of pregnancy, the respiratory system adapts in response to physiological and anatomical demands related to fetal growth and development as well as maternal metabolic needs (see Table 4-3). Pulmonary function is not compromised in a normal pregnancy.

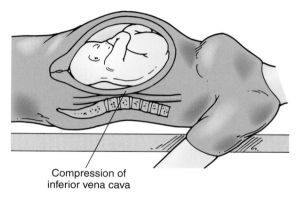

Compression of
inferior vena cava

Figure 4–6 Supine hypotension compression of the inferior vena cava by the gravid uterus while in the supine position reduces venous blood return to the heart causing maternal hypotension.

Physiological changes occur to accommodate the additional requirements for oxygen delivery and carbon dioxide removal in mother and fetus during pregnancy.

Physiological changes include:

- Tidal volume increases 35%–50%
- Slight respiratory alkalosis
  - *Decrease in PCO_2 leads to an increase in pH (more alkaline) and decrease in bicarbonate.*
  - *This change promotes transport of carbon dioxide away from the fetus.*
- Increases in estrogen, progesterone, and prostaglandins cause vascular engorgement and smooth muscle relaxation resulting in edema and tissue congestion, which can lead to:
  - *Dyspnea*
  - *Nasal and sinus congestion*
  - *Epistaxis (nosebleeds)*

Anatomical changes include:

- Diaphragm is displaced upward approximately 4 cm.
- Increase in chest circumference of 6 cm with an increase in the costal angle of greater than 90 degrees
- There is a shift from abdominal to thoracic breathing as the pregnancy progresses (see Fig. 4-5).
- These anatomical changes may contribute to the physiological dyspnea that is common during pregnancy.

PATIENT EDUCATION (SEE TABLE 4-4)

- Educate and reassure the woman about normal respiratory changes and suggest symptom relief measures.
- Encourage the woman to stand and stretch, taking a deep breath, periodically throughout the day and stretch and take a deep breath periodically throughout the night.

Renal System

The kidneys undergo change during pregnancy as they adapt to perform their basic functions of regulating fluid and electrolyte balance, eliminating metabolic waste products, and helping to regulate blood pressure (see Table 4-3). *Physiological* changes include:

- Renal plasma flow increases.
- Glomerular filtration rate (GFR) increases.
- Renal tubular reabsorption increases.
- Proteinuria and glucosuria can normally occur in small amounts related to tubal reabsorption threshold of protein and glucose being exceeded due to increased volume.
  - *Even though a small amount of proteinuria and glucosuria can be normal, it is important to assess and monitor for pathology.*
- Shift in fluid and electrolyte balance
  - *The need for increased fluid and electrolytes results in alteration of regulating mechanisms including the renin–angiotensin–aldosterone system and antidiuretic hormone.*
- Positional variation in renal function
  - *In the supine and upright maternal position, blood pools in the lower body, causing a decrease in cardiac output, GFR, and urine output; also causing excess sodium and fluid retention.*
  - *A left lateral recumbent maternal position can:*
    - Maximize cardiac output, renal plasma volume, and urine output
    - Stabilize fluid and electrolyte balance
    - Minimize dependent edema
    - Maintain optimal blood pressure

These changes support the increased circulatory and metabolic demands of the pregnancy because the renal system secretes both maternal and fetal waste products.

Anatomical changes include:

- Renal pelvis dilation with increased renal plasma flow
- Ureter alterations
  - *Become elongated, tortuous, and dilated*
- Bladder alterations
  - *Bladder capacity increases and bladder tone decreases related to progesterone effect on smooth muscle of the bladder causing relaxation and stretching.*
- Urinary stasis
  - *Progesterone reduces the tone of renal structures, allowing for pooling of urine.*
  - *Stasis promotes bacterial growth and increases the woman's risk for urinary tract infections and pyelonephritis.*
- Hyperemia of bladder and urethra related to increased vascularity that results in pelvic congestion; edematous mucosa is easily traumatized.
- Most women experience urinary symptoms of frequency, urgency, and nocturia beginning early in pregnancy and continuing to varying degrees throughout the pregnancy. These symptoms are primarily a result of the systemic hormonal changes of pregnancy and may also be attributed to anatomical changes in the renal system and other body system changes during pregnancy, but are not generally indicative of infection. Urinary tract infections are common in pregnancy and may be asymptomatic (see Critical Component: Urinary Tract Infection).

CRITICAL COMPONENT

Urinary Tract Infection

The most common bacterial infection during pregnancy is a urinary tract infection (UTI). Physiological changes that occur in the renal system during pregnancy predispose pregnant women to urinary tract infections. Symptoms of a UTI include urinary frequency, dysuria, urgency, and sometimes pus or blood in the urine. Treatment includes anti-infective medication for a 7- to 10-day period. If untreated, the infection can lead to pyelonephritis or premature labor.

PATIENT EDUCATION (SEE TABLE 4-4)

- Educate the woman on reasons for increased frequency of urination during first and third trimesters.
- Teach signs and symptoms of a urinary tract infection and advise her to seek prompt treatment if she experiences them.
- Encourage UTI prevention measures such as:
  - Emptying bladder frequently
  - Wiping front to back
  - Washing hands before and after urination
  - Urinating after intercourse
  - Maintaining adequate hydration with at least 8 glasses of liquid a day
  - Teach and encourage Kegel exercises and instruct to wear perineal pad if needed.

Gastrointestinal System

The gastrointestinal (GI) system adapts in its anatomy and physiology during pregnancy in support of maternal and fetal nutritional requirements (see Table 4-3). The adaptations are related to hormonal influences as well as the impact of the enlarging uterus on the GI system as pregnancy progresses.

Most pregnant women (90%) experience some degree of nausea and vomiting in pregnancy (NVP). For the majority of affected women, the symptoms are an expected part of pregnancy and tolerated well; however, about a third of affected women experience significant distress. As the pregnancy progresses, NVP symptoms usually diminish; 60% of cases resolve by 12 weeks' gestation and 90% have symptom improvement by 16 weeks' gestation (Tan & Omar, 2011). It is important to identify women with significant NVP so they can be successfully treated.

Additional alterations in nutritional patterns commonly seen in pregnancy include:

- Increase in appetite and intake
- Cravings for specific foods
  - *Pica is a craving for and consumption of nonfood substances such as starch and clay. It can result in toxicity due to ingested substances or malnutrition from replacing nutritious foods with nonfood substances.*
- Avoidance of specific foods

Anatomical and *physiological* changes include:

- Uterine enlargement displaces the stomach, liver, and intestines as the pregnancy progresses.

- By the end of pregnancy, the appendix is situated high and to the right along the costal margin.
- The GI tract experiences a general relaxation and slowing of its digestive processes during pregnancy, contributing to many of the common discomforts of pregnancy such as heartburn, abdominal bloating, and constipation.
- Hemorrhoids (varicosities in the anal canal) are common in pregnancy due to increased venous pressure and are exacerbated by constipation. 30%–40% of pregnant women experience hemorrhoidal discomfort, pruritis, and/or bleeding.
- Gallstones: Progesterone-induced relaxation of smooth muscle results in distention of gallbladder and slows emptying of bile; bile stasis and elevated levels of cholesterol contribute to formation of gallstones.
- Pruritus: Abdominal pruritus may be an early sign of cholestasis.
- Ptyalism: Increase in saliva
- Bleeding gums and periodontal disease
  - *Increased vascularity of the gums can result in gingivitis.*

PATIENT EDUCATION (SEE TABLE 4-4)

- Reassure of normalcy and self-limiting nature of nausea and vomiting of pregnancy and suggest measures to prevent and relieve.
- Advise the woman to maintain good oral hygiene and continue routine preventative dental care.
- Encourage the woman to eat a high-fiber diet with adequate hydration and physical activity to prevent constipation and hemorrhoids.
- Instruct on preventive and relief measures for heartburn, flatulence, constipation, and hemorrhoids.

Musculoskeletal System

Significant adaptation occurs in the musculoskeletal system as a result of pregnancy (see Table 4-3). Hormonal shifts are responsible for many of these changes. Mechanical factors attributable to the growing uterus also contribute to musculoskeletal adaptation.

Anatomical and *physiological* changes include:

- Altered posture and center of gravity related to distention of the abdomen by the expanding uterus and reduced abdominal tone that shifts the center of gravity forward.
  - *A shift in the center of gravity places the woman at higher risk for falls.*
- Altered gait ("pregnant waddle"): Hormonal influences of progesterone and relaxin soften joints and increase joint mobility.
- Lordosis: Abnormal anterior curvature of the lumbar spine. The body compensates for the shift in center of gravity by developing an increased curvature of the spine.
- Joint discomfort: Hormonal influences of progesterone and relaxin soften cartilage and connective tissue, leading to joint instability.
- Round ligament spasm: Estrogen and relaxin increase elasticity and relaxation of ligaments, and abdominal distention stretches round ligaments causing spasm and pain.
- **Diastasis recti:** This is the separation of the rectus abdominis muscle in the midline caused by the abdominal distention. It is a benign condition that can occur in the third trimester.
- The impact of all of the musculoskeletal adaptations in pregnancy resulting in numerous common discomforts of pregnancy can sometimes be reduced if the woman maintains a normal body weight and exercises regularly prior to and throughout her pregnancy.

PATIENT EDUCATION (SEE TABLE 4-4)

- Discuss musculoskeletal system changes during pregnancy.
- Encourage good posture and body mechanics to prevent symptoms of pain.
- Teach symptom relief measures for back or ligament pain.
- Encourage gentle abdominal strengthening exercises.

Integumentary System

The integumentary system includes the skin and related structures such as hair, nails, and glands. Hormonal influences are primary factors in integumentary system adaptations during pregnancy, with mechanical factors associated with the enlarging uterus playing a lesser role in changes associated with this body system (see Table 4-3).

Anatomical and physiological changes include:

- Hyperpigmentation: Estrogen and progesterone stimulate increased melanin deposition of light brown to dark brown pigmentation.
  - *Linea nigra: Darkened line in midline of abdomen* (**Fig. 4-7**)
  - *Melasma (chloasma), also referred to as mask of pregnancy, is a brownish pigmentation of the skin over the cheeks, nose, and forehead. This occurs in 50%–70% of pregnant women and is more common in darker skinned women. It usually occurs after the 16th week of pregnancy and is exacerbated by sun exposure.*
- **Striae** (stretch marks): Stretching of skin due to growth of breast, hips, abdomen, and buttocks plus the effects of estrogen, relaxin, and adrenocorticoids may result in tearing of subcutaneous connective tissue/collagen (see Fig. 4-7).
- Varicosities, spider nevi, and palmer erythema: Vascular changes related to hormonally induced increased elasticity of vessels and increased venous pressure from enlarged uterus.
- Hot flashes and facial flushing: Caused by increased blood supply to skin, increase in basal metabolic rate, progesterone-induced increased body temperature, and vasomotor instability.
- Oily skin and acne: Effects of increase in androgens.
- Sweating: Thermoregulation process at the level of skin increased in response to increases in thyroid activity, basal metabolic rate (BMR), metabolic activity of fetus, and increased maternal body weight.
- Although none of these integumentary system adaptations is seen universally, each alteration is seen commonly, is

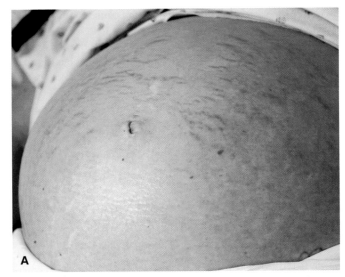

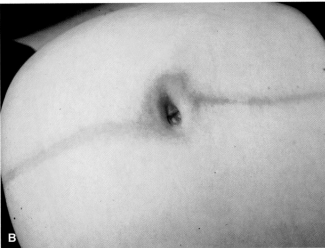

Figure 4-7   Pregnant abdomen with striae (A) and linea nigra (B).

not of pathological significance, and typically resolves or regresses significantly after pregnancy.

PATIENT EDUCATION (SEE TABLE 4-4)

- Offer reassurance as skin pigmentation and/or other changes occur.
- Discuss normalcy of striae in pregnancy and encourage good weight control.
- Suggest maintaining skin comfort with daily bathing, lotions, oatmeal baths, non-binding clothing.
- Advise to limit sun exposure and wear sunscreen.

Endocrine System

Endocrine system adaptations are essential for maintaining the stability of both the woman and her pregnancy and for promoting fetal growth and development. Endocrine glands mediate the many metabolic process adaptations in pregnancy.

There are general endocrine system alterations as a result of pregnancy as well as pregnancy-specific endocrine adaptations related to the placenta that develop once conception has occurred (See Table 4-3).

Physiologic changes include:

- Significant alterations in pituitary, adrenal, thyroid, parathyroid, and pancreatic functioning occur in pregnancy. For example, the hormonal production activity and size of the thyroid gland increase during pregnancy in support of maternal and fetal physiological needs, and there is an increase in pancreatic activity during pregnancy to meet both maternal and fetal needs related to carbohydrate metabolism.

Pregnancy-specific hormones

- The hormones of pregnancy are responsible for most of the physiological adaptations and physical changes seen throughout the entire pregnancy. The placental hormones are initially produced by the corpus luteum of pregnancy. Once implantation occurs, the fertilized ovum and chorionic villi produce hCG.
- The function of the high hCG level in early pregnancy is to maintain the corpus luteum and its production of progesterone and, to a lesser extent, estrogen until the placenta develops and takes over this function.
- After the development of a functioning placenta, the placenta produces most of the hormones of pregnancy, including estrogen, progesterone, human placental lactogen (hPL), and relaxin.
- Each of these hormones plays a role in the physiology of pregnancy, resulting in specific alterations in nearly all body systems, as described in this chapter, to support maternal physiological needs, maintenance and progression of the pregnancy, and fetal growth and development. (See Table 4-3 for details on pregnancy hormones.)

Immune System

Every aspect of the body's very complicated immune system undergoes adaptation during pregnancy in order to maintain a tenuous balance between preservation of maternal–fetal well-being through normal immune responses on the one hand, and the necessary alterations of the maternal immune system required for maintenance of the pregnancy on the other. This adaptive process involves the maternal immune system becoming tolerant of the "foreign" fetal system so that the fetus is not rejected and, further, so that the fetus is protected from infection. Immune function changes in pregnancy are far-reaching and beyond the scope of this chapter. This is also a relatively new body of science that is not fully understood.

ANTEPARTAL NURSING CARE: PHYSIOLOGY-BASED NURSING ASSESSMENT AND NURSING ACTIONS

Prenatal Assessment

The **prenatal period** is the entire time period during which a woman is pregnant through the birth of the baby. It is a time of transition in the life of a family as they prepare for the birth of a child. This time period affords an opportunity for positive change in all aspects of health and health maintenance behaviors. During ongoing interactions, the nurse places emphasis on health education and health promotion involving the woman in her care. The holistic view of health inherent in nursing care for the childbearing woman and her family contributes to a unique situation in which the antepartal patient has ready access to health information, support, and guidance to help her achieve the healthiest possible pregnancy and the best possible outcome for mothers and babies (Barron, 2014). The impact of this **prenatal care** (health care related to pregnancy) and the possibility for positive change it engenders can extend well beyond the antepartal period into the life of the new family. Prenatal nursing care and interventions also contribute to the woman's and family's ability to make informed choices about the health care of the entire family throughout the childbearing cycle, choices based on an integration of information provided by the nurse with the family's personal values, preferences, and beliefs. One of the Healthy People 2020 Objectives is to increase by nearly 10% the proportion of women who receive early and adequate prenatal care from 70%–78% (United States Department of Health and Human Services, 2010). **Family-centered maternity care** is a model of obstetrical care based on a view of pregnancy and childbirth as a normal life event, a life transition that is not primarily medical but rather developmental.

■ The initial prenatal visit parallels a preconception health care visit (see Table 4-1). It also includes information about the health and health history of the father of the baby (age, blood type and Rh status, current health status and history of any chronic or past medical problems, genetic history, occupation, lifestyle factors impacting health, and his involvement in the woman's life and with her pregnancy).

■ The focus of patient education and anticipatory guidance shifts toward pregnancy-related health concerns, but the basic components of the visit as well as the emphasis on health maintenance and health promotion remain the same. Prenatal visits also include specific assessment of the pregnancy and fetal status. Some of these components are uniform across all prenatal visits, and others are specific to one or more trimesters of the pregnancy.

■ Subsequent prenatal visits are more abbreviated than the initial visit, with nursing care and interventions focused on current pregnancy status and patient needs, always with an emphasis on patient education and anticipatory guidance (see **Table 4-5** and Clinical Pathway).

■ The standard accepted frequency of prenatal care visits in a low-risk population in the United States results in approximately 14–16 prenatal visits per pregnancy. However, available evidence suggests that a schedule with reduced frequency of prenatal visits for this population is not associated with an increase in adverse maternal or perinatal outcomes and may be associated with increased levels of patient satisfaction. In spite of this evidence, the routine remains unchanged for the present (Villar, Carrolli, Khan-Neelofer, Piaggio, & Gulmezoglo, 2007; Walker, McCully, & Vest, 2001).

■ The efficacy of the current model for individual prenatal care visits has been questioned as well (see Evidence-Based Practice: Centering Pregnancy).

Evidence-Based Practice: Centering Pregnancy

The generally accepted model of individual prenatal care currently in use in the United States lacks a scientific basis; there is also some question as to its effectiveness in meeting public health objectives in care provision to a healthy population (Walker & Rising, 2004). A group model of prenatal care delivery, Centering Pregnancy, is designed to promote individual responsibility for health in pregnancy; provide appropriate prenatal assessment and risk screening; and provide education, social support, and a sense of community, all in a cost-effective and efficient manner. In one early pilot study, perinatal outcomes were comparable to the traditional care control group, and women reported satisfaction with their care, with 96% of the Centering Pregnancy participants preferring this alternative model to a traditional model of prenatal care (Rising, 1998). Subsequent research has shown positive benefits, including higher birth weights in a low socioeconomic status population (Ickovics et al., 2003); fewer missed prenatal appointments, preterm births, and low birth weight babies, and increased rates of breastfeeding in an adolescent population (Grady & Bloom, 2004); and increased knowledge about pregnancy in the Centering Pregnancy group compared to the traditional care group (Baldwin, 2006).

Essential elements of the Centering Pregnancy model of group prenatal care include:

1. Health Assessment occurs within the group space.
2. Participants are involved in self-care activities.
3. A facilitated leadership style is used.
4. Each session has an overall plan.
5. Attention is given to general content outline.
6. There is stability of group leadership.
7. Group conduct honors the contribution of each member.
8. The group is conducted in a circle.
9. Opportunity for socializing is provided.
10. The composition of the group is stable, not rigid (Rotundo, 2011).

Advantages of the Centering Pregnancy model of care include: focus on the normalcy of pregnancy, increased time with the care provider during the pregnancy, a perceived benefit for both the care provider and the pregnant woman, efficiency for the care provider in providing important prenatal education content, development of social connections between group members, social support for participants in managing the normal challenges of pregnancy, and validation of the woman's experience of pregnancy by a peer group (Rotundo, 2011). Benefits of group prenatal care include:

■ Improved birth outcomes
■ Improved patient satisfaction
■ Improved patient knowledge and readiness for labor and infant care
■ Higher breastfeeding initiation rates
■ Improvement in racial disparities with regard to maternal outcomes
■ No increase in antenatal service costs

Sources: Baldwin, 2006; Grady & Bloom, 2004; Ickovics et al., 2003, 2007; Rising, 1998; Rotundo, 2011; Walker & Rising, 2004.

TABLE 4–5   PRENATAL CARE: CONTENT AND TIMING OF ROUTINE PRENATAL VISITS

	HISTORY AND PHYSICAL ASSESSMENT	LABORATORY/DIAGNOSTIC STUDIES IN NORMAL PREGNANCY (RECOMMENDED TIMING)
First Trimester		

Initial visit	Comprehensive health and risk assessment (see Table 4-1)
	
	Current pregnancy history
	
	Complete physical and pelvic examination
	
	Determine EDD
	
	Nutrition assessment including 24-hour diet recall
	
	Psychosocial assessment (see Chapter 5)
	
	Assessment for intimate partner violence
		• Blood type and Rh factor
		• Antibody screen
		• Complete blood count (CBC) including:
		  • Hemoglobin
		  • Hematocrit
		  • Red blood cell count (RBC)
		  • White blood cell count (WBC)
		  • Platelet count
		• RPR, VDRL (syphilis serology)
		• HIV screen
		• Hepatitis B screen (surface antigen)
		• Genetic screening based on:
		  • Family history
		  • Racial/ethnic background (e.g., sickle cell disease, Tay-Sachs)
		• Rubella titer
		• PPD (tuberculosis screen)
		• Urinalysis
		• Urine culture and sensitivity
		• Pap smear
		• Gonorrhea and Chlamydia cultures
		• Ultrasound

Return visit (4 weeks after initial visit)	Chart review Interval history Focused physical assessment: Vital signs, urine, weight, fundal height Clinical pelvimetry	
Second Trimester		
Return visits (Every 4 weeks)	Chart review Interval history Nutrition follow-up Focused physical assessment: Vital signs, urine dipstick for glucose, albumin, ketones, weight, fundal height, FHR, fetal movement, Leopold maneuver, edema Pelvic exam or sterile vaginal examination if indicated Confirm established due date.	• Triple screen or quad screen • Ultrasound • Screening for gestational diabetes at 24–28 weeks • Hemoglobin and hematocrit • Antibody screen if Rh-negative • Administration of RhoGAM if Rh-negative and antibody screen negative

TABLE 4–5 PRENATAL CARE: CONTENT AND TIMING OF ROUTINE PRENATAL VISITS—cont'd		
	HISTORY AND PHYSICAL ASSESSMENT	LABORATORY/DIAGNOSTIC STUDIES IN NORMAL PREGNANCY (RECOMMENDED TIMING)
Third Trimester		
RETURN VISITS (Every 2 weeks until 36 weeks, then weekly until 40 weeks; typically twice weekly after 40 weeks)	Chart review Interval history Nutrition follow-up Focused physical assessment: Vital signs, urine dipstick for glucose, albumin, ketones, weight, fundal height, FHR, fetal movement (i.e., kick counts), Leopold maneuver, edema Pelvic exam or sterile vaginal examination if indicated	Group B *Streptococcus* screening: Vaginal and rectal swab cultures done at 35–37 weeks' gestation to determine presence of GBS bacterial colonization before the onset of labor in order to anticipate intrapartum antibiotic treatment needs (CDC, 2010) Additional screening testing: • H&H if not done in second trimester • Repeat GC, Chlamydia, RPR, HIV, HbSAg (if indicated and not done in late second trimester) • 1-hour glucose challenge test 24–28 weeks

Goals of Prenatal Care

■ Maintenance of maternal fetal health
■ Accurate determination of gestational age
■ Ongoing assessment of risk status and implementation of risk-appropriate intervention
■ Build rapport with the childbearing family
■ Referrals to appropriate resources

Nursing Actions

■ Provide for comfort and privacy.
■ Use therapeutic communication techniques during the interview and conversation.
■ Demonstrate sensitivity toward the patient related to the personal nature of the interview and conversation.
■ Obtain the woman's identifying information (initial prenatal visit).
■ Obtain a complete health history (initial prenatal visit) or an interval history (subsequent visits) (see Tables 4-1 and 4-4 and Clinical Pathway).
■ Conduct a Review of Systems (initial prenatal visit).
■ Obtain blood pressure, temperature, pulse, respirations, weight, height (initial prenatal visit), and BMI (initial prenatal visit).
■ Assess urine specimen for protein, glucose, and ketones.
■ Assess for absence or presence of edema.
■ Provide anticipatory guidance for the patient before and during the physical examination (initial prenatal visit and subsequent visits when indicated).

■ Assist with physical and pelvic examination as needed (initial prenatal visit and subsequent visits when indicated).
■ Assist with obtaining specimens for laboratory or diagnostic studies as ordered (initial prenatal visit and subsequent visits when indicated).
■ Provide teaching about procedures as needed (initial prenatal visit and subsequent visits when indicated).
■ Provide anticipatory guidance related to the plan of care and appropriate follow-up, including how and when to contact care provider with warning signs or symptoms (see Critical Components).
■ Provide teaching appropriate for the woman, her family, and her gestational age.
■ Assess the woman's understanding of the teaching provided.
■ Allow time for the woman to ask questions.
■ Document, according to agency protocol, all findings, interventions, and education provided.
■ Assess for intimate partner violence (see Critical Component: Intimate Partner Violence).

First Trimester

It is best to begin prenatal care in the first trimester. Current reports from the National Center for Health Statistics indicate that 70.8% of women who gave birth began prenatal care within the first 3 months of pregnancy, but 7.1% of all women received late (care beginning in the third trimester of pregnancy) or no care (Martin, Hamilton, Sutton, Ventura, Mathews, Kimeyer, & Osterman, 2010). The percentage of women with timely prenatal care declined (down 2%), and

CRITICAL COMPONENT

Intimate Partner Violence (Abuse)

Intimate partner violence (IPV) against women consists of actual or threatened physical or sexual violence and psychological and emotional abuse. IVP crosses all ethnic, racial, religious, ethnic, and socioeconomic levels. Pregnancy does not protect women from abuse. Homicide is the most likely cause of death in pregnant or recently pregnant women, and a significant portion of those homicides are committed by their intimate partners (Association of Women's Health, Obstetrics and Neonatal Nursing [AWHONN], 2007). Based on the Abuse Assessment Screen, 16% or one in six pregnant women reported physical or sexual abuse during pregnancy (McFarlane, Parker, & Moran, 2007), seriously impacting maternal and fetal health and infant birth weight. Men who abuse pregnant women jeopardize the safety of the woman and infant. Pregnancy is often the only time a woman may come into frequent contact with a health provider. Research has documented that three simple screening tools can reliably identify abused women. Those questions are:

Within the last year have you been hit, slapped, kicked, or otherwise physically hurt by someone?

Since you have been pregnant have you been hit, slapped, kicked, or otherwise physically hurt by someone?

Within the last year, has anyone forced you to have sexual activities?

Assessment for abuse during pregnancy with education, advocacy, and referral to community resources should be standard for all pregnant women. AWHONN advocates for universal screening for domestic violence for all pregnant women and recommends the ABCs of patient care to guide nurses caring for victims of abuse (AWHONN, 2007).

Learn and practice the ABCs of patient care:

A: Alone. Reassure the woman that she is not alone, that there have been others in her position before, and that help is available.

B: Belief. Articulate your belief in the victim—that you know the abuse is not her fault and that no one deserves to be hurt or mistreated.

C: Confidentiality. Ensure the confidentiality of the information that is being provided and explain the implication of mandatory reporting laws, where applicable.

D: Documentation. Descriptive documentation with photographs, taken with the woman's permission, and a verbatim account from the patient's perspective is helpful to accurately capture and record the nature and extent of injuries.

E: Education. Education about community resources can be life-saving. Know where you can refer a woman for help and have information about local shelters readily available. Also ask if she knows how to obtain a restraining order.

S: Safety. One of the most dangerous times for women is the point at which they decide to leave. Tell the woman to call 911 if she is in imminent danger and to consider alerting neighbors to call the police if they hear and/or see signs of conflict.

(AWHONN, 2007; Campbell & Furniss, 2002; McFarlane, Parker, & Moran, 2007)

---

the percentage of women with late or no care increased (up 6%) (Martin et al., 2010). Additionally, current government statistics reflect a decrease in timely prenatal care and increase in late or no prenatal care in the United States, and disparities exist among ethnic groups (i.e., Hispanics and African Americans being less timely in accessing care as compared to Euro Americans). Specifically, non-Hispanic white women (76.2%) were markedly more likely than non-Hispanic black (59.2%) and Hispanic (64.7%) mothers to begin care in the first trimester of pregnancy.

During the initial prenatal visit, the woman learns the frequency of follow-up visits and what to expect from her prenatal visits as the pregnancy progresses (see Table 4-5 and clinical pathway). If the patient is seen for her initial prenatal visit early in the first trimester, she may have more than one visit during that trimester. Subsequent visits are similar to those described for the second trimester. If the woman presents late for prenatal care and is in her second or third trimester at her initial prenatal visit, the nurse may need to modify typical patient education content to meet the current needs of the patient and her family.

At every prenatal care encounter, it is imperative that the nurse provides a relaxed environment for the woman and her family, one in which the childbearing family feels comfortable asking questions and sharing personal details about their lives related to the health of the woman, her fetus, and the developing family.

Components of Initial Prenatal Assessment (see Table 4-5 and Clinical Pathway)

- History of current pregnancy:
  - *First day of last normal menstrual period (LNMP) and degree of certainty about the date*
  - *Regularity, frequency, and length of menstrual cycles*
  - *Recent use or cessation of contraception*
  - *Woman's knowledge of conception date*
  - *Signs and symptoms of pregnancy*
  - *Whether the pregnancy was intended*
  - *The woman's response to being pregnant*
- Obstetrical history, detail about all previous pregnancies:
  - *TPAL*
  - *Whether abortions, if any, were spontaneous or induced*
  - *Dates of pregnancies*
  - *Length of gestation*
  - *Type of birth experiences (e.g., induced or spontaneous labors, vaginal or cesarean births, use of forceps or vacuum-assist, type of pain management)*
  - *Complications with pregnancy, or labor and birth*

- *Neonatal outcomes including Apgar scores, birth weight, neonatal complications, feeding method, health and development since birth*
- *Pregnancy loss and assess grieving status*
- Physical and pelvic examinations:
  - *The bimanual component of the pelvic examination enables the examiner to palpate internally the dimensions of the enlarging uterus. This information assists with dating the pregnancy, either confirming an LMP-based EDD or providing information in the absence of a certain LMP. In the absence of a certain LMP or with conflicting data about gestational age, a decision may be made to perform an ultrasound examination of the pregnancy in order to determine an EDD. It is important to determine an accurate EDD as early as possible in a pregnancy because numerous decisions related to timing of interventions and management of pregnancy are based on gestational age as determined by the EDD.*
  - *Clinical pelvimetry (measurement of the dimensions of the bony pelvis through palpation during an internal pelvic examination) may be performed during the initial pelvic examination. Its purpose is to identify any variations in pelvic structure that might inhibit or preclude a fetus passing through the bony pelvis during a vaginal birth.*
- Assessment of uterine growth:
  - *Uterine growth after 10–12 weeks' gestation is assessed by measuring the height of the fundus with the use of a centimeter measuring tape. The zero point of the tape is placed on the symphysis pubis and the tape is then extended to the top of the fundus. The measurement should approximately equal the number of weeks pregnant. Instruct the woman to empty her bladder before the measurement because a full bladder can displace the uterus (Fig. 4-8).*
  - *Maternal position and examiner uniformity are variables that render this evaluation somewhat imprecise, but it is useful as a gross measure of progressive fetal growth as well as to help identify a pregnancy that is growing outside the optimal or normal range, either too large or too small for its gestational age. This serves as a screening tool for fetal growth.*
- Assessment of fetal heart tones:
  - *Fetal heart tones are auscultated with an ultrasound Doppler in the first trimester, initially heard by 10 and 12 weeks' gestation. The normal fetal heart rate (FHR) baseline is between 110 bpm to 160 bpm.*
- Comprehensive laboratory and diagnostic studies:
  - *Laboratory studies are ordered or obtained at the initial prenatal visit to establish baseline values for follow-up and comparison as the pregnancy progresses (see Table 4-5 and clinical pathway).*
  - *Ultrasound might be performed during the first trimester to confirm intrauterine pregnancy, viability, and gestational age.*

PATIENT EDUCATION

- General information about physical changes (see Table 4-3)
- General information about common discomforts of pregnancy
  - Relief measures for normal discomforts in early pregnancy are discussed based on patient need (Table 4-4)
- General information about fetal development: By the end of the first trimester the fetus is 3 inches in length and weighs 1 to 2 ounces, all organ systems are present, the head is large, and the heartbeat is audible with Doppler.
- General health maintenance/health promotion information:
  - *Avoid exposure to tobacco, alcohol, and recreational drugs.*
  - *Avoid exposure to environment hazards with teratogenic effects.*
  - *Obtain input from the care provider before using medications, complementary and alternative medicine (CAM), and nutritional supplements.*
  - *Reinforce safety behaviors (e.g., seat belt, sunscreen).*
  - *Recognize the need for additional rest.*
  - *Maintain daily hygiene.*
  - *Decrease the risk for urinary tract infections (UTI) and vaginal infections by wiping from front to back, wearing cotton underwear, maintaining adequate hydration, voiding after intercourse, and not douching.*
  - *Maintain good oral hygiene: Gentle brushing of teeth and flossing; continue routine preventative dental care.*
  - *Exercise 30 minutes each day: Avoid risk for trauma to abdomen, avoid overheating, and maintain adequate hydration while exercising.*
  - *Establish daily Kegel exercises routine to maintain pelvic floor muscle strength and decrease risk of urinary incontinence and uterine prolapse.*
  - *Travel is safe in low-risk pregnancy: Need to stop more frequently to stretch and walk to decrease risk of thrombophlebitis; take copy of prenatal record.*
  - *Use coping strategies for stress such as relaxation and meditation.*
  - *Communicate with partner regarding changes in sexual responses: Sexual responses/desires change throughout pregnancy. Couples need to talk openly about these changes and explore different sexual positions that accommodate the changes of pregnancy.*
- Warning/danger signs that need to be reported to the care provider (see Critical Component: Warning/Danger Signs of the First Trimester)

CRITICAL COMPONENT

Warning/Danger Signs of the First Trimester

- Abdominal cramping or pain indicates possible threatened abortion, UTI, appendicitis.
- Vaginal spotting or bleeding indicate possible threatened abortion.
- Absence of fetal heart tone indicates possible missed abortion.
- Dysuria, frequency, urgency indicate possible UTI.
- Fever, chills indicate possible infection.
- Prolonged nausea and vomiting indicate possible hyperemesis gravidarum; increased risk of dehydration.

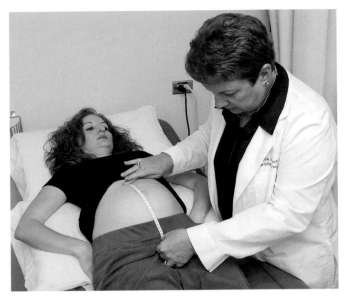

Figure 4–8 Fundal height measurement during prenatal visit.

Nutritional Assessment and Education

Nutrition should be discussed at all prenatal visits to reinforce the importance of appropriate weight gain as both excessive and inadequate weight gain in pregnancy are associated with poor perinatal outcomes.

■ Discuss appetite, cravings, or food aversions.
■ Obtain a 24-hour diet recall and review for obvious deficiencies.
■ Based on the woman's pre-pregnancy BMI and IOM guidelines (**Boxes 4-1** and **4-3**):
  ■ *Assist the woman to set weight gain goals with a recommended weight gain of between 1 to 5 pounds during the first trimester.*
  ■ *Discuss distribution of weight gain during pregnancy (Box 4-4).*
  ■ *Encourage the woman to eat a variety of unprocessed foods from all food groups, including fresh fruits, vegetables, whole grains, lean meats or beans, and low-fat dairy products.*
  ■ *For more detailed information on nutritional needs during pregnancy, or to design a personalized daily food plan tailored to personal life circumstances, refer her to www.choosemyplate.gov/mypyramidmoms*
  ■ *MyPyramid For Moms (Fig. 4-9) outlines the recommended daily food group amounts for each trimester.*
■ Encourage the woman to drink 8–10 glasses of fluid per day and limit caffeine to 200 mg per day.
■ Certain types of fish (king mackerel, shark, swordfish, and tilefish) should be avoided due to high levels of methylmercury; however, most other fish and seafood are safe as long as fully cooked.
■ Advise on prevention of food borne illnesses:
  ■ *Wash hands frequently.*

BOX 4–3 NEW RECOMMENDATIONS FOR TOTAL AND RATE OF WEIGHT GAIN DURING PREGNANCY, BY PRE-PREGNANCY BMI

The impact of pre-pregnancy weight and gestational weight gain on perinatal outcomes is significant and is directly related to infant birth weight, morbidity, and mortality. The current evidence suggests that inadequate weight gain and/or an underweight pre-pregnancy weight increase risk for poor fetal growth and low birth weight. At the other end of the spectrum, excessive weight gain and/or an overweight or obese pre-pregnancy weight increase the risk for poor maternal and neonatal outcomes and may have far-reaching implications for long-term health and development of chronic disease. Pre-pregnancy weight and BMI as well as gestational weight gain have increased nationally. The new recommendations for maternal weight gain in a singleton pregnancy are individualized based on pre-pregnancy BMI.

PRE-PREGNANCY BMI	TOTAL WEIGHT GAIN RECOMMENDED IN POUNDS	RATES OF WEIGHT GAIN* 2ND AND 3RD TRIMESTER MEAN (RANGE) IN LBS/WEEK
Underweight (<18.5)	28–40	1 (1–1.3)
Normal weight (18.5–24.9)	25–35	1 (0.8–1)
Overweight (25.0–29.9)	15–25	0.6 (0.5–0.7)
Obese ≥30.0)	11–20	0.5 (0.4–0.6)

*Calculations assume a 1.1–4.4 lbs weight gain in the first trimester

World Health Organization (WHO); Institute of Medicine (2009).

BOX 4–4 MATERNAL WEIGHT GAIN DISTRIBUTION

Baby	7 1/2 pounds
Placenta	1 1/2 pounds
Amniotic Fluid	2 pounds
Breasts	2 pounds
Uterus	2 pounds
Body Fluids	4 pounds
Blood	4 pounds
Maternal Stores of Protein, Fat, and Other Nutrients	7 pounds

Your Pregnancy & Birth, 4th edition, 2005. The American College of Obstetricians and Gynecologists (ACOG), Washington, D.C.

■ *Thoroughly rinse all raw vegetables and fruits before eating.*
■ *Cook eggs and all meats, poultry, or fish thoroughly, and sanitize all areas that come in contact with these during food preparation.*
■ *Foods to avoid:*
  ■ Unpasteurized juices or dairy products
  ■ Raw sprouts of any kind
  ■ Soft cheeses like Brie or feta (if unpasteurized)

What Should I Eat?

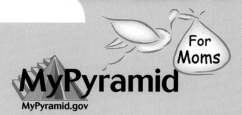

MyPyramid
For Moms
MyPyramid.gov

When you are pregnant, you have special nutritional needs. Follow the MyPyramid Plan below to help you and your baby stay healthy. The Plan shows different amounts of food for different trimesters, to meet your changing nutritional needs.

Food Group	1st Trimester	2nd and 3rd Trimesters	What counts as 1 cup or 1 ounce?	Remember to...
	Eat this amount from each group daily.*			
Fruits	2 cups	2 cups	1 cup fruit or juice ½ cup dried fruit	*Focus on fruits—* Eat a variety of fruits.
Vegetables	2½ cups	3 cups	1 cup raw or cooked vegetables or juice 2 cups raw leafy vegetables	*Vary your veggies—* Eat more dark-green and orange vegetables and cooked dry beans.
Grains	6 ounces	8 ounces	1 slice bread 1 ounce ready-to-eat cereal ½ cup cooked pasta, rice, or cereal	*Make half your grains whole—*Choose whole instead of refined grains.
Meat & Beans	5½ ounces	6½ ounces	1 ounce lean meat, poultry, or fish ¼ cup cooked dry beans ½ ounce nuts or 1 egg 1 tablespoon peanut butter	*Go lean with protein—* Choose low-fat or lean meats and poultry.
Milk	3 cups	3 cups	1 cup milk 8 ounces yogurt 1½ ounces cheese 2 ounces processed cheese	*Get your calcium-rich foods—*Go low-fat or fat-free when you choose milk, yogurt, and cheese.

*These amounts are for an average pregnant woman. You may need more or less than the average. Check with your doctor to make sure you are gaining weight as you should.

In each food group, choose foods that are low in "extras"—solid fats and added sugars.

Pregnant women and women who may become pregnant should not drink alcohol. Any amount of alcohol during pregnancy could cause problems for your baby.

Most doctors recommend that pregnant women take a prenatal vitamin and mineral supplement every day **in addition to** eating a healthy diet. This is so you and your baby get enough folic acid, iron, and other nutrients. But don't overdo it. Taking too much can be harmful.

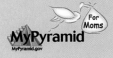

Get a MyPyramid Plan for Moms designed just for you.
Go to www.MyPyramid.gov for your Plan and more.
Click on "Pregnancy and Breastfeeding."

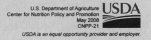

U.S. Department of Agriculture
Center for Nutrition Policy and Promotion
May 2008
CNPP-21
USDA is an equal opportunity provider and employer.

Figure 4–9 USDA What Should I Eat? MyPyramid For Moms. U.S. Department of Agriculture. MyPyramid.gov Web site. Washington, DC.

■ Refrigerated, smoked seafood
■ Unheated deli meats or hot dogs
■ *For more detailed advice on food safety during pregnancy, refer to the FDA Web site: http://www.fda.gov/Food/ResourcesForYou/HealthEducators/ucm081819.htm*

Second Trimester

Subsequent or return prenatal visits begin with a chart review from the previous visit(s) and an interval history. This history includes information about the pregnancy since the previous prenatal visit (see Table 4-5 and Clinical Pathway).

Components of Second-Trimester Prenatal Assessments

■ Focused physical assessment
■ Vital signs
  ■ *Vital signs within normal limits; slight decrease in blood pressure toward end of second trimester*
■ Weight
  ■ *Average weight gain per week depending on pre-pregnancy BMI (Box 4-3)*
■ Urine dipstick for glucose, albumin, and ketones
  ■ *Mild proteinuria and glucosuria are normal.*
■ FHR
  ■ *Able to auscultate FHR with Doppler; rate 110–160 bpm* (**Fig. 4-10**)
■ Fetal movement
  ■ *Assess for* **quickening** *(when the woman feels her baby move for the first time).*
■ **Leopold's maneuvers** (palpation of the abdomen) to identify the position of the fetus in utero (Chapter 8)
  ■ *Examiner able to palpate fetal parts.*

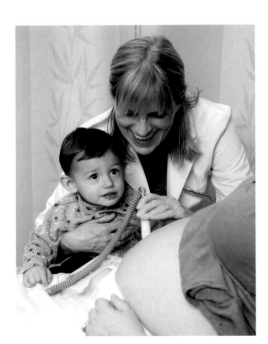

Figure 4–10 A nurse-practitioner listening to fetal heart tone with a pregnant mom and her toddler.

■ Presence of edema
  ■ *Slight lower body edema is normal due to decreased venous return.*
  ■ *Upper body edema, especially of the face, is abnormal and needs further evaluation.*
■ Fundal height measurement
  ■ *Fundal height should equal weeks of gestation.*
■ Confirm established due date:
  ■ *Quickening occurs around 18 weeks' gestation (usually between 18 and 20 weeks' gestation, but sometimes as early as 14–16 weeks' gestation in a multigravida and occasionally as late as 22 weeks' gestation in some primigravidas).*
  ■ *Ultrasound around 20 weeks' gestation to confirm EDD and scan fetal anatomy*
■ Laboratory and diagnostic studies:
  ■ *Triple screen or quad screen blood tests at 15–20 weeks' gestation (Chapter 6): Screening tests for neural tube defect and Trisomy 21are not diagnostic. Amniocentesis is recommended if screening tests are positive.*
  ■ *Screening for gestational diabetes: 1-hour glucose challenge test recommended between 24 and 28 weeks. 3-hour glucose tolerance test (GTT) is ordered if 1-hour screen is elevated.*
  ■ *Hemoglobin and hematocrit between 28 and 32 weeks to identify anemia and the need for iron supplement. This is the time in pregnancy when the hemoglobin and hematocrit are likely to be at their lowest, so the result provides the care provider with valuable information for management of late pregnancy.*
  ■ *Syphilis serology if prevalent or as indicated*
  ■ *Antibody screen for Rh-negative women*
■ Administer RhoGAM to Rh-negative women with negative antibody screen results.
  ■ *RhoGAM is administered at 28 weeks' gestation to help prevent isoimmunization and the resulting risk of hemolytic disease in fetuses in subsequent pregnancies (see Medication: Rho (D) Immune Globulin (RhoGAM)).*

Medication

Rho (D) Immune Globulin (RhoGAM)

■ Indication: Administered to Rh-negative women prophylactically at 28 weeks' gestation to prevent isoimmunization from potential exposure to Rh-positive fetal blood during the normal course of pregnancy. Also administered with likely exposure to Rh-positive blood, such as with pregnancy loss, amniocentesis, or abdominal trauma.
■ Specific mechanism of action: Prevents production of anti-Rho (D) antibodies in Rho (D) negative women exposed to Rho (D) positive blood. Prevention of antibody response and hemolytic diseases of the newborn (erythroblastosisfetalis) in future pregnancies of women who have conceived an Rho (D)-positive fetus.
■ Adverse reactions: Pain at IM site; fever
■ Route/dosage: 1 vial standard dose (300 mcg) IM at 28 weeks' gestation

(Deglin & Vallerand, 2011)

PATIENT EDUCATION

- Information on fetal development during the second trimester
  - *At 20 weeks' gestation, the fetus is 8 inches long, weighs 1 pound, and is relatively long and skinny.*
- General health maintenance/health promotion topics
- Nutritional follow-up and reinforcement
  - *Recommend increase in daily caloric intake by 340/kcal/day during second trimester (IOM, 2006)*
  - *Offer counseling and guidance on dietary intake or physical activity as needed*
- Information on physical changes during the second trimester (see Table 4-4)
- Relief measures for normal discomforts commonly experienced during the second trimester (see Table 4-4)
- Reinforce warning/danger signs that need to be reported to care provider (see Critical Component: Warning/Danger Signs of the Second Trimester)
- Signs and symptoms of preterm labor (PTL)
  - *Rhythmic lower abdominal cramping or pain*
  - *Low backache*
  - *Pelvic pressure*
  - *Leaking of amniotic fluid*
  - *Increased vaginal discharge*
  - *Vaginal spotting or bleeding*
- Signs and symptoms of hypertensive disorders
  - *Severe headache that does not respond to usual relief measures*
  - *Visual changes*
  - *Facial or generalized edema*
- Information about the benefits and risks of procedures and tests with goal of enabling the woman to make informed decisions about what procedures she will choose based on her knowledge of the available options coupled with her and her family's values and beliefs.

CRITICAL COMPONENT

Warning/Danger Signs of the Second Trimester

- Abdominal or pelvic pain indicates possible PTL, UTI, pyelonephritis, or appendicitis.
- Absence of fetal movement once the woman is feeling daily movement indicates possible fetal distress or death.
- Prolonged nausea and vomiting indicates possible hyperemesis gravidarum; at risk for dehydration.
- Fever and chills indicates possible infection.
- Dysuria, frequency, and urgency indicate possible UTI.
- Vaginal bleeding indicates possible infection, friable cervix due to pregnancy changes, placenta previa, abruptio placenta, or PTL.

Third Trimester

The focused assessment includes all aspects of the second trimester assessment and may also include a pelvic examination to identify cervical change, depending on weeks of gestation and maternal symptoms. Assessment of pregnancy in the third trimester becomes more frequent and involved than in previous return visits as the pregnancy advances and the fetus nears term (see Table 4-5 and Clinical Pathway).

Components of Third Trimester Assessments

- Chart review
- Interval history
- Focused assessment (e.g., fundal height)
- Assessment of fetal well-being
  - *Auscultation of FHR*
  - *Record woman's assessment of "kick counts"*
    - Daily **fetal movement count (kick counts)** is a maternal assessment of fetal movement by counting fetal movements in a period of time to identify potentially hypoxic fetuses. Maternal perception of fetal movement was one of the earliest tests of fetal well-being and remains an essential assessment of fetal health. The pregnant woman is instructed to palpate the abdomen and track fetal movements daily by tracking fetal movements for 1 or 2 hours.
    - In the 2-hour approach recommended by ACOG, maternal perception of at least 10 distinct fetal movements within 2 hours is considered reassuring; once movement is achieved, counts can be discontinued for the day.
    - In the 1-hour approach, the count is considered reassuring if it equals or exceeds the established baseline; in general 4 movements in 1 hour is reassuring.
      - *Define fetal movements or kick counts to include: kicks, flutters, swishes, or rolls.*
      - *Instruct mother to keep journal or documentation of the time it takes to feel fetal movement.*
      - *Instruct mother to perform counts at same time every day.*
      - *Instruct mother to monitor time intervals it takes and to contact HCP immediately for deviations from normal (e.g., no movements or decreased movements).*
    - Decreased fetal activity should be reported to the provider as further evaluation of the fetus, such as a non-stress test or biophysical profile, is indicated.
    - Pelvic examination to identify cervical change, depending on weeks of gestation and maternal symptoms
- Leopold's maneuvers to identify the position of the fetus in utero (Chapter 8)
- Screening for Group B Streptococcus (GBS)
  - *A quarter to a third of all women are colonized with GBS in the lower gastrointestinal or urogenital tract (typically asymptomatic).*
  - *GBS infection in a newborn, either early-onset (first week of life) or late-onset (after first week of life), can be invasive and severe, with potential long-term neurological sequella.*
  - *Vaginal and rectal swab cultures are done at 35–37 weeks' gestation to determine presence of GBS bacterial colonization before the onset of labor in order to anticipate intrapartum antibiotic treatment needs (CDC, 2010).*

■ Laboratory tests and screening
  ■ *1-hour glucose test at 24–28 weeks' gestation (may have already been done in 2nd trimester)*
  ■ *H & H (if not recently done in second trimester)*
  ■ *Repeat gonorrhea culture (GC), Chlamydia, syphilis test by rapid plasma reagin (RPR) if indicated and not screened in second trimester, human immunodeficiency virus (HIV), and hepatitis B surface antigen (HbSAg) tests as indicated*

PATIENT EDUCATION

- ■ Information about fetal growth during the third trimester
  - ■ *At term fetus is about 17–20 inches in length, weighs between 6–8 pounds, increased deposits of subcutaneous fat, has established sleep and activity cycles*
- ■ General health maintenance/health promotion topics
- ■ Nutritional follow-up and reinforcement
- ■ *Recommend increase in daily caloric intake by 452/kcal/day during third trimester (IOM, 2006)*
- ■ *Offer counseling and guidance on dietary intake or physical activity as needed*
- ■ Information on physical changes during the third trimester (Table 4-4)
- ■ Relief measures for normal discomforts commonly experienced during the third trimester (see Table 4-4).
- ■ Reinforce warning/danger signs that need to be reported to care provider (see Critical Component: Warning/Danger Signs of the Third Trimester)

CRITICAL COMPONENT

Warning/Danger Signs of the Third Trimester

- ■ Abdominal or pelvic pain (PTL, UTI, pyelonephritis, appendicitis)
- ■ Decreased or absent fetal movement (fetal hypoxia or death)
- ■ Prolonged nausea and vomiting (dehydration, hyperemesis gravidarum)
- ■ Fever, chills (infection)
- ■ Dysuria, frequency, urgency (UTI)
- ■ Vaginal bleeding (infection, friable cervix due to pregnancy changes or pathology, placenta previa, placenta abruptio, PTL)
- ■ Signs/symptoms of PTL: Rhythmic lower abdominal cramping or pain, low backache, pelvic pressure, leaking of amniotic fluid, increased vaginal discharge
- ■ Signs/symptoms of hypertensive disorders: Severe headache that does not respond to usual relief measures, visual changes, facial or generalized.

■ Travel limitations may be suggested in the last month.
■ Discussion of preparation for labor and birth
  ■ *Attend childbirth classes.*
  ■ *Discuss the method of labor pain management.*
  ■ *Develop birth plan; list preferences for routine procedures.*
■ Signs of impending labor
■ Discussion of true versus false labor
■ Instruction on when to contact the doctor or midwife
■ Instructions on when to go to the birthing unit
■ Discussion on parenting and infant care
  ■ *Attend parenting classes*
  ■ *Select the method of infant feeding*
  ■ *Select the infant health care provider*
  ■ *Preparation of siblings*

Quality and Safety Education in Nursing (QSEN): Informatics

Informatics is the use of information and technology to communicate, manage knowledge, mitigate error, and support decision making. The Association of Women's Health, Obstetric and Neonatal Nurses (AWHONN) recognizes the vital role of informatics and health information technology (HIT) in health care delivery. AWHONN supports standard data collection across the perinatal setting. Additionally, AWHONN recognizes the critical need for interoperability and archiving in data collection systems. Hospital- and institution-wide HIT systems should incorporate specialty specific data (e.g., obstetric outpatient records) into patient records. To accomplish the efficient use of HIT in the perinatal setting, nurses must be involved in the product selection, development, implementation, evaluation, and improvement of information systems. (Association of Women's Health, Obstetric and Neonatal Nurses (2011) JOGNN, 40, 383–385; 2011. DOI: 10.1111/j.1552-6909.2011.01246.)

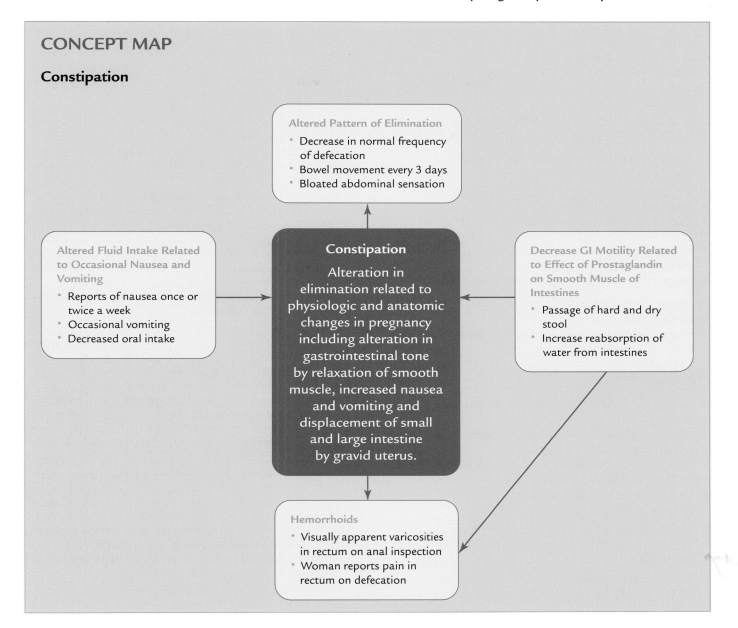

CONCEPT MAP

Constipation

Altered Pattern of Elimination
- Decrease in normal frequency of defecation
- Bowel movement every 3 days
- Bloated abdominal sensation

Altered Fluid Intake Related to Occasional Nausea and Vomiting
- Reports of nausea once or twice a week
- Occasional vomiting
- Decreased oral intake

Constipation
Alteration in elimination related to physiologic and anatomic changes in pregnancy including alteration in gastrointestinal tone by relaxation of smooth muscle, increased nausea and vomiting and displacement of small and large intestine by gravid uterus.

Decrease GI Motility Related to Effect of Prostaglandin on Smooth Muscle of Intestines
- Passage of hard and dry stool
- Increase reabsorption of water from intestines

Hemorrhoids
- Visually apparent varicosities in rectum on anal inspection
- Woman reports pain in rectum on defecation

Problem No. 1: Altered pattern of elimination
Goal: Resumption of typical bowel patterns
Outcome: Patient will resume her normal bowel patterns.

Nursing Actions

1. Assess prior bowel patterns before pregnancy, including frequency, consistency, shape, and color.
2. Auscultate bowel sounds.
3. Assess prior experiences with constipation.
4. Explore prior successful strategies for constipation.
5. Explain contributing factors to constipation in pregnancy.
6. Teach strategies for dealing with constipation, including diet, exercise, and adequate fluid intake.
7. Encourage high-fiber foods and fresh fruits and vegetables.
8. Encourage dietary experimentation to evaluate what works for her.
9. Establish regular time for bowel movement.
10. Discuss rationale for strategies.
11. Explore with the woman and discuss with the care provider use of stool softener and/or bulk laxative.
12. Encourage the patient to discuss concerns about constipation by asking open-end questions.

Problem No. 2: Altered fluid intake related to nausea and vomiting

Goal: Normal fluid intake

Outcome: Normal fluid intake and decreased nausea and vomiting

Nursing Actions

1. Assess factors that increase nausea and vomiting.
2. Suggest small frequent meals.
3. Decrease fluid intake with meals.
4. Avoid high-fat and spicy food.
5. Explore contributing factors to nausea in pregnancy.
6. Teach strategies for dealing with nausea in pregnancy.
7. Encourage the woman to experiment with strategies to alleviate nausea.
8. Suggest vitamin B_6 or ginger to decrease nausea.

Problem 3: Decreased gastric motility

Goal: Increased motility

Outcome: Patient has normal bowel movement.

Nursing Actions

1. Provide dietary information to increase fiber and roughage in diet.
2. Review high-fiber foods, for example, pears, apples, prunes, kiwis, and dried fruits.
3. Bran cereal in the morning and instruct woman to check labels for at least 4–5 grams of fiber per serving.
4. Discuss strategies to increase fluid intake.
5. Drink warm liquid upon rising.
6. Encourage exercise to promote peristalsis.
7. Reinforce relationship of diet, exercise, and fluid intake on constipation.

Problem 4: Discomfort with defecation because of hemorrhoids

Goal: Decreased pain with bowel movement

Outcome: Patient will have decreased pain and maintain adequate bowel function.

Nursing Actions

1. Reinforce strategies to avoid constipation.
2. Encourage the woman to not avoid defecation.
3. Instruct the woman to avoid straining on evacuation.
4. Discuss care of hemorrhoids, including TUCKS pads and hemorrhoid creams.
5. Discuss use of stool softeners.
6. Recommend that the woman support a foot on a foot stool to facilitate bowel evacuation.
7. Reinforce relationship of diet, exercise, and fluid intake on constipation.

TYING IT ALL TOGETHER

As a nurse in an antenatal clinic you are part of an interdisciplinary team that is caring for Margarite Sanchez during her pregnancy. Margarite is a 28-year-old G3 P1 Hispanic woman here for her first prenatal care appointment. By her LMP she is at 8 weeks' gestation. Margarite reports some spotting 2 weeks ago that prompted her to do a home pregnancy test that was positive. The spotting has stopped. She tells you that she is very tired throughout the day, has some nausea in the morning and breast tenderness. She is happy to be pregnant but a bit surprised.

Outline the aspects of your initial assessment.

Outline for Margarite what laboratory tests are done during this first prenatal visit and rationale for the tests.

Detail the prenatal education and anticipatory guidance appropriate to the first trimester of pregnancy.

What teaching would you do for Margarite's discomforts of pregnancy?

Discuss nursing diagnosis, nursing activities, and expected outcomes related to this woman.

At 18 weeks' gestation Margarite comes to the clinic for a prenatal visit. She states she thinks she felt her baby move for the first time last week and that the pregnancy now feels real to her. She states she feels "Great! The nausea and fatigue are gone." She is concerned she is not eating enough protein as she has little interest in red meat but eats beans and rice at dinner. She remembers discussing with you at her first visit some screening tests for problems with the baby but now is unsure how they are done and what they are for.

Outline for Margarite nutritional needs during pregnancy, highlighting protein requirements.

Outline for Margarite the screening tests that are done in the second trimester and what they are for.

Detail the prenatal education and anticipatory guidance appropriate to the second trimester of pregnancy.

Discuss nursing diagnosis, nursing activities, and expected outcomes related to this woman.

Margarite comes to your clinic for a prenatal visit and is now at 34 weeks' gestation. She states she feels well but has some swelling in her legs at the end of the day, a backache at the end of the day, and difficulty getting comfortable to fall asleep. She is also having difficulty sleeping as she gets up to go to the bathroom two or three times a night.

She remembers from her first pregnancy some things she should be aware of that indicate a problem at the end of pregnancy but is not sure what they are.

Detail the prenatal education and anticipatory guidance appropriate to the third trimester of pregnancy.

What teaching would you do for Margarite's discomforts of pregnancy?

What warning signs would you reinforce with Margarite at this point in her pregnancy?

Discuss nursing diagnosis, nursing activities, and expected outcomes specific to Margarite.

■ ■ ■ **Review Questions** ■ ■ ■

1. The appropriate recommended weight gain during pregnancy for a woman with a normal BMI is:
   A. 10–15 lbs.
   B. 6–20 lbs.
   C. 21–25 lbs.
   D. 25–35 lbs.

2. The purpose of preconception care is to:
   A. Prevent unwanted pregnancies
   B. Improve perinatal outcomes
   C. Facilitate desired pregnancy
   D. Screen for sexually transmitted diseases

3. Presumptive signs of pregnancy are:
   A. All the objective signs of pregnancy
   B. Those perceived by the healthcare provider
   C. Physiological changes perceived by the woman herself
   D. Those attributed to the fetus.

4. Physiological changes in pregnancy:
   A. Involve primarily reproductive organs
   B. Are protective of the woman and/or fetus
   C. Are most profound in the first trimester
   D. Primarily impact the musculoskeletal system

5. Intimate partner violence:
   A. Consists of physical abuse
   B. Decreases during pregnancy
   C. Crosses all ethnic, racial, religious, and socioeconomic levels
   D. Primarily impacts maternal health

6. RhoGAM would be administered during pregnancy at 28 weeks' gestation to women with the following:
   A. Blood type O+
   B. Blood type A+
   C. Blood type O–
   D. Blood type AB

7. Blood volume increases during pregnancy by:
   A. 20%–30%
   B. 30%–40%
   C. 40%–50% (correct answer)
   D. 50%–60%

8. A woman presents for prenatal care at 10 weeks' gestation reporting nausea and vomiting. Self-care and relief measures include:
   A. Suggest a high protein diet
   B. Suggest avoiding eating early in the day
   C. Suggest increasing fluid intake
   D. Suggest small, frequent meals

9. A woman who gets pregnant within 45 days of delivering a baby is at a higher risk for:
   A. Iron deficiency anemia (correct answer)
   B. Periodontal disease
   C. Urinary stasis
   D. Striae gravidarum

10. Treatment with IV antibiotics is indicated for patients with all of the following except:
    A. History of group B streptococcus (GBS) in the urine during pregnancy
    B. Scheduled for cesarean delivery prior to rupture of membranes or labor with a history of positive GBS (correct answer)
    C. GBS status unknown with a history of an infant with invasive GBS infection
    D. Screened negative for GBS at 37 weeks, now in labor with temperature >100.4° F (38° C)

11. Which of the following lab results indicates anemia?
    A. Hemoglobin 11.2
    B. Hemoglobin 10(correct answer)
    C. Hematocrit 34%
    D. Hematocrit 38%

12. Which hormone is responsible for maintaining pregnancy by relaxing smooth muscles leading to decreased uterine activity and decreasing the risk of spontaneous abortion?
    A. Estrogen
    B. Human chorionic gonadatropin (hCG)
    C. Progesterone (correct answer)
    D. Oxytocin

13. Softening of the cervix that occurs in the second month of pregnancy is known as:
    A. Hegar's sign
    B. Braxton's sign
    C. Goodell's sign (correct answer)
    D. Chadwick's sign

14. Using Naegele's rule, calculate the EDD for a patient with a LMP of 10 March.
    A. December 3
    B. December 7
    C. December 10
    D. December 17

References

American Academy of Pediatrics/American College of Obstetricians and Gynecologists. (2007). Appendix D: Standard terminology for reporting of reproductive health statistics in the United States. *Guidelines for perinatal care* (6th ed.). Elk Grove Village, IL: American Academy of Pediatrics; Washington, DC: American College of Obstetricians and Gynecologists.

American Dietetic Association and the American Society for Nutrition. (2009). Position of the American Dietetic Association and American Society for Nutrition: Obesity, reproduction, and pregnancy outcomes. *Journal of the American Dietetic Association, 109*(5), 918–927.

American College of Obstetricians and Gynecologists (ACOG). (2005). *Your pregnancy and birth* (4th ed.). Washington, DC: ACOG.

Association for Women's Health, Obstetric and Neonatal Nurses (AWHONN). (2007). *Universal screening for domestic violence.* Washington, DC: Author.

Baldwin, K. A. (2006). Comparison of selected outcomes of center-ing pregnancy versus traditional prenatal care. *Journal of Midwifery & Women's Health, 51*(4), 266–272.

Barron, M. (2014). Antenatal care. In K. Simpson, & P. Creehan, *Perinatal Nursing*. Philadelphia: Lippincott Williams & Wilkins.

Bernstein, H. B., & Weinstein, M. Normal pregnancy and prenatal care (2010). In A. Decherney & L. Nathan (Eds.), *Current Diagnoses and Treatment in Obstetrics and Gynecology*. New York: McGraw-Hill.

Blackburn, S. T. (2007). *Maternal, fetal, & neonatal physiology: A clinical perspective* (3rd ed.). St. Louis, MO: W. B. Saunders.

Blackburn, S. T. (2014) Physiologic changes of pregnancy. In K. Simpson, & P. Creehan, *Perinatal Nursing*. Philadelphia: Lippincott Williams & Wilkins.

Jack, B, Atrash, H., Coonrod, D., Moos, M., O'Donnell, J., Johnson, K. (2008). The clinical content of preconception care: An overview and preparation of this supplement. *American Journal of Obstetrics & Gynecology, 199*(6), Supplement B, S266–S279.

Campbell, J., & Furniss, K. (2002). *Violence against women: Identification, screening and management of intimate partner vio-lence*. Washington, DC: Association of Women's Health, Obstetric and Neonatal Nurses.

Centers for Disease Control and Prevention (CDC). (1992). Recommendations for the use of folic acid to reduce the number of cases of spina bifida and other neural tube defects. *MMWR Recommendations and Reports, 41*(RR-14), 001.

Centers for Disease Control and Prevention (CDC). (2006). Recommendations to Improve Preconception Health and Health Care—United States. *MMWR Recommendations and Reports, 55*(RR-6), 1–23.

Centers for Disease Control and Prevention (CDC). (2010). Prevention of perinatal group B streptococcal disease: Revised guidelines from CDC. *MMWR Recommendations and Reports, 59*(RR-10), 1–23.

Cunningham, E. G., Leveno, K. J., Bloom, S. L., et al. Obesity and pregnancy complications (2010). In A. Fried & K. Davis (Eds.), *Williams Obstetrics* (23rd ed.). New York: McGraw-Hill.

Deglin, J., &Vallerand, A. (2011). Davis's drug guide for nurses (12th ed.). Philadelphia: F.A. Davis.

Frey, K., Navarro, S., Kotelchuck, M., & Lu, M. (2008). The clini-cal content of preconception care: preconception care for men. *American Journal of Obstetrics & Gynecology, -199*(6), Supplement B, S389–S395.

Gardner, S. L., & Hernandez, J. A. (2011). Initial nursery care. In S. L. Gardner (Ed.), Merenstein & Gardner's Handbook of neonatal intensive care (7th ed., pp. 78–112). St. Louis, MO: Mosby.

Grady, M. A., & Bloom, K. C. (2004). Pregnancy outcomes of ado-lescents enrolled in a Centering Pregnancy program. *Journal of Midwifery & Women's Health, 49*(5), 412–420.

Gussler, J., & Arensberg, M. B. (2011). Impact of maternal obesity on pregnancy and lactation: the health care challenge, *Nutrition Today, 46*(1), 6–11.

Ickovics, J. R., Kershaw, T. S., Westdahl, C., Schindler-Rising, S. S., Klima, C., Reynolds, H., & Magriples, U. (2003). Group pre-natal care and preterm birth weight: Results from a matched cohort study at public clinics. *Obstetrics & Gynecology, 102*(5), Part 1, 1051–1057.

Ickovics, J. R., Kershaw, T. S., Westdahl, C., Magriples, U., Massey, Z., Reynolds, H., & Rising, S. S. (2007). Group prena-tal care and perinatal outcomes. *Obstetrics & Gynecology, 110*(2), 330–339.

Institute of Medicine. (2006). *Dietary reference intakes: The essen-tial guide to nutrient requirements*. Washington, DC: National Academies Press.

Institute of Medicine. (2009). *Weight gain during pregnancy: Reexamining the guidelines*. Washington, DC: National Academies Press.

Kahn, D. A., & Hoos, B. J. (2010). Maternal physiology during pregnancy: Introduction. In A. Decherney & L. Nathan (Eds.), *Current Diagnoses and Treatment in Obstetrics and Gynecology*. New York: McGraw-Hill.

Mattson, S., & Smith, J. (2011). *Core curriculum for maternal-newborn nursing* (4th ed.). St. Louis, MO: Elsevier.

Martin, J. A., Hamilton, B. E., Sutton, P. D., Ventura, S. J., Mathews, T. J., Kimeyer, S., & Osterman, M. J. (2010). Births: Final data for 2007. *National vital statistics reports, 58*(24). Hyattsville, MD: National Center for Health Statistics.

McFarlane, J., Parker, B., & Moran, B. (2007). *Abuse during preg-nancy: A protocol for prevention and intervention* (3rd ed.). White Plains, NY: March of Dimes.

Ogden, C. L., Carroll, M. D., Kit, B. K., & Flegal, K. M. (2012). *Prevalence of obesity in the United States, 2009–2010*. NCHS data brief, no. 82. Hyattsville, MD: National Center for Health Statistics. Retrieved from http://www.cdc.gov/obesity/data/adult.html

Rising, S. S. (1998). Centering pregnancy: An interdisciplinary model of empowerment. *Journal of Nurse-Midwifery, 43*(1), 46–54.

Rotundo, G. (2011). Centering pregnancy: the benefits of group prenatal care. *Nursing for Women's Health, 15*(6), 507–518.

Tan, P. C., & Omar, S. Z. (2011). Contemporary approaches to hyperemesis during pregnancy. *Current Opinion in Obstetrics and Gynecology, 23*, 87–93.

U.S. Department of Agriculture. *Health and nutrition information for pregnancy and breastfeeding women*. Retrieved from www.choosemyplate.gov/pregnancy-breastfeeding/pregnancy-nutritional-needs.html

United States Department of Health and Human Services. (2010). *Healthy People 2020*, Office of Disease Prevention and Health Promotion Publication number 80132.

United States Department of Health and Human Services, Food and Drug Administration. *Food: Resources for Health Educators*. Retrieved from www.fda.gov/Food/ResourcesForYou/HealthEducators/ucm081819.html

Villar, J., Carroli, G., Khan-Neelofur, D., Piaggio, G., & Gulmezoglu, M. (2007). Patterns of routine antenatal care for low-risk pregnancy. *Cochrane Database of Systematic Reviews, 2*, 2007. Oxford: Update Software.

Walker, D. S., & Rising, S. S. (2004/2005). Revolutionizing prenatal care: New evidence-based prenatal care delivery models. *Journal of the New York State Nurses Association*, Fall/Winter, 18–21.

Whitaker, R. C. (2004). Predicting preschooler obesity at birth: The role of maternal obesity in early pregnancy. *Pediatrics 14*, 29–36.

World Health Organization. *BMI Classification*. Retrieved from http://apps.who.int/bmi/index.jsp?introPage=intro_3.html

CLINICAL PATHWAY FOR PRENATAL CARE: CONTENT AND TIMING OF ROUTINE PRENATAL VISITS FOR NORMAL PREGNANCY

Focus of Care	Initial Prenatal Visit	First Trimester	Second Trimester	Third Trimester
Frequency of Prenatal visits	Initial visit	Return visit (4 weeks after initial visit) and then every 4 weeks	Return visit every 4 weeks	Return visits every 2 weeks until 36 weeks, then weekly until 40 weeks; twice weekly after 40 weeks
Assessments	Comprehensive health and risk assessment Current pregnancy • First day of LMP • Regularity, frequency, and length of menstrual cycles • Recent use or cessation of contraception • Woman's knowledge of conception date • Determine EDD • Signs and symptoms of pregnancy • Inquire whether the pregnancy was intended • Assess the woman's response to being pregnant Obstetrical history • TPAL • Date of pregnancies • Length of gestation • Type of birth experiences • Complications with previous pregnancies • Prior pregnancy losses • Neonatal outcomes including Apgar scores Medical history Family history Social history • Smoking • Alcohol • Substance use Sexual history and practices Complete physical assessment • Vital signs • Urine • Pelvic examination	Chart review Interval history since last visit Focused physical assessment: • Weeks gestation • Blood pressure • Urine dipstick for glucose, albumin, ketones • Weight including cumulative weight gain or loss • Fundal height measurement • Fetal heart tones • Clinical pelvimetry	Chart review Interval history Nutrition follow-up Focused physical assessment: • Blood pressure and vital signs • Urine dipstick for glucose, albumin, ketones • Weight • Fundal height measurement • Fetal heart tones • Fetal movement – note beginning of fetal movement (quickening) • Leopold maneuver • Edema Pelvic exam or sterile vaginal examination if indicated Re-evaluate pregnancy risk status	Chart review Interval history Nutrition follow-up Focused physical assessment: • Vital signs • Urine dipstick for glucose, albumin, ketones • Weight • Fundal height measurement • Leopold maneuver • Edema • Pelvic exam or sterile vaginal examination if indicated • Assessment of fetal well-being • FHR • Fetal movement (i.e., kick counts)

Continued

CLINICAL PATHWAY FOR PRENATAL CARE: CONTENT AND TIMING OF ROUTINE PRENATAL VISITS FOR NORMAL PREGNANCY—cont'd

Focus of Care	Initial Prenatal Visit	First Trimester	Second Trimester	Third Trimester
	Nutrition assessment • Height and weight to calculate BMI • 24-hour diet recall Physical activity level Psychosocial assessment (see Chapter 5) Depression Assessment for intimate partner violence			
Laboratory and Diagnostic Studies	Blood type and Rh factor Antibody screen Complete blood count (CBC) including: • Hemoglobin • Hematocrit • Red blood cell count (RBC) • White blood cell count (WBC) • Platelet count (See Appendix C for normal laboratory values in pregnancy.) RPR, VDRL (syphilis serology) HIV screen Hepatitis B screen (surface antigen) Genetic screening based on family history racial or ethnic background (e.g., sickle cell disease, Tay-Sachs) Rubella titer PPD (tuberculosis screen) Urinalysis Urine culture and sensitivity Pap smear Gonorrhea and *Chlamydia* cultures Ultrasound	Review labs	Triple screen or quad screen at 15–20 weeks Ultrasound as indicated Screening for gestational diabetes with 1- hour glucose challenge test at 24–28 weeks Hemoglobin and hematocrit (See Appendix C for normal laboratory values in pregnancy.) Antibody screen if Rh-negative around 26–28 weeks • Administration of RhoGAM at 28 weeks if Rh-negative and antibody screen negative	Group B Streptococcus screening: • Vaginal and rectal swab cultures done at 35–37 weeks on all pregnant women Additional screening testing: H&H if not done recently in second trimester (See Appendix C for normal laboratory values in pregnancy.) Repeat if indicated (and not done in late second trimester): • GC • Chlamydia • RPR • HIV • HbSAg 1-hour glucose challenge test 24–28 weeks Ultrasound as indicated
Prenatal Education and Anticipatory Guidance	Provide information to the woman and her support person on the following: • Physical changes and common discomforts to expect during first trimester	Same as for initial visit	Provide information to the woman and her support person on the following: • Physical changes and common discomforts to	Provide information to the woman and her support person on the following: • Physical changes and common discomforts to

CLINICAL PATHWAY FOR PRENATAL CARE: CONTENT AND TIMING OF ROUTINE PRENATAL VISITS FOR NORMAL PREGNANCY—cont'd

Focus of Care	Initial Prenatal Visit	First Trimester	Second Trimester	Third Trimester
	• Relief measures for common discomforts • Fetal development • General health maintenance/health promotion • Warning/Danger signs to report to care provider • Nutrition, prenatal vitamins, and folic acid • Exercise • Self-care and modifying behaviors to reduce risks • Physiology of pregnancy • Course of care		expect during second trimester • Relief measures for common discomforts • Fetal development and growth during second trimester • Reinforce warning/danger signs to report to care provider • Nutritional follow-up and recommendation of increase in daily caloric intake by 340 kcal/day • Follow-up on physical activity as needed • Follow-up on modifiable risk patterns • Begin teaching on preparing for birth	expect during third trimester • Relief measures for normal and common discomforts • Fetal development and growth during third trimester • Reinforce warning/danger signs to report to care provider • Nutritional follow-up and recommendation of increase in daily caloric intake by 452 kcal/day • Follow-up on modifiable risk patterns Teach fetal movement kick counts Continue teaching and preparing the couple for delivery • Discussion on attending childbirth preparation classes • Teach signs of impending labor • Discuss true vs. false labor • Instruction on when to contact the care provider or go to birthing unit • Discussion on attending parenting classes • Select the method of infant feeding • Select the infant health care provider • Preparation of siblings

The Psycho-Social-Cultural Aspects of the Antepartum Period

5

EXPECTED STUDENT OUTCOMES

On completion of this chapter, the student will be able to:

☐ Describe expected emotional changes of the pregnant woman and appropriate nursing responses to these changes.

☐ Identify the major developmental tasks of pregnancy as they relate to maternal, paternal, and family adaptation.

☐ Identify critical variables that influence adaptation to pregnancy, including age, parity, and social and cultural factors.

☐ Identify nursing assessments and interventions that promote positive psycho-social-cultural adaptations for the pregnant woman and her family.

☐ Analyze critical factors in preparing for birth, including choosing a provider, birth setting, and creating a birth plan.

☐ Identify key components of childbirth preparation education for expectant families.

☐ Analyze and critique current evidence-based research in the area of psycho-social-cultural adaptation to pregnancy.

Nursing Diagnoses

☐ At risk for anxiety and fear related to:
- ■ unknown processes of pregnancy
- ■ changes in roles related to pregnancy
- ■ changes in family dynamics
- ■ changes in body image

☐ Knowledge deficit related to pregnancy emotional/physical changes

☐ At risk for impaired adjustment related to role changes in pregnancy

☐ At risk for interrupted family processes related to developmental stressors of pregnancy

☐ At risk for impaired communication related to cultural differences between family and health care providers

☐ Risk for ineffective coping related to inadequate social support during pregnancy

Nursing Outcomes

The pregnant woman and her family will:

☐ Be able to communicate effectively with health care providers

☐ Verbalize decreased anxiety

☐ Verbalize appropriate family dynamics

☐ Report increasing acceptance of changes in body image

☐ Seek clarification of information about pregnancy and birth

☐ Demonstrate knowledge regarding expected changes of pregnancy

☐ Develop a realistic birth plan

☐ Exhibit acceptance of roles as parents

☐ Identify appropriate support systems

☐ Receive positive and effective social support

☐ Express satisfaction with health care providers' sensitivity to traditional beliefs and practices of her culture.

Don't have time to read this chapter? Want to reinforce your reading? Need to review for a test?
Listen to this chapter on Davis*Plus*.

MATERNAL ADAPTATION TO PREGNANCY

The news of pregnancy confers profound and irrevocable changes in a woman's life and the lives of those around her. With this news, the woman begins her journey towards becoming a mother. Less visible than the physical adaptations of pregnancy, but just as profound, the pregnant woman's psychological adaptations and development of her identity as a mother are crucial aspects of the childbearing cycle. Psychological, cultural, and social variables all significantly influence this process. Psychosocial support for the pregnant woman and her family is a distinct and major nursing responsibility during the antepartum period. This chapter presents the expected emotional changes a woman and her family must navigate to achieve a positive adaptation to pregnancy. Factors influencing these changes are also described.

Successful adaptation to the maternal role requires important psychological work. Although becoming a mother has been noted to occur on a long-term continuum, the psychological groundwork is laid during the course of each woman's individual experience during pregnancy. The pregnant woman is able to use the 9 months available to her to restructure her psychological and cognitive self towards motherhood. Motherhood, an irrevocable change in a woman's life, progressively becomes part of a woman's total identity (Koniak-Griffin, Logsdon, Hines, & Turner, 2006; Mercer, 1995, 2004).

Maternal Tasks of Pregnancy

Maternal tasks of pregnancy were first identified in the psychoanalytic literature (Bibring, Dwyer, Huntington, & Valenstein, 1961), then further explored and outlined by classic maternity nurse researchers Reva Rubin, Ramona Mercer, and Regina Lederman. Rubin's research has provided a framework and core knowledge base from which researchers and clinicians have worked. Rubin identified significant maternal tasks women undergo during the course of pregnancy on their journey towards motherhood (1975, 1984).

- Ensuring a safe passage for herself and her child refers to the mother's knowledge and care-seeking behaviors to ensure that both she and the newborn emerge from pregnancy healthy.
- Ensuring social acceptance of the child by significant others refers to the woman engaging her social network in the pregnancy.
- Attaching or "binding-in" to the child refers to the development of maternal-fetal attachment.
- Giving of oneself to the demands of being a mother refers to the mother's willingness and efforts to make personal sacrifices for the child.

Building on Rubin's work, Regina Lederman (1996, 2009) identified seven dimensions of maternal role development. These are:

- Accepting the pregnancy

This task focuses on the woman's adaptive responses to the changes that occur related to pregnancy growth and development (Lederman, 1996). These responses include:

- *Responding to mood changes*
- *Responding to ambivalent feelings.*
- *Responding to nausea, fatigue, and other physical discomforts of the early months of pregnancy.*
- *Responding to financial concerns*
- *Responding to increased dependency needs*

Expected findings:

- *Desire and/or acceptance of pregnancy (see Critical Component: Ambivalent Feelings Toward Pregnancy)*
- *Predominately happy feelings during pregnancy*
- *Little physical discomfort or a high tolerance for the discomfort*
- *Acceptance of body changes*
- *Minimal ambivalent feelings and conflict regarding pregnancy by the end of her pregnancy*
- *A dislike of being pregnant but a feeling of love for the unborn child.*

CRITICAL COMPONENT

Ambivalent Feelings Toward Pregnancy

It is common for women to experience ambivalent feelings toward pregnancy during the first trimester. These feelings decrease as pregnancy progresses. Ambivalence that continues into the third trimester may indicate unresolved conflict. When evaluating ambivalence it is important to assess:

- The reason for the ambivalence
- The intensity of the ambivalence

- Identification with the motherhood role

Accomplishment of this task is influenced by the woman's acceptance of pregnancy and the relationship the woman has with her own mother. Women who have accepted their pregnancy and who have a positive relationship with their own mothers have an easier time accomplishing this task (Lederman, 1996). Accomplishment of this task is also influenced by the woman's degree of fears about labor related to helplessness, pain, loss of control, and loss of self-esteem (Lederman, 1996). Vivid dreams are common during pregnancy, which allows the woman to envision herself as a mother in various situations. A woman often rehearses or pictures herself in her new role in different scenarios (Rubin, 1975). The motherhood role is progressively strengthened as she attaches to the fetus. Events that facilitate fetal attachment:

- Hearing the fetal heartbeat
- Seeing the fetus move during an ultrasound examination
- Feeling the fetus kick or move
- Fetal attachment influences the woman's sense of her child and her sense of being competent as a mother.

Expected Findings:
The woman:

■ *Moves from viewing herself as a woman-without-child to a woman-with-child*
■ *Anticipates changes motherhood will bring to her life*
■ *Seeks company of other pregnant women*
■ *Is highly motivated to assume the motherhood role*
■ *Actively prepares for the motherhood role*

■ Relationship to her mother
   ■ *A woman's relationship with her mother is an important determinant of adaptation to motherhood. Unresolved mother-daughter conflicts re-emerge and can confront women during pregnancy (Lederman, 1996).*

Four components important to the woman's relationship with her own mother are:

■ *Availability of the woman's mother to her in the past and in the present*
■ *The mother's reaction to her daughter's pregnancy*
■ *The mother's relationship to her daughter*
■ *The mother's willingness to reminisce with her daughter about her own childbirth and child-rearing experiences*

Expected Findings

■ *The woman's mother was available to her in the past and continues to be available during the pregnancy (Fig. 5-1).*
■ *The woman's mother accepts the pregnancy, respects her autonomy, and acknowledges her daughter becoming a mother.*
■ *The woman's mother relates to her daughter as an adult versus as a child.*

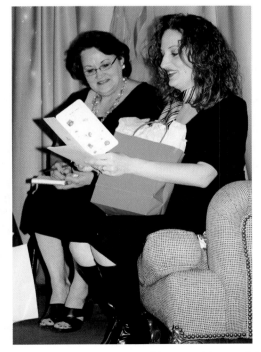

Figure 5-1 Pregnant woman and her mother participating in baby shower.

■ *The woman's mother reminisces about her own childbearing and child-rearing experiences.*

■ Re-ordering relationships with her partner

Pregnancy has a dramatic effect on a couple's relationship. Some couples view pregnancy and childbirth as a growth experience and as an expression of deep commitment to their bond, while others view it as an added stressor to a relationship already in conflict. The partner's support during pregnancy enhances the woman's feelings of well-being and is associated with earlier and continuous prenatal care (Lederman, 1996, 2009). Feeling loved and valued and having her child accepted by her partner are two major contributors to positive adaptation (Cannella, 2006; Orr, 2004). Assessment of the relationship between the couple includes:

■ *The partner's concern for the woman's needs during pregnancy*
■ *The woman's concerns for her partner's needs during pregnancy*
■ *The varying desire for sexual activity among pregnant women*
■ *The effect pregnancy has on the relationship (e.g., does it being them closer together or cause conflict?)*
■ *The partner's adjustment to his or her new role.*

Expected Findings

■ *The partner is understanding and supportive of the woman.*
■ *The partner is thoughtful and "pampers" the woman during pregnancy.*
■ *The partner is involved in the pregnancy.*
■ *The woman perceives that her partner is supportive.*
■ *The woman is concerned about her partner's needs of making emotional adjustments to the pregnancy and new role. Women in relationships with established open communication about sexuality are likely to have less difficulty with changes in sexual activity.*
■ *Couples indicate that they are growing closer to each other during pregnancy.*
■ *The partner is happy and excited about the pregnancy and prepares for the new role.*

■ Preparation for labor

Preparation for labor means preparation for the physiological processes of labor as well as the psychological processes of separating from the fetus and becoming a mother to the child. Preparation for labor and birth occur by taking classes, reading, fantasizing, and dreaming about labor and birth (Lederman, 1996, 2009). The degree of preparation for labor and birth has an effect on the woman's level of anxiety and fear. The more prepared a woman feels, the lower the level of anxiety and fear.

Expected Findings

■ *The woman attends childbirth classes and reads books about labor and birth.*
■ *The woman mentally rehearses (fantasizes) the labor and birthing process.*
■ *The woman has dreams about labor and birth.*
■ *The woman develops realistic expectations of labor and birth.*

■ *The pregnant woman may engage in a flurry of activity known as "nesting behavior," hurrying to finish preparing for the newborn's arrival (Driscoll, 2008).*

■ Prenatal fear of loss of control in labor

Loss of control includes two factors (Lederman 1996, 2009):

■ *Loss of control over the body*
■ *Loss of control over emotions*

The degree of fear is related to:

■ *The woman's degree of trust with the medical and nursing staff, her partner, and other support persons*
■ *The woman's attitude regarding the use of medication and anesthesia for labor pain management*

Expected Findings

■ *The woman perceives individual attention from medical staff.*
■ *The woman perceives that she is being treated as an adult and her questions and concerns are addressed by the medical staff.*
■ *The woman perceives that the nursing staff is compassionate, understanding, and available.*
■ *The woman perceives that she is being supported by her partner and family/friends.*
■ *The woman has realistic expectations regarding management of labor pain and these expectations are met.*

■ Prenatal fear of loss of self-esteem in labor

Some women have fears that they will lose self-esteem in labor and "fail" during labor (Lederman, 2009). When a woman feels a threat to her self-esteem, it is important to assess the following areas (Lederman, 2009):

■ *The source of the threat*
■ *The response to the threat*
■ *The intensity of the reaction to the threat*

Behaviors that reflect self-esteem are:

■ *Tolerance of self*
■ *Value of self and assertiveness*
■ *Positive attitude regarding body image and appearance*

Expected Findings

■ *Able to develop realistic expectations of self during labor and birth and an awareness of risks and potential complications*
■ *Able to identify and respect her own feelings*
■ *Able to assert herself in acquiring information needed to make decisions*
■ *Able to recognize her own needs and limitations*
■ *Able to adjust to the unexpected and unknown*
■ *Able to recover from threats quickly*

As the woman prepares to experience labor, give birth, and take on the maternal role, the process of maternal adaptation to pregnancy is completed. With the dominating physical discomforts of the third trimester, most women become impatient for labor to begin. There is relief and excitement about going into labor. The mother is ready and eager to deliver and hold her baby. She has prepared for her future as a mother (Rubin, 1984).

Nursing Actions

During the antepartal period, the nurse can take on a variety of roles: teacher, counselor, clinician, resource person, role model (see Critical Component: Nursing Actions That Facilitate Adaptation to Pregnancy).

■ Nursing actions should be focused on health promotion, individualized care, and prevention of individual and family crises (Driscoll, 2008; Matson & Smith, 2004; Lederman, 2009).

Factors That Influence Maternal Adaptation

The ability of the woman to adapt to the maternal role is influenced by a variety of factors, including parity, maternal age, sexual orientation, single parenting, multiple gestation (twins, triples), socioeconomic factors, and abuse.

Multiparity

■ Multigravidas may have the benefit of experience, but it should not be assumed that they need less help than a first-time mother. They know more of what to expect in terms of pain during labor, postpartum adaptation, and the many added responsibilities of motherhood, but they may need time to process and develop strategies for integrating a new member into the family.

■ Pregnancy tasks may be more complex. Giving adequate attention to all of her children and supporting sibling adaptation are unique challenges faced by the multigravida. She may spend a great deal of time working out a new relationship with the first child, and grieve for the loss of their special relationship. She also has to consider the financial issues associated with feeding, clothing, and providing for another child while at the same time maintaining a relationship with her partner and continuing her career, whether inside or outside the home (Jordan, 1989).

Maternal Age

■ Adolescent Mothers

Adolescents who have an unintended pregnancy face a number of challenges, including abandonment by their partners, increased adverse pregnancy outcomes, and inability to complete school education, which may ultimately limit their future social and economic opportunities (Ehiri, Meremikwu, & Meremikwu, 2005). The major developmental task of adolescence is to form and become comfortable with a sense of self. Pregnancy presents a challenge for teenagers who, as expectant parents, must cope with the conflicting developmental tasks of pregnancy and adolescence at the same time. Achieving a maternal identity is very difficult for an adolescent who is in the throes of evolving her own identity as an adult capable of psychosocial independence from her family. Although she may achieve

CRITICAL COMPONENT

Nursing Actions That Facilitate Adaptation to Pregnancy

First Trimester:

- Begin psychosocial assessment at initial contact; assess woman's response to pregnancy; assess stressors in woman's life. It allows the nurse to determine whether there are issues that may require referrals, and to begin to develop the plan of care.
- Promote pregnancy and birth as a family experience; encourage family and father or partner participation in prenatal visits; encourage questions from father and family members about the pregnancy. It is important to offer an inclusive model of care that acknowledges the needs of the family as well as the individual. Pregnancy significantly affects all family members. Meeting with family members provides additional information to the nurse, and helps to complete the family assessment. Positive family support is associated with positive maternal adaptation.
- Assess learning needs. It allows the nurse to provide individualized information.
- Offer anticipatory guidance regarding normal developmental stressors of pregnancy, such as ambivalence during early pregnancy, feelings of vulnerability, mood changes, and active dream/fantasy life. It allows the nurse to emphasize normalcy, health, universality, strengths, and developmental concepts, to decrease anxiety.
- Assess for increased anxieties and fear; if anxieties seem greater than normal, refer to psych care provider. Excessive anxiety and stress, and prenatal depression have a negative impact on the course of a woman's pregnancy and also affect the physiology of the developing fetus. Specialized intervention is needed.
- Listen, validate, provide reassurance, and teach expected emotional changes. Educate partner and family members, and stress normalcy of feelings to decrease anxiety and ensure the woman feels "heard" and validated.
- If appropriate, discuss common phases through which expectant fathers progress through pregnancy. Be aware of phases of paternal adaptation when counseling parents about expected changes of pregnancy; provide anticipatory guidance regarding potential communication conflicts. This will acknowledge the partner as a significant participant in the pregnancy process, and assist in improving communication and decreasing stress in the relationship.

Second Trimester:

- Encourage verbalization regarding possible grief process during pregnancy related to body image changes, loss of old life, changing relationships with family and friends. The woman may be more anxious about body changes in the second trimester. The woman may begin to have fears or phobias. The nurse needs to acknowledge and validate the woman's feelings, and help the woman work towards resolving any conflicting feelings.
- Discuss normal changes in sexual activity and provide information and acknowledge the woman's sexuality.
- Encourage "tuning in" to fetal movements; discuss fetal capacities for hearing, responding to interaction, and maternal activity. This will encourage the attachment process, and help empower the woman with increased involvement in care.
- Reinforce to partner and family the importance of giving the expectant mother extra support; give specific examples of ways to help (helping her eat well, helping with heavy work, giving extra attention). This will encourage family and partner participation in the pregnancy process and promote support for the woman. A well-supported woman will likely have a more positive adaptation to pregnancy.

Third Trimester

- Encourage attendance at childbirth classes to promote knowledge and decrease fears.
- Discuss preparations for birth, parenthood; explore expectations of labor. The woman will begin to focus more on the impending birth during the third trimester, and her learning needs will be more focused on this area. It is important to provide anticipatory information and guidance.
- Assess partner's comfort level with labor coach role and reassure as needed; stress that help in labor will be available; encourage presence of second support person if appropriate. The woman's partner may not feel comfortable providing labor support, and it is important to discuss prior to the onset of labor so all roles can be clarified.
- Refer to appropriate educational materials on parenthood. Encourage discussions of plans, expectations with partner. Give anticipatory guidance regarding the realities of infant care, breastfeeding, and so on. This will promote communication and planning with the expectant parents, as well as a positive transition to parenthood.
- If psychosocial complications develop, plan for appropriate referrals to coordinate with social workers, nutritionist, and community agencies to ensure continuity of psychosocial assessment and provide appropriate support during the woman's pregnancy.
- Help expectant mother identify and use support systems to promote positive adaptation to pregnancy, birth, and postpartum. To anticipate the need for postpartum support, and decrease the risk of postpartum depression.

(Driscoll, 2008; Lederman, 2009; Simpson & Creehan, 2008; Mattson & Smith, 2010)

the maternal role, research indicates that she functions at a lower level of competence than do older women (Mercer, 2004). The younger she is, the more difficulty the adolescent woman has with body image changes, acknowledging the pregnancy, seeking health care, and planning for the changes that pregnancy and parenting will bring. Delayed entry into prenatal care is common. There is also a higher rate of abuse among pregnant adolescents (Montgomery, 2003; Porter, 2011). Successful adaptation to pregnancy and parenthood may greatly depend on the age of the adolescent (**Fig. 5-2**).

  ■ *Comprehensive and community-based health care programs for adolescents have been shown to be effective in*

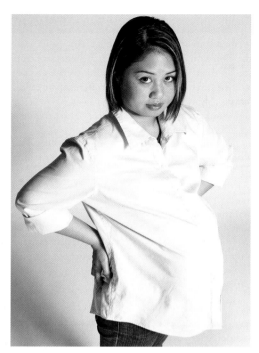

Figure 5–2 Pregnant adolescent. *(Photo courtesy of Randi Willis and Gwen Ortiz.)*

improving outcomes for the teen mother and her infant. Examples include programs that have been implemented in schools, clinics, community agencies, or home visitation programs. Additionally, higher levels of support and higher self-esteem are associated with a more positive adaptation to mothering for adolescents (Key et al., 2008; Logsdon, Gagne, Hughes, Patterson, & Rakestraw, 2005; Schaffer, Jost, Pederson, & Lair, 2008; Porter & Holness, 2011).

■ *Early adolescence can be defined as the period between 11 and 15 years. Adolescents in this phase of life are self-centered and oriented towards the present. Additionally, there is a greater likelihood that pregnancy at this age is a result of abuse or coercion. Moving into the maternal role is a difficult challenge for this age group. Grandmothers will play a significant role in caring for the infant as well as providing guidance to their daughter regarding mothering skills. (Mercer, 1995; Montgomery 2003; Pinazo-Hernandis & Tompkins, 2009).*

■ *Middle adolescence is defined as the period between 14 and 16 years. During this time, the adolescent will be more capable of abstract thinking and understanding consequences of current behaviors.*

■ *By age 17–20, as adolescents mature into late adolescence, these skills will be further developed and eventually mastered. The older pregnant adolescent is more likely to be a capable and active participant in health care decisions (DeVito, 2010; Montgomery, 2003).*

■ Older Mothers

In North America, increasing numbers of women have delayed childbearing until after the age of 30–35. The majority of women in this age group deliver at term without adverse outcomes. However, even with good prenatal care, there is an increased incidence of adverse perinatal outcomes. Chronic diseases that are more common in women over 35 may affect the pregnancy. Older mothers are also more likely to have miscarriages, fetal chromosomal abnormalities, low birth weight infants, premature births, and multiple births. In women over 40, the risk increases for placenta previa, placenta abruptio, caesarean deliveries, and gestational diabetes. In fact, 49.5% of babies of women over the age of 40 are delivered by caesarean section (Bayrampour & Heaman, 2010; CDC, 2009; Joseph, Allen, Dodds, Turner, Scott, & Liston, 2005). The more mature woman is better equipped psychosocially to assume the maternal role. However, she also might have increased difficulty with the changing roles in her life, experiencing heightened ambivalence. She might have difficulty balancing a career with the physical and psychological demands of pregnancy. The sometimes unpredictable nature of pregnancy, labor, and life with a newborn may challenge a woman who may have developed a predictable life over which she has much control (Carolan, 2005; Dobrzykowski & Stern, 2003; Schardt, 2005). Older mothers are more commonly from a higher socioeconomic background and have a greater number of years of education. They are more likely to be established in a career, their relationships, and their lifestyles. Pregnancy is often chosen and planned. Sometimes it culminates after infertility treatments and may involve extensive use of reproductive technologies. Pregnant women in this age group are highly motivated to seek information about childbirth and parenting from books, friends, and electronic resources.

Lesbian Mothers

Little research has been conducted on the process of maternal adaptation to pregnancy in lesbian women. Although the developmental tasks of pregnancy are likely to be similar, the lesbian woman faces unique obstacles and challenges in today's health care environment. Healthy People 2020 has added new objectives relating to improving the health, safety, and well-being of lesbian, gay, bisexual, and transgender (LGBT) individuals (U.S. DHHS, 2010).

■ Lesbian women may be more likely to lack social support, particularly from their families of origin. They may be exposed to additional stress due to homophobic attitudes, in particular in the health care system.

■ Finding supportive health care providers with whom they are comfortable disclosing sexual orientation is an important need identified by lesbian women (**Fig. 5-3**). Heteronormative health care environments in which parents are assumed to be a man and a woman present barriers to care for all same-sex couples. The role of the woman's partner and legal considerations of the growing family will also affect the lesbian experience of pregnancy (McManus, Hunter, & Renn, 2006; Rondahl, 2009; Ross, 2005).

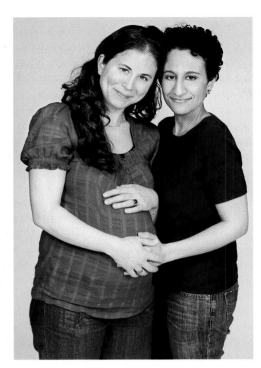

Figure 5–3 Lesbian pregnant couple. *(Photo courtesy of Gwen Ortiz and Randi Willis.)*

- Lesbian mothers most commonly plan their pregnancies, conceiving through donor insemination. In addition, it has been observed that many lesbian couples participate in a relatively equal division of child care. These factors can combine to help decrease the stress a lesbian mother might experience and act as protection from perinatal depression (Ross, 2005).
- Nursing assessments of lesbian women should be adapted accordingly. Nurse needs to strive toward the use of inclusive language and avoid making assumptions about a woman's gender orientation without further information. Birth partners who are not the biologic fathers experience the same fears, questions, and concerns. Birth partners need to be kept informed, supported, and included in all activities in which the mother desires their participation.

Single Parenting

The literature reports a higher degree of stress for pregnant single women (e.g., greater anxiety; less tangible reliable support from family and friends) (Logsdon, 2000; Simpson & Creehan, 2008).

- Single mothers may live at or below the poverty level, facing greater financial challenges, resulting in a higher risk of depression. Single women engage in the maternal tasks of pregnancy and face more complex tasks and a variety of challenges. With the initial news, the decision must be made whether or not to proceed with the pregnancy.
  - *Telling the family may cause concern.*

- *Issues regarding legal guardianship in the event she is incapacitated must be considered.*
  - *Putting the father's name on the birth certificate is another decision she must make.*
- The reasons surrounding the pregnancy and the presence or absence of strong support persons can significantly influence her adaptation (Beeber & Canuso, 2005). Initial assessments are crucial for providing appropriate care:
  - *Is the woman single by choice?*
  - *Is she a single mother by accident? (i.e., death of partner following conception, separation, divorce)*
  - *Did she get pregnant by a casual acquaintance?*

Multigestational Pregnancy

A multiple gestation pregnancy (twins, triples, etc.) places added psychosocial stressors on the family unit. The diagnosis shocks many expectant parents, and they may need additional support and education to help them cope with the changes they face. The increased risk for adverse outcomes results in increased fears and anxieties for the pregnant woman.

- If the woman is found to be carrying more than three fetuses, the parents may receive counseling regarding selective reduction of the pregnancies to reduce the incidence of premature birth and allow the remaining fetuses to grow to term gestation.
  - *This situation poses an ethical dilemma and emotional strain for many parents, particularly if they have been attempting to achieve pregnancy for a lengthy time (Begley, 2000; Collopy, 2004; Damato, 2004; Maifeld, Hahn, Titler, Marita, & Mullen, 2003).*

Socioeconomic Factors

The resources of the family to meet the needs for food, shelter, and health care play a crucial role in how a family responds to pregnancy.

- Financial barriers have been identified as the one of the most important factors contributing to maternal inability to receive adequate prenatal care.
- Immigrant women face significant economic barriers. Women in this group are often marginalized, and many may work in low-income service oriented jobs. Access to health care may be particularly limited (Driscoll, 2008; Jentsch, Durham, Hundley, & Hussein, 2007; Meleis, 2003).
- The elimination of these health care disparities resulting from low income has been noted as one of the major goals of Healthy People 2020 (U.S. DHHS, 2010).

The Abused Woman

Pregnancy can often be a trigger for beginning or increased abuse, or intimate partner violence (IPV) (see Chapters 4 and 7). Yet, pregnancy offers a unique opportunity for health care providers to recognize abuse and to intervene appropriately.

- Screen all pregnant women for abuse. For further information on IPV, refer to Chapters 4 and 7.

Military Deployment

Military deployment can significantly influence adaptation to pregnancy. Thousands of women of childbearing age are serving and being deployed in the U.S. military. Women currently comprise more than 14% of active duty forces. Although women are excluded from serving in direct combat roles in the military, they serve in positions that put them in the direct line of fire and may cause significant stress (e.g., convoy driver, patrol).

■ For women veterans, pregnancy can exacerbate mental health conditions (Mattocks et al., 2010) (see Evidence-Based Practice: Women in the Military). Since the Veterans Health Administration (VHA) does not provide pregnancy care, pregnant veterans may also be faced with fragmentation between the VHA and non-VHA care providers, putting them at further risk for poor outcomes.

■ Women with deployed partners may also have more difficulty with accepting the pregnancy, and experience greater conflict. There is evidence, however, that on-base community support can have a positive effect on pregnancy acceptance for these women (Weis et al., 2008; Weis & Ryan, 2012).

■ The Centering Pregnancy model of care, implemented at various military treatment facilities, also shows promise for offering effective group support for military spouses (Foster, Alviar, Neumeier, & Wootten, 2012).

Evidence-Based Practice: Women in the Military

Mattocks, K., et al. (2010). Pregnancy and mental health among women veterans returning from Iraq and Afghanistan. *Journal of Women's Health, 19*(12), 2166–2159.

Little is known about mental health problems or treatment among pregnant women veterans. Veterans may experience significant stress during military service that can have lingering effects.

This study was conducted to determine the prevalence of mental health problems among veterans who received pregnancy related care in the Veterans Health Administration (VHA) system.

Data was collected and analyzed from the Defense Manpower Data Center deployments roster of military discharges from October 2001 to April 2008, resulting in a cohort of 43,078 female veterans. Pregnancy and mental health conditions were quantified according to VHA codes.

Results indicate that veterans with a pregnancy were twice as likely to have a diagnosis of depression, anxiety, post-traumatic stress disorder, bipolar disorder, or schizophrenia as those without a pregnancy.

Limitations of the study are that only women who received VHA care were included. Women veterans seeking care outside the VHA system were not included.

Results point to the need for further study to understand the overlap between pregnancy and mental health conditions in VHA patients, and the impact of mental health treatment on pregnancy outcomes among women veterans

---

Nursing Actions

■ Assess adaptation to pregnancy at every prenatal visit. Early assessment and intervention may prevent or greatly reduce later problems for the pregnant woman and her family.

■ Identify areas of concern, validate major issues, and make suggestions for possible changes.

■ Refer to the appropriate member of the health care team.

■ Establish a trusting relationship, as women may be reluctant to share information until one has been formed (e.g., questions asked at the first prenatal visit bear repeating with ongoing prenatal care).

■ Use psychosocial health assessment screening tools.

  ■ *A variety of screening tools can be used to assess adaptation to pregnancy and to identify risk factors. Psychosocial assessment reported in the literature ranges from a few questions asked by the health care provider to questionnaires and risk screening tools focusing on a specific area such as depression or abuse (Beck, 2002; Carroll et al., 2005; Midmer, Carroll, Bryanton, & Stewart, 2002; Priest, Austin, & Sullivan, 2006; Spietz & Kelly, 2003).*

  ■ *The Antenatal Psychosocial Health Assessment (ALPHA) form, developed in Ontario, Canada, has been demonstrated to be a useful evidence-based prenatal tool that can identify women who would benefit from additional support and intervention (**Box 5-1**) (Carroll et al., 2005; Midmer et al., 2002).*

PATERNAL ADAPTATION DURING PREGNANCY

The news of a pregnancy has a profound effect on the man. Men have fears, questions, and concerns regarding the pregnancy, his partner, and his transition to fatherhood. Each

---

BOX 5–1   ANTENATAL PSYCHOSOCIAL HEALTH ASSESSMENT (ALPHA)

The Antenatal Psychosocial Health Assessment is an evidence-based prenatal tool that can help providers identify women who would benefit from additional support and intervention. This tool assesses the following areas:

Social support
Recent stressful life events
Couple's relationship
Onset of prenatal care
Plans for prenatal education
Feelings toward pregnancy after 20 weeks
Relationship with parents in childhood
Self-esteem
History or psychiatric/emotional problems
Depression in this pregnancy
Alcohol/drug use
Family violence

Source: Carroll, Reid, Biringer, Midmer, Glazier, Wilson, et al. (2005).

Patient-Centered Care

Definition: Recognize the patient or designee as the source of control and full partner in providing compassionate and coordinated care based on respect for patient's preferences, values, and needs.

This chapter explores the influence of culture on values and beliefs, the effects of pregnancy on the woman as well as on members of the immediate and extended family, and variables that influence the woman's adaptation to pregnancy.

We explore many topics related to patient and family empowerment, barriers to culturally competent care, and how to remove those barriers.

We describe how diverse cultural, ethnic, and social backgrounds function as sources of patient, family, and community values.

We explore patient-centered care with sensitivity and respect for the diversity of human experience.

There is an emphasis on women's choices in choosing a provider and place of birth, and developing a birth plan.

Nursing actions are focused on providing autonomy and choices based on the respect for the woman's preferences, values, and needs. Health promotion, individualized care, and a family-centered approach are all crucial components of nursing care.

man brings to pregnancy a unique history with which he begins his own experience of becoming a father. Some men relish the role and look forward to actively nurturing a child. Others may be more detached or even hostile to the idea of fatherhood.

Fathers' Participation

Changing cultural and professional attitudes have encouraged fathers' participation in the birth experience.

■ Some fathers respond well to this expectation, wishing to explore every aspect of pregnancy, childbirth, and parenting (May, 1980).
■ Others are more task oriented and view themselves as managers. They may direct the woman's diet and rest periods and act as coaches during childbirth but remain detached from the emotional aspects of the experience.
■ Some men are more comfortable as observers and prefer not to participate.
■ In some cultures, men view pregnancy and childbirth as exclusively a woman's domain, and may be removed from the experience completely.
■ In high-risk populations, increased paternal involvement can be one way to potentially improve birth outcomes and reduce health care disparities. Fatherhood initiatives and employment assistance are examples of programs that can promote paternal involvement (Alio et al., 2010; Alio, Bond, Padilla, Heidelbaugh, Lu, & Parker, 2011; Misra, Caldwell, Young, & Abelson, 2010).

Effect of Pregnancy on Fathers

Concerns about the well-being of his partner are heightened, and worries may be present about whether he and his partner will be good parents.

■ Increased emphasis on his role as provider causes a reevaluation of lifestyle and job or career status.
  ■ *There may be anxiety about providing financial stability for his growing family.*
■ Changes in relationships and roles will challenge expectant fathers, creating the potential for distancing from their partners.
  ■ *There may be a higher risk for infidelities.*
■ With the focus of prenatal care on the woman and the growing fetus, the man may struggle at times to feel that he is relevant in the pregnancy (Widarsson et al., 2012).
■ Some fathers may find themselves without models to assist them in taking on the role of active and involved parent (Genesoni & Tallandini, 2009; Hanson et al., 2009).
■ Men may experience pregnancy-like symptoms and discomforts similar to those of their pregnant partner, such as nausea, weight gain, or abdominal pains. This is referred to as **Couvade Syndrome** (Brennan, 2007).
■ Abuse may begin or escalate with the news of pregnancy.

Paternal Developmental Tasks

There is evidence that paternal adaptation involves unique developmental tasks for fathers (**Table 5-1**). May's classic research (1982) on men identified three phases that fathers experience as the pregnancy progresses:

■ The announcement phase
■ The moratorium phase
■ The focusing phase

These experiences unfold concurrently but in a distinctly different manner than the pregnant woman's adaptive experience.

Nursing Actions

■ Explore the man's response to news of pregnancy.
■ Reassure that ambivalence is common in the early months of pregnancy.
■ Reassure normalcy of pregnancy-like symptoms (Couvade Syndrome).
■ Encourage attendance in childbirth classes (i.e., provide resources for classes, discuss advantages of attending classes).
■ Encourage the man to negotiate his role in labor with his partner.
■ Explore his attitudes and expectations of pregnancy, childbirth, and parenting (see Critical Component: Nursing Actions That Facilitate Adaptation to Pregnancy).

TABLE 5–1   PATERNAL ADAPTATION TO PREGNANCY

ANNOUNCEMENT PHASE Men may react to the news of pregnancy with joy, distress, or a combination of emotions, depending on whether the pregnancy is planned or unwanted.	Occurs as the news of the pregnancy is revealed. It may last from a few hours to several weeks. It is very common at this phase for men to feel ambivalence. The main developmental task is to accept the biologic fact of pregnancy. Men will begin to attempt to take on the expectant father role.
MORATORIUM PHASE During this phase, many men appear to put conscious thought of the pregnancy aside for some time, even as their partners are undergoing dramatic physical and emotional changes right before their eyes.	This can cause potential conflict when women attempt to communicate with their partners about the pregnancy. Sexual adaptation will be necessary as well; men may fear hurting the fetus during intercourse. Feelings of rivalry may surface as the fetus grows larger and the woman becomes more preoccupied with her own thoughts of impending motherhood. Men's main developmental task during this phase is to accept the pregnancy. This includes accepting the changing body and emotional state of his partner, as well as accepting the reality of the fetus, especially when fetal movement is felt.
FOCUSING PHASE The focusing phase begins in the last trimester. Men will be actively involved in the pregnancy and their relationship with the child.	Men begin to think of themselves as fathers. Men participate in planning for labor and delivery, and the newborn. Men's main developmental task is to negotiate with their partner the role they are to play in labor and to prepare for parenthood.

Source: May, 1982.

SEXUALITY IN PREGNANCY

Sexuality in pregnancy occurs on a wide continuum of responses for women. Some women feel more beautiful and desirable with advancing pregnancy and others unattractive and ungainly. The sexual relationship can be significantly affected during pregnancy. Physical, emotional, and interactional factors all play a part in the woman's and her partner's sexual response during pregnancy (Crooks & Baur, 2010).

■ The desire for sexual activity varies among pregnant women. Sexual desire can vary even in the same woman at different times during the pregnancy.
  ■ *During the first trimester, fatigue, nausea, and breast tenderness may affect sexual desire.*
  ■ *During the second trimester, there may be an increase in desire as a result of increased sense of well-being and the pelvic congestion associated with this time in pregnancy.*
  ■ *During the third trimester, sexual interest may once again decrease as the enlarging abdomen creates feelings of awkwardness and bulkiness.*
■ Women in relationships with established open communication about sexuality are less likely to have difficulty with changes in sexual activity.
■ It may be necessary for a couple to modify intercourse positions for the pregnant woman's comfort.
  ■ *The side-by-side, woman-above, and rear-entry positions are generally more comfortable than the man-above positions.*
■ Nonsexual expression of affection is important as well.

■ Common concerns related to sexual activity include:
  ■ *Fears about hurting the fetus during intercourse or causing permanent anomalies as a result of sexual activity.*
  ■ *Fear the birth process will drastically change the woman's genitals.*
■ Changes in body shape and body image will influence both partners' desire for sexual expression.

Nursing Actions

■ Discuss fears and concerns related to sexual activity.
■ Encourage communication between partners and discuss possible changes with couples.
  ■ *Encourage the couple to verbalize fears and to ask questions.*
  ■ *Use humor and encourage the couple to use humor to relieve anxiety or embarrassment.*
■ Advise pregnant women that there are no contraindications to intercourse or masturbation to orgasm provided the woman's membranes are intact, there is no vaginal bleeding, and she has no current problems or history of premature labor (Crooks & Baur, 2010).
■ Review sexual positions to increase comfort for couple with advancing pregnancy.
■ Discuss alternative forms of sexual expression.

FAMILY ADAPTATION DURING PREGNANCY

The **family** is a basic structural unit of the community and constitutes one of society's most important institutions. It is a key target for perinatal assessment and intervention.

This primary social group assumes major responsibility for the introduction and socialization of children, and forms a potent network of support for its members. An understanding of the different family structures and the life cycle of the family and the related developmental tasks can assist the nurse in the development of nursing care during pregnancy.

■ The family has traditionally been defined as "the fundamental social group in society typically consisting of one or two parents and their children" (Friedman, Bowen, & Jones, 2003).
■ The structure of families varies widely among and within cultures. Social scientists now commonly recognize that families exist in a variety of ways, and that during the course of their lives, children may indeed belong to several different family groups.

Changing Structures of the Family

The U.S. census data indicates major shifts in the configuration of families over the past several decades. A woman's family is the primary support during the childbearing years and has a direct influence on her emotional and physical health. It is essential that the nurse identify the woman's definition of family and provide care on that basis. Nurses must support all types of families (**Fig. 5-4**). The variety of family configurations includes (Friedman, 2003):

■ The nuclear family: a father, mother, and child living together but apart from both sets of grandparents.
■ The extended family: three generations, including married brothers and sisters and their families.
■ Single parent family: divorced, never married, separated, or widowed man or woman and at least one child.
■ Three generational families: any combination of first, second and third generation members living within a household.
■ Dyad family: couple living alone without children.
■ Stepparent family: one or both spouses have been divorced or widowed and have remarried into a family with at least one child.

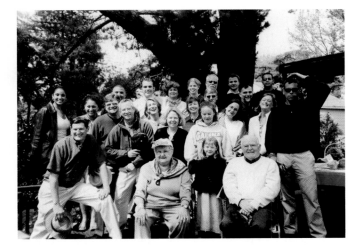

Figure 5–4 Multicultural family.

■ Blended or reconstituted family: a combination of two families with children from one or both families and sometimes children of the newly married couple.
■ Cohabiting family: an unmarried couple living together.
■ Gay or lesbian family: a homosexual couple living together with or without children; children may be adopted, from previous relationships, or conceived via artificial insemination.
■ Adoptive family: single persons or couples who have at least one child who is not biologically related to them and to whom they have legally become parents.

Family theorists have identified eight stages in the life cycle of a family that provide a framework for nurses caring for childbearing families (Duvall, 1985, Friedman, et al., 2003):

■ Beginning families
■ Childbearing families
■ Families with preschool children
■ Families with school-aged children
■ Families with teenagers
■ Families launching young adults
■ Middle-aged parents
■ Family in retirement

Each of these stages has developmental tasks that the family needs to accomplish to successfully move to the next stage.

Developmental Tasks

The events of pregnancy and childbirth are considered a developmental (maturational) crisis in the life of a family, i.e., those changes associated with normal growth and development.

■ All family members are significantly affected.
  ■ *Previous life patterns may be disturbed and there may be a sense of disorganization.*
■ Certain developmental tasks have been identified which a family must face and master to successfully incorporate a new member into the family unit and allow the family to be ready for further growth and development. The developmental tasks for the childbearing family are:
  ■ *Acquiring knowledge and plans for the specific needs of pregnancy, childbirth, and early parenthood*
  ■ *Preparing to provide for the physical care of the newborn*
  ■ *Adapting financial patterns to meet increasing needs*
  ■ *Realignment of tasks and responsibilities*
  ■ *Adjusting patterns of sexual expression to accommodate pregnancy*
  ■ *Expanding communication to meet emotional needs*
  ■ *Reorienting of relationships with relatives*
  ■ *Adapting relationships with friends and community to take account of the realities of pregnancy and the anticipated newborn*

The accomplishment of these tasks during pregnancy lays the groundwork for later adaptation required when the newborn is added to the family unit (Duvall, 1985; Friedman, et al., 2003).

Nursing Actions

- Assess knowledge related to pregnancy, childbirth, and early parenting.
- Assess progress in developmental tasks of pregnancy.
- Explore patterns of communication related to emotional needs, responsibilities, and new roles.
- Include the entire family; assessments and interventions must be considered in a family-centered perspective.
- Provide education and guidance related to pregnancy, childbirth, and early parenting (see Critical Component: Nursing Actions That Facilitate Adaptation to Pregnancy).

GRANDPARENT ADAPTATION

Grandparents are often the first family members to be told about the pregnancy. They must make complex adjustments to the news. When it is their first grandchild, most grandparents are delighted. A first pregnancy is also undeniable evidence that they are growing older, and some may respond negatively, indicating that they are not ready to be grandparents.

- New parents recognize that the tie to the future represented by the fetus is of special significance to grandparents.
- Grandparents provide a unique sense of family history to expectant parents that may not be available elsewhere. They can be a valuable resource and can strengthen family systems by widening the circle of support and nurturance.
- Grandparents may also be called upon for more long-term help. Teen pregnancy, parents' incarceration, substance abuse, child abuse, and death or mental illnesses of the parents are examples of situations where grandparents may have to assume the care and upbringing of the newborn.
- The demands of helping to raise their grandchild may create added stressors in their lives that they may not have anticipated. Community and home-based multigenerational parent support interventions may address some of these concerns (Sadler & Clemmens, 2004; Pinazo-Hernandis, & Tompkins, 2009).

Nursing Actions

- Assess the grandparents' response to pregnancy.
- Explore grandparents as a resource during pregnancy and early parenting.

SIBLING ADAPTATION

Sharing the spotlight with a new brother or sister can be a major crisis for a child. The older child often experiences a sense of loss or feels jealous at being "replaced" by the new sibling. During pregnancy, areas of change that impact siblings the most involve maternal appearance, parental behavior, and changes in the home environment such as sleeping arrangements.

- Sibling adaptation is greatly influenced by the child's age and developmental level, and the attitude of the parents.
  - *Children under the age of 2 are usually unaware of the pregnancy and do not understand explanations about the future arrival of the newborn.*
  - *Children from 2–4 years of age may respond to the obvious changes in their mother's body but may not remember from month to month why the changes are occurring. This age group is particularly sensitive to the disruptions of the physical environment. Therefore, if the parents plan to change the sibling's sleeping arrangements to accommodate the new baby, these arrangements should be implemented well in advance of the birth. Children still sleeping in a crib should be moved to a bed at least 2 months before the baby is due.*
  - *Children ages 4–5 often enjoy listening to the fetal heartbeat and may show interest in the development of the fetus. As pregnancy progresses, they may resent the changes in their mother's body that interfere with her ability to lift and hold them, or engage in physical play.*
  - *School-age children ages 6–12 are usually enthusiastic and keenly interested in the details of pregnancy and birth. They have many questions and are eager to learn. They often plan elaborate welcomes for the newborn and want to be able to help when their new sibling comes home (Fortier, Carson, Will, & Shubkagel, 1991).*
  - *Adolescent responses to pregnancy will vary according to their developmental status. They may be uncomfortable with the obvious evidence of their parents' sexuality or be embarrassed by the changes in their mother's appearance. They may be fascinated and repelled by the birth process all at once. Older adolescents may be somewhat indifferent to the changes associated with pregnancy but also may respond in a more adult fashion by offering support and help.*
- Expectant parents should make a special effort to prepare and include the older child as much as their developmental age allows. Preparation must be carried out at the child's level of understanding and readiness to learn (**Box 5-2**).
- Some children may express interest in being present at the birth. If siblings are to attend the birth, they should participate in a class that prepares them for the event. During the labor and birth, a familiar person who has no other role should be available to explain what is taking place and to comfort or remove them if the situation becomes overwhelming.

Nursing Actions

- Explore with parents strategies for sibling preparation (see Box 5-2).
- Assess adaptation to pregnancy at every prenatal visit. Early assessment and intervention may prevent or greatly reduce later problems for the pregnant woman and her family.

■ Discuss strategies to facilitate sibling adaptation based on the child's age and development.

■ Facilitate discussion of the birth plan if parents want the children present during the sibling's birth.

DIFFICULTIES WITH ADAPTATION TO PREGNANCY

Women may present with psychosocial issues and concerns that are beyond the realm of the perinatal nurse. Nurses need to be aware of community mental health resources and be prepared to collaborate with psychiatric or mental health specialties, social services, or community agencies. Mental health issues during pregnancy can create problems for the pregnant woman across several dimensions.

■ Difficulty with taking on the maternal role, making the necessary transitions to parenthood, and mourning losses associated with that time before pregnancy are all potential areas of concern.

■ Prenatal depression, maternal stress, and anxiety all exert biochemical influences that significantly impact the

developing fetus and contribute to adverse birth outcomes that have long-term consequences (e.g., low birth weight, shorter gestational age, adverse neonatal behavioral responses) (Lederman, 2009).

■ When assessing mood, emotional states, and anxiety, the nurse should consider three aspects: frequency, duration, and intensity. If the woman is having difficulty functioning in her daily life and having difficulty coping, a referral is necessary (Simpson & Creehan, 2008; Lederman, 2009).

Nursing Actions

■ Assess adaptation to pregnancy at every prenatal visit. Early assessment and intervention may prevent or greatly reduce later problems for the pregnant woman and her family.

■ Assess the woman's *mood, anxiety, and emotional state* and consider three aspects: frequency, duration, and intensity of patients' emotional response.

■ Assess the woman's support system and coping mechanism.

■ Discuss expectations about pregnancy, childbirth, and parenting.

■ Identify areas of concern, validate major issues, and make suggestions for possible changes.

■ Refer to the appropriate member of the health care team.

■ Establish a trusting relationship, as women may be reluctant to share information until one has been formed (e.g., questions asked at the first prenatal visit bear repeating with ongoing prenatal care).

■ Make appropriate referrals to other health professionals when needed.

PSYCHOSOCIAL ADAPTATION TO PREGNANCY COMPLICATIONS

The majority of the time, pregnancy progresses with few problems and results in generally positive outcomes. However, with the diagnosis of pregnancy complications, normal concerns and anxieties of pregnancy are exacerbated even more. Uncertainty of fetal outcome can interfere with parental attachment.

■ Response to pregnancy complications depends on:
   ■ *Pregnancy condition*
   ■ *Perceived threat to mother or fetus*
   ■ *Coping skills*
   ■ *Available support*

■ Disequilibrium, feelings of powerlessness, increased anxiety and fear, and a sense of loss are all responses to the news of a pregnancy complication.

■ The pregnant woman may distance herself emotionally from the fetus as she faces varying levels of uncertainty about the pregnancy, impacting attachment (Gilbert, 2010).

■ Events such as antepartal hospitalization or activity restrictions may contribute to a greater incidence of depression in the pregnant woman.

BOX 5–2   TIPS FOR SIBLING PREPARATION

Pregnancy:

■ Take the child on a prenatal visit. Let the child listen to the fetal heartbeat and feel the baby move.

■ Take the child to the homes of friends who have babies to give them an opportunity to see firsthand what babies are like.

■ Take the child on a tour of the hospital or birthing center; if available, enroll in a sibling preparation class, it age appropriate.

After the Birth:

■ Encourage parents to be sensitive to the changes the sibling is experiencing; that jealousy and a sense of loss are normal feelings at this time.

■ Plan for high-quality, uninterrupted time with the older child.

■ Encourage older children to participate in care of their sibling, i.e., bringing a diaper, singing to the baby, sitting with Mom during infant feeding times.

■ Teach a parent to be watchful when the older child is with the newborn; natural expressions of sibling jealousy may involve rough handling, slapping or hitting, throwing toys, etc.

■ Reassure parents that regressive behaviors in the very young child may be a normal part of sibling adjustment (i.e., return to diapers, wanting to breastfeed or take a bottle, tantrums), and with consistent attention and patience the behaviors will decrease.

■ Praise the child for acting age appropriately; show the child how and where to touch the baby.

■ In the hospital: encourage sibling visitation; call older children on the phone; have visitors greet the older child before focusing on the newborn.

■ Give a gift to the new sibling from the newborn; let the sibling select a gift for the baby before delivery to bring to the newborn after the birth.

■ The risk of crisis for the pregnant woman and her family clearly increases due to an unpredictable or uncertain pregnancy outcome (Durham, 1998).

■ How a woman and her family respond to this additional stress is crucial in determining whether a crisis will develop.

■ *Having a realistic perception of the event, adequate situational support, and positive coping mechanisms are all factors that help a woman maintain her equilibrium and avoid crisis.*

■ *Poor self-esteem, lack of confidence in the mothering role, and an inability to communicate concerns to health care providers and close family members are all factors that increase the risk of crisis.*

Nursing Actions

When caring for a pregnant woman with complications, the first priority is to re-establish and maintain physiologic stability. However, nurses must also be able to intervene to promote psychosocial adaptation to the news of pregnancy complications (Giurgescu et al., 2006; Lederman, 2011; Mattson & Smith, 2010) (see Concept Map: Maternal Adaptation to Pregnancy Complications). The following actions can assist to reduce or limit the detrimental effects of complications on individual or family functioning:

■ Provide frequent and clear explanations about the problem, planned interventions, and therapy.

■ Assess and encourage the use of the woman's support systems.

■ Support individual adaptive coping mechanisms.

■ Make appropriate referrals when additional assistance is needed.

Social Support During Pregnancy

Social support refers to that support given by someone with whom the expectant mother has a personal relationship. It involves the primary groups of most importance to the individual woman. During pregnancy, the predominant sources of support for the woman are her spouse or partner, and the woman's mother. A high-quality relationship with one's partner has a positive effect on physical and emotional well-being (Logsdon, 2000; Ngui, 2009; Lederman, 2011). Social support takes several forms: material, emotional, informational, and comparison support have all been identified as important types of support for the pregnant woman.

■ Material (aka instrumental) support consists of practical help such as assistance with chores, meals, and managing finances.

■ Emotional support involves support that gives affection, approval, and encouragement feelings of togetherness.

■ Informational support consists of sharing information, helping women investigate new sources of information.

■ Comparison support consists of help given by someone in a similar situation. Their shared information is useful and credible because they are experiencing or have experienced the same events in their lives.

Social Support Research

Research from several disciplines provides evidence for the importance of social support for the pregnant woman's health, positive adaptation to pregnancy, and the prevention of pregnancy complications. It is a naturally occurring resource that can prevent health problems and complications and promote health. Receiving adequate help from others enhances self-esteem and feelings of being in control (see Evidence-Based Practice: Measurable Outcomes of Social Support Intervention). Women who have little support during pregnancy are more likely to begin prenatal care late and experience depression during pregnancy and postpartum (Beeber & Canuso, 2005; Giurgescu et al., 2006; Logsdon, 2000; Logsdon et al., 2005; Orr, 2004; Mercer, 1995; Tilden, 1983; Lederman 2009).

■ Social support benefits the expectant mother the most when it matches the pregnant woman's expectations, referred to as perceived social support. It is important that the woman identify and clarify her expectations and needs for support. Perceived support expectations that do not materialize for the pregnant woman can lead to increased distress and problems with adaptation to pregnancy (Ngai, 2010).

■ Pregnant women frequently need social support that differs from that they receive. Nurses can advise the pregnant woman how best to use her existing support networks or how to expand her support network so her needs are met. Nurses have the opportunity and responsibility to help women explore potential sources of support such as childbirth education classes, church, work, or school. High-risk populations including adolescents, women with pregnancy complications, and low-income women may need particular direction from nurses in obtaining adequate support (Beeber & Canuso, 2005; Logsdon et al., 2005).

■ A woman's cultural background also influences the amount of social support received and who provides this support. Women in cultures that value individualism, self-sufficiency, and independence may have more difficulty receiving social support than those from a culture that values interdependence and collectivism (Meleis, 2003).

■ Recent immigrants face many challenges in obtaining needed social support. The disruption of lifelong attachments can cause anxieties and a sense of disorientation. Language barriers and socioeconomic struggles are additional stressors facing immigrant women, creating a higher risk for depression (Zelkowitz et al., 2004). Their families, experiencing the same difficulties, may not be able to provide sufficient support. Further research is needed in the area of examining the impact of culture on social support.

■ Social support is not considered professional support, although professionals can provide supportive actions such as counseling, teaching, role modeling, or problem solving. When expectant mothers have no other means of support, some community programs will employ para-professionals to visit expectant mothers, providing education and social support. Programs which capitalize on the skills of experienced mothers living in the communities may be less expensive and more culturally sensitive than purely hospital-based programs led by teams of health care professionals. Additionally, post-delivery follow-up programs offering home-based social support may also have important benefits for socially disadvantaged mothers and children (Cannella, 2006; Dawley & Beam, 2005; Logsdon, 2000; Logsdon et al., 2005).

Evidenced-Based Practice: Measurable Outcomes of Social Support Interventions

There is substantial evidence that social support interventions improve pregnancy outcomes on the following factors:

Attachment to infant and improved interactions with infant
Compliance with health care regimen
Improved functional status
Improved coping
Improved birth outcomes (fewer LBW infants)
Increased incidence of breastfeeding
Reduced physical symptoms
Reduced loneliness
Satisfaction with support
Satisfaction with intimate relationships

Source: Logsdon, 2000.

Assessing Social Support

Assessing social support is a crucial component of prenatal care. The following areas of assessment should be addressed when planning care:

■ Who is available to help provide support? Who is available to provide each type of support (material, emotional, informational, and comparison)? Is the support adequate in each category?
■ With whom does the pregnant woman have the strongest relationships, and what type of support is provided by these individuals?
■ Is there conflict in relationships with support providers?
■ Is there potential for improvement of the woman's support network? Should members who provide more stress than support be deleted? Should new members be added?
■ Who are the people living with the pregnant woman?
■ Who assists with household chores?
■ Who assists with child care and parenting activities?
■ Who does the pregnant woman turn to when problems occur or during a crisis?

Nursing Actions

The nurse has an important role in promoting social support during pregnancy (Logston, 2000). Due to the strong evidence that social support improves pregnancy outcomes, the following nursing actions are recommended:

■ Provide opportunities for the woman to ask for support, and rehearse with her appropriate language to use in asking for support.
■ Invite key support providers to attend prenatal and postpartum visits.
■ Facilitate supportive functioning and interactions within the family.
■ Encourage the pregnant woman to interact with other pregnant or postpartum women she knows.
■ Suggest church, health clubs, work and/or school as sites to meet women with similar interests and concerns.
■ Provide information regarding community resources.

CHILDBEARING AND CULTURE

Childbirth is a time of transition and celebration in all cultures (Callister, 2014). **Culture** is a distinct way of life that characterizes a particular community of people. It has a significant influence on a client's perspective on health. Every culture has a set of behaviors, beliefs, and practices that influence women and their families profoundly during childbearing. Culture can affect how women think, make decisions, and act. A culturally responsive nurse recognizes these influences and considers them carefully when planning care (Amidi-Nouri, 2011; Moore, Moos, & Callister, 2010). See **Box 5-3** for further cultural information.

■ It is critical that nurses acquire the knowledge and skills to provide quality care to culturally divergent groups. Expectations of nursing practice will increasingly demand sensitivity to the cultural needs of families and competence in providing care.
■ All nursing care is given within the context of many cultures: that of the patient, nurse, health care system, and the larger culture of the society. A holistic approach to care will provide the most effective outcomes (Meleis, 2003).

Statistics of the U.S. Population

The U.S. Census Bureau identifies five major groups in the United States: African American/Blacks, American Indian/Alaska Native, Asian American/Pacific Islander, Hispanic/Latino, and white/Caucasian. The Arab-American and Jewish populations together comprise another 2%–3% of the total population (Semenic, Callister, & Feldman, 2004; U.S. Census, 2010). From a global perspective, the movement of immigrants, refugees, and diplomatic and military personnel and their families worldwide has resulted in increasingly diverse populations. Although the U.S. Census has classified these populations primarily by race, it is important to recognize that many may also identify with their country of origin, or ethnicity. Indeed, the 2010 U.S. Census has expanded its classifications in an attempt to achieve greater clarity and includes Hispanic/Latino as a population as well as an option to select multiple races (**Table 5-2**).

BOX 5–3   RESOURCES FOR FURTHER CULTURAL INFORMATION

Africa online: www.africaonline.com/site
Alliance for Hispanic Health: www.hispanichealth.org
American immigration resources on the Internet: www.theodora.com/resource.html
Arab topics: www.al-bab.com
Asian and Pacific Islander American health forum: www.apiahf.org
AT&T Language Line: www.languageline.com
Gay & Lesbian Medical Association: www.glma.org
Hmong studies Internet resource center: www.hmongstudies.com/HmongStudiesJournal
Indian Health Services: www.ihs.gov
Office of Minority Health: www.omhrc.gov
Transcultural Nursing Society: www.tcns.org

TABLE 5–2	U.S. NATIONAL POPULATION BY RACE AND ETHNICITY, 2010 CENSUS	
GROUP	EXAMPLES OF ETHNIC ORIGIN	PERCENT OF U.S. POPULATION
White	Europe, North Africa	72.4
African American/ Black	Africa, West Indies, Dominican Republic, Haiti, Jamaica	12.6
Asian American	China, Japan, Korea, Philippines, Vietnam, Cambodia, Laos, India, Pakistan	4.8
American Indian/ Alaska Native	Navajo, Cherokee, Aleut	0.9
Hispanic or Latino		16.3
Native Hawaiian and other Pacific Islander	Fiji, Tonga, American Samoa	0.2
Some other race		6.2
Two or more races		2.9

Culturally Based Behavioral Practices

Cultural practices can be viewed from a variety of dimensions, which nurses need to consider when planning care (Moore, Moos, & Callister, 2010).

■ Decision Making

Are decisions made by the woman alone or by others such as her partner, extended family, male elders, spiritual leaders?

■ Concept of Time

Is the culture past, present, or future oriented? This may affect the woman's understanding about the need for specific time commitments, such as prenatal care appointments.

The dominant U.S. culture is future oriented, which means people act today with expectations for future rewards. Cultures that are not future oriented may not see the need for preventative care.

■ Communication

Verbal communication may be challenging due to language barriers, meanings of words in different cultures, or how willing a client is to disclose personal information.

Cultures may have different practices regarding such nonverbal communication practices as eye contact, personal space, use of gestures, facial expressions, and appropriate touching.

■ Religion

May have a powerful influence on sexual attitudes and behaviors.

■ Worldview

A client's understanding of how human life fits into the larger picture.

How is illness explained? Examples include ancestral displeasure, body imbalance, breach of taboo, evil eye, germ theory, spirit possession.

■ Modesty and Gender

What are the norms for interaction between men and women?

Some cultures accept public exposure of the human body, while in others, women are expected to cover almost all their bodies.

Common Themes for the Childbearing Family

During the prenatal period, preventing harm to the fetus and ensuring a safe and easy birth are common themes through various cultures. Common themes influencing labor and delivery include general attitudes toward birth, preferred positions, methods of pain management, and the role of family members and the health care provider.

■ The postpartum period is generally considered to be a time of increased vulnerability for both mothers and babies, influencing care of the new mother as well as infant care practices related to bathing, swaddling, feeding, umbilical cord care, and circumcision (Lauderdale, 2011; Mattson, 2010).
■ Pregnancy and childbirth may elicit certain customs and beliefs during pregnancy about acceptable and unacceptable practices which have implications for planning nursing care and interventions. All of these beliefs must be taken into consideration when assessing and promoting adaptation to pregnancy (**Box 5-4**).
■ **Prescriptive behavior** is an expected behavior of the pregnant woman during the childbearing period.
■ **Restrictive behavior** describes activities during the childbearing period which are limited for the pregnant woman.

BOX 5–4 EXAMPLES OF CULTURAL PRESCRIPTIONS, RESTRICTIONS, AND TABOOS

Prescriptive Beliefs

Remain active during pregnancy to aid the baby's circulation.

Remain happy to bring the baby joy and good fortune.

Drink chamomile tea to ensure an effective labor.

Soup with ginseng root is a good general strength tonic.

Pregnancy cravings need to be satisfied or the baby will be born with a birthmark.

Sleep flat on your back to protect the fetus from harm.

Attach a safety pin to an undergarment to protect the fetus from cleft lip or palate.

Restrictive Beliefs

Do not have your picture taken because it might cause stillbirth.

Avoid sexual intercourse during the third trimester because it will cause respiratory distress in the newborn.

Coldness in any form may cause arthritis or other chronic illness.

Avoid seeing an eclipse of the moon; it will result in a cleft lip or palate.

Do not reach over your head or the cord will wrap around the baby's neck.

Taboos

Avoid funerals, and visits from widows or women who have lost children because they will bring bad fortune to the baby.

Avoid hot and spicy foods as they can cause overexcitement for the pregnant woman.

An early baby shower will invite the evil eye and should be avoided.

Avoid praising the newborn; it will call the attention of the gods to the vulnerable infant.

Source: Adapted from Lauderdale, 2007.

BOX 5–5 EXAMPLES OF CULTURAL PRACTICES/ BELIEFS AFFECTING CHILDBEARING

Sons are highly valued.

Umbilical cord should be saved.

Circumcision should be performed on the eighth day of life.

Placenta should be buried.

Colostrum is harmful and should be avoided.

Technology is highly valued.

May avoid eye contact and limit touch.

Pregnancy requires medical attention to ensure health.

Father's participation in labor and birth is not expected.

The polarity of yin/yang as major life force; health requires a balance between yin (cold) and yang (heat).

Source: Adapted from Moore, Moos, & Callister, 2010.

■ **Taboos** are cultural restrictions believed to have serious supernatural consequences.

Cultural practices can also be classified as functional (enhances well-being), neutral (does not harm or help), or non-functional (potentially harmful). Nurses must be able to differentiate among these beliefs and practices, and respect functional and neutral practices even if they differ from their own beliefs (**Box 5-5**).

Nurses need to keep in mind that few cultural customs related to pregnancy are dangerous; although they might cause a woman to limit her activity and her exposure to some aspects of life, they are rarely harmful to herself or her fetus. When encountering non-functional practices, the nurse should first try to understand the meaning of the practice for the woman and her family and then work carefully to bring about change. An example of a non-functional practice would be the ingestion of clay during pregnancy (Lauderdale, 2011; Moore, Moos, & Callister, 2010).

Barriers to Culturally Sensitive Care

Cultural health disparities are created when nurses and other care providers fail to understand the importance of client beliefs about health and illness (Moore, Moos, & Callister, 2010). Nurses' attitudes can create barriers to culturally competent care. **Ethnocentrism,** the belief that the customs and values of the dominant culture are preferred or superior in some way, creates obstacles that can make culturally sensitive care challenging to implement. **Stereotyping,** the assumption that everyone in a group is the same as everyone else in the group, also creates barriers. Contributing to barriers is:

■ Lack of diversity of health care providers
  ■ *Only 16% of registered nurses come from racial or ethnic minority backgrounds (U.S. DHHS, 2010).*
■ There is strong evidence that the quality of health care varies as a function of race, ethnicity, and language (Amidi-Nouri, 2011; Meleis, 2003; Moore, Moos, & Callister, 2010).
■ Mainstream models of obstetric care as practiced in North America can present a strange and confusing picture to many women from different ethnic backgrounds. The predominant culture's emphasis on formal prenatal care, technology, hospital deliveries, and a bureaucratic health care system presents barriers to care for many groups.
  ■ *Protocols, a strange environment, and health care providers who only speak English all create barriers that confuse, intimidate, and result in inadequate access to care.*
  ■ *Health literacy, or a person's ability to obtain and use health information, may also be affected by language, cultural traditions, and beliefs. Groups with low or marginal health literacy skills may not be able to gather and process health information in a useful way (Ferguson, 2008).*
  ■ *These obstacles to health care significantly contribute to health care disparities, or differences in care experienced by one population compared with another population. (For further information on health care disparities, see Chapter 1.)*
  ■ *Disparities also may occur in gender, age, economic status, religion, and sexual preference.*

Culturally Responsive Nursing Practice

Nurses have an obligation to provide to patients and their families effective, understandable, and respectful care in a manner that is compatible with their cultural beliefs, practices, and preferred language. The goal is to gain knowledge to create an environment in which a trusting relationship with the client can be developed (see Box 5-3).

■ Mandates from professional health care accrediting bodies and government agencies provide evidence of increased commitment to providing culturally appropriate health care. Examples of these directives include:

   ■ *The Joint Commission for Accreditation of Health Care Organizations (JCAHCO) mandated plan of patient care includes cultural and spiritual assessments and interventions (Andrews & Boyle, 2003).*

   ■ *The American Association of Colleges of Nursing (AACN) has stated that nursing graduates should have the knowledge and skills to provide holistic care that addresses the needs of diverse populations. AACN has also published specific end-of-program cultural competencies for baccalaureate nursing education (AACN, 2008).*

   ■ *Cultural competence is addressed explicitly in the DHHS Healthy People 2020 focus area of health communications, stating that cultural sensitivity is necessary for effective communication with individuals and the public to stimulate systems change and to influence health behavior (US DHSS, 2010).*

   ■ *The U.S. DHHS office of minority health has published 14 National Standards for Culturally and Linguistically Appropriate Services (CLAS Standards) (U.S. DHHS, 1999).*

■ Culturally sensitive nursing practice (see Critical Component: Strategies for Nurses: Improving Culturally Responsive Care):

   ■ *If the nurse is willing to maintain an open attitude and sensitivity to differences, the chances of providing culturally competent care increase greatly.*

Cultural practices or beliefs may not apply to all individuals, and a great deal of diversity will be found among women of any ethnic group. Educational background, family heritage, social class, economic factors, work/occupational experience, urban/rural origin, length of time in the United States (or place of migration), and a variety of individual characteristics or choices such as sexual orientation, disability, and strength of ethnic identity will all influence how women experience health and illness (Machado, 2001; Meleis, 2003).

It is also important to recognize that socioeconomic factors may be blended with culturally influenced patterns of behavior. Variations that appear to be cultural may actually be a reflection of socioeconomic conditions in which many minority groups live. This arises in part because ethnic minorities tend to be poorer than European Americans, are overrepresented among the very poor, and have fewer opportunities for education and upward mobility. The economic gap accentuates differences, and soon the assumption is made that observed differences are cultural in origin (May, 1994).

Cultural Assessment

When considering cultural aspects of care (Andrews & Boyle, 2011; Moore, Moos, & Callister, 2010), the nurse caring for expectant families must answer a variety of questions to individualize care:

■ What is the woman's predominant culture? To what degree does the client identify with the cultural group?
■ What language does the client speak at home? What are the styles of nonverbal communication (for example, eye contact, space orientation, touch)?
■ How does the woman's culture influence her beliefs about pregnancy and childbirth? Is pregnancy considered a state

---

CRITICAL COMPONENT

Strategies for Nurses: Improving Culturally Responsive Care

■ Maintain an open attitude.
■ Recognize yourself as a part of the diversity in society and acknowledge your own belief system.
■ Examine the biases and assumptions you hold about different cultures.
■ Avoid preconceptions and cultural stereotyping.
■ Explore and acknowledge historical and current portrayals of racial and ethnic groups in society.
■ Develop an understanding of how racial or ethnic differences affect the quality of health care.
■ Acknowledge the power you have to use professional privilege positively or negatively.
■ Recall your commitment to "individualized care," "respect," and "professionalism."
■ Identify who the client calls "family."
■ Include notes on cultural preferences and family strengths and resources as part of all intake and ongoing assessments, and nursing care plans and care maps.

■ Use the cultural wisdom (beliefs, values, customs, and habits) of the client to shape his or her participation in health practices and care plans.
■ Seek out client-friendly teaching and assessment tools.
■ Review the literature to generate a culture database.
■ Read literature from other cultures.
■ Participate in professional development/continuing education programs which address cultural competence.
■ Recognize all care is given within the context of many cultures.
■ Develop linguistic skills related to your client population.
■ Learn to use nonverbal communication in an appropriate way.
■ Learn about the communication patterns of various cultures.
■ Advocate for organizational change.
■ Understand and apply the various regulatory standards (CLAS, AACN, etc.).
■ Promote cultural practices that are helpful, tolerate practices that are neutral, and work to educate women to avoid practices that are potentially harmful.

(Callister, 2014; Amidi-Nouri, 2011; Moore, Moos, & Callister, 2010)

of illness or health? How does the culture explain illness? Are there particular attitudes towards age at the time of pregnancy? Marriage? Who would be an acceptable father or partner? What is considered acceptable in terms of pregnancy frequency?

■ Are there cultural prescriptions, restrictions, or taboos related to certain activities, dietary practices, or expressions of emotion? What does the pregnant woman consider to be normal practice during pregnancy, birth, postpartum?

■ How does the woman interpret and respond to experiences of pain?

■ How is modesty expressed by men and women?

■ Are there culturally defined expectations about male-female relationships?

■ What is the client's educational background? Does it affect her knowledge level concerning the health care delivery system, teaching/learning, written material given?

■ How does the client relate to persons outside her cultural group? Does she prefer a caregiver with the same cultural background?

■ What is the role of religious beliefs related to pregnancy and childbirth?

■ How are childbearing decisions made, and who is involved in the decision making process?

■ How does the woman's predominant culture view the concept of time? (Cultures may be past, present, or future oriented.)

■ How does the woman's culture explain illness? (Examples: ancestral displeasure, germ theory, etc.)

Nursing Actions

With the increasing diverse patient population, it is imperative nurses provide culturally sensitive care. Professionals must acknowledge belief and value systems different from their own, and consider these differences when delivering care to childbearing women and their families (Callister, 2008; Leininger, 1991; Moore, Moos, & Callister, 2010; Purnell & Paulanka, 2008).

■ Enhance communication
  ■ *Greet respectfully*
  ■ *Establish rapport*
  ■ *Demonstrate empathy and interest*
  ■ *Listen actively*
■ Emphasize the woman's strengths; consider each woman's individuality regarding how she conforms to traditional values and norms.
■ Respect functional and neutral practices.
■ If proposed practices are non-functional, work with the woman and her support network to bring about change.
■ Accommodate cultural practices as appropriate.
■ Identify who the client calls "family."
■ Determine who the family decision makers are and include them.
■ Provide an interpreter when necessary (**Box 5-6**).
■ Recognize that a patient agreeing and nodding "yes" to the nurse's instruction or questions may not always guarantee comprehension.
■ Use nonverbal communication and visual aids in an appropriate way.

■ When providing patient education, include family and elicit support from the established caretakers in the family (i.e., grandmother, aunt, etc.).

■ Demonstrate how scientific and folk practices can be combined to provide optimal care.

PLANNING FOR BIRTH

Planning and preparing for childbirth requires many decisions by the woman and her family during pregnancy (i.e., choosing a provider, choosing a place of birth, planning for the birth, and preparing for labor through education). These choices affect how the woman approaches her pregnancy and can contribute significantly to a positive adaptation.

Choosing a Provider

One of the first decisions a woman makes is who will be her care provider during her pregnancy and birth. This important decision also influences where her birth will take place.

Physicians

Obstetricians and family practice physicians attend approximately 91% of births in the United States. Most physicians care for their patients in a hospital setting.

■ Care often includes pharmacologic and medical management of problems as well as use of technologic procedures.

■ Their practice includes both low- and high-risk patients.

Midwives

The focus of midwifery care is on non-interventionist care, with an emphasis on the normalcy of the birth process.

■ Midwives care for women in hospital settings, alternative birth centers, or a home setting.

■ In many countries, midwives are the primary providers of care for healthy pregnant women, and physicians are consulted when medical or surgical intervention is required (Kennedy & Shannon, 2004).

■ Nurse-midwives are registered nurses with advance training in care of obstetric patients. They provide care for

---

BOX 5-6   WORKING WITH AN INTERPRETER

A trained medical interpreter should be used for medical interpretations. A friend or family member may not understand terms used by the health care provider. A woman may be discussing issues she wants to keep private. The interpreter can be a valuable member of the health care team.

The nurse should be alert to the client's nonverbal cues and ask the patient to repeat information that she needs to recall later.

Many nursing schools and health care institutions may prohibit nursing students from interpreting, for example, to obtain consent for a procedure, because limited knowledge about the procedure may lead the student to give inaccurate information.

Source: Adapted from Moore, Moos, & Callister, 2010.

about 10% of births in the United States and Canada, usually seeing low-risk patients. Nurse-midwives practice with physicians or independently with a contracted health care provider agency for physician backup.

■ Lay midwives manage about 1% of the births in the United States and Canada, with the majority taking place in the home setting. Their training varies greatly, from being self-taught to having formal training and licensing.

■ Direct entry midwives are trained in midwifery schools or universities as a profession distinct from nursing. Increasing numbers of midwives in the United Kingdom and Ireland fall into this category.

■ Given the variations in midwifery training and knowledge, pregnant women considering midwifery care may need education and information regarding the experience and credentials of the midwife providing their care in order to make informed decisions (**Box 5-7**).

Choosing a Place of Birth

Hospitals

■ In the United States, approximately 99% of all births take place in hospital settings.

■ Hospital maternity services can vary greatly, from traditional labor and delivery rooms with separate newborn and postpartum units to in-hospital birth centers.

■ Labor, delivery, and recovery rooms (LDRs) may be available in which the expectant mother is admitted, labors, gives birth, and spends the first 2 hours of recovery.

■ In labor, delivery, recovery, postpartum units (LDRPs), the mother remains in the same room for her entire hospital stay.

Birth Centers

■ Free-standing birth centers are usually built in locations separate from the hospital but may be located nearby in case transfer of the woman or newborn is needed.

■ Only women at low risk for complications are included in care.

■ Birth centers are usually staffed by nurse-midwives or physicians who also have privileges at the local hospital.

■ They offer homelike accommodations, with emergency equipment available but stored out of view.

Home Births

■ Home births are popular in European countries such as Sweden and the Netherlands, with rigorous screening policies in place to ensure that only low-risk women are having home births, and are attended by trained midwives (deJong, 2009).

■ In developing countries, home birth may occur due to the lack of hospitals or adequate birthing facilities.

■ In the United States, home births account for less than 1% of births. In the North American medical community, many have concluded that home birth exposes the mother and fetus to unnecessary danger. Consequently, a woman seeking a home birth may find it more challenging to find

---

BOX 5–7   PROFESSIONAL POSITION STATEMENT: AWHONN POSITION STATEMENT ON MIDWIFERY

AWHONN supports the practice of the certified nurse-midwife as a primary care provider who is prepared to independently manage most aspects of women's health care. The certified nurse-midwife's practice should include appropriate professional consultation, collaboration, and referral as indicated by the health status of the patient and applicable state and federal laws.

Background

AWHONN identifies a wide range of disparate educational requirements and certification standards in the United States that fall under the umbrella category of midwifery. The following titles are attributed to midwives without prior nursing credentials who are not graduates of ACNM-accredited programs: direct entry, lay, licensed, or professional. Direct entry midwives cover the spectrum from the doctorally prepared European midwife to the self-taught, beginning practitioner.

The wide range of what is actually meant by the designation "midwife" can easily confuse consumers, health care institutions, and legislators. Definitions of various certification levels are:

■ CNM: Certified Nurse-Midwife (administered by ACNM)
■ CM: Certified Midwife (administered by ACNM)
■ CPM: Certified Professional Midwife [administered by NARM (North American Registry of Midwives)]. Also referred to as *direct entry, lay,* or *licensed midwife.*
■ Midwives with a state license or permit (administered on a state-by-state basis). Also referred to as *direct entry, lay,* or *licensed midwife.*
■ Midwives without formal credentials (no administrative oversight). Also referred to as *direct entry* or *lay midwife.*

Individual state-by-state laws govern the practice of midwifery in the United States. Certified nurse-midwives and certified midwives often practice in collaboration and consultation with other health care professionals to provide primary, gynecological, and maternity care to women in the context of the larger health care system. Certified nurse-midwives may have prescriptive privileges, admitting privileges to hospitals, and may own and/or manage freestanding practices. The scope of practice for a direct entry, or lay, midwife who is not ACC accredited is typically limited to the practice of home birth or birth center options for women, but varies according to state-by-state regulations.

Source: Association of Women's Health, Obstetric and Neonatal Nurses (AWHONN). (2000b). Policy position statement: Midwifery. *Washington, DC: Author.*

---

a qualified health care provider willing to give prenatal care and attend the birth.

■ Home births allow the expectant family to be in control of the experience, and the mother may be more relaxed than in the hospital environment. It may be less expensive, and there may be decreased risk of serious infection.

■ If home birth is the woman's choice, the following criteria will promote a safe home birth experience:

  ■ *The woman must be comfortable with her decision.*

  ■ *The woman should be in good health; home birth is not for high-risk pregnancy.*

■ *The woman should have access to a good transportation system in case of transfer to the hospital.*

■ *The woman should be attended by a well-trained health care provider with adequate medical supplies and resuscitation equipment (Romano, 2010; deJong, 2009).*

The Birth Plan

A birth plan is a tool by which parents can explore their childbirth options and choose those that are most important to them. A written birth plan can help women clarify their desires and expectations and communicate those desires with their care providers (Lothian, 2006).

■ Birth plans typically emphasize specific requests for labor and immediate post-delivery care. Some involve expectations surrounding postpartum and newborn care as well.

■ The birth plan document can be inserted into the woman's prenatal record or hospital chart as a way of communicating with care providers.

The Doula

The word "doula" comes from ancient Greek and means "woman's servant" (ICEA, 1999). A **doula** is an individual who provides support to women and their partners during labor, birth, and postpartum. The doula does not provide clinical care.

■ Continuous support by a trained doula during labor has been associated with shorter labors, decreased need for analgesics, decreased need for many forms of medical interventions, and increased maternal satisfaction (Campbell, Lake, Falk, & Backstrand, 2006; Hodnett, Gates, Hofmeyr, & Sakala, 2011; Pascali-Bonaro & Kroeger, 2004).

■ Pregnant women should be made aware of the benefits of doula care.

■ Many hospitals have implemented doula services that are either free or fee-based. (Mottl-Santiago, Walker, Ewan, Vragovic, Winder, & Stubblefield, 2008).

Childbirth Education

The roots of prenatal education began in the early 1900s with classes in maternal hygiene, nutrition, and baby care taught by the American Red Cross in New York City. Childbirth education as we know it today developed as a consumer response to the increasing medical control and technologic management of normal labor and birth during the 1950s and 1960s in Europe and North America. Early proponents of childbirth education such as Lamaze, Bradley, and Dick-Read focused primarily on the prevention of pain in childbirth. Methods of "natural childbirth" (Dick-Read), "psychoprophylaxis" (Lamaze), and "husband coached childbirth" (Bradley) attained great popularity among middle-class groups. Childbirth education has evolved since that time towards a more eclectic approach. The focus has shifted away from rigid techniques to embrace a philosophy that "affirms

the normalcy of birth, acknowledges women's inherent ability to birth their babies, and explores all the ways that women find strength and comfort during labor and birth" (Lamaze International, 2009; Walker, 2009). The content of childbirth education classes has also greatly expanded, assisting women and their families to make informed decisions about pregnancy and birth based on knowledge of their options and choices.

■ Specialized classes have been developed to meet the needs of specific groups as well (e.g., classes for breastfeeding; sibling preparation; and refresher, or prenatal/postpartum exercise, online childbirth preparation). Programs have been developed for adolescents, mothers expecting twins, and mothers older than 35. Nurses and childbirth educators have played an important role in the development of these innovative education programs.

■ Professional organizations including International Childbirth Education Association (ICEA), Lamaze International, and Association of Women's Health, Obstetrics and Neonatal Nursing (AWHONN) have all published position papers that delineate expectations of basic components of prenatal education. Through the development of position papers as well as teacher training and certification programs, these organizations have ensured that childbirth educators have a sound knowledge base and specific competencies.

■ The Healthy People 2020 Maternal Infant and Child Health goals include an objective that commits to increasing the proportion of pregnant women who attend a formal series of prepared childbirth classes (U.S. DHHS, 2010).

■ The overall goal of childbirth education is to promote the competence of expectant parents in meeting the challenges of childbirth and early parenting. The focus is on promoting healthy pregnancy and birth outcomes and facilitating a positive transition to parenting.

■ Class content typically includes the physical and emotional aspects of pregnancy, childbirth and early parenting, coping skills, and labor support techniques (**Box 5-8**).

■ Values clarification and informed decision making are emphasized, as well as the promotion of wellness behaviors, and healthy birth practices. Pregnant women are encouraged to identify their own unique goals for childbirth (Green & Hotelling, 2009; Lothian, 2011).

■ Class formats have evolved to meet the varied needs of expectant families and may include a traditional weekly series, one-day intensives, or online classes.

Childbirth classes remain a popular and well-established component of care during the childbearing years. However, the evidence regarding the effects of antenatal education remains inconclusive. As the body of research on childbirth and childbirth education increases and as more childbirth educators use research findings as a basis for their teaching, evidence-based practice will be enhanced (see Evidence-Based Practice: Effectiveness of Antenatal Education).

Evidence-Based Practice: Effectiveness of Antenatal Education

Gagnon, A. J., & Sandall, J. (2007). Individual or group antenatal education for childbirth or parenthood, or both. Cochrane Database of Systematic Reviews 2007, Issue 3. Art. No.: CD002869.

A great deal of research has attempted to assess the effectiveness of antenatal education in preparing women for pregnancy, birth, and child care. Researchers have attempted to link attendance at childbirth classes with a variety of outcomes, including shorter labors, higher Apgar scores, decreased incidence of cesarean sections, decreased anxiety, breastfeeding success, pain management, maternal satisfaction, infant care competencies, and teaching methods (Gagnon & Sandall, 2007). The majority of the evidence has been inconclusive. Difficulties with sample size, poorly designed methodologies, and lack of funding have persistently hindered the creation of an evidence-based body of knowledge. The effects of general antenatal education for childbirth or parenthood, or both, remain largely unknown. Despite its popularity, more research is needed to determine the effects and benefits of childbirth education in a variety of populations and programs, and to ensure that effective ways of helping health professionals support pregnant women and their partners in preparing for birth and parenting are investigated so that the resources used meet the needs of parents and their newborn infants.

■ In addition to classes, there are books, pamphlets, magazines, and videos aimed at childbearing women and their families. The Internet is also a widely used resource for information and advice, as are mobile phone device applications. (Jordan, 2011) (see Patient Education: Mobile Phone Education: Text4Baby).

PATIENT EDUCATION

Mobile Phone Education: Text4Baby

Text4Baby is an innovative educational program offering perinatal education via text messages. It is estimated that over 90% of American households have cell phones, with the majority of those phones with text messaging capabilities. The program was developed through a collaboration of public and private agencies, including the National Healthy Mothers Healthy Babies Coalition, Voxiva, Johnson & Johnson, the Department of Health & Human Services, and Office of Science and Technology. Message content was reviewed by an interdisciplinary panel of experts to ensure the information reflected evidence-based practice.

Once signed up for the service, women will receive three free SMS text messages each week timed to their due dates. The program provides vital health information to pregnant women and new mothers. Examples of topics include nutrition, seasonal flu prevention and treatment, mental health topics, risks of tobacco use, oral health, and safe infant sleeping. Women can sign up for the program by texting BABY to 511411 (or by texting BEBE for Spanish).

Jordan, E., Ray, E., Johnson, P., & Evans, W. (2011).Using text messaging to improve maternal and newborn health. *AWHONN Nursing for Women's Health, 15*(3). 206–212.

BOX 5–8   PERINATAL EDUCATION: SAMPLE CONTENT IN A CHILDBIRTH PREPARATION CLASS

Introduction
Introductions
Overview of childbirth education: Rationale and pain theory
Physical and emotional changes of pregnancy; fetal development
Nutrition, exercise, and self-care during pregnancy
Introduction to breathing and relaxation techniques

Labor
Signs of labor
Stages and phases of labor and delivery
Labor support techniques; the role of the support person in labor
Practice of breathing and relaxation techniques

Birth Plans
Labor review, incorporating labor support techniques and non-pharmacological comfort strategies
Birth options and birth plans: Developing advocacy skills
Pharmacological interventions
Practice of breathing and relaxation techniques
Hospital tour

Variations in Labor
Variations of labor: back labor, prodromal labor, precipitous labor
Cesarean delivery
Medical procedures (IVs, episiotomy, assisted delivery, EFM, Pitocin, epidurals)
Practice of relaxation and breathing techniques

Newborn
Review of labor; practice of relaxation and breathing techniques
Newborn care
Breastfeeding

Postpartum
Postpartum and transition to parenthood
Community resources for new parents

■ Nurses need to be aware of these powerful influences on the health-related decisions of childbearing women and their families. The quality of information and advice varies widely. For a list of reliable Internet resources for parent education, see **Box 5-9**.

BOX 5–9   INTERNET RESOURCES FOR EXPECTANT FAMILIES

Babycenter: www.babycenter.com
Childbirth Connection: www.childbirthconnection.org
Doulas of North America: www.dona.org
Healthy Mothers, Healthy Babies Coalition: www.hmhb.org
ICEA (International Childbirth Education Association): www.icea.org
La Leche League: www.lalecheleague.org
Lamaze International: www.lamaze.org
March of Dimes: www.marchofdimes.com
American College of Nurse Midwives: www.Mymidwife.org
AWHONN Patient Education: www.Health4women.org

CONCEPT MAP

Maternal Adaptation to Pregnancy Complications

Frustration
- Woman expresses anger or aggression
- Withdrawal from pregnancy or partner

Fear
- Woman states she is afraid of fetal death
- Woman states she is afraid of newborn disability
- Woman is crying

Pregnancy Complication
Woman diagnosed with high risk pregnancy

Anxiety
- Unexpected pregnancy complication
- Unanticipated interruption in normal pregnancy

Threat to Self-Esteem
- Woman feels lack of self-confidence related to pregnancy
- Woman reports feeling she has failed as a woman
- Woman feels little confidence to be a mother

Problem No. 1: Fear related to uncertain fetal outcome
Goal: Decreased fear
Outcome: Patient will express decreased fear related to uncertain fetal outcome.

Nursing Actions

1. Provide time for the patient and family to express their concerns regarding fetal outcome.
2. Encourage the woman to vent apprehension, uncertainty, anger, fear, and/or worry.
3. Discuss prior pregnancy outcomes if applicable.
4. Explain pregnancy complication, management, and reason for each treatment.
5. Help the woman to obtain needed social support.
6. Refer the family to community or hospital resources such as social worker, case manager, or chaplain services as needed.
7. Provide contact information for the woman and family as issues arise.

Problem No. 2: Impaired self-esteem related to pregnancy complication
Goal: Improved self-esteem
Outcome: Patient will express improved self-esteem.

Nursing Actions

1. Encourage verbalization of feelings.
2. Practice active listening.
3. Provide emotional support.
4. Encourage the patient to participate in decision making.
5. Make needed referrals to social services and mental health specialists.

Problem 3: Anxiety related to unexpected pregnancy complication
Goal: Decreased anxiety
Outcome: Patient verbalizes that she feels less anxious.

Nursing Actions

1. Be calm and reassuring in interactions with patient and family.
2. Explain all information repeatedly related to complication.
3. Provide autonomy and choices.
4. Encourage patient and family to verbalize their feelings regarding diagnosis by asking open-end questions.
5. Explore past coping strategies.
6. Explore with the woman spiritual practices and beliefs.

Problem 4: Frustration related to pregnancy complication
Goal: Positive pregnancy adaptation
Outcome: Patient demonstrates adaptation to pregnancy.

Nursing Actions

1. Allow the woman to express her feelings related to loss of normal pregnancy.
2. Allow the woman to express her feelings related to not having a normal birth.
3. Allow the woman to express her feelings related to uncertainty of fetal outcome.
4. Provide choices related to management when possible.

TYING IT ALL TOGETHER

As a nurse in an antenatal clinic, you are part of an interdisciplinary team that is caring for Margarite Sanchez during her pregnancy. Margarite is 10 weeks pregnant and is a 28-year-old G3 P1 Hispanic woman. She began prenatal care at 8 weeks' gestation visit. She works in a day-care center. She has a 2-year-old son. José, her husband, has not accompanied her to her second prenatal appointment as he is in his busy season at work in landscaping. Margarite reports they are pleased about the pregnancy although planned to wait another year or two before attempting another pregnancy. Margarite was seen for some spotting at 6 weeks' gestation that has resolved. Marguerite tells you has she has been irritable and short tempered with her husband and son, particularly at the end of the day when she feels exhausted. She states she is relieved the spotting stopped but is not sure she feels ready to be a mother of two children. Her mother lives four blocks away and they speak on the phone daily and see each other several times a week. She is very involved in her parish, and the women in her church study group all know she is pregnant and are all certain the baby is a girl.

Detail the aspects of your psychosocial assessment at 10 weeks' gestation.

Discuss the rationale for the assessment.

Discuss the nursing diagnosis, nursing activities, and expected outcomes related to this problem.

Discuss the importance of the pregnant woman's mother during pregnancy.

Suggest two interventions that could help to prepare Margarite's 2-year-old son during the pregnancy.

■ ■ ■ Review Questions ■ ■ ■

1. Signs of possible maladaptation to pregnancy include:
   A. Denial of fears about childbirth and unrealistic expectations about birth
   B. Excessive maternal weight gain and limiting physical activity
   C. Denial of physical symptoms of pregnancy and emotional lability
   D. Changes in couple's interactions and sexual activity

2. Nursing interventions that facilitate adaptation to pregnancy in the first trimester focus on:
   A. Physiological changes in pregnancy
   B. Promoting pregnancy and birth as a family experience
   C. Readiness for parenting
   D. Partners' role during labor and birth

3. Ambivalent feelings toward pregnancy in the third trimester may indicate:
   A. Normal expected finding
   B. Unresolved conflict
   C. Depression
   D. Unwanted pregnancy

4. Prescriptive behavior is:
   A. Behavior during the childbearing period that is limited for pregnant women
   B. Expected behavior for pregnant women
   C. Behavior that is restricted for pregnant women that has supernatural consequences
   D. An unacceptable practice that has implications for pregnant women

5. Measurable outcomes of social support interventions during pregnancy include:
   A. Improved coping and functional status
   B. Improves relationship with mother
   C. Reduced stress
   D. Reduced depression

6. When conducting a psychosocial assessment, it is important to determine the ____, _____, and ____ of mood or emotional disturbances.
   A. Anxiety, depression, level
   B. Coping, support, distress
   C. Frequency, duration, intensity
   D. Acceptance, avoidance, character

7. To facilitate adaptation to pregnancy during the first trimester, an appropriate nursing action would be to:
   A. Encourage the woman to sign up for prepared childbirth classes
   B. Assess the woman's response to pregnancy
   C. Encourage the woman to "tune in" to fetal movement
   D. Give anticipatory guidance regarding breastfeeding

8. When caring for a woman who speaks limited English, the appropriate method for translating information is:
   A. Using a trained medical interpreter
   B. Asking a student nurse who speaks the woman's primary language to translate
   C. Providing printed material for the woman to take home
   D. Asking for a family member to translate

9. While planning care for the lesbian client, it is most important for the nurse to include a goal that addresses the need for:
   A. Referrals to a perinatal social worker on admission to the hospital
   B Establishing a trusting relationship with health care providers
   C. Providing counseling to lesbian mothers regarding legal issues they may face with parenting
   D. Choosing a name for the infant and obtaining supplies for the new baby

10. According to May's research, it is during the _____ phase that many expectant fathers appear to put conscious thought of their partner's pregnancy aside.
   A. Announcement
   B. Transition
   C. Moratorium
   D. Developing

References

Amidi-Nouri, A. (2011). Culturally Responsive Nursing Care. In A. Berman & S. Snyder, *Kozier & Erb's Fundamentals of Nursing* (9th ed.). San Francisco: Pearson.

Alio, A., Salihu, H., Komosky, J., Richman, A., & Marty, P. (2010). Feto-infant Health and Survival: Does Paternal Involvement Matter? *Maternal Child Health Journal, 14*, 931–937.

Alio, A., Bond, M., Padilla, Y., Heidelbaugh, J., Lu, M., & Parker, W. (2011). Addressing Policy Barriers to Paternal Involvement during Pregnancy. *Maternal Child Health Journal, 15*, 425–430.

American Association of Colleges of Nursing. (2008). *The Essentials of Baccalaureate Education for Professional Nursing Practice.* Retrieved from: http://aacn.nche.edu/education-resources/BaccEssentials08.pdf

Andrews, M., & Boyle, C. (2011). *Transcultural concepts in nursing care* (6th ed.). Philadelphia: Lippincott Williams & Wilkins.

Association of Women's Health, Obstetric and Neonatal Nurses (AWHONN). (2000a). *Nurse providers of perinatal education: Competencies and program guide.* Washington, DC: Author.

Association of Women's Health, Obstetric and Neonatal Nurses (AWHONN). (2000b). *Policy position statement: Midwifery.* Washington, DC: Author.

Barron, M. (2008). Antenatal Care. In K. Simpson & P. Creehan (Eds.), *AWHONN Perinatal Nursing* (3rd ed., pp. 88–124). Philadelphia: Lippincott Williams & Wilkins.

Bayrampour, H., & Heaman, M. (2010). Advanced Maternal Age and the Risk of Cesarean Birth: A Systematic Review. *Birth, 37*(3), 219–226.

Beck, C. (2002). Revision of the Postpartum Depression Predictors Inventory. *Journal of Obstetric, Gynecologic, and Neonatal Nursing, 31*(4), 394–402.

Beeber, L., & Canuso, R. (2005). Strengthening social support for the low income mother: Five critical questions and a guide for intervention. *Journal of Obstetric, Gynecologic, and Neonatal Nursing, 34*(6), 769–776.

Begley, A. (2000). Preparation for practice in the new millennium: a discussion of the moral implications of multifetal pregnancy reduction. *Nursing Ethics, 7*(2), 99–112.

Bibring, G., Dwyer, T., Huntington, D., & Valenstein, D. (1961). A study of the psychological processes in pregnancy and of the early mother-child relationships. *Psychoanalytic Study of the Child, 16*(9), 9–24.

Brennan, A., Ayers, S., Ahmed, H., & Marshall-Lucette, S. (2007). A critical review of the Couvade syndrome: the pregnant male. *Journal of Reproductive and Infant Psychology, 25*(3), 173–189.

Callister, L. (2014). Integrating cultural beliefs and practices into the care of childbearing women. In K. Simpson & P. Creehan (Eds.), *AWHONN Perinatal Nursing* (4th ed., pp. 41–70). Philadelphia: Lippincott Williams & Wilkins.

Campbell, D., Lake, M., Falk, M., & Backstrand, J. (2006). A randomized trial of continuous support in labor by a lay doula. *Journal of Obstetric, Gynecologic, and Neonatal Nursing, 35*(4), 456–464.

Cannella, B. (2006). Mediators of the relationship between social support and positive health practices in pregnant women. *Nursing Research, 55*(6), 437–445.

Carolan, M. (2005). "Doing it properly": the experience of first time mothering over 35 years. *Health Care for Women International, 26*(9), 764–87.

Carroll J., Reid A., Biringer A., Midmer D., Glazier, R., Wilson, L., Permaul, J., Pugh, P., Chalmers, B., Seddon, F., & Stewart, D. (2005). Effectiveness of the Antenatal Psychosocial Health Assessment (ALPHA) form in detecting psychosocial concerns: a randomized controlled trial. *CMAJ: Canadian Medical Association Journal, 173*(3), 253–259.

Collopy, K. (2004). "I couldn't think that far": infertile women's decision making about multifetal reduction. *Research in Nursing and Health, 27*(2), 75–86.

Crooks, R., & Baur, K. (2010). *Our Sexuality* (11th ed.). Menlo Park, NJ: Benjamin Cummings Publishing Company.

Damato, E. (2003). Predictors of prenatal attachment in mothers of twins. *Journal of Obstetric, Gynecologic, and Neonatal Nursing, 33*(4), 436–445.

Dawley, K., & Beam, R. (2005). "My Nurse taught me how to have a healthy baby and be a good mother:" Nurse home visiting with pregnant women 1888 to 2005. *Nursing Clinics of North America, 40*, 803–815.

de Jonge, A., van der Goes, B., Ravelli, A., Amelink-Verburg, M., Mol, B., Nijhuis, J., Bennebroek Gravenhorst, J., & Buitendijk, S. (2009). Perinatal mortality and morbidity in a nationwide cohort of 529,688 low-risk planned home and hospital births. *BJOG: An International Journal of Obstetrics and Gynaecology, 116*, 1177–1184.

DeVito, J. (2010). How Adolescent Mothers Feel About Becoming a Parent. *The Journal of Perinatal Education, 19*(2), 25–34.

Dobrzykowski, T., & Stern, P. (2003). Out of sync: a generation of first-time mothers over 30. *Health Care for Women International, 24*(3), 242–253.

Driscoll, J. (2008). Psychosocial Adaptation to Pregnancy and Postpartum. In K. Simpson & P. Creehan (Eds.), *AWHONN Perinatal Nursing* (3rd ed., pp. 78–87). Philadelphia: Lippincott Williams & Wilkins.

Durham, R. (1998). Strategies women engage in when analyzing preterm labor at home. *Journal of Perinatology, 19*, 61–69.

Duvall, E. (1985). Marriage and Family Development. New York: Harper & Row.

Ehiri, J., Meremikwu, A., & Meremikwu, M. (2005). Interventions for preventing unintended pregnancies among adolescents. (Protocol) *Cochrane Database of Systematic Reviews 2.*

Ferguson, B. (2008). Health literacy and health disparities: The role they play in maternal and child health. *Nursing for Women's Health, 12*(4), 290–298.

Fortier, J., Carson, V., Will, S., & Shubkagel, B. (1991). Adjustment to a newborn: Sibling preparation makes a difference. *Journal of Obstetric, Gynecologic, and Neonatal Nursing, 20*(4), 73–78.

Foster, G., Alviar, A., Neumeier, R., & Wootten, A. (2012). A tri-service perspective on the implementation of a centering pregnancy model in the military. *Journal of Obstetric, Gynecologic, and Neonatal Nursing, 41*(2), 315–321.

Friedman, M., Bowden, V., & Jones, E. (2003). *Family nursing: Research, theory, and practice* (5th ed.). Upper Saddle River, NJ: Prentice Hall.

Gagnon, A. (2007). Individual or group antenatal education for childbirth/parenthood (Cochrane Review). In *The Cochrane Library*, Issue 4, 2006, Oxford: Update Software.

Genesoni, L., & Tallandini, M. (2009). Men's Psychological Transition to Fatherhood: An Analysis of the Literature, 1989–2008. *Birth, 36*(4), 305–317.

Gilbert, E. (2010). *Manual of high risk pregnancy and delivery* (5th ed.). St. Louis, MO: C.V. Mosby.

Giurgescu, C., Penckofer, S., Maurer, M., & Bryant, F. (2006). Impact of uncertainty, social support, and prenatal coping on the psychological well-being of high risk pregnant women. *Nursing Research, 55*(5), 356–65.

Green, J., & Hotelling, B. (2009). *Healthy Birth Practices.* Lamaze International. Retrieved from: http://lamaze.org

Hanson, S., Hunter, L., Bormann, J., & Sobo, E. (2009). Paternal fears of childbirth: A literature review. *The Journal of Perinatal Education, 18*(4), 12–20.

Hodnett, E. D., Gates, S., Hofmeyr, G., & Sakala, C. (2011). Continuous support for women during childbirth (Cochrane Review). In *The Cochrane Library*, Issue 2, 2011, Oxford: Update Software.

International Childbirth Education Association (ICEA). (1999). Position paper: The role and scope of the doula. *International Journal of Childbirth Education, 14*(1), 38–45.

Jentsch, B., Durham, R., Hundley, V., Hussein, J. (2007) Creating Consumer Satisfaction in Maternity Care: The neglected needs of migrants, asylum seekers and refugees. *International Journal of Consumer Studies, 31*, 128–134.

Jordan, E., Ray, E., Johnson, P., & Evans, W. (2011). Using text messaging to improve maternal and newborn health. *AWHONN Nursing for Women's Health, 15*(3), 206–212.

Jordan, P. (1989). Support behaviors identified as helpful and desired by second time parents over the perinatal period. *Maternal Child Nursing Journal, 18*(2), 133–145.

Joseph, K., Allen, A., Dodds, L., Turner, L., Scott, H., & Liston, R. (2005). The perinatal effects of delayed childbearing. *Obstetrics and Gynecology, 105*(6), 1410–1418.

Kennedy, H., & Shannon, M. (2004). Keeping Birth Normal: Research findings on midwifery care during childbirth. *Journal of Obstetric, Gynecologic, and Neonatal Nursing, 33*(5), 554–560.

Key, J. D., Gebregziabher, M. G., Marsh, L. D., & O'Rouke, K. M. (2008). Effectiveness of an intensive school-based intervention for teen mothers. *Journal of Adolescent Health, 42*, 394–400.

Koniak-Griffin, D., Logsdon, C., Hines-Martin, V., & Turner, C. (2006). Contemporary mothering in a diverse society. *Journal of Obstetric, Gynecologic, and Neonatal Nursing, 35*(5), 671–678.

Lamaze International. (2009). *Position Paper—Lamaze For the 21st Century.* Retrieved from http://lamaze.org

Lauderdale, J. (2011). Transcultural perspectives in childbearing. In M. Andrews & J. Boyle (Eds.), *Transcultural concepts in nursing care* (6th ed., pp. 95–131). Philadelphia: Lippincott Williams & Wilkins.

Lederman, R. (2011). Preterm birth prevention: a mandate for psychosocial assessment. *Issues in Mental Health Nursing, 32*, 163–169.

Lederman, R. (1996). *Psychosocial adaptation in pregnancy* (2nd ed.). New York: Springer.

Lederman, R., & Weis, K. (2009). *Psychosocial adaptation in pregnancy: Seven Dimensions of Maternal Role Development* (3rd ed.). New York: Springer.

Leininger, M. (Ed.). (1991). *Culture care diversity & universality: A theory of nursing.* New York: National League for Nursing Press.

Logsdon, C. (2000). *Social Support for Pregnant and Postpartum Women.* AWHONN: Washington, DC.

Logsdon, C., Gagne, P., Hughes, T., Patterson, J., & Rakestraw, V. (2005). Social support during adolescent pregnancy: piecing together a quilt. *Journal of Obstetric, Gynecologic, & Neonatal Nursing, 34*(5), 606–614.

Lothian, J. (2011). Lamaze breathing: what every pregnant woman needs to know. *The Journal of Perinatal Education, 20*(2), 118–120.

Lothian, J. (2006). Birth plans: the good, the bad, and the future. *Journal of Obstetric, Gynecologic, & Neonatal Nursing, 35*(2), 295–303.

Machado, G. (2001). Cultural sensitivity and stereotypes. *Journal of Multicultural Nursing and Health, 7*(2), 13–15.

Maifeld, M., Hahn, S., Titler, M., Marita, G., & Mullen, M. (2003). Decision making regarding multifetal reduction. *Journal of Obstetric, Gynecologic, & Neonatal Nursing, 32*(3), 357–369.

Mattocks, K., Skanderson, M., Goulet, J., Brandt, C., Womack, J., Krebs, E., Desai, R., Justice, A., Yano, E., & Haskell, S. (2010). Pregnancy and mental health among women veterans returning from Iraq and Afghanistan. *Journal of Women's Health, 19*(12), 2159–2166.

Mattson, S., & Smith, J. (Eds.). (2010). *Core Curriculum for Maternal Newborn Nursing* (4th ed.). St. Louis, MO: Elsevier Saunders.

May, K. (1980). A typology of detachment/involvement styles adopted by first time expectant fathers. *Western Journal of Nursing Research, 2*, 443–453.

May, K. (1982). Three phases of father involvement in pregnancy. *Nursing Research, 31*(6), 337–342.

May, K., & Mahlmeister, L. (1994). *Maternal & neonatal nursing, family centered care.* Philadelphia: Lippincott Williams & Wilkins.

McManus, A., Hunter, L., & Renn, H. (2006). Lesbian experiences and needs during childbirth: Guidance for health care providers. *Journal of Obstetric, Gynecologic, & Neonatal Nursing, 35*(1), 13–23.

Meleis, A. (2003). Theoretical consideration of health care for immigrant and minority women. In P. St. Hill, J. Lipson, & A. Meleis (Eds.), *Caring for women cross culturally.* Philadelphia: F.A. Davis.

Mercer, R. (1995). *Becoming a mother.* New York: Springer.

Mercer, R. (2004). Becoming a mother versus maternal role attainment. *Journal of Nursing Scholarship, 36*(3), 226–233.

Midmer, D., Carroll, J., Bryanton, J., & Stewart, D. (2002). From research to application: The development of an antenatal psychosocial health assessment tool. *Canadian Journal of Public Health, 93*(4), 291–296.

Misra, D. P., Caldwell, C., Young, A. A., & Abelson, S. (2010). Do fathers matter? Paternal contributions to birth outcomes and racial disparities. *American Journal of Obstetrics and Gynecology, 202*, 99–100.

Montgomery, K. (2003). Nursing care for pregnant adolescents. *Journal of Obstetric, Gynecologic, and Neonatal Nursing, 32*(2), 249–256.

Moore, M., Moos, M., & Callister, L. (2010). *Cultural Competence: An Essential Journey for Perinatal Nurses*. White Plains, NY: March of Dimes Foundation.

Mottl-Santiago, J., Walker, C., Ewan, J., Vragovic, O., Winder, S., & Stubblefield, P. (2008). A hospital-based doula program and childbirth outcomes in an urban, multicultural setting. *Maternal and Child Health Journal, 12*(3), 372–377.

Ngai, F., Chan, S., & Ip, W. (2010). Predictors and correlates of maternal role competence and satisfaction. *Nursing Research, 59*(3), 185–93.

Orr, S. (2004). Social support and pregnancy outcome: a review of the literature. *Clinical Obstetrics & Gynecology, 47*(4), 842–55.

Pascali-Bonaro, D., & Kroeger, M. (2004). Continuous female companionship during childbirth: a crucial resource in times of stress or calm. *Journal of Midwifery & Women's Health, 49*(4), 19–27.

Pinazo-Hernandis, S., & Tompkins, C. (2009). Custodial grandparents: The state of the art and the many faces of this contribution. *Journal of Intergenerational Relationships, 7*(2–3), 137–143.

Porter, L., & Holness, N. (2011). Breaking the repeat teen pregnancy cycle: How nurses can nurture resilience in at-risk teens. *AWHONN Nursing for Women's Health, 15*(5), 369–381.

Price, S., Lake, M., Breene, G., Carson, G., Quinn, C., & O'Donnor, T. (2007). The spiritual experience of high-risk pregnancy. *Journal of Obstetric, Gynecologic, and Neonatal Nursing, 36*(1), 63–69.

Priest, S., Austin, M., & Sullivan, E. (2006). Antenatal psychosocial screening for prevention of antenatal and postnatal anxiety and depression (Protocol). In *The Cochrane Library*, Issue 1, 2006, Oxford: Update Software.

Purnell, L., & Paulanka, B. (2008). *Guide to culturally competent health care (*3rd ed.). Philadelphia: F.A. Davis Company.

Romano, A. (2010). Safe and healthy birth: the importance of data. *The Journal of Perinatal Education, 19*(4), 52–58.

Rondahl, G., Bruhner, E., & Lindhe, J. (2009). Heteronormative communication with lesbian families in antenatal care, childbirth and postnatal care. *Journal of Advanced Nursing, 65*(11), 2337–2344.

Ross, L. (2005). Perinatal mental health in lesbian mothers: a review of potential risk and protective factors. *Women & Health, 41*(3), 113–28.

Rubin, R. (1975). Maternal Tasks in pregnancy. *Maternal-Child Nursing Journal, 4*(3), 143–153.

Rubin, R. (1984). *Maternal Identity and the Maternal Experience.* New York: Springer.

Sadler, L., & Clemmens, D. (2004). Ambivalent grandmothers raising teen daughters and their babies. *Journal of Family Nursing, 10*(2), 211–231.

Schaffer, M. A., Jost, R., Pederson, B. J., & Lair, M. (2008). Pregnancy-free club: A strategy to prevent repeat adolescent pregnancy. *Public Health Nursing, 25*(4), 304–311.

Schardt, D. (2005). Delayed childbearing: Underestimated psychological implications. *International Journal of Childbirth Education, 20*(3), 34–37.

Semenic, S., Callister, L., & Feldman, P. (2004). Giving birth: The voices of orthodox Jewish women living in Canada. *Journal of Obstetric, Gynecologic, and Neonatal Nursing, 33*(1), 80–87.

Simpson, K., & Creehan, P. (Eds.). (2008). AWHONN Perinatal Nursing, 3rd Edition, Philadelphia: Lippincott.

Tilden, V. (1983). The relation of life stress and social support to emotional disequilibrium during pregnancy. *Research in Nursing and Health, 6,* 167–174.

U.S. Census Bureau. (2010). *National Population by Race, United States, 2010.* Retrieved from: http://2010.census.gov/2010census/data/

U.S. Department of Health and Human Services, Health Resources and Services Administration. (2010). *The registered nurse population: Findings from the National Sample Survey of Registered Nurses.* Washington, DC: Author.

U.S. Department of Health and Human Services, Health Resources and Services Administration. (2010). Healthy People 2020 Objectives. Washington, DC: Author. Retrieved from http://healthypeople.gov/2020/topicsobjectives

U.S. Department of Health and Human Services, Office of Minority Health. (1999). *National standards for culturally and linguistically appropriate services (CLAS).* Retrieved from http://omhrc.gov/clas/index.htm

Walker, D., Visger, J., & Rossie, D. (2009). Contemporary childbirth education models. *Journal of Midwifery and Women's Health, 54*(6), 469–476.

Weis, K., Lederman, R., Lilly, A., & Schaffer, J. (2008). The relationship of military imposed marital separations on maternal acceptance of pregnancy. *Research in Nursing & Health, 31,* 196–207.

Weis, K., & Ryan, T. (2012). Mentors offering maternal support: a support intervention for military mothers. *Journal of Obstetric, Gynecologic, and Neonatal Nursing, 42*(2), 303–314.

Widarsson, M., Kerstis, B., Sundquist, K., Engström, G., & Sarkadi, A. (2012). Support needs of expectant mothers and fathers: a qualitative study. *The Journal of Perinatal Education, 21*(1), 36–44.

Zelkowitz, P., Schinazi, J., Katofsky, L., Saucier, J., Valenzuela, M., Westreich, R., & Dayan, J. (2004). Factors associated with depression in pregnant immigrant women. *Transcultural Psychiatry, 41*(4), 445–464.

Antepartal Tests

6

Nursing Diagnosis

- Knowledge deficit related to antenatal tests
- Anxiety related to antenatal tests
- Risk of fetal injury or death related to invasive antenatal tests

Nursing Outcomes

- The pregnant woman and her family will verbalize understanding of antenatal tests.
- The pregnant woman will be able to make informed decisions.
- Complications of antenatal tests will be identified promptly and appropriate nursing interventions will be initiated.

INTRODUCTION

This chapter presents various antenatal tests offered to pregnant women. The focus of the chapter is on tests for at-risk and/or high-risk pregnancies. Common maternal conditions indicating need for antenatal tests are presented in Table 6-1. The purpose, indication, basic procedure, interpretation, advantages, risks, and nursing actions are outlined. Specifics on procedures are not detailed as they may vary from institution to institution. Routine tests performed during pregnancy are presented in Chapter 4. Antenatal tests are often performed as outpatient procedures, such as ultrasound, amniocentesis, and non-stress tests. Antenatal tests may also be performed during an antenatal hospitalization for a high-risk pregnancy. The nurse's role and responsibility related to antenatal tests may vary based on the inpatient or outpatient setting. Nursing care may be provided before, during, and/or after a procedure.

ASSESSMENT FOR RISK FACTORS

The nurse needs to assess for factors that place the woman and/or her fetus at risk for adverse outcomes:

- **Biophysical factors** originate from the mother or fetus and impact the development or function of the mother or fetus. They include genetic, nutritional, medical, and obstetric issues (**see Table 6-1**).
- **Psychosocial factors** are maternal behaviors or lifestyles that have a negative effect on the mother or fetus. Examples include smoking, caffeine use, alcohol/drug use, and psychological status.
- **Sociodemographic factors** are variables that pertain to the woman and her family and place the mother and the fetus at increased risk. Examples include access to prenatal care, age, parity, marital status, income, and ethnicity.
- **Environmental factors** are hazards in the workplace or the general environment that impact pregnancy outcomes.

TABLE 6–1	COMMON MATERNAL CONDITIONS INDICATING NEED FOR ANTENATAL TESTS
PREEXISTING MEDICAL CONDITIONS	Hypertensive disorder
	Renal disease
	Pulmonary or cardiac disease
	Autoimmune disease
	Type 1 diabetes
PREGNANCY-RELATED CONDITIONS	Pregnancy-related hypertension
	Decreased fetal movement
	Hydramnios, oligohydramnios, polyhydramnios
FETAL CONDITIONS	Intrauterine growth restriction
	Multiple gestation
	Postterm pregnancy
	Previous unexplained fetal demise
	Rh Isoimmunization Fetal anomalies

[handwritten annotation: excess amniotic fluid]

Source: American Academy of Pediatrics and the American College of Obstetricians and Gynecologists (2002). *Guidelines for perinatal care* (6th ed.). Washington, DC: Author.

Various environmental substances can affect fetal development. Examples include exposure to chemicals, radiation, and pollutants.

The underlying mechanism for how some risk factors impact pregnancy outcomes is not fully understood. Many risk factors appear to have a combined or cumulative effect. Identification of risk factors for poor perinatal outcomes is essential to minimize maternal and neonatal morbidity and mortality. Risk factors are described in more detail in Chapters 7, 10, 14, and 17 as they relate specifically to pregnancy, labor, the postpartum period, and the neonate.

THE NURSE'S ROLE IN ANTEPARTAL TESTING

The nurse's role during antepartal testing varies based on the specific test. In general, it includes assessment of risk factors and providing information and emotional support and comfort to women undergoing antenatal tests. Many women having antenatal tests are at high risk for fetal and maternal complications and are anxious and vulnerable. In some instances, the nurse assists or performs the antenatal test, but in most instances this requires advanced competencies (i.e., ultrasound).

To provide appropriate support to families, nurses need to understand (Barron, 2014; Gilbert, 2011; Torgerson, 2001):

■ The variety of tests available during pregnancy (see Critical Component: Antepartal Screening and Diagnostic Tests)
■ The risks and benefits of tests/procedures
■ The indications for the test/procedure
■ The interpretation of findings

■ The nursing care associated with the test/procedure
■ The physical and psychological benefits, limitations, and implications of the test/procedure

Nursing Actions for Women Undergoing Antenatal Testing

■ Establish a trusting relationship.
■ One of the main functions of nursing is to promote informed decisions and prevent uninformed decisions by patients.
■ Assess for factors that place the woman and/or her fetus at risk for adverse outcomes.
■ Provide information regarding the test.
  ■ *Explain how the test/procedure is performed.*
  ■ *Explain potential risks and benefits.*
  ■ *Explain what the woman can expect during the test/ procedure.*
  ■ *Explain what the test measures.*
  ■ *Encourage questions.*
  ■ *Encourage and foster open communication with providers.*
  ■ *Provide online resources for further information (Box 6–1).*
■ Provide comfort.
  ■ *Assist woman into a comfortable position.*
  ■ *Preserve the woman's modesty by closing doors and exposing only the portions of her body necessary for the test/procedure.*
■ Reassure the woman and her significant other.
  ■ *Address the woman's and her significant other's concerns regarding the test/procedure such as type of discomfort or pain she may experience and effects on her and/or her unborn child.*
  ■ *If she prefers, encourage the woman's significant others to be with her during procedures.*
■ Provide psychological support to the woman and her significant other (**Fig. 6–1**).
  ■ *Incorporate understanding of cultural and social issues.*
  ■ *Remain with the woman and her significant other during the test/procedure.*
  ■ *Assess for anxiety and provide care to reduce the level of anxiety.*
  ■ *Allow client to vent feelings and frustrations with the discomfort, time-consuming demands, and limitations imposed by high-risk pregnancy and antenatal testing.*
  ■ *Allow the woman to express feelings related to high-risk pregnancy.*
  ■ *Encourage expression and exploration of feelings.*
■ Document the woman's response and the results of tests.
■ Report results of tests to providers.
■ Schedule appropriate follow-up.
■ Reinforce information given by the woman's provider regarding the results of the tests and need for further testing, treatment, or referral.

BIOPHYSICAL ASSESSMENT

Since the 1970s, the fetus has become more accessible with the refinement of new technology such as ultrasound. Fetal physiological parameters that can now be assessed include

BOX 6–1 INFORMATIVE ONLINE RESOURCES

American College of Obstetrics and Gynecology (ACOG): http://acog.net
Association of Women's Health, Obstetrics and Neonatal Nursing (AWHONN): http://awhonn.org
Gene Testing: http://genetests.org
March of Dimes: http://marchofdimes.com/gyponline
National Society of Genetic Counseling: http://nsgc.org

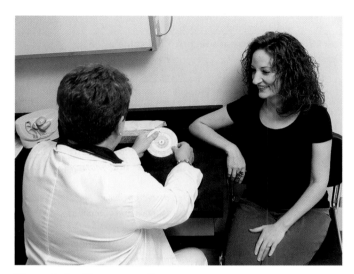

Figure 6–1 Nurse counseling a pregnant woman.

fetal movement, urine production, and observing fetal structures and blood flow. Tests used in biophysical assessment of the fetus are ultrasonography, umbilical artery Doppler flow, and magnetic resonance imaging (MRI).

Ultrasonography

Definition

Ultrasonography is the use of high-frequency sound waves to produce an image of an organ or tissue (**Fig. 6-2**). It is the most common diagnostic test during pregnancy (Cunningham et al., 2010).

Ultrasound use varies based on trimester (**Table 6-2**) and is commonly used to obtain vital information:

■ Gestational age
■ Fetal growth
■ Fetal anatomy
■ Placental abnormalities and location
■ Fetal activity
■ Amount of amniotic fluid
■ Visual assistance for some invasive procedures such as amniocentesis.

A **standard ultrasound** is one that is used for evaluating fetal presentation, amniotic fluid volume, cardiac activity, placental position, gestational age measurements, and fetal number (Fig. 6-3A). Other categories of ultrasound include

CRITICAL COMPONENT

Antepartal Screening and Diagnostic Tests
Screening Test

A screening test is a test designed to identify those who are not affected by a disease or abnormality. Some screening tests are offered to all pregnant women and include multiple marker screening and ultrasound. Other screening tests are reserved for high-risk pregnancies to provide information on fetal status and well-being. If the results of screening tests indicate an abnormality, further testing is indicated. Screening tests include:

■ Amniotic fluid index
■ Biophysical profile
■ Contraction stress test
■ Daily fetal movement count
■ Multiple marker screening: Alpha–fetoprotein screening, triple marker, and quad marker
■ Non-stress test
■ Ultrasonography
■ Umbilical artery Doppler flow
■ Vibroacoustic stimulation

Diagnostic Tests

Diagnostic tests help to identify a particular disease or provide information which aids in the making of a diagnosis. Most fetal diagnostic tests are reserved for high-risk pregnancies where there is increased risk to fetus for developmental or physical problems. Prenatal diagnosis is the science of identifying structural or functional anomalies or birth defects in the fetus (Cunningham et al., 2010).

Diagnostic tests include:

■ Amniocentesis
■ Chorionic villi sampling
■ Magnetic resonance imaging
■ Percutaneous umbilical blood sampling
■ Ultrasonography

limited obstetric ultrasound and specialized ultrasound, which usually are done after a standard ultrasound when deemed necessary for further fetal evaluation. **Limited ultrasound** can be used to measure amniotic fluid volume, to evaluate interval growth, to evaluate the cervix, to confirm fetal cardiac activity or fetal presentation as an adjunct to ultrasound guided amniocentesis or external version, for confirmation of embryonic number, for measurement of crown-rump length, or for confirmation of a yolk sac or uterine sac with assisted reproductive technology. **Specialized ultrasounds** include those involving fetal Doppler assessment, performance of biophysical profile (BPP), assessment of amniotic fluid, fetal echocardiography, or measurement of additional fetal structures (AAP & ACOG, 2007).

Timing

Standard ultrasounds are typically done in the first trimester to confirm pregnancy and calculate gestational age. Additional ultrasounds may be done at other times as needed.

TABLE 6–2   INDICATIONS FOR ULTRASOUND BY TRIMESTER OF PREGNANCY

FIRST TRIMESTER	SECOND TRIMESTER	THIRD TRIMESTER
Confirm intrauterine pregnancy.	Confirm the due date.	Confirm gestational age.
Confirm fetal cardiac activity.	Confirm fetal cardiac activity.	Confirm fetal viability.
Detect multiple gestation (number and size of gestational sacs).	Confirm fetal number, position, fetal size, amnionicity, and chronionicity.	Detect placental abruption, previa, or maturity.
Assessment of amnionicity and chronionicity of multiples.	Confirm placental location.	Detect fetal position, congenital anomalies, IUGR.
Visualization during chorionic villus sampling.	Confirm fetal weight and gestational age.	Assess biophysical profile (BPP).
Estimate gestational age.	Detect fetal anomalies (best after 18 weeks) or intrauterine growth restriction (IUGR).	Assess amniotic fluid volume (AFI).
Evaluate uterine structures.	Visualize for amniocentesis.	Perform Doppler flow studies.
Detect missed abortion, tubal, or ectopic pregnancy.	Evaluate uterine and cervical structures.	Visualize for diagnostic tests and external version.
Define cause of vaginal bleeding.	Evaluate vaginal bleeding.	Evaluate vaginal bleeding.

Procedures

■ Transvaginal ultrasound
  ■ *Is generally performed in the first trimester for earlier visualization of the fetus.*
  ■ *The woman is in a lithotomy position.*
  ■ *A sterile covered probe/transducer is inserted into the vagina.*
■ Abdominal ultrasound (**Fig. 6-2**)
  ■ *A full bladder is necessary to elevate the uterus out of the pelvis for better visualization when abdominal ultrasound is performed during the first half of pregnancy.*

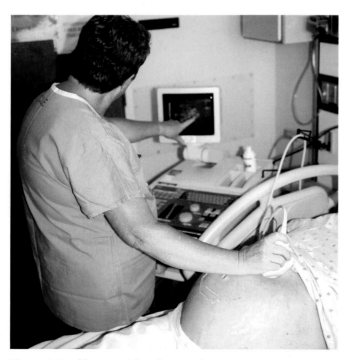

Figure 6–2   Nurse explains ultrasound to a pregnant woman having an ultrasound test.

  ■ *The woman is in a supine position.*
  ■ *Transmission gel and transducer are placed on the maternal abdomen.*
  ■ *The transducer is moved over the maternal abdomen to create an image of the structure being evaluated.*

Interpretation of Results

■ Post-procedure interpretation is typically done by a practitioner such as a radiologist, obstetrician, or nurse-midwife. After specialized training, nurses can perform limited obstetrical ultrasound (**Box 6-2**).
■ Ultrasound for gestational age is determined through measurements of fetal–crown rump length, biparietal diameter, and femur length. It is most accurate when performed before 20 weeks' gestation (AAP & ACOG, 2007).
■ Normal findings for the fetus are appropriate gestational age, size, viability, position, and functional capacities.
■ Normal findings for the placenta are expected size, normal position and structure, and an adequate amniotic fluid volume.
■ Abnormal findings should be referred for further testing and management of fetal anomalies (AAP & ACOG, 2007).

Advantages

■ Accurate assessments of gestational age, fetal growth, and detection of fetal and placental abnormalities
■ Noninvasive
■ Provides information on fetal structures and status

Risks

■ None, but controversy exists on the use of routine ultrasound for low-risk pregnant women as there is no evidence it improves outcomes.

BOX 6–2   AWHONN ULTRASOUND GUIDELINES

The Association of Women's Health, Obstetric and Neonatal Nurses (AWHONN) has developed guidelines for the didactic and clinical preparation for nurses who perform limited obstetric ultrasound. A minimum of 8 hours of didactic content is recommended in the following areas: (1) ultrasound physics and instrumentation; (2) patient education; (3) nursing accountability; (4) documentation; (5) image archiving; (6) legal and ethical issues; (7) lines of authority and responsibility (AWHONN, 2010).

Currently there are no certification requirements for nurses performing limited ultrasound. Appropriate institutional policies, didactic and clinical education, and evaluation components are needed to ensure competence for nurses to perform limited ultrasound.

Assessing the number of fetuses
Assessing for the presence or absence of fetal cardiac activity
Assessing fetal presentation
Assessing placental location
Assessing amniotic fluid
Biophysical profile

Source: Association of Women's Health, Obstetric and Neonatal Nurses (AWHONN). (2010). *Ultrasound Examinations Performed by Nurses in Obstetric Gynecologic and Reproductive Medicine Settings: Clinical Competencies and education guide:* (3rd ed.). Washington, DC: Author.

Nursing Actions

■ Explain the procedure to the woman and her family. Explain that ultrasound uses sound waves to produce an image of the baby.
■ Assess for latex allergies with transvaginal ultrasound.
■ For transvaginal, have patient put on gown and undress from waist down. For abdominal ultrasound, only the lower abdomen needs to be exposed.
■ Inform the woman that a sterile sheathed probe is used for transvaginal ultrasound and is inserted into the vagina. Inform her that she may feel pressure, but no pain is usually felt.
■ Position patient in lithotomy for transvaginal ultrasound and supine for abdominal ultrasound.
■ Provide comfort measures to the woman during the procedure such as a pillow under her head and a warm blanket above and below her abdomen.
■ Be sensitive to cultural and social as well as modesty issues.
■ Provide emotional support.
■ Schedule appropriate follow-up.
■ Document ultrasound examination according to the institutional policy.

Three-Dimensional and Four-Dimensional Ultrasound

Definition

Three-dimensional (3D) ultrasound and four-dimensional (4D) ultrasound are more advanced types of trans-abdominal ultrasounds that take thousands of images at once to produce a 3D or 4D image. They allow for visualization of complex facial movements and features, as well as the branching of placental stem vessels, and connection of the umbilical vessels to the chorionic plate of the placenta (**Fig. 6-3B**). Current recommendations are that 3D ultrasound be used only as an adjunct to conventional ultrasonography.

Purpose

■ Standard determination of gestational age, fetal size, presentation, and volume of amniotic fluid
■ Determination of complications such as vaginal bleeding, ventriculomegaly, hydrocephaly, and congenital brain defects
■ Diagnosis of fetal malformations, uterine or pelvic abnormalities, hypoxic ischemic brain injury, and inflammatory disorders of the brain (Torgersen, 2011).

Timing

■ 3D and 4D ultrasounds are ordered as needed for further evaluation of possible fetal anomalies such as face and cardiac and skeletal.

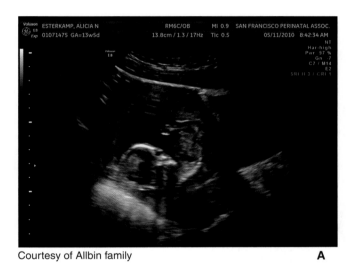

Courtesy of Allbin family   A

Figure 6–3A   2D Ultrasound picture.

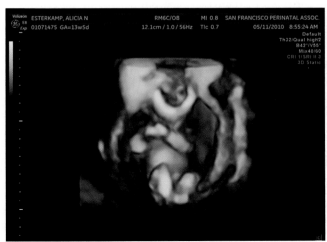

Courtesy of Allbin family   B

Figure 6–3B   3D Ultrasound picture.

■ 3D and 4D ultrasounds are most commonly requested by the patient to see a more life-like picture of their developing baby in-utero.

Procedure

■ See abdominal ultrasound.

Interpretation of Results

■ Same as ultrasound

Advantages

■ More detailed assessment of fetal structures
■ 3D presentation of placental blood flow
■ Measurement of fetal organs
■ 4D ultrasound allows for evaluation of brain morphology and identification of brain lesions.

Risks

■ Same as standard ultrasound

Nursing Actions

■ Same as standard ultrasound

Umbilical Artery Doppler Flow

Definition

Umbilical artery Doppler flow is a noninvasive screening technique that uses advanced ultrasound technology to assess resistance to blood flow in the placenta. It evaluates the rate and volume of blood flow through the placenta and umbilical cord vessels using ultrasound. This assessment is commonly used in combination with other diagnostic tests to assess fetal status in intrauterine growth restricted (IUGR) fetuses.

Purpose

■ Assesses placental perfusion
■ Used in combination with other diagnostic tests to assess fetal status in intrauterine growth restricted (IUGR) fetuses
■ Not a useful screening tool for determining fetal compromise and therefore is not recommended to the general obstetric population (Harman, 2009).

Procedures

■ The woman is assisted into a supine position.
■ Transmission gel and transducer are placed on the woman's abdomen.
■ Images are obtained of blood flow in the umbilical artery.

Interpretation of Results

■ The directed blood flow within the umbilical arteries is calculated using the difference between systolic and diastolic flow (Gilbert, 2011).
■ As peripheral resistance increases, diastolic flow decreases and the systolic/diastolic increases. Reversed end-diastolic flow can be seen with severe cases of intrauterine growth restriction (AAP & ACOG, 2007).

■ Umbilical artery Doppler is considered abnormal if the systolic/diastolic (S/D) ratio is above the 95th percentile for gestational age, or a ratio above 3.0, or the end-diastolic flow is absent or reversed (Cunningham, Leveno, Blooms, Hauth, Rouse, & Spong, 2010).

Advantages

■ Noninvasive
■ Allows for assessment of placental perfusion

Risks

■ None

Nursing Actions

■ Explain the procedure to the woman and her family. The Doppler test evaluates the blood flow through the placenta and umbilical cord vessels using ultrasound.
■ Address questions and concerns.
■ Provide comfort measures.
■ Provide emotional support.
■ Schedule appropriate follow-up.

Magnetic Resonance Imaging

Definition

Magnetic resonance imaging (MRI) is a diagnostic radiological evaluation of tissue and organs from multiple planes. During pregnancy, it is used to visualize maternal and/or fetal structures for detailed imaging when screening tests indicate possible abnormalities. It is most commonly performed for suspected brain abnormality.

Purpose

■ Scan tissue and organs.

Procedure

■ The woman is instructed to remove all metallic objects before the test.
■ The woman is placed in a supine position with left lateral tilt on the MRI table.
■ The woman's abdominal area is scanned.

Interpretation

■ Interpretation of the study is done by a radiologist.

Advantages

■ Provides very detailed images of fetal anatomy; particularly useful for brain abnormalities and complex abnormalities of thorax, gastrointestinal, and genitourinary systems.

Risks

■ No known harmful effects

Nursing Actions

■ Nurses are involved in the pre- and post-procedure.
■ Explain the procedure to the woman and her family. The MRI is used to see maternal and/or fetal structures for detailed pictures.
■ Address questions and concerns.

BIOCHEMICAL ASSESSMENT

Biochemical assessment involves biological examination and chemical determination. Procedures used to obtain biochemical specimens include chorionic villi sampling, amniocentesis, percutaneous blood sampling, and maternal assays. More than 15% of pregnancies are at sufficient risk to warrant invasive testing (Queenan, Hobbins, & Spong, 2005).

Chorionic Villus Sampling

Definition

Chorionic villus sampling (CVS) is aspiration of a small amount of placental tissue (chorion) for chromosomal, metabolic, or DNA testing. This test is used for chromosomal analysis between 10 and 12 weeks' gestation to detect fetal abnormalities caused by genetic disorders. It tests for metabolic disorders such as cystic fibrosis but does not test for neural tube defects (NTDs).

Timing

- Preformed during first or second trimester, ideally at 10–13 weeks' gestation.

Procedure

- The woman is in a supine position or lithotomy position depending on route of insertion.
- A catheter is inserted either transvaginally through the cervix using ultrasonography to guide placement, or abdominally using a needle and ultrasongraphy to guide placement as well.
- A small biopsy of chorionic (placental) tissue is removed.
- The villi are harvested and cultured for chromosomal analysis and processed for DNA and enzymatic analysis as indicated (**Fig. 6-4**).

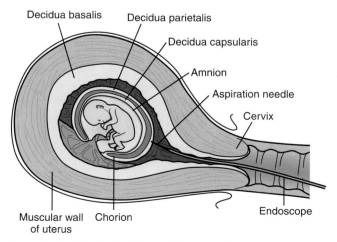

Figure 6–4 Chorionic villi sampling procedure.

Interpretation of Results

- Results of chromosomal studies are available within 1 week.
- Detailed information is provided on specific chromosomal abnormality detected.

Advantages

- Can be performed earlier than amniocentesis, but is not recommended before 10 weeks (AAP & ACOG, 2007)
- Examination of fetal chromosomes

Risks

- There is a 7% fetal loss rate due to bleeding, infection, and rupture of membranes.
- 10% of women experience some bleeding after the procedure.

Nursing Actions

- Review the procedure with the woman and her family. This test obtains amniotic fluid to test for fetal abnormalities caused by genetic problems.
- Instruct the woman in breathing and relaxation techniques she can use during the procedure.
- Assist the woman into the proper position.
  - *Lithotomy for transvaginal aspiration*
  - *Supine for transabdominal aspiration*
- Provide comfort measures.
- Provide emotional support.
- Recognize anxiety related to test results.
- Label specimens.
- Assess fetal and maternal well-being post-procedure. Fetal heart rate is auscultated twice in 30 minutes.
- Instruct the woman to report abdominal pain or cramping, leaking of fluid, bleeding, fever, or chills to the care provider.
- Administer RhoGAM to Rh-negative women post-procedure as per order to prevent antibody formation in Rh-negative women.

Amniocentesis

Definition

Amniocentesis is a diagnostic procedure in which a needle is inserted through the maternal abdominal wall into the uterine cavity to obtain amniotic fluid. It is commonly performed for genetic testing, assessment of fetal lung maturity, and assessment of hemolytic disease in fetus or for intrauterine infection.

Risk factors for fetal genetic disorders include advanced maternal age (older than 35 years of age), history of genetic disorders, positive screening test such as a positive alpha-fetoprotein, and known or suspected hemolytic disease in the fetus.

Timing

- Usually preformed between 14 and 20 weeks' gestation.

Procedure

- Detailed ultrasound is performed to take fetal measurements and locate the placenta to choose a site for needle insertion.
- A needle is inserted transabdominally into the uterine cavity using ultrasonography to guide placement (**Fig. 6-5**).
- Amniotic fluid is obtained.

Interpretation of Results

- Amniocentesis has an accuracy rate of 99% (Gilbert, 2011).
- Amniotic fluid sample is sent to a lab for cell growth, and results of chromosomal studies are available within 2 weeks.
- Elevated bilirubin levels indicate fetal hemolytic disease.
- A positive culture indicates infection.
- If the purpose of the test is to determine fetal lung maturity, lecithin/sphingomyelin (L/S) ratio, phosphatidyl glycerol (PG), lamellar body count (LBC), results are interpreted as follows (Torgerson, 2011):
  - *L:S ratio >2:1 indicates fetal lung maturity.*
  - *L:S ratio <2:1 indicates fetal lung immaturity in increased risk of respiratory distress syndrome.*
  - *Positive PG indicates fetal lung maturity.*
  - *Negative PG indicates immature fetal lungs.*
  - *A LBC of ≥50,000/μL is highly indicative of fetal lung maturity.*
  - *A LBC of ≤15,000/μL highly indicative of fetal lung immaturity.*
  - *LBC results can be hindered by the presence of meconium, vaginal bleeding, vaginal mucous, or hydramnios.*

Advantages

- Examines fetal chromosomes for genetic disorders
- Direct examination of biochemical specimens

Risks

- Less than 1% fetal loss rate after 15 weeks' gestation; increases to 2%–5% earlier in gestation (AAP & ACOG, 2007)
- Trauma to the fetus or placenta

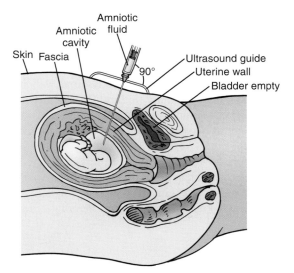

Figure 6–5   Amniocentesis procedure.

- Bleeding
- Preterm labor
- Maternal infection
- Rh sensitization from fetal blood into maternal circulation

Nursing Actions

- Review the procedure with the woman and assure her that precautions are followed during the procedure with ultrasound visualization of fetus to avoid fetal or placental injury (Leeuwen, Kranpitz, & Smith, 2006).
- Explain that in the amniocentesis procedure a needle is inserted through the abdomen into the womb to obtain amniotic fluid for testing.
- Explain that during needle aspiration discomfort will be minimized with the use of a local anesthetic.
- Explain that a full bladder may be required for ultrasound visualization if the woman is less than 20 weeks' gestation.
- Instruct the woman in breathing and relaxation techniques she can use during the procedure.
- Provide comfort measures.
- Provide emotional support.
- Recognize anxiety related to test results.
- Prep abdomen with an antiseptic such as betadine if indicated.
- Label specimens.
- Assess fetal and maternal well-being post-procedure, monitoring and evaluating the FHR.
- Instruct the woman to report abdominal pain or cramping, leaking of fluid, bleeding, decreased fetal movement, fever, or chills to the care provider.
- Instruct woman not to lift anything heavy for 2 days.
- Administer Rho(D) immune globulin (RhoGAM) to Rh-negative women post-procedure as per order to prevent antibody formation in the Rh-negative women.

Delta OD 450

Definition

Delta OD 450 is a diagnostic evaluation of amniotic fluid obtained via amniocentesis to predict life-threatening anemia in the fetus during the second and third trimester. This test is often done when alloimmunization exists, due to the increase risk for severe fetal anemia from RBC hemolysis. Studies have determined that Umbilical Artery Doppler Flow is a safer option in the management of RH-alloimmunized pregnancies than Delta OD 450 (Oepkes et al., 2006). Umbilical Artery Doppler Flow is a non-invasive procedure which can measure the peak velocity of systolic blood flow in the middle cerebral artery of the fetus, and therefore does not involve the risks associated with amniocentesis.

Timing

- Second and third trimester

Procedure

- Amniotic fluid is collected via amniocentesis and used in a lab to determine whether there is a deviation of optical density (OD) at 45 nm.

Advantages

■ Early evaluation and detection leads to early intervention, including fetal intrauterine transfusion, to increase chances of fetal survival.

Risks

■ Membrane rupture
■ Infection
■ Worsening sensitization
■ Fetal loss

Nursing Actions

■ See amniocentesis above.

Fetal Blood Sampling/Percutaneous Umbilical Blood Sampling

Definition

Fetal blood sampling/percutaneous umbilical blood sampling (PUBS), or **cordocentesis,** is the removal of fetal blood from the umbilical cord. The blood is used to test for metabolic and hematological disorders, fetal infection, and fetal karyotyping. It can also be used for fetal therapies such as red blood cell and platelet transfusions.

Timing

■ Usually used after ultrasound has detected an anomaly in the fetus.
■ May be done as early as 11 weeks but is generally done in the second trimester to evaluate results of potential diagnoses and make further recommendations for medical management if necessary (Gilbert, 2011).

Procedure

■ A needle is inserted into the umbilical vein at or near placental origin and a small sample of fetal blood is aspirated (**Fig. 6-6**).
■ Ultrasound is used to guide the needle.

Interpretation of Results

■ Results are usually available within 48 hours.
■ Interpretation of studies is based on the indication for the procedure.
■ Biochemical testing on the blood may include a complete blood count with a differential analysis, anti-1 and anti-I cold agglutinin, ß-hCG, factors IX and VIIIC, and AFP levels (Gilbert, 2011).

Advantages

■ Direct examination of fetal blood sample

Risks

■ Complications are similar to those for amniocentesis and include cord vessel bleeding or hematomas, maternal–fetal hemorrhage, fetal bradycardia, and risk for infection.
■ The overall procedure-related fetal death rate is 1.4% but varies depending on induction (Cunningham et al., 2010).

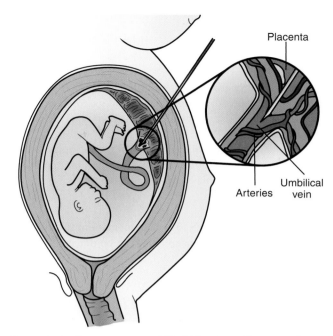

Figure 6–6   Percutaneous umbilical blood sampling procedure.

Nursing Actions

■ Nurses may be involved in the pre- and post-procedure.
■ Explain the procedure to the woman and her family. During PUBS fetal blood is removed from the umbilical cord.
■ Address questions and concerns.
■ Position client in a lateral or wedged position to avoid supine hypotension during fetal monitoring tests.
■ Have terbutaline ready as ordered in case uterine contractions occur during procedure (Torgersen, 2011).
■ Assess fetal well-being post-procedure for 1–2 hours via external fetal monitoring.
■ Educate patient on how to count fetal movements for when she goes home (Gilbert, 2011).

MATERNAL ASSAYS

Alpha-Fetoprotein/α_1-Fetoprotein/Maternal Serum Alpha-Fetoprotein

Definition

Alpha-fetoprotein (AFP) is a glycoprotein produced in the fetal liver, gastrointestinal tract, and yolk sac in early gestation. Assessing for the levels of AFP in the maternal blood is a screening tool for certain developmental defects in the fetus such as fetal NTDs and ventral abdominal wall defects. Because 95% of NTDs occur in the absence of risk factors, routine screening is recommended (Cunningham et al., 2010).

Timing

■ 15–20 weeks' gestation

Procedure

■ Maternal blood is drawn and sent to the lab for analysis.

Interpretation of Results

■ Increased levels are associated with defects such as NTDs, anencephaly, omphalocele, and gastroschisis.
■ Decreased levels are associated with trisomy 21 (Down syndrome).
■ Abnormal findings require additional testing such as amniocentesis, chorionic villus sampling, or ultrasonography to make a particular diagnosis.

Advantages

■ 80%–85% of all open NTDs and open abdominal wall defects and 90% of anencephalies can be detected early in pregnancy (AAP & ACOG, 2007).

Risks

■ There is a high false-positive rate (meaning the test results indicate an abnormality in a normal fetus) that can result in increased anxiety for woman and her family related to identification of a potential defect as they wait for results of additional testing. High false positives can occur with low birth weight, oligohydramnios, multifetal gestation, decreased maternal weight, and underestimated fetal gestational age. False low levels can also occur as a result of fetal death, increased maternal weight, and overestimated fetal gestational age (Gilbert, 2011).

Nursing Actions

■ Educate the woman about the screening test. The AFP test is a maternal blood test that evaluates the levels of AFP in the maternal blood to screen for certain fetal abnormalities.
■ Support the woman and her family, particularly if results are abnormal.
■ Assist in scheduling diagnostic testing when results are abnormal.
■ Provide information on support groups if a NTD occurs.

Multiple Marker Screen

Definition

Triple marker screening combines all three chemical markers—AFP, human chorionic gonadotropin (hCG), and estriol levels—with maternal age to detect some trisomies and NTDs. It is sometimes used as an alternative to amniocentesis. **Quad screen** adds inhibin-A to the triple marker screen to increase detection of trisomy 21 to 80% (Queenan, Hobbins, & Spong, 2005).

Timing

■ 15–16 weeks' gestation

Procedure

■ Maternal blood is drawn and sent to the lab for analysis.

Interpretation

■ Low levels of maternal serum alpha-fetoprotein (MSAFP) and unconjugated estriol levels suggest an abnormality.
■ hCG and inhibin-A levels are twice as high in pregnancies with trisomy 21.
■ Decreased estriol levels are an indicator of NTDs.

Advantages

■ 60%–80% of cases of Down syndrome can be identified.
■ 85%–90% of open NTDs are detected.

Risks

■ None

Nursing Actions

■ Educate the woman about the test. This is a maternal blood test that assesses for the levels of chemicals in the maternal blood to screen for certain developmental abnormalities.
■ Provide emotional support for the woman and her family.
■ Assist in scheduling additional testing if needed.
■ Provide information on support groups if a NTD occurs.

TESTS OF FETAL STATUS AND WELL-BEING

The assessment of fetal status is a key component of perinatal care. A variety of methods are available for ongoing assessment of fetal well-being during pregnancy (AWHONN, 2008):

■ Daily fetal movement count (kick counts)
■ Non-stress test (NST)
■ Vibroacoustic stimulation (VAS)
■ Contraction stress test (CST)
■ Amniotic fluid index (AFI)
■ Biophysical profile (BPP)

The goal of fetal testing is to reduce the number of preventable stillbirths and to avoid unnecessary interventions. The purpose of antenatal testing is to validate fetal well-being or identify fetal hypoxemia and to intervene before permanent injury or death occurs (AWHONN, 2008; Torgerson, 2011). In most clinical situations a normal test result indicates that intrauterine fetal death is highly unlikely in the next 7 days and is highly reassuring (AAP & ACOG, 2007). In most pregnancies, when indicated, testing begins by 32–34 weeks (Cunningham et al., 2010).

Daily Fetal Movement Count

Definition

Daily fetal movement count (kick counts) is a maternal assessment of fetal movement by counting fetal movements in a period of time to identify potentially hypoxic fetuses. Maternal perception of fetal movement was one of the earliest and easiest tests of fetal well-being and remains an essential assessment of fetal health. Fetal activity is diminished in the compromised fetus, and cessation of fetal movement has been documented preceding fetal demise (AWHONN, 2008).

Timing

■ Kick counts have been proposed as a primary method of fetal surveillance for all pregnancies after 28 weeks' gestation. However, many women may begin feeling fetal movement around 16–20 weeks (Gilbert, 2011).

Procedure

■ The pregnant woman is instructed to palpate her abdomen and track fetal movements daily for 1–2 hours.

Interpretation

■ In the 2-hour approach, maternal perception of 10 distinct fetal movements within 2 hours is considered normal and reassuring; once movement is achieved, counts can be discontinued for the day.
■ In the 1-hour approach, the count is considered reassuring if it equals or exceeds the established baseline; in general 4 movements in 1 hour is reassuring.
■ Reports of decreased fetal movement should be reported to the provider and is an indication for further fetal assessment such as a non-stress test or biophysical profile.
■ Fewer than four fetal movements in 2 hours should be reported to provider (Barron, 2014).

Advantages

■ Done by pregnant women
■ Inexpensive, reassuring, and relatively easily taught to pregnant women

Risks

■ None

Nursing Actions

■ Teach the woman how to do kick counts and provide a means to record them. Instruct the woman to lie on her side while counting movements. Explain that maternal assessment of fetal movement by counting fetal movements is an important evaluation of fetal well-being.
■ If fetal movement is decreased, the woman should be instructed to have something to eat, rest, and focus on fetal movement for 1 hour. Four movements in 1 hour is considered reassuring.
■ Instruct the woman to report decreased fetal movement below normal, as decreasing fetal movements are an indication for further assessment by care providers.

Non-Stress Test

Definition

The **non-stress test (NST)** is a screening tool that uses electronic fetal monitoring (EFM) to assess fetal condition or well-being (**Fig. 6-7**). The heart rate of a physiologically normal fetus with adequate oxygenation and intact autonomic nervous system accelerates in response to movement (AWHONN, 2008). The NST records accelerations in the fetal heart rate (FHR) in relation to fetal activity. It is the most widely accepted method of evaluating fetal status, particularly for high-risk pregnant women with complications such as hypertension, diabetes,

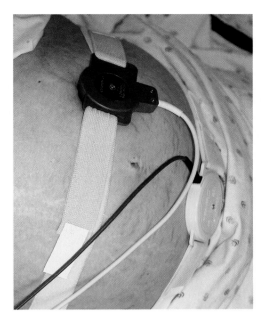

Figure 6-7 Monitoring for a non-stress test.

multiple gestation, trauma and/or bleeding, woman's report of lack of fetal movement, and placental abnormalities.

Procedure

■ The FHR is monitored with the external FHR transducer until reactive (up to 40 minutes), while running a FHR contraction strip for interpretation.
■ Monitor FHR and fetal activity for 20–30 minutes (placement of EFM and interpretation of EFM are described in Chapter 9).

Interpretation

■ The NST is considered reactive when the FHR increases 15 beats above baseline for 15 seconds twice or more in 20 minutes.
■ In fetuses less than 32 weeks' gestation two accelerations peaking at least 10 bpm above baseline and lasting 10 seconds in a 20-minute period is reactive (AWHONN, 2008).
■ Nonreactive NST is one without sufficient FHR accelerations in 40 minutes and should be followed up with further testing such as a BPP (AAP & ACOG, 2007).
■ Presence of repetitive variable decelerations that are >30 seconds requires further assessment of amniotic fluid (Cunningham et al., 2010).

Advantages

■ Noninvasive, easily performed, and reliable indicator of fetal well-being

Risks

■ No indicated risks
■ NST has a high false-positive rate, 80%–90%, but does have a low false-negative rate of less than 1% (APA & ACOG, 2007).

Nursing Actions

- Explain the procedure to the woman and her family. The NST uses electronic fetal monitoring (EFM) to assess fetal well-being.
- Have the patient void prior to the procedure and lie in a semi-Fowler's or lateral position.
- Provide comfort measures.
- Provide emotional support.
- Interpret FHR and accelerations; report results to the care provider.
- Document the date and time the test was started, the patient's name, the reason for the test, and the maternal vital signs.
- Schedule appropriate follow-up; the typical interval for testing is biweekly or weekly depending on indication.

Vibroacoustic Stimulation

Definition

Vibroacoustic stimulation (VAS) is a screening tool that uses auditory stimulation (using an artificial larynx) to assess fetal well-being with EFM when NST is nonreactive. Vibroacoustic stimulation may be effective in eliciting a change in fetal behavior, fetal startle movements, and increased FHR variability. VAS is only used when the baseline rate is determined to be within normal limits. When deceleration or bradycardia is present, VAS is not an appropriate intervention (Gilbert, 2011).

Procedure

- VAS is conducted by activating an artificial larynx on the maternal abdomen near the fetal head for 1 second in conjunction with the NST. This can be repeated at 1-minute intervals up to 3 times.

Interpretation

- The NST using VAS is considered reactive when the FHR increases 15 beats above baseline for 15 seconds twice in 20 minutes.

Advantages

- Using VAS to stimulate the fetus has reduced the incidence of nonreactive NSTs and reduced the time required to conduct NSTs.

Risks

- No adverse effects reported
- Not recommended as a routine procedure in high-risk pregnancies

Nursing Actions

- Explain the procedure to the woman and her family. The test uses a buzzer (in auditory stimulation) to assess fetal well-being.
- Provide comfort measures.
- Provide emotional support.

- Interpret FHR and accelerations and conduct VAS appropriately. Report results to physician or midwife and document.
- Schedule appropriate follow-up.

Contraction Stress Test

Definition

The **contraction stress test (CST)** is a screening tool to assess fetal well-being and uteroplacental function with EFM in women with nonreactive NST at term gestation. The purpose of the CST is to identify a fetus that is at risk for compromise through observation of the fetal response to intermittent reduction in utero placental blood flow associated with stimulated uterine contractions (UCs) (AWHONN, 2008).

Procedure

- Monitor FHR and fetal activity for 20 minutes.
- If no spontaneous UCs, contractions can be initiated in some women by having them brush the nipples for 10 minutes.
- If nipple stimulation is unsuccessful, UCs can be stimulated with oxytocin via IV until 3 UCs in 10–20 minutes lasting 40 seconds occur. (Placement of EFM and interpretation of EFM are described in Chapter 9.)

Interpretation

- The CST is considered negative or normal when there are no significant variable decelerations or no late decelerations in a 10-minute strip with 3 UCs > 40 seconds assessed with moderate variability.
- The CST is positive where there are late decelerations of FHR with 50% of UCs usually assessed with minimal or absent variability.
- A positive result has been associated with an increased rate of fetal death, fetal growth restriction, lower 5-minute Apgar scores, cesarean section, and the need for neonatal resuscitation due to neonatal depression (Harman, 2009). This requires further testing such as BPP.
- The CST is equivocal or suspicious when there are intermittent late or variable decelerations, and further testing may be done or the test repeated in 24 hours.

Advantages

- Negative CSTs are associated with good fetal outcomes.

Risks

- CST has a high false-positive rate which can result in unnecessary intervention.
- Cannot be used with women who have a contraindication for uterine activity.

Nursing Actions

- Explain the procedure to the woman and her family. The CST stimulates contractions to evaluate fetal reaction to the stress of contractions.
- Have patient void before testing.
- Position patient in a semi-Fowler's position.

- Monitor vitals before and every 15 minutes during the test.
- Provide comfort measures.
- Provide emotional support.
- Correctly interpret FHR and contractions.
- Safely administer oxytocin (i.e., avoid uterine tachysystole). Uterine tachysystole is defined as more than five uterine contractions in 10 minutes, fewer than 60 seconds between contractions, or a contraction greater than 90 seconds with a late deceleration occurring (Gilbert, 2011).
- Recognize adverse effects of oxytocin.
- Schedule appropriate follow-up.

Amniotic Fluid Index

Definition

The **amniotic fluid index (AFI)** is a screening tool that measures the volume of amniotic fluid with ultrasound to assess fetal well-being and placental function. The amniotic fluid level is based on fetal urine production, which is the predominate source of amniotic fluid and is directly dependent on renal perfusion (Queenan, Hobbins, & Spong, 2005). In prolonged fetal hypoxemia, blood is shunted away from fetal kidneys to other vital organs. Persistent decreased blood flow to the fetal kidneys results in reduction of amniotic fluid production and oligohydramnios. In conjunction with NST, AFI is a strong indicator of fetal status, as it is accurate in detecting fetal hypoxia.

Procedure

- Ultrasound measurement of pockets of amniotic fluid in four quadrants of the uterine cavity via ultrasound.

Interpretation of Results

- Average measurement in pregnancy is 8–24 cm (Cunningham et al., 2010).
- Abnormal AFI is below 5 cm. An AFI ≤ 5 cm is indicative of **oligohydramnios.** Oligohydramnios is associated with increased prenatal mortality and a need for close maternal and fetal monitoring.
- Represented graphically: decreased uteroplacental perfusion→ decreased fetal renal blood flow→decreased urine production→oligohydramnios
- An AFI above 24 cm is **polyhydramnios,** which may indicate fetal malformation such as NTDs, obstruction of fetal gastrointestinal tract, or fetal hydrops.

Advantages

- AFI is a reflection of placental function and perfusion to the fetus as well as overall fetal condition.

Risks

- None

Nursing Actions

- Explain the procedure to the woman and her family. This test measures the amount of amniotic fluid with ultrasound to assess fetal well-being and how well the placenta is working.
- Provide comfort measures.
- Provide emotional support.
- Schedule appropriate follow-up.
- Special training in obstetric ultrasound is required for evaluation of amniotic fluid volume (see Box 6-2).

Biophysical Profile

Definition

The **biophysical profile (BPP/BPA)** is an ultrasound assessment of fetal status along with an NST. It involves evaluation of fetal status through ultrasound observation of various fetal reflex activities that are central nervous system (CNS) controlled and sensitive to fetal hypoxia. If fetal oxygen consumption is reduced, the immediate fetal response is reduction of activity regulated by the CNS. The BPP includes assessment of fetal breathing movement, gross body movement, fetal tone, amniotic fluid volume, and heart rate reactivity. The BPP provides improved prognostic information because physiological parameters associated with chronic and acute hypoxia are evaluated. It is indicated in pregnancies involving increased risk of fetal hypoxia and placental insufficiency such as maternal diabetes and hypertension. Some controversy exists related to this test as a Cochrane Review concluded that available evidence from randomized clinical trials provides no support for the use of BPP as a test of fetal well-being in high-risk pregnancies (Alfirevic & Neilson, 2006).

Procedure

- BPP consists of an NST with the addition of 30 minutes of ultrasound observation for four indicators: fetal breathing movements, fetal movement, fetal tone, and measurement of amniotic fluid.
  - *Assess fetal breathing movements: One or more episodes of rhythmic breathing movements of 30 seconds or movement within 30 minutes is expected.*
  - *Assess fetal movement: Three or more discrete body or limb movements in 30 minutes are expected.*
  - *Assess fetal tone: One or more fetal extremity extension with return to fetal flexion or opening and closing of the hand is expected.*
  - *Assess amniotic fluid volume: A pocket of amniotic fluid that measures at least 2 cm in two planes perpendicular to each other is expected.*

Interpretation

- A score of 2 (present) or 0 (absent) is assigned to each of the five components.
- A total score of 8/10 is reassuring.
- A score of 6/10 is equivocal and may indicate the need for delivery depending on gestational age.
- A score of 4/10 means delivery is recommended because of a strong correlation with chronic asphyxia (AAP & ACOG, 2007).
- A score of 2/10 or less prompts immediate delivery.
- Fetal activity decreases or stops to reduce energy and oxygen consumption as fetal hypoxemia worsens. Decreased activity occurs in reverse order of normal development.

■ Fetal activities that appear earliest in pregnancy (tone and movement) are usually the last to cease, and activities that are the last to develop are usually the first to be diminished (FHR variability).

Advantages

■ Lower false-positive rate

Risks

■ None

Nursing Actions

■ Explain the procedure to the woman and her family. The BPP is an ultrasound evaluation of fetal status and involves observation of various fetal reflex activities with ultrasound and fetal monitoring.
■ Provide comfort measures.
■ Provide emotional support.
■ Special training in obstetric ultrasound is required for interpretation of ultrasound components of the test (see Box 6-2).
■ Schedule appropriate follow–up; the typical interval for testing is 1 week but for specific pregnancy complications may be biweekly.

Modified Biophysical Profile

Definition

The **modified BPP** combines an NST as an indicator of short-term fetal well-being and AFI as an indicator of long-term placental function to evaluate fetal well-being. It is indicated in high-risk pregnancy related to maternal conditions or pregnancy-related conditions (see Table 6-1).

Procedure

■ A modified BPP combines the use of an NST with an AFI.

Interpretation

■ A modified BPP is considered normal when the NST is reactive and the AFI is greater than 5 cm. An AFI less than or equal to 5 is indicative of oligohydramnios. Oligohydramnios is associated with increased perinatal mortality, and decreased amniotic fluid may be a reflection of acute or chronic fetal asphyxia (Feinstein, Torgesen, & Atterbury, 2003).

Advantages

■ Less time to complete
■ Predictive of fetal well-being

Risks

■ None

Nursing Actions

■ Explain the procedure to the woman and her family. A modified BPP is an NST and measurement of the amount of amniotic fluid.

■ Provide comfort measures.
■ Provide emotional support.
■ Special training in ultrasound is required for interpretation of amniotic fluid volume (see Box 6-2).
■ Schedule appropriate follow-up; the typical interval for testing is 1 week but for specific pregnancy complications may be biweekly.

■ ■ ■ Review Questions ■ ■ ■

1. Assessment for risk factors includes:
   A. Cultural factors
   B. Medical and obstetrical issues
   C. Religion
   D. Sexual preference

2. The nurse's role in antepartal testing includes:
   A. Interpreting results
   B. Obtaining consent
   C. Explaining how and why test is performed
   D. Referring the woman's question to a physician

3. Screening tests are designed to:
   A. Be offered to all pregnant women
   B. Identify those not affected by a disease
   C. Identify a particular disease
   D. Make a specific diagnosis

4. Specialized ultrasounds are involved in all the following except:
   A. Maternal assays
   B. BPP
   C. Assessment of amniotic fluid
   D. Measurement of fetal structures

5. Amniocentesis done after 15 weeks is associated with a fetal death rate of:
   A. Less than 1%
   B. Less than 5%
   C. Greater than 1%
   D. Approximately 5%

6. What lamellar body count (LBC) value is highly indicative of fetal lung maturity?
   A. 20,000
   B. 35,000
   C. 55,000
   D. 40,000

7. Umbilical Artery Doppler Flow can replace which antepartal test?
   A. Amniocentesis
   B. Chorionic Villus Sampling
   C. Multiple Marker Screen
   D. Delta OD 450

8. Daily fetal movement counts are done:
   A. Only in high-risk pregnancies
   B. By care providers during prenatal visits
   C. As soon as the pregnancy is confirmed
   D. To identify potentially hypoxic fetuses

9. A FHR that increases 15 beats above baseline for 15 seconds twice in 20 minutes is considered:
   A. Category III
   B. Reactive
   C. Nonreactive
   D. Negative

10. What BPP score would indicate the need for immediate delivery of the fetus?
    A. 6
    B. 2
    C. 12
    D. 4

References

Alfirevic, Z., & Neilson, J. (2006). Biophysical profile for fetal assessment in high risk pregnancies. (Cochrane Review). Cochrane Library, Issue 1, 2006. Oxford: Update Software.

American Academy of Pediatrics and the American College of Obstetricians and Gynecologists. (2002). *Guidelines for perinatal care* (6th ed.). Washington, DC: Author.

Association of Women's Health, Obstetric and Neonatal Nurses (AWHONN). (2010). *Ultrasound Examinations Performed by Nurses in Obstetric Gynecologic and Reproductive Medicine Settings: Clinical Competencies and education guide* (3rd ed.). Washington, DC: Author.

Association of Women's Health, Obstetric and Neonatal Nurses (AWHONN). (2008). *Fetal heart rate monitoring: Principles and practice* (4th ed.). Washington, DC: Author.

Barron, M. Antenatal tests. In Simpson, K., & Creehan, P., & Association of Women's Health, Obstetrics and Neonatal Nursing. (2014). *Perinatal Nursing.* Philadelphia: Lippincott.

Cunningham, F., Leveno, K., Bloom, S., Hauth, J., Rouse, D., & Spong, C. (2010). *Williams obstetrics* (23rd ed.). New York: McGraw-Hill.

Feinstein, N., Torgersen, K., & Atterbury, J. (2003). *AWHONN's fetal heart monitoring principles and practices* (3rd ed.). Washington, DC: Association of Women's Health, Obstetric and Neonatal Nurses.

Gilbert, E. (2011). *Manual of high risk pregnancy and delivery* (6th ed.). St. Louis, MO: C. V. Mosby.

Harman, C. R. (2009). Assessment of fetal health. In R. Creasy, R. Resnick, J. Iams, C. J. Lockwood, & T. R. Moore (Eds.), *Creasy & Resnik's maternal-fetal medicine: Principles and practice* (6th ed., pp. 361–395). Philadelphia: Saunders

Leeuwen, A., Kranpitz, T., & Smith, L. (2006). *Davis's comprehensive handbook of laboratory and diagnostic tests with nursing implications.* Philadelphia: F.A. Davis.

Oepkes, D., Seaward, P. G., Vandenbussche, F. P. H., Windrim, R., Kingdom, J., Beyene, J., Kanhai, H., Ohlsson, A., & Ryan, G. (2006). Doppler ultrasonography versus amniocentesis to predict fetal anemia. *New England Journal of Medicine, 355*, 156–164.

Queenan, J., Hobbins, J., & Spong, C. (2005). *Protocols in high risk pregnancies.* Malden, MA: Blackwell.

Torgersen, K. L (2011). Antepartal Fetal Assessment. In Mattson, S., & Smith, J. (Ed). Core Curriculum for Maternal-Newborn Nursing, 4th ed., pp 161-200, St Louis: Elsevier Saunders.

Torgerson, K. L. (2011). Maternal and fetal health. In Mattson, S., & Smith, J. (Ed.), *Lippincott manual for nursing practice* (8th ed., pp. 1174–1199). Philadelphia: Lippincott Williams & Wilkins.

High-Risk Antepartum Nursing Care

EXPECTED STUDENT OUTCOMES

On completion of this chapter, the student will be able to:

☐ Define key terms.
☐ Describe the primary complications of pregnancy and the related nursing and medical care.
☐ Demonstrate understanding of knowledge related to preexisting medical complications of pregnancy and related management.
☐ Identify potential antenatal complications for the woman, the fetus, and the newborn.
☐ Describe the key aspects of discharge teaching for women with antenatal complications.

Nursing Diagnosis

▪ Risk of maternal injury related to pregnancy complications
▪ Risk of maternal injury related to preexisting medical conditions
▪ Risk of fetal injury related to complications of pregnancy

Nursing Outcomes

▪ The woman will understand management of a pregnancy complication and warning signs.
▪ The woman will give birth without serious complications.
▪ The woman will give birth to a healthy infant without complications.

INTRODUCTION

This chapter presents information on key complications that can occur during pregnancy and on preexisting medical conditions that have the potential to be exacerbated by pregnancy. An overview of each complication is presented, including underlying pathophysiology, risk factors, and risks posed to the woman and fetus and typical medical management and nursing actions.

The nature of perinatal nursing is unpredictable, and pregnancy complications can arise abruptly, resulting in rapid deterioration of maternal and fetal status. It is imperative that nurses understand the underlying physiological mechanisms of pregnancy, the impact of complications on maternal and fetal well-being, and current interventions to optimize maternal and fetal outcomes.

GESTATIONAL COMPLICATIONS

Although most pregnant women experience a normal pregnancy, various complications can develop during pregnancy that affect maternal and fetal well-being. When women

experience pregnancy complications, astute assessment, rapid intervention, and a collaborative team approach are essential to optimize maternal and neonatal outcomes. In this section, complications related to pregnancy are presented along with the physiological and pathological basis for the most common complications of pregnancy. Nursing care and appropriate management are discussed.

Preterm Labor and Birth

Preterm labor (PTL) is the onset of labor before 37 weeks' gestation. **Preterm birth (PTB)** refers to gestational age at birth of less than 37 weeks. According to an Institute of Medicine report (2007), preterm birth is a complex cluster of problems with a set of overlapping factors of influence. Its causes may include individual level behavioral and psychosocial factors, neighborhood characteristics, environmental exposures, medical conditions, infertility treatments, biological factors, and genetics. Many of these factors occur in combination, particularly in those who are socioeconomically disadvantaged or who are members of racial and ethnic minority groups (Berhman & Stith Butler, 2007). Most preterm births are a result of spontaneous preterm labor; however, between 20% and 25% of preterm births are intentional, necessary, and indicated for problems such as hypertension, preeclampsia, hemorrhage, and intrauterine growth restriction (IUGR) where early delivery would improve either maternal or fetal status.

A **preterm/premature infant** is born after 20 weeks and before 37 completed weeks of gestation (**Fig. 7-1**). More specific classifications of prematurity include (PeriStats, 2012):

■ **Late preterm infant:** An infant born between 34 and 36 weeks of gestation

■ **Very preterm infant:** An infant born before 32 completed weeks of gestation

■ **Low birth weight infant (LBW):** An infant who weighs less than 2,500 grams at delivery, regardless of gestational age; among low birth weight infants, two thirds are preterm.

■ **Very low birth weight infant:** An infant who weighs less than 1,500 grams at birth

■ **Extremely low birth weight infant:** An infant who weighs less than 1,000 grams at birth

During the last 20 years, the preterm birth rate has increased more than 28%, from 9.6% in 1983 to 11.0% in 1993 to 12.3% in 2003, and to 12.2% (over 500,00 infants per year) in 2009 (Martin, Hamilton, Ventura, Osterman, Kirmeyer, Mathews, & Wilson, 2011; March of Dimes, 2012). Between 1999 and 2009, the rate of infants born preterm in the United States increased more than 3%.

Prematurity is the number one cause of neonatal mortality and the number two cause of infant mortality in the United States. Data indicated hospital charges for premature infants that year totaled more than $18 billion in immediate costs of neonatal intensive care and the morbidity associated with prematurity, such as respiratory distress syndrome, intraventricular hemorrhages, and necrotizing enterocolitis (March of Dimes, 2006b). The annual societal economic cost (medical, educational, and lost productivity) associated with preterm birth in the United States was over $26 billion. The average first-year medical costs, including both inpatient and outpatient care, were about 10 times greater for preterm ($32,325) than for term infants ($3,325).

Long-term sequelae for preterm infants include cerebral palsy, hearing and vision impairment, and chronic lung disease. Long-term costs include not only health care costs but also special education costs for learning problems, costs of developmental services, and health care costs for long-term sequelae associated with prematurity. The goals of Healthy People 2020 and the March of Dimes are to reduce the preterm birth rate from 12.2% to 11.4% (March of Dimes, 2012).

Pathophysiological Pathways of Preterm Labor

Spontaneous preterm birth may be characterized by a syndrome composed of several components including uterine (preterm labor), chorioamnionic-decidual (premature rupture of membranes), and cervical (cervical insufficiency) (Owens & Harger, 2007). Yet the specific causes of spontaneous preterm labor and delivery are largely unknown. Preterm labor is characterized as a series of complex interactions of factors. No single factor acts alone, but multiple factors interact to initiate a cascade of events that result in preterm labor and birth (Reedy, 2014). The pathways to preterm birth are thought to be multicausal, and contributing factors include (Iams, 2007; March of Dimes, 2006a) (**Fig. 7-2**):

■ Uterine overdistention
  ■ *Prostaglandin can be produced, stimulating the uterus to contract when overdistended from multiple gestation, or polyhydramnios, or uterine abnormalities.*
■ Decidual activation
  ■ *From hemorrhage*
  ■ *From fetal-decidual paracrine system*
  ■ *From upper genital tract infection*
■ Premature activation of the normal physiological initiators of labor, activation of the maternal-fetal hypothalamic–pituitary adrenal (HPA) axis
■ Inflammation and infection in the decidua, fetal membranes, and amniotic fluid are associated with preterm birth.
  ■ *Inflammatory cytokines or bacterial endotoxins can stimulate prostaglandin release resulting in cervical ripening, contractions, and weakening and rupture of membranes.*

Psychosocial factors are also hypothesized to contribute to a stress response that results in uterine contractions (UCs). Studies of chronic and catastrophic stress exposures are suggestive of an association between stress and preterm birth (IOM, 2008).

Because we do not know what triggers normal labor at term, it is difficult to know what causes preterm labor. Extensive research has been conducted over the past three decades to predict which women are at risk to deliver preterm so that intensive interventions can be implemented to prevent prematurity. Risk factors predict only about half the women who will deliver preterm.

Risk Factors for Preterm Labor and Birth

Despite its use for decades, risk factor assessment alone has a limited utility for identifying who will deliver preterm (March of Dimes, 2011). Fifty percent of women who deliver preterm

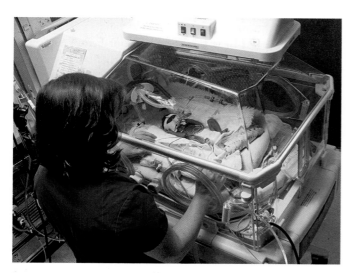

Figure 7–1 Premature infant in the NICU.

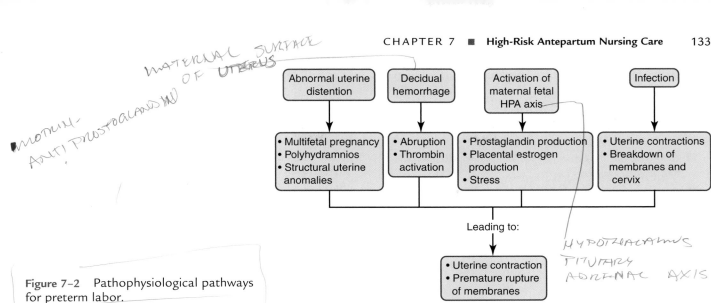

MATERIAL SURFACE OF UTERUS

MOTRIN - ANTI PROSTAGLANDIN

Abnormal uterine distention
- Multifetal pregnancy
- Polyhydramnios
- Structural uterine anomalies

Decidual hemorrhage
- Abruption
- Thrombin activation

Activation of maternal fetal HPA axis
- Prostaglandin production
- Placental estrogen production
- Stress

Infection
- Uterine contractions
- Breakdown of membranes and cervix

Leading to:
- Uterine contraction
- Premature rupture of membranes

HYPOTHALAMUS PITUITARY ADRENAL AXIS

Figure 7–2 Pathophysiological pathways for preterm labor.

have no risk factors. Seventy percent of women who are at risk for preterm delivery go on to deliver at term. Research indicates it is a complex interplay of multiple risk factors (PeriStats, 2008).

A host of behavioral, psychosocial, socio-demographic, and medical/pregnancy conditions, and biological factors are associated with risk for preterm birth (March of Dimes, 2011). The most consistently identified risk factors include a history of preterm birth; for example, the additive risk associated with multiple prior preterm births is especially evident when early preterm births are considered. Women with one prior preterm delivery <35 weeks have a 16% recurrence risk, those with two early preterm deliveries have a 41% risk, and those with three prior preterm deliveries have a 67% risk of subsequent preterm birth before 35 weeks (NIH, DHHS, 2008).

Common risk factors include (Freda, Patterson, & Wieczorek, 2004; Goldstein, 2007):

- Prior preterm birth (single most important factor reoccurrence rates of up to 40%) *#1*
- History of second trimester loss
- History of incompetent cervix
- Cerclage *(SURG INTERVENTION → CERVIX CLOSED)*
- IVF pregnancy
- Multiple gestation (50% of twins delivered preterm, ≥90% higher multiples delivered preterm)
- Uterine/cervical abnormalities, diethylstilbestrol (DES) exposure
- Hydramnios or oligohydramnios
- Infection, especially genitourinary infections and periodontal disease
- Premature rupture of membranes
- Short pregnancy interval (less than 9 months)
- Pregnancy associated problems such as hypertension, diabetes, and vaginal bleeding
- Chronic health problems such as hypertension, diabetes, or clotting disorders
- Inadequate nutrition, low BMI, low pre-pregnancy weight, or poor weight gain
- Age younger than 17 or older than 35 years old

UTI - SILENT D/T FREQ

- Late or no prenatal care
- Obesity, high BMI, or excessive weight gain
- Low BMI
- Working long hours, long periods of standing
- Ancestry and ethnicity
  - *Preterm birth rates are highest for African American infants (17.8% vs. 12.2%) (March of Dimes, 2012).*
- Maternal unmarried status is associated with an increased risk of preterm birth as well as low birth weight and small for gestational age (Shah, Zao, & Ali, 2011).
- Preterm birth is more likely in the presence of intimate partner violence (IPV), mental health issues, substance abuse, and other psychosocial stressors (March of Dimes, 2011).
  - *Maternal exposure to domestic violence is associated with significantly increased risk of low birth weight and preterm birth. Inadequate prenatal care, higher incidences of high-risk behaviors, direct physical trauma, stress, and neglect are postulated mechanisms (Shah & Shah, 2010).*
- Lack of social support
- Smoking, alcohol, and illicit drug use
- Lower education and socioeconomic status, poverty

Most preterm births (75%) are a result of spontaneous preterm labor (40%) and/or preterm premature rupture of membrane (PPROM) (35%) and related diagnoses (Iams, 2007; Owen & Harger, 2007; Creasy, Resnik, & Iams, 2004). However, more than 20% of preterm births are clinically indicated for complications (intentional preterm birth).

Prediction and Detection of Preterm Labor

Early detection of pregnant women who will give birth prematurely has been extensively research since the 1970s with few definitive findings. No screening methods have been found to be consistently effective.

Tests for preterm birth prediction include biomarkers for decidual-membrane separation, such as fetal fibronectin; proteomics to identify inflammatory activity; and genomics for susceptibility for preterm birth. Since 1998, cervical length, bacterial vaginosis, and the presence of fetal fibronectin in cervicovaginal fluid have been identified as factors most strongly linked to risk of spontaneous preterm births (March of Dimes, 2011).

■ Uterine contraction monitoring and cervical change has a 40% false positive rate.
■ Transvaginal cervical ultrasonography
    ■ *In symptomatic women a cervical length of >30 mm reliably excludes preterm labor.*
    ■ *A cervical length of <20 mm has strong positive predictive value.*
■ Fetal fibronectin has a low positive predictive value but a high negative predictive value, thereby making it a useful test to predict those women who will NOT deliver preterm.

Risks for the Woman Related to Preterm Labor and Birth

■ Complications related to bed rest and treatment with tocolytics

Risks for the Fetus and Newborn Related to Preterm Labor and Birth

■ Complications of prematurity and long term sequelae associated with prematurity (see Chapter 17)

Assessment Findings

Criteria for the diagnosis of preterm labor have varied, and there is not universal agreement on criteria.

■ Persistent uterine contractions (see Critical Component: Diagnosis of Preterm Labor) >6h + 1 or ↓
■ Dilated to 1 cm or greater or 80% effaced or ROM
■ Positive biochemical marker
    ■ *Fetal fibronectin (fFN) is an extracellular matrix protein that acts as glue that attaches the fetal membranes to the underlying uterine decidua (Iams, 2007). It is detected via immunoassay; a positive test is greater than 50 ng/mL. A negative fFN has a high negative predictive value (up to 95%) that the woman will not deliver in 7–14 days. It has a poor positive predictive value (25%–40%), which limits its ability to predict women who will deliver preterm (Iams, 2007; Simpson & Creehan, 2008). In other words, fFN is better at predicting who will not deliver preterm than who will deliver preterm.*

CRITICAL COMPONENT

Diagnosis of Preterm Labor

The diagnosis of preterm labor is made when the following criteria are met:

■ Gestational age of >20 weeks and <37 weeks
■ Documented regular uterine contractions (UCs) >6/hour *and* at least one of the following:
    ■ Rupture of membranes (ROM)
    ■ Cervical change: Cervix >1 cm dilated or 80% effaced (criteria for cervical dilation varies)

Medical Management

Current interventions to stop preterm labor have not been proven to be effective (Cunningham et al., 2010; Goldstein, 2007). The cornerstones of management of preterm labor are still administration of medications to stop uterine contractions and bed rest. Although there is little evidence to support these strategies and despite recommendations to the contrary (ACOG, 2012), they are still commonly used. Typically management is focused on delaying delivery for several days (optimal is 72 hours) to give glucocorticoids (corticosteroids) time to facilitate fetal lung maturity. Medical management includes:

■ **Tocolytic drugs** are medications that are used to suppress uterine contractions in preterm labor. There are no clear "first-line" tocolytic drugs to manage preterm labor. Clinical circumstances and physician preferences should dictate treatment (ACOG, 2003). These agents have drawbacks and potential serious adverse effects (**Table 7-1**). A review of evidence on tocolytic therapy revealed a small improvement in pregnancy prolongation and that extended use has little or no value (Berkman et al., 2003).
■ Tocolytic drugs may prolong pregnancy for 2 to 7 days, which may allow for administration of steroids to ⊃x in 24h improve fetal lung maturity and the consideration of maternal transport to a tertiary care facility.
■ Neither maintenance treatment with tocolytic drugs nor repeated acute tocolysis improve perinatal outcome; neither should be undertaken as a general practice (ACOG, 2012).
■ Current management now is focused on delaying delivery for several days to give corticosteroids time to work and to treat Group B *Streptococcus* infections. Using tocolytic drugs to delay delivery for a few days is well documented. However, their impact on decreasing prematurity is yet unproved (Creasy, Resnik, & Iams, 2004). Terbutaline pump therapy has not been shown to decrease the risk of preterm birth by prolonging pregnancy (Nanda, Cook, Gallo, & Grimes, 2002). Bed rest, hydration, and pelvic rest do not appear to improve the rate of preterm birth and should not be routinely recommended (ACOG, 2013; Goldstein, 2007).
■ Despite extensive evidence, bed rest is not effective; bed rest is a widely used first step in the treatment of preterm labor. Current evidence based on systematic reviews of research on bed rest during pregnancy highlights potential adverse effects on the woman and her family (Maloni, 1993, 1998; Sosa, Althabe, Belizán, & Bergel, 2004):
    ■ *Muscle atrophy*
    ■ *Cardiovascular deconditioning*
    ■ *Maternal weight loss*
    ■ *Stress for the woman and her family*
■ Intravenous hydration is a common strategy to reduce preterm uterine contractions because it increases vascular volume and may help to decrease contractions. It should be used with caution due to the potential for pulmonary edema when tocolytic agents are used. There has been no evidence that hydration can avert PTB.
■ Antibiotics are commonly used to treat genital urinary infections, but prophylactic antibiotic treatment is not

TABLE 7-1 COMMON TOCOLYTIC DRUGS

DRUG	PHARMACOLOGY AND ACTION	DOSAGE AND ADMINISTRATION	MATERNAL EFFECTS AND CONTRAINDICATIONS	FETAL EFFECTS	NURSING CONSIDERATIONS
MAGNESIUM SULFATE (MgSO₄)	Depresses myometrium contractility, relaxes smooth muscle of the uterus. It has not been proven to have either short- or long-term effectiveness as a tocolytic agent.	Administered continuous IV infusion via a pump. Initial loading dose of 4–6 g in 20 minutes, then 2 g/hr. Therapeutic level at 5–8 mg/dL in maternal serum levels, or as tolerated by the patient.	Flushing, lethargy, headache, muscle weakness, diplopia, dry mouth, pulmonary edema, cardiac arrest. Respiratory depression can occur with serum levels above 9 mg/dL. Contraindications include myasthenia gravis.	Lethargy, hypotonia, respiratory depression, demineralization with prolonged use. No demonstrable effect on the neonate. Evidence suggests MgSO₄ given before early preterm birth may reduce risk of cerebral palsy.	Monitor FHR and UCs. Monitor serum magnesium levels. Signs and symptoms of maternal toxicity include: • Absent DTRs, respiratory rate < 14 breaths/min, severe hypotension and muscle relaxation, decreased level of consciousness • Assess lungs for signs and symptoms of pulmonary edema. Check I&O for fluid overload or output of <30 mL/hr. For details of care of the woman and Magnesium Sulfate see Critical Component: Care of the Woman on Magnesium Sulfate.
PROSTAGLANDIN SYNTHESIS INHIBITORS Indomethacin Naproxen Fenoprofen	Depresses synthesis of prostaglandins Effective in delaying delivery 48+ hours; because of fetal side effects generally used short term and before 32 weeks.	Indomethacin 50 mg orally loading dose, then 25–50 mg orally every 6 hours Contraindications include significant renal or hepatic impairment (for indomethacin), active peptic ulcer disease (for ketorolac), coagulation disorders or thrombocytopenia,	Nausea, heartburn GI upset; serious side effects are uncommon.	Constriction of ductus arteriosus, pulmonary hypertension, reversible decrease in renal function with oligohydramnios, intraventricular hemorrhage, hyperbilirubinemia, necrotizing enterocolitis Serious fetal side effects include constriction of the patent ductus arteriosus, neonatal pulmonary hypertension, oligohydramniosis, and	Monitor FHR and UCs. Treat nausea and heartburn.

Continued

TABLE 7-1 COMMON TOCOLYTIC DRUGS—cont'd

DRUG	PHARMACOLOGY AND ACTION	DOSAGE AND ADMINISTRATION	MATERNAL EFFECTS AND CONTRAINDICATIONS	FETAL EFFECTS	NURSING CONSIDERATIONS
		nonsteroidal anti-inflammatory drug (NSAID)-sensitive asthma, other sensitivity to NSAIDs (for sulindac).		intraventricular hemorrhages.	
CALCIUM CHANNEL BLOCKERS Nifedipine Nicardipine	Inhibits smooth muscle contractions of uterus by blocking calcium availability for muscle contraction. As effective or superior as other agents in delaying delivery 48–72 hours.	10–20 mg PO every 4–6 hours	Flushing, headache, dizziness, nausea, transient hypotension. Caution should be used in patients with renal disease and hypotension when administering calcium channel blockers. In addition, concomitant use of calcium channel blockers and is potentially harmful and has resulted in cardiovascular collapse. Flushing, headache, nausea, transient tachycardia and hypotension Contraindications include cardiac disease; should not be used concomitantly with . • Terbutaline	None noted as yet Limited clinical evidence on fetal effects may decrease uteroplacental blood flow.	Monitor FHR and UCs. Monitor maternal blood pressure and heart rate and may hold dose for blood pressure <90/50 or heart rate >120.
BETA-ADRENERGIC AGONISTS Terbutaline The U.S. Food and Drug Administration (FDA) notified health care professionals that injectable terbutaline should not be used in pregnant women for prevention or prolonged treatment (beyond 48–72 hours) of preterm	Beta 2 adrenergic effects to suppress uterine activity Can delay delivery for 3 days. Given IV or SQ. Oral use of drugs has not demonstrated any improvement in preterm birth or preterm labor.	Terbutaline IV/SQ IV maximum dose 0.08 mg/min SQ; 0.25 mg every 3–4 hours Ritodrine IV maximum dose .350 mg/min	Cardiac or cardiopulmonary arrhythmias, pulmonary edema, myocardial ischemia, hypotension, tachycardia Highest rates of serious maternal side effects including tachycardia, cardiac arrhythmia, myocardial ischemia and pulmonary edema, elevation in maternal glucose, hypokalemia • Ritodrine	• Terb Fetal tachycardia, hyperinsulinemia, hyperglycemia, myocardial and septal hypertrophy, myocardial ischemia • Mild fetal tachycardia, conflicting reports on incidence of Ritodrine Neonatal tachycardia, hypoglycemia, Hypocalcemia,	Monitor FHR and UCs. Monitor I&O for fluid overload. Auscultate lungs for pulmonary edema. Monitor maternal HR and may hold dose for heart rate >120. Monitor blood glucose. Life-threatening complications are pulmonary edema,

labor in either the hospital or outpatient setting because of the potential for serious maternal heart problems and death. In addition, oral terbutaline should not be used for prevention or any treatment of preterm labor because it has not been shown to be effective and has similar safety concerns. FDA is requiring the addition of a new Boxed Warning and Contraindication to the terbutaline drug labels to warn health care professionals about these risks.

Ritodrine

Metabolic hyperglycemia, hyperinsulinemia, hypokalemia, antidiuresis, altered thyroid function, physiological tremor, palpitations, nervousness, nausea or vomiting, fever, hallucinations

Contraindications include cardiac arrhythmias (for terbutaline) and poorly controlled thyroid disease and diabetes mellitus (for Ritodrine).

hyperbilirubinemia, hypotension, intraventricular hemorrhage

IVH

myocardial failure, and fluid overload.

Contraindicated in women with cardiac disease.

Sources: Gilbert (2011); Deglin & Vallerand (2007); Reedy (2014); (ACOG, 2012); (ACOG, 2010).

recommended (Creasy, Resnik, & Iams, 2004). Antibiotics do not appear to prolong gestation and should be reserved for group B streptococcal prophylaxis in patients in whom delivery is imminent (ACOG, 2012).

- **Progesterone** supplementation may be useful to prevent preterm birth for women with a history of spontaneous preterm birth (ACOG, 2008; Meis, Klebanoff, Thom, Dombrowski, Sibai, Moawad, Spong, Hauth, Miodovnik, Varner, Leveno, Caritis, Iams, Wapner, Conway, O'Sullivan, Carpenter, Mercer, Ramin, Thorp, Peaceman, & Gabbe, 2003). Use of 17-alpha-hydroxyprogesterone-caproate at 250 mg/week beginning at 16 weeks to 36 weeks of gestation is considered safe (Meis, 2007). It is not recommended for prophylactic use in multiple gestation.
- Neonatal neuroprophylaxis with intravenous magnesium sulfate administration is recommended to reduce microcapillary brain hemorrhage in premature birth of the neonate (Doyle, Crowther, Middleton, Marret, & Rouse, 2009). Magnesium sulfate tocolysis with a loading bolus and maintenance dose is given to the mother for 12 hours to protect the fetal brain and can be repeated whenever preterm delivery is imminent.
- **Corticosteroid therapy,** with antenatal steroids, is currently recommended to women at risk of preterm birth (see Medication: Corticosteroids). Betamethasone is one antenatal steroid given to women to accelerate fetal lung maturity, thereby decreasing the severity of respiratory distress syndrome and other complications of prematurity in the neonate. Treatment with antenatal corticosteroids reduces the risk of neonatal respiratory distress syndrome, cerebroventricular hemorrhage, necrotizing enterocolitis, and infectious morbidity in the neonate when used between 24 and 34 weeks' gestation (Roberts & Dalziel, 2006).
  - *The short-term benefits for babies of less respiratory distress and fewer serious health problems in the first few weeks after birth support the use of repeat dose(s) of prenatal corticosteroids for women still at risk of **preterm birth** seven days or more after an initial course. These benefits were associated with a small reduction in size at birth. The current available evidence reassuringly shows no significant harm in early childhood, although no benefit (Crowther, McKinlay, Middleton, & Harding, 2011).*
- If UCs decrease to fewer than five per hour, then women are often transferred to less acute antenatal units for further observation for several days. If they remain stable, they may be discharged to home undelivered. Discharge instructions typically include bed rest or activity restriction, self-monitoring of uterine activity, and signs and symptoms of preterm labor, and may include oral tocolytics or use of terbutaline pump therapy, but these are no longer commonly used. There has been no demonstrated benefit to maintenance tocolytic therapy (Cunningham et al., 2010).
- Contraindications to treating preterm labor include:
  - *Active hemorrhage*
  - *Severe maternal disease*
  - *Fetal compromise*
  - *Chorioamnionitis*
  - *Fetal death*
  - *Previable gestation and PPROM*

- General contraindications for tocolysis include severe preeclampsia, placental abruption, intrauterine infection, lethal congenital or chromosomal abnormalities, advanced cervical dilatation, myasthenia gravis, concurrent treatment with nifedipine, terbutaline use in the previous 4 hours, and evidence of fetal compromise or placental insufficiency (ACOG, 2012). Myocardial compromise or cardiac conduction defects, renal disease, and hypertensive disease are indications for precautionary use.

Medication

Corticosteroids

Betamethasone

- Indication: Given to women at 24 and 34 weeks' gestation with signs of preterm labor or at risk to deliver preterm
- Action: Stimulate the production of more mature surfactant in the fetal lungs to prevent respiratory distress syndrome in premature infants
- Adverse reactions: Will raise blood sugar and may require temporary insulin coverage to maintain euglycemia in diabetic women
- Route and dose: Betamethasone 12 mg IM every 24 hours × 2 doses

(Deglin & Vallerand, 2009; Goldstein, 2007; ACOG, 2012)

Nursing Actions

Nurses can provide expertise in directing patient care, stabilizing the woman and fetus, counseling, coordinating care, and providing patient teaching (Grey, 2006; March of Dimes, 2006b). Immediate care, including assessment and stabilization, occurs in labor and delivery. If uterine activity decreases, generally to fewer than 5 UCs/hr, and there is no further cervical change, women are often moved to a less intensive care setting than a labor and delivery unit. Once moved to an antenatal high-risk unit, they are often observed for several days and, if stable, discharged to home undelivered.

Immediate care:

- Review the prenatal record for risk factors and establish gestational age through history and ultrasound (ultrasound early in pregnancy is more reliable for gestational age).
- Assess the woman and fetus for signs and symptoms of:
  - *Vaginal and urinary infection*
  - *Rupture of membranes*
    - A sterile speculum exam may be performed to assess for ferning of the amniotic fluid.
  - *Vaginal bleeding or vaginal discharge*
  - *Dehydration*
- Assess fetal heart rate (FHR) and uterine contractions.
  - *Report fetal tachycardia or increased uterine contractions to the health care provider.*
- Obtain vaginal and urine cultures as per orders.
- Obtain fFN as per orders.
  - *This should be obtained before the sterile vaginal exam. Contraindicated if ROM, bleeding, sexual intercourse, or prior collection in the last 24 hours.*

- Maintain strict input and output (I&O).
- Provide oral or IV hydration.
  - *May restrict total intake to 3,000 mL/24 hr if on tocolytics.*
- Administer tocolytic agents as per protocol.
  - *Monitor for adverse reactions (see Table 7–1).*
- Administer glucocorticoids (betamethasone) as per orders.
- Position the patient on her side to increase uteroplacental perfusion and decrease pressure on the maternal inferior vena cava.
- Assess vital signs per protocol for tocolytic administered.
  - *Report to the provider blood pressure greater than 140/90 mm Hg or less than 90/50 mm Hg; heart rate greater than 120; temperature greater than 100.4°F (38°C).*
- Auscultate lungs for evidence of pulmonary edema.
- Assess cervical status with a sterile vaginal exam unless contraindicated by ROM or bleeding (may be done by the health care provider to minimize multiple exams); cervical ultrasound may be done (cervical length of less than 30 mm is clinically significant).
- Facilitate a clear understanding of the treatment plan and the woman and family's involvement in clinical decision making.
- Notify the care provider of findings.

Continuing care once stable:

- Provide emotional support to the woman by providing opportunities to discuss her feelings. Women often feel guilt that they caused the preterm labor, are concerned for the infant's health, and have anxiety and sadness over loss of "normal" newborn and normal pregnancy labor and delivery (see Critical Component: Nursing Actions to Promote Adaptation to Pregnancy Complications).
- Facilitate a clear understanding of the treatment plan and the woman and family's involvement in clinical decision making.
- Facilitate consultations with the neonatal staff regarding neonatal survival rates, the anticipated care of the newborn, treatments, complications, and possible long-term disabilities. The family may be taken on a tour of NICU.
- Monitor the woman's response to treatment including FHR baseline and variability and uterine contractions, maternal vital signs, woman's response to tocolytics, increase in vaginal discharge, or ROM.
- Assessment of women on tocolytics is based on tocolytic used and is detailed in Table 7-1, but generally includes monitoring of blood pressure and pulse and auscultation of lungs for pulmonary edema. Watch for:
  - *Shortness of breath, chest tightness or discomfort, cough, oxygen saturation less than 95%, increased respiratory and heart rates*
  - *Changes in behavior such as apprehension, anxiety, or restlessness*
- Encourage a side-lying position to enhance placental perfusion.
- Evaluate laboratory reports such as urine and cervical cultures.
  - *White blood cell (WBC) counts are elevated in women who have received corticosteroids; therefore, elevated WBCs are not indicative of infection.*

- Provide ongoing reassurance and explanations to the woman and her family.
- Explain the purpose and side effects of the medication.
- Set short-term goals such as completion of a gestational week or milestones.
- Facilitate family interactions and visiting by having flexible visiting policies.
- Facilitate a clear understanding of the treatment plan and the woman's involvement in clinical decision making.
- Assist with passive limb exercises for women on bed rest to decrease muscle deterioration.
- Assist with hygiene and self-care based on orders for activity.
- Provide diversional activities that interest the woman.

CRITICAL COMPONENT

Nursing Activities to Promote Adaptation to Pregnancy Complications

Pregnancy complications represent a threat to both the woman and fetus's health and to the emotional well-being of the family. Assessment of emotional status and coping of the entire family is necessary to provide comprehensive care. Implementing individualized plan of care will facilitate the family's transition during an often unexpected and frightening experience (Gilbert, 2011). Responses to high-risk pregnancy can include:

- Anxiety related to unmet needs
- Threats to self-esteem; the woman may feel she has somehow failed as a woman and/or is failing as a mother.
- Self-blaming commonly occurs for real or imagined wrongdoing.
- Frustration often occurs when goals of having a healthy pregnancy, a normal birth, and a healthy baby are impeded by a pregnancy complication.
- Conflict can occur when competing and opposing goals are presented during a high-risk pregnancy.
- Crisis occurs when the woman and her family are threatened by a pregnancy complication and an uncertain outcome.

Some general nursing actions include:

- Provide time for the woman and family to express their concerns, which may include apprehension, fear, anger, and frustration. Talking can help them identify, analyze, and understand their experience and fears.
- Provide information repeatedly with patient and significant other(s) to facilitate a realistic appraisal of events.
- Explain high-risk conditions, procedures, diagnostic tests, and treatment plan in layman's terms.
  - *Provide ongoing updates.*
  - *Clarify misconceptions.*
- Facilitate referrals related to the condition, which may include social services and chaplain services to enhance family coping and provide resources.
- Practice active listening.
- Self-blaming commonly occurs for real or imagined wrongdoing. Discussing with the woman the underlying causes of a complication may help to alleviate these feelings.
- Encourage the woman and her family to participate in decision making and care to provide autonomy.
- If patient is hospitalized, have flexible guide lines for the family to minimize separation.

Discharge Plan

All plans should be decided with the woman's and family's strengths, needs, and goals in mind and with their participation (March of Dimes, 2006b) (**Fig. 7-3**). Discharge teaching should include:

- Warning signs and how and when to call the provider (**Box 7-1**)
- A clear understanding of the treatment plan including use of tocolytics and bed rest/activity restriction (**Box 7-2**)

Programs have demonstrated some improvement in outcomes with nurse phone or home care follow-up (Freda, Patterson, & Wieczorek, 2004; Gilbert, 2007). Typically, women treated for preterm labor are sent home without follow-up at home except for weekly prenatal visits. Topics

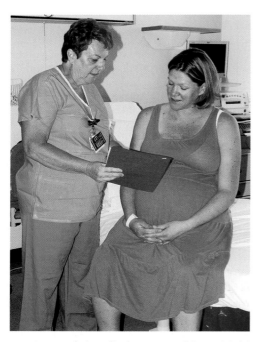

Figure 7–3　Nurse doing discharge teaching with high-risk pregnant woman in the hospital.

BOX 7–1　WARNING SIGNS OF PRETERM LABOR

Call your doctor or midwife or the hospital for any of the following:

- Your bag of waters breaks.
- Your baby stops moving.
- You have more than _____ contractions in an hour.
- You have a low backache, menstrual-like cramps, pelvic pressure, or intestinal cramps with or without diarrhea.
- You have increased discharge from your vagina.
- You have a fever higher than 100.4°F (38°C).
- You feel "something is not right."

　MD or midwife number is _____
　Hospital labor and delivery number is _____

BOX 7–2　HOME CARE INSTRUCTIONS FOR PRETERM LABOR

Baby movements and contractions	Lie on your side for 1 hour and count the number of times your baby moves. If your baby does not move _____ times, call your doctor or midwife. 　While lying on your side place your fingertips on your abdomen and feel for tightening. If you have more than _____ contractions in 1 hour, call your doctor or midwife.
Activity restrictions	Indicate restrictions on physical activity and be specific.
Sexual relations	Indicate restrictions on sexual relations.
Diet	Small meals and snacks may be easier to tolerate, and be sure to include foods high in fiber, calcium, and iron.
Fluids	Drink at least eight 8-ounce glasses of fluid a day including water, milk, and juices.
Medication schedule	Per discharge orders with teaching related to specific medications may include: tocolytic, prenatal vitamin (PNV), iron sulfate, stool softeners

that should be discussed include (Durham, 1998; Maloni, 1998):

- Effects of activity restriction on the woman and family, including emotional distress (see Evidence-Based Practice: Cochrane Review on Social Support during at-risk Pregnancy)
- Maternal anxiety about the health of the woman and fetus
- Child care difficulties when on bed rest and plan for at home
- Financial and career difficulties
- Physical activity restrictions may include restricted sexual activity.

Preterm Premature Rupture of Membranes/Chorioamnionitis

Preterm premature rupture of membranes (PPROM) is rupture of membranes with a premature gestation (<37 weeks). It occurs in about 3% of pregnancies yet is responsible for about 30% of all preterm births. **Premature rupture of membranes** is defined as rupture of the chorioamniotic membranes before the onset of labor but at term. Adding to the confusion is **prolonged rupture of membranes**, which is greater than 24 hours (PROM). This section focuses on those women that have rupture of membranes preterm (PPROM) because it accounts for approximately one third of premature births. Once the membranes rupture preterm, most women go into labor within a week. The term **latency** refers to the time from membrane rupture to delivery. **Previable PROM** is rupture of membranes (ROM) before 23–24 weeks,

[handwritten: Premature Rupture of membranes]

preterm PROM remote from term is from 24–32 weeks' gestation, and **preterm PROM near term** is 31–36 weeks' gestation (Mercer, 2007).

Premature rupture of membranes is a multifactorial, although choriodecidual, infection and inflammation appears to be an important factor especially with preterm PROM at earlier gestations (Mercer, 2007). Bacterial infections are thought to weaken the membranes leading to rupture, but in most cases the cause is unknown.

Risk Factors for Preterm PROM

- Previous preterm PROM or preterm delivery
- Bleeding during pregnancy
- Hydramnios
- Multiple gestation (up to 15% in twins, up to 20% in triplets)
- Sexually transmitted infections (STIs)
- Cigarette smoking

Risks for the Woman

- Maternal infection (i.e., chorioamnionitis)
- Preterm labor and birth
- Increased rates of cesarean birth

Risks for the Fetus and Newborn

- Fetal or neonatal sepsis
  - *The earlier the fetal gestation at ROM, the greater the risk for infection*
  - *The membranes serve as a protective barrier that separates the sterile fetus and fluid from the bacteria-laden vaginal canal.*
- Preterm delivery and complications of prematurity
- Hypoxia or asphyxia because of umbilical cord compression due to decreased fluid
- Fetal deformities if preterm PROM before 26 weeks' gestation

Assessment Findings

- Confirmed premature gestational age by prenatal history and ultrasound
- Confirmed rupture of membranes with speculum exam and positive ferning test *[handwritten: not nitrazine (false + w/ sperm)]*
- Oligohydramnios on ultrasound may be seen but is not diagnostic.

Medical Management

The risk of perinatal complications changes drastically with gestational age at membrane rupture. Therefore, a gestational age–based approach is appropriate for medical management (Mercer, 2007). Medical treatment is aimed at balancing the risks of prematurity and the risks of infections. Unless near term gestation premature PROM, management is aimed at prolonging gestation for the woman who is not in labor, not infected, and not experiencing fetal compromise. Conservative management refers to treatment directed at continuing the pregnancy. According to ACOG (2007), guidelines for management include:

- Patients with PROM between 34–36 weeks should be managed as if they were at term with induction of labor and treatment for group B streptococcal prophylaxis recommended.
- Patients with PROM before 32 weeks of gestation should be cared for expectantly until 33 completed weeks of gestation if no maternal or fetal contraindications exist.
  - *A 48-hour course of intravenous ampicillin and erythromycin followed by 5 days of amoxicillin and erythromycin is recommended during expectant management of preterm PROM remote from term to prolong pregnancy and to reduce infectious and gestational age–dependent neonatal morbidity. Although antibiotics have been unsuccessful for the treatment of women with intact membranes, adjunctive antibiotic therapy is recommended for women who are managed expectantly after preterm PROM.*
- All women with preterm PROM and a viable fetus, including those known to be carriers of group B streptococci and those who give birth before carrier status can be delineated, should receive intrapartum chemoprophylaxis to prevent vertical transmission of group B streptococci regardless of earlier treatments.
- A single course of antenatal corticosteroids should be administered to women with preterm PROM before 32 weeks of gestation to reduce the risks of respiratory distress syndrome (RDS), perinatal mortality, and other morbidities.
- Delivery is recommended when preterm PROM occurs at or beyond 34 weeks of gestation.
- With preterm PROM at 32–33 completed weeks of gestation, labor induction may be considered if fetal pulmonary maturity has been documented.
- Digital cervical examinations should be avoided in patients with PROM unless they are in active labor or imminent delivery is anticipated.
- Monitor for infection, labor, and fetal compromise.
- Assess for fetal lung maturity with LS ratio/phosphatidyl glycerol (PG).
- Administer prophylactic antibiotic therapy to reduce maternal and fetal infections.
- The use of tocolytics is controversial, as is the use of corticosteroids to accelerate lung maturity, but they appear to improve outcomes when used before 32 weeks' gestation and in conjunction with prophylactic antibiotic therapy (Mercer, 2007; Creasy, Resnik, & Iams, 2004).
- With previable PROM before 24 weeks' gestation, recommendations include:
  - *Patient counseling about risks to fetus*
  - *Expectant management or induction of labor*
  - *Group B streptococcal prophylaxis is not recommended.*
  - *Corticosteroids are not recommended.*
  - *Antibiotics—there are incomplete data on use in prolonging latency.*

Nursing Actions

- Assess FHR and uterine contractions.
- Assess for signs of infection including:
  - *Maternal and/or fetal tachycardia*
  - *Maternal fever 100.4°F (38°C) or greater*

■ *Uterine tenderness*
■ *Malodorous fluid or vaginal discharge*
■ Monitor for labor and for fetal compromise.
■ Provide antenatal testing including non-stress tests (NSTs) and biophysical profiles (BPPs).
■ See Critical Component: Nursing Activities to Promote Adaptation to Pregnancy.

Evidence-Based Practice: Cochrane Review on Social Support During At-Risk Pregnancy

Hodnett, E. (2010). Support during pregnancy for women at increased risk of low birthweight babies. *Cochrane Database Of Systematic Reviews*, (6), Accessed November 23, 2012.

Programs offering additional support during pregnancy were not effective in reducing the number of babies born too early and babies with low birth weights. Babies born to mothers in socially disadvantaged situations are more likely to be small and so have health problems. Programs providing emotional support, practical assistance, and advice have been offered in addition to usual care.

Randomized trials of additional support during at-risk pregnancy by either a professional (social worker, midwife, or nurse) or specially trained layperson, compared to routine care. They defined additional support as some form of emotional support (e.g., counseling, reassurance, sympathetic listening) and information or advice, or both, either in home visits or during clinic appointments, and could include tangible assistance (e.g., transportation to clinic appointments, assistance with care of other children at home).

The review of 17 randomized controlled trials, involving 12,264 women, found that women who received additional support during pregnancy were less likely to be admitted to the hospital for pregnancy complications and to have a cesarean birth. However, the additional support did not reduce the likelihood of giving birth too early or that the baby was smaller than expected.

Authors' Conclusions

Pregnant women need the support of caring family members, friends, and health professionals. While programs which offer additional support during pregnancy are unlikely to prevent the pregnancy from resulting in a low birth weight or preterm baby, they may be helpful in reducing the likelihood of antenatal hospital admission and caesarean birth.

Incompetent Cervix

Incompetent cervix is classically defined as a mechanical defect in the cervix that results in painless cervical dilation in the second trimester that can progress to ballooning of the membranes into the vagina and delivery of a premature fetus (Cunningham et al., 2010). When undiagnosed, it can result in repeated second trimester abortions. Currently there is more discussion of **cervical insufficiency**, a process of premature cervical ripening, and the notion of cervical competency existing of reproductive performance on a continuum rather than all or none, competent versus incompetent (Owen & Harger, 2007).

The cause of cervical incompetence is unclear, but it is associated with previous cervical trauma such as cervical dilation and curettage or cauterization, and abnormal cervical development from genetics or diethylstilbestrol (DES) exposure in utero, infection and inflammation, and/or local or systemic hormonal effects.

Risks to the Woman

■ Repeated second trimester or early third trimester births
■ Recurrent pregnancy losses (e.g., spontaneous abortions)
■ Preterm delivery
■ Rupture of membranes/infection

Risk to the Fetus and Newborn

■ Preterm birth and consequences of prematurity

Assessment Findings

■ Woman reports pelvic pressure and increased mucoid vaginal discharge.
■ Shortened cervical length or funneling of the cervix, although use of ultrasound to diagnose cervical incompetence is not currently recommended (Cunningham et al., 2010).
■ Obstetrical history of second trimester cervical dilation or fetal losses
■ Live fetus and intact membranes

Medical Management

■ Obtain transcervical ultrasound to evaluate cervix for cervical length, and funneling may be done but is not diagnostic.
■ Cervical cultures for chlamydia, gonorrhea, and other cervical infections
■ Treatment of incompetent cervix is **cerclage,** which is a type of purse string suture placed cervically to reinforce a weak cervix (**Fig. 7-4**).
    ■ *Prophylactic cerclage may be placed in women with a history of unexplained recurrent painless dilation and second trimester birth, generally between 12 and 16 weeks of gestation.*
    ■ *Rescue cerclage is placed after the cervix has dilated with no perceived contractions, up to about 24 weeks of gestation (Cunningham et al., 2010).*
■ Administer antibiotics or tocolytics, but this has not been demonstrated to be effective and is controversial in perioperative period (Owen & Harger, 2007).
■ Remove sutures if membranes rupture, infection occurs, or labor develops.

Postoperative Nursing Actions

■ Monitor for uterine activity with palpation.
■ Monitor for vaginal bleeding and leaking of fluid/rupture of membranes.
■ Monitor for infection.
    ■ *Maternal fever*
    ■ *Uterine tenderness*
■ Administer tocolytics to suppress uterine activity as per orders.

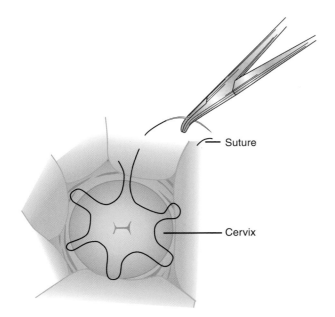

Figure 7-4 Cerclage.

■ Discharge teaching may include teaching patient to:
  ■ *Monitor for signs and symptoms of uterine activity, rupture of membranes, bleeding, infection*
  ■ *Modify activity and pelvic rest for a week*

Multiple Gestation

Multiple gestation pregnancies are pregnancies with more than one fetus. In 2009, 3.5% of all live births were multiple births, and 96.5% were singleton births in the United States. Over 3 decades, the twin birth rate rose 74% (Martin, Hamilton, & Osterman, 2012). An increase in multiple births is related to increasing maternal age and greater use of infertility treatment. They are more common now because of the use of ovulation-stimulating drugs and assisted reproductive technology (ART). Approximately one third of twins are monozygotic (from one egg) and two thirds are dizygotic (from two eggs) (Fig. 7-5A & B).

■ **Monozygotic twins** are from one zygote that divides in the first week of gestation. They are genetically identical and similar in appearance and always have the same gender.
■ **Dizygotic twins** result from fertilization of two eggs. Dizygotic twins may be the same or differing genders. If the fetuses are of differing gender, they are dizygotic and therefore dichorionic.

Either of these processes can be involved in the development of higher order multiples.

The rate of twin specific complications varies in relation to zygosity and chorionicity. There are two principal placental types, **monochorionic** (one chorion) and **dichorionic** (two chorions). About 20% of twins are monochorionic, and it indicates monozygotic twins. There are increased rates of perinatal mortality and neurological injury in monochorionic, diamniotic twins compared with dichorionic pairs (**Fig. 7-5A**).

Only 1% of monozygotic twins are **monoamniotic** that share the same amniotic sac. Because they share the same sac, monoamniotic twins have a fetal mortality rate of 50%–60% due to entangling of umbilical cords (Creasy, Resnik, & Iams, 2004) (**Fig. 7-5B**). **Conjoined twins** may result from an aberration in the twinning process ascribed to incomplete splitting of an embryo into two separate twins (Cunningham et al., 2010).

Although multiple gestations are only about 3% of births in the United States, they contribute disproportionately to maternal, fetal, and neonatal morbidity and mortality (Cunningham et al., 2010). Risks for both the fetus and the woman increase with increased number of fetuses (Creasy, Resnik, & Iams, 2004). Compared with women with twins, women with triplets or higher order multiples (HOM) are at even higher risk of pregnancy related morbidities and mortality (Bowers, 2014).

Risks for the Woman

■ Preterm labor and delivery rate is 50% or greater related to over distension of the uterus.
■ Premature prolonged rupture of membranes related to over distension of the uterus occurs up to 15% in twins and up to 20% in triplets.
■ Hypertensive disorders and preeclampsia, which tend to develop earlier and be more severe, are related to enlarged placenta.
■ Gestational diabetes often occurs due to physiological changes related to supporting multiple fetuses.
■ Antepartum hemorrhage, abruptio placenta, placenta previa
■ Anemia related to dilutional anemia
■ Pulmonary edema related to increase cardiac workload
■ Cesarean birth

Risks for the Fetus and Newborn

■ Increase in fetal morbidity and mortality due to sharing uterine space and placental circulation
  ■ *Increased perinatal mortality (threefold higher than in singleton pregnancy)*
  ■ *Intrauterine fetal death of one fetus after 20 weeks' gestation increases the risks to the surviving fetus(es).*
■ Delivery before term is the major reason for increased morbidity and mortality in twins. Rate of preterm delivery (50% higher in twins and >90% higher in multiples; i.e., triplets or higher). As the number of fetuses increases, the duration of gestation decreases.
■ Increase of low birth weight neonates (20% higher than singleton)
■ Increase of intrauterine growth restriction (IUGR) and discordant growth (weight of one fetus differs significantly from the others, usually ≥25%) related to placental insufficiency.
  ■ *Discordant growth and twin-to-twin transfusions from sharing a placenta occurs.*
  ■ *Vascular anastomosis between twins can occur with monochorionic twin placentas. Most of these vascular*

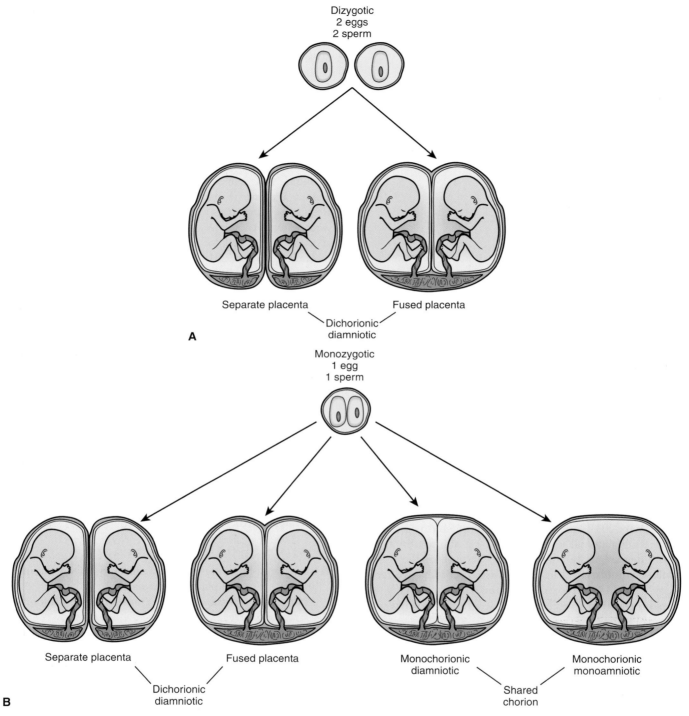

Figure 7–5   *A.* Monozygotic twins. *B.* Dizygotic twins.

communications are hemodynamically balanced and do not impact fetal development and perfusion.

■ *In twin-to-twin transfusion syndrome, blood is transfused from donor twin to recipient twin. Twin-to-twin transfusion is due to an imbalance in blood flow through the vasculature of the placenta because of arteriovenous anastomosis in the placenta. This results in overperfusion of one twin and can result in circulatory overload and* *heart failure and underperfusion and anemia of the co-twin.*

■ Increase of congenital, chromosomal, and genetic defects, in particular structural defects with monozygotic twins

Assessment Findings

■ Nearly every maternal system is affected by the physiological changes that occur in multiple gestations. These changes are greater in multiple pregnancies than in singleton pregnancies (Cunningham, 2010; Simpson & Creehan, 2008).

■ Elevation of human chorionic gonadotropin (hCG) may contribute to increased nausea and vomiting gonadotropin (hCG) and alpha-fetoprotein.
■ Ultrasound confirmation of multiple gestation
■ Chorionicity can be determined in the first trimester.
■ Fundal height and size greater than dates and palpation of excessive number of fetal parts during Leopold's maneuver
■ Maternal blood volume expansion is greater than 50%–60%, an additional 500 cc rather than 40%–50% with singleton gestation.
■ Increased cardiac output is increased an additional 20% and increased stroke volume.
■ Uterine growth is substantially greater, and uterine content may be up to 10 L and weigh in excess of 20 pounds.
■ Increased uterine size, which leads to increased susceptibility to uterine hypotensive syndrome and PTL and PPROM.
  ■ *This displaces lungs and can result in increased dyspnea and shortness of breath.*
■ Increased plasma volume 50%–100% (results in dilutional anemia)
■ Increased iron-deficiency anemia
■ Increased lower back and ligament pain
■ Increased dermatosis

Antepartal Medical Management

A woman pregnant with multiple fetuses needs ongoing, frequent surveillance of the pregnancy because of the increased rates of complications, including:

■ Ultrasound for discordant fetal growth and IUGR, as well as placental sites, dividing membranes, congenital anomalies, and gender(s)
■ Genetic testing for anomalies
■ Monitor for preterm labor and prevent preterm birth (Cunningham et al., 2010)
  ■ *Corticosteroids for fetal lung maturity are effective in reducing RDS and other complications of prematurity.*
  ■ *Studies demonstrate routine use of bed rest does not prolong pregnancy.*
  ■ *There is no evidence that tocolytic therapy improves outcomes.*
  ■ *Prophylactic cerclage has not been shown to be effective.*
■ Monitor for maternal anemia.
■ Fetal surveillance including NST, BPP
■ Monitor for hypertension and preeclampsia.
■ Monitor for hydramnios.
■ Monitor for antepartal hemorrhage.
■ Monitor for intrauterine fetal demise.
■ Nutritional consult
■ Consultation with perinatologist if complications occur

Intrapartum Medical Management

Many complications of labor and birth are encountered more often in multiple gestation deliveries including preterm labor, uterine contractile dysfunction, abnormal presentation, umbilical cord prolapse, abruption, and post-partum hemorrhage.

■ Type and crossmatch blood immediately available.
■ Ultrasound to confirm placental location and fetal positions
■ Continuous electronic fetal monitoring (EFM) of all fetuses
■ Cesarean birth access should be immediately available, including anesthesia, obstetricians, circulating nurse, and scrub personnel.
■ Agents for hemorrhagic management available, including medications and blood products
■ The neonatal team available should be sufficient for all infants.
■ Birth mode varies with fetal presentations, maternal and fetal health, and preference of the mother and the clinician (See Chapter 10):
  ■ *Vaginal birth for both infants*
  ■ *Cesarean birth for both*
  ■ *Combined vaginal and cesarean birth if first fetus is born vaginally and second fetus needs to be delivered by cesarean birth for malpresentation or category II or III fetal heart rate patterns.*
■ Triplets and higher multiples are delivered by cesarean birth.

Nursing Actions

■ Assess for the following possible complications:
  ■ *Preterm labor, however, uterine contractions as preterm labor can be more difficult to identify in women pregnant with multiple gestations because of more discomfort, stretching, and pressure with multiple fetuses, and overdistention of the uterus results in more uterine irritability (Gilbert, 2011).*
  ■ *Hypertension or preeclampsia*
  ■ *Antepartal hemorrhage*
■ Conduct antepartal surveillance including NST, amniotic fluid index (AFI), and BPP.
■ Provide information to the woman and her family regarding signs and symptoms of preterm labor, preeclampsia, and other possible complications related to multiple gestations.
■ Facilitate nutritional consult. The woman has an increased need for iron, calcium, and magnesium to support growth of multiple fetuses.
■ Provide emotional support to the woman and family. The woman and her family often experience an increase of stress related to fear of pregnancy loss, high-risk pregnancy, and potential complications during pregnancy and delivery, and anxiety related to caring for more than one infant.
■ Explain plan for PNC and antenatal testing and follow up related to multiple gestation.
■ Assess woman's and her partner's response to twin diagnosis and adaptation to multiple gestation
  ■ *Acknowledge feeling of distress and fear toward pregnancy.*
  ■ *Provide family with information on multiple and support groups.*
■ Provide psychological support appropriate to family's response.

- Discuss the plan of care for delivery. Cesarean birth is often recommended for multiples.
- Facilitate referrals such as perinatologist, neonatologist, and social worker.

Hyperemesis Gravidarum

Hyperemesis gravidarum is vomiting during pregnancy that is so severe it leads to dehydration, electrolyte, and acid–base imbalance, starvation ketosis, and weight loss. Hyperemesis appears to be related to rapidly rising serum levels of pregnancy related hormones such as chorionic gonadotropin (hCG), progesterone, and estrogen levels. An association has been noted with *H. pylori*, but evidence is inconclusive (ACOG, 2004). Other factors may include a psychological component related to ambivalence about the pregnancy, but this is controversial. Regardless of the cause, a woman experiencing hyperemesis presents in the clinical situation severely dehydrated and physically and emotionally debilitated, sometimes in need of hospitalization to manage profound and prolonged nausea and vomiting (ACOG, 2004; Gilbert, 2011; Queenan, Hobbins, & Spong, 2005).

Assessment Findings

- Vomiting that may be prolonged, frequent, and severe
- Weight loss, acetonuria, and ketosis
- Signs and symptoms of dehydration including:
  - *Dry mucous membranes*
  - *Poor skin turgor*
  - *Malaise*
  - *Low blood pressure*

Medical Management

- Treatment of nausea and vomiting of pregnancy with vitamin B_6 or vitamin B_6 plus doxylamine is safe and effective and should be considered first-line pharmacotherapy (ACOG, 2004; Matthews, Dowswell, Haas, Doyle, & O'Mathúna, 2010).
- Intravenous hydration should be used for the patient who cannot tolerate oral liquids for a prolonged period or if clinical signs of dehydration are present. Correction of ketosis and vitamin deficiency should be strongly considered. Dextrose and vitamins, especially thiamine, should be included in the therapy when prolonged vomiting is present.
- In refractory cases of nausea and vomiting of pregnancy, the following medications have been shown to be safe and efficacious in pregnancy: antihistamine H_1 receptor blockers, phenothiazines, and benzamides (ACOG, 2004).
- Laboratory studies to monitor kidney and liver function
- Correction of ketosis and vitamin deficiency should be strongly considered. Dextrose and vitamins, especially thiamine, should be included in the therapy when prolonged vomiting is present.

Nursing Actions

- Assess factors that contribute to nausea and vomiting.
- Reduce or eliminate factors that contribute to nausea and vomiting, such as eliminating odors.

- Treatment of nausea and vomiting of pregnancy with ginger has shown beneficial effects and can be considered as a nonpharmacological option.
- In refractory cases of nausea and vomiting of pregnancy, use antiemetics as ordered.
- Early treatment of nausea and vomiting of pregnancy is recommended to prevent progression to hyperemesis gravidarum.
- Provide emotional support.
- Provide comfort measures such as good oral hygiene.
- Provide IV hydration with vitamins and electrolytes as per orders.
- Check weight daily.
- Monitor I&O and specific gravity of urine to monitor hydration.
- Monitor nausea and vomiting.
- Monitor laboratory values for fluid and electrolyte imbalances.
- Ensure that the woman remains NPO until vomiting is controlled, then slowly advance the diet as tolerated.
- Facilitate nutritional and dietary consult.
- Determine the woman's food preferences and provide them.
- Minimizing fluid intake with meals can decrease nausea and vomiting.
- Explore complementary therapies to manage hyperemesis, such as traditional Chinese medicine, hypnotherapy, and acupuncture (see Chapter 4). In a recent Cochrane Review on nausea and vomiting in pregnancy, 27 trials, with 4041 women, were reviewed covering many interventions, including acupressure, acustimulation, acupuncture, ginger, vitamin B_6, and several antiemetic drugs (Matthews, Dowswell, Haas, Doyle, & O'Mathúna, 2010). Evidence regarding the effectiveness of P6 acupressure, auricular (ear) acupressure, and acustimulation of the P6 point was limited. Acupuncture (P6 or traditional) showed no significant benefit to women in pregnancy. The use of ginger products may be helpful to women, but the evidence of effectiveness was limited and not consistent. There was only limited evidence from trials to support the use of pharmacological agents including vitamin B_6, and anti-emetic drugs to relieve mild or moderate nausea and vomiting.

DIABETES MELLITUS

Diabetes mellitus is a chronic metabolic disease characterized by hyperglycemia as a result of limited or no insulin production.

- **Type 1 diabetes** is a result of autoimmunity of beta cells of the pancreas resulting in absolute insulin deficiency and is managed with insulin.
- **Type 2 diabetes** is characterized by insulin resistance and inadequate insulin production. This is the most prevalent form of diabetes, and the rates are increasing as it is linked to increased rates of obesity. It is typically controlled with diet, exercise, and oral glycemic agents. Oral hypoglycemic agents are not recommended for use during pregnancy in type 2 diabetic women (Gilbert, 2011).

■ Women with diabetes in pregnancy can be divided into two groups: pregestational and gestational diabetics.

Diabetes in Pregnancy

For many of the complications of pregnancy, and particularly for diabetes, medical management is continually under investigation and recommendations for treatment are changing. This chapter provides a general discussion of diabetes in pregnancy and then considers pregestational diabetes, followed by a discussion of gestational diabetes. Many of the same principles apply in the approach to both conditions. Diabetes in pregnancy is categorized into two groups:

■ Women with diabetes in pregnancy can be divided into two groups: pregestational and gestational diabetes.
■ Pregestational diabetes (either type 1 or type 2 diabetes)
■ Gestational diabetes mellitus (GDM) is glucose intolerance that had not previously been present prior to pregnancy.

Some of the normal physiological changes in pregnancy present challenges for managing diabetes in pregnancy. The physiological changes that accompany pregnancy produce a state of insulin resistance. To spare glucose for the developing fetus, the placenta produces several hormones that antagonize insulin:

■ Human placental lactogen
■ Progesterone
■ Growth hormone
■ Corticotropin-releasing hormone

These hormones shift the primary energy sources to ketones and free fatty acids.

Most pregnant women maintain a normal glucose level in pregnancy despite increasing insulin resistance by producing increased insulin. Whether preexisting or gestational diabetes, the risk of the perinatal morbidity and mortality for the woman and neonate are significant.

For preexisting or gestational diabetes, the treatment goals are the same and management strategies are similar:

■ Maintain euglycemia control.
■ Minimize complications.
■ Prevent prematurity.

Overall, diabetes in pregnancy is a complex health problem that requires a multidisciplinary approach to facilitate a healthy outcome for both the woman and her baby. Care for women with diabetes should begin before conception and for GDM at the time of diagnosis. The goal of preconception care is to maintain the lowest possible glycosylated hemoglobin (HbA$_1$C) without episodes of hypoglycemia, and the care should include (Mattson & Smith, 2011):

■ Assessment and education regarding current diabetes self-management skills
■ Exploration of strategies to improve adherence to treatment regimen
■ Involvement of the woman and her family in the treatment regimen (essential in improving adherence to treatment regimen)
■ Establishment of mutual goals for glycemic controls and self-monitoring

TESTED @ BEGINNING 2 △

Pregestational Diabetes

The incidence of pregestational diabetes is approximately 1% of all pregnancies and affects 10,000–14,000 women annually (ACOG, 2005). Women with preexisting pregestational diabetes have a fivefold increase in the incidence of major fetal anomalies of the heart and central nervous system (CNS). The precise mechanism for teratogenesis in diabetic women is not well understood but is believed to be related to hyperglycemia and deficiencies in membrane lipids and prostaglandin pathways. The quality of diabetic control throughout pregnancy is key in the prevention of major complications of diabetes and the associated risks for diabetes during pregnancy (Gilbert, 2011).

Risks for the Woman

■ Hypoglycemia or hyperglycemia
■ Diabetic ketoacidosis (DKA, 1%), especially in second trimester
■ Hypertensive disorders and preeclampsia (10%–15% risk)
■ Metabolic disturbances related to hyperemesis, nausea, and vomiting of pregnancy
■ Preterm labor (25% risk)
■ Spontaneous abortion (30+% risk)
■ Polyhydramnios/oligohydramnios: Polyhydramnios related to fetal anomalies and fetal hyperglycemia (20% risk). Oligohydramnios related to decreased placental perfusion.
■ Cesarean delivery
■ Exacerbation of chronic diabetes-related conditions such as: heart disease, retinopathy, nephropathy, and neuropathy
■ Infection related to hyperglycemia (80% risk): urinary tract infection, chorioamnionitis, and postpartum endometritis
■ Induction of labor

BACTERIA NEED SUGAR

Risks for the Fetus and Newborn

■ Congenital defects including cardiac, skeletal, neurological, genitourinary, and gastrointestinal related to maternal hyperglycemia during organogenesis (first 6–8 weeks of pregnancy)
■ Growth disturbances, macrosomia related to fetal hyperinsulinemia
■ Hypoglycemia related to fetal hyperinsulinemia
■ Hypocalcemia and hypomagnesemia
■ Intrauterine growth restriction related to maternal vasculopathy and decreased maternal perfusion
■ Asphyxia related to fetal hyperglycemia and hyperinsulinemia
■ Respiratory distress syndrome related to delayed fetal lung maturity
■ Polycythemia (hematocrit <65%) related to increased fetal erythropoietin
■ Hyperbilirubinemia related to polycythemia and red blood cell breakdown
■ Prematurity because of maternal complications
■ Cardiomyopathy related to maternal hyperglycemia

■ Birth injury related to macrosomia
■ Stillbirth in poorly controlled maternal diabetes, especially after 36 weeks' gestation

Assessment Findings

■ Pregestational diabetes, history type 1 or type 2 diabetes
■ Abnormal blood glucose levels
■ HbA1C test to determine the average blood glucose levels over the last 4–8 weeks
■ Cardiac, renal, and ophthalmic function assessment and evaluation

Self-Management

Comprehensive self-management of diabetes is complex yet essential for successful pregnancy outcomes:

■ Self-monitoring of blood glucose (SMBG) by checking blood glucose levels 4–8 times per day (before and after meals and at bedtime) in pregnancy. This is the most important parameter for determining metabolic control. **Table 7-2** indicates glycemic goals for pregnancy.
■ Self-monitoring of urine ketone. Self-testing is done by testing the first void specimen for ketones, when blood glucose level is greater than 200 mg/dL, during maternal illness, and/or when glucose control is altered. Moderate to large amounts of ketones is an indication of inadequate food intake. Moderate to large amounts of ketone should be reported to care provider.
■ Record keeping of blood glucose levels, food intake, insulin, and activity need to be maintained for appropriate management of treatment regimen.
■ Exercise is beneficial for glycemic control and overall well-being. Generally, exercise three times a week for at least 20 minutes is recommended, but some contraindications such as hypertension and preeclampsia do exist.
■ Review signs and symptoms of maternal hypoglycemia for the prevention and management of hypoglycemic episodes. Patients should keep a source of fast-acting carbohydrate with them at all times (hard candy or fruit juice).

Medical Nutritional Therapy

Medical nutritional therapy (MNT) is a cornerstone of diabetes management for all diabetic women, and the goal is to provide adequate nutrition, prevent diabetic ketoacidosis, and promote euglycemia. MNT needs to be individualized and continually adjusted based on blood glucose values and insulin regimen and the woman's lifestyle. A registered dietitian should meet with the woman regularly to assess and reevaluate the nutritional needs of the woman.

Medical Management

Preconception care for women with preexisting diabetes is key to a successful pregnancy and decreasing risks to the woman and her fetus. Achieving euglycemic control for 1–2 months is recommended, achieving a HbA$_1$C less than 7%. Pregnancies complicated by preexisting diabetes are managed by a multidisciplinary team including a perinatologist, diabetes nurse educator, and dietitian. Screening at diagnosis of pregnancy may include kidney, heart, and thyroid function and ophthalmic exams. Additional diagnostic testing is typically done related to the fetus, including regular ultrasound examinations, intensive prenatal care schedule, and antenatal testing. The insulin needs of type 1 diabetic women increase such that by the end of pregnancy, insulin requirements may be two to three times that of pre-pregnancy levels and may require three or four injections per day of Humulin insulin.

Delivery Issues

Timing of delivery is a tremendous challenge in pregnancies complicated by diabetes. At term, the risk of stillbirth increases, as does that of macrosomia. In contrast, intervention may place the woman at risk for prolonged labor and operative deliveries. Thus it is necessary for care providers to determine the pregnancies that should be allowed to go into spontaneous labor and those in need of labor induction. Most guidelines state that diabetes in pregnancy is not an automatic indication for scheduled cesarean delivery (Cunningham et al., 2010).

Complicating the issue of when and how to deliver is the fact that infants of diabetic women (IDM) have delayed pulmonary lung maturity and are at risk for respiratory distress syndrome (RDS). Excess maternal glucose levels result in excess insulin production by the fetus in utero, which is known to result in delayed surfactant production thus interfering with fetal lung maturity (Mattson & Smith, 2011).

The following are general recommendations for intrapartal care:

■ Evaluate fetal lung maturity by checking if amniotic fluid is positive for phosphatidylglycerol, to try to avert RDS in the newborn who is less than 38 weeks' gestation. The lecithin/sphingomyelin (L/S) ratio is not a specific indicator for fetal lung maturity in diabetic women.
■ Maintain maternal plasma glucose levels at 70–110 mg/dL during labor.
■ Administer intravenous insulin when necessary to achieve desired glucose levels.

Nursing Actions

Extensive teaching is needed for women with diabetes in pregnancy. For type 1 diabetic pregnant women, this means

TABLE 7–2 BLOOD GLUCOSE GOALS	
TIMING	BLOOD GLUCOSE (mg/dL)
AM Fasting	<90
Premeal	<105
1-Hour Postprandial	<140
Mean Blood Glucose	<100
Source: Mattson & Smith, 2011.	

learning about the effects pregnancy has on the management of diabetes and the adjustments required to the prior diabetic management regimen. The pregnancy represents new stressors and challenges for diabetic women and their families. Women may feel vulnerable and anxious related to their health and that of their fetus.

■ Provide information on:
 ■ *Physiological changes in pregnancy and the impact on diabetes*
 ■ *Changes in insulin requirements during pregnancy with advancing gestation*
■ Assist the woman in arranging for dietary counseling with a dietitian.
■ Dietary counseling should include the woman's preferences and pregnancy requirements.
■ Review self-monitoring of blood glucose, urine ketones, signs and symptoms of hyper- and hypoglycemic episode, dietary intake, and activity.
■ Emphasize the importance of record keeping of dietary intake, urine ketones, glucose levels and activity.
■ Instruct the woman to bring records to prenatal appointments to be reviewed by the primary health care provider.
■ Review signs and symptoms, and treatment of hyperglycemia based on the individualized treatment plan.
■ Review signs and symptoms, and treatment of hypoglycemia (blood glucose <70 mg/dL) including:
 ■ *Diaphoresis; tachycardia; shakiness; cold, clammy skin; blurred vision; extreme fatigue; mental confusion and irritability; somnolence; and pallor (Daley, 2014)*
 ■ *Ingest 10–15 g of carbohydrate for blood glucose of 60 mg/dL to raise blood glucose by 30–40 mg/dL in 30 minutes.*
■ Review signs and symptoms of diabetic ketoacidosis, including:
 ■ *Abdominal pain, nausea and vomiting, polyuria, polydipsia, fruity breath, leg cramps, altered mental status, and rapid respirations (Daley, 2014)*
■ Care for women admitted to the hospital in diabetic ketoacidosis during pregnancy should be provided by nurses with experience in intensive care and obstetrics. The goals of care include fluid resuscitation, restoration of electrolyte balance, reduction of hyperglycemia, and treatment of underlying cause such as infection (Gilbert, 2010).
■ Provide information on when and how to call the care provider:
 ■ *Glucose levels greater than 200 mg/dL, moderate ketones in urine, persistent nausea and vomiting, decreased fetal movement, and other indicators based on individualized plan of care (Daley, 2014)*
■ Provide information on management of nausea, vomiting, and illness:
 ■ *The glucose level should be checked every 1–2 hours, urine ketones checked every 4 hours; insulin should still be given with vomiting (Daley, 2014)*
■ Provide an expected plan of prenatal care, antenatal tests, and fetal surveillance.
■ Provide an expected plan for labor and delivery.

■ Assist the woman in arranging to meet with a diabetic nurse educator:
 ■ *Ideally, women are referred to a diabetic nurse educator to help them to learn self-care management of diabetes and to facilitate regulation of diabetes in pregnancy.*
■ Emphasize that changes in the management plan may be necessary every few weeks due to the physiological changes of pregnancy.
■ Arrange for antenatal testing:
■ Antenatal testing generally starts at 28 weeks' gestation and includes NST and BPP.

Gestational Diabetes Mellitus

Metabolic changes during pregnancy lower glucose tolerance. Blood glucose levels rise and more insulin is produced in response. As the pregnancy develops, insulin demands increase. For the majority of pregnant women, this is a normal physiological process.

However, some women develop glucose intolerance resulting in gestational diabetes (Alwan, Tuffnell, & West, 2011). **Gestational diabetes mellitus (GDM)** is defined as any degree of glucose intolerance with the onset or first recognition in pregnancy (ACOG, 2011; American Diabetes Association [ADA], 2004). This definition applies whether the GDM is controlled only with diet and exercise or with insulin as well. When medical nutrition therapy is inadequate to control glucose in GDM, insulin is required. Approximately 7% of pregnancies are complicated by GDM, resulting in more than 200,000 cases annually (ADA, 2004). Pregnancy is a condition characterized by progressive insulin resistance that begins mid-pregnancy and progresses throughout the gestation. Insulin resistance during pregnancy stems from a variety of factors, including alterations in growth hormone and cortisol secretion (insulin antagonists), human placental lactogen secretion (which is produced by the placenta and affects fatty acids and glucose metabolism, promotes lipolysis, and decreases glucose uptake), and insulinase secretion (which is produced by the placenta and facilitates metabolism of insulin). In addition, estrogen and progesterone also contribute to a disruption of the glucose insulin balance. Increased maternal adipose deposition, decreased exercise, and increased caloric intake also contribute to this state of relative glucose intolerance (Hoffert Gilmartin, Ural, & Repke, 2008).

Two main contributors to insulin resistance are:

■ Increased maternal adiposity
■ Insulin desensitizing hormones produced by the placenta

The placenta produces human chorionic somatomammotropin (HCS), cortisol, estrogen, and progesterone. HCS stimulates pancreatic secretion of insulin in the fetus and reduces peripheral uptake of glucose in the woman. It has been proposed that, as the placenta increases in size with increasing gestation, so does the production of these hormones, leading to a progressive insulin-resistant state. Women with deficient insulin secretory capacity develop GDM. Because maternal insulin does not cross the placenta, the fetus is exposed to maternal hyperglycemia and in response the fetus produces more insulin, which promotes growth and subsequent macrosomia.

The American Association of Obstetricians and Gynecologists recommends routine screening for all pregnant women at 24–28 weeks of gestation, with a nonfasting 1-hour 50-g oral glucose tolerance test (ACOG, 2011). A positive test is a result of 130 mg/dL or 140 mg/dL depending on the criteria used (Griffith & Conway, 2004). For women who test positive, a 3-hour glucose tolerance test is done after the woman ingests a 100-g glucose load; plasma glucose levels are drawn at 1, 2, and 3 hours post glucose load. If two or more glucose levels are above these thresholds, a diagnosis of GDM is made: fasting ≥95 mg/dL, 1-hour ≥180 mg/dL, 2-hour ≥155 mg/dL, and 3-hour ≥140 mg/dL (ACOG, 2011). Less stringent criteria have been proposed and may be used by some institutions or providers.

Risks Factors for GDM

■ No known risk factors are identified in 50% of patients with GDM.
■ History of fetal macrosomia
■ Strong family history of diabetes
■ Obesity

Risks for the Woman

■ Hypoglycemia and DKA
■ Preeclampsia
■ Cesarean birth
■ Development of nongestational diabetes

Risks for the Fetus and Newborn

■ Macrosomia is the most common morbidity (15%–45%) (Perkins, Dunn, & Jagasia, 2007).
    ■ *Macrosomia places the fetus at risk for birth injuries such as brachial plexus injury.*
■ Hypoglycemia during the first few hours post-birth
■ Hyperbilirubinemia
■ Shoulder dystocia
■ Respiratory distress syndrome
■ The magnitude of fetal–neonatal complications is proportional to the severity of maternal hyperglycemia.
■ Risks of GDM for newborns are similar to risks with pregestational diabetes, except they are not at risk for congenital anomalies. Risks for newborns born to GDM are similar to the risks for newborns born to pregestational diabetic women, except GDM newborns are not at risk for congenital anomalies.

Assessment Findings

■ Abnormal glucose screening results

Medical Management

■ GDM may be managed by care providers with consultation and referral as appropriate.
■ For most women with GDM, the condition is controlled with diet and exercise.

■ Up to 40% of women with GDM may need to be managed with insulin.
■ Oral hypoglycemic agents may be used, but there is not agreement on their recommended use during pregnancy.
■ Cesarean birth is recommended for estimated fetal weight >4,500 g.
■ Women with GDM need to be monitored for type 2 diabetes after the birth. About one third of women will have recurrent GDM in subsequent pregnancies (Griffith & Conway, 2004).

Nursing Actions

■ The cornerstone of management of GDM is glycemic control. For women diagnosed during pregnancy with GDM, this means learning many complex skills and management strategies to maintain a healthy pregnancy.
■ Teach the woman to test glucose four times a day, one fasting and three postprandial checks/day (suggested glucose control is to maintain fasting glucose less than 95 mg/dL before meals, and between 120–135 mg/dL after meals) (Hoffert, Gilmartin, Ural, & Repke, 2008). (**Fig. 7-6** and Table 7-2)
■ Provide information on effects of elevated glucose on developing fetus and rationale for managing euglycemic glucose levels.
■ Encourage active participation in management and decision making.
■ Teach the woman to monitor fasting ketonuria levels in the morning.
■ Teach proper self-administration of insulin (site selection, insulin onset, peak, duration, administration). For the gestational diabetic, consider that it may be the first insulin administration time related to the pregnancy. Unlike for women with preexisting diabetes, this can create a tremendous change in lifestyle. Successful self-administration of insulin requires patience, support and

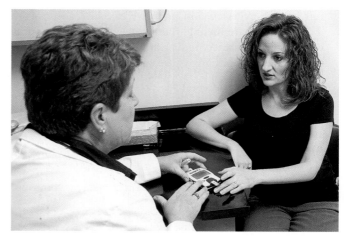

Figure 7–6 Blood glucose levels need to be checked regularly for any woman who has diabetes at any time during pregnancy.

encouragement, and reassurance by the nurse educator (Kendrick, 2004).

■ Teach the woman signs and symptoms and treatment for hypoglycemia, hyperglycemia, and diabetic ketoacidosis outlined above.

■ Reinforce diet management. The recommended overall dietary ratio is 33%–40% complex carbohydrates, 35%–40% fat, and 20% protein. This calorie distribution will help 75%–80% of GDM women become normoglycemic.

■ Reinforce plan of care related to self-management and fetal surveillance.

■ Exercise has been shown to improve glycemic control. The mechanism of this improvement is mostly secondary to increasing tissue sensitivity to insulin. Walking 10–15 minutes after a meal is beneficial and can be managed by most pregnant women. Typically exercising three or more times a week for at least 15–30 minutes duration is recommended.

PREGNANCY HYPERTENSION

Hypertension is identified as systolic pressure 140 mm Hg or greater or diastolic pressure 90 mm Hg or greater. Hypertensive disorders of pregnancy have a 12%–22% occurrence rate, are the most common complication of pregnancy, and are the second leading cause of maternal death and contribute to neonatal morbidity and mortality. Hypertension is directly responsible for 17.6% of maternal deaths in the United States. Hypertension during pregnancy has increased more than 50% since 1990 (ACOG, 2012; Cunningham et al., 2010; Martin, Hamilton, Ventura, Osterman, Kirmeyer, Mathews, & Wilson, 2011; National High Blood Pressure Education Working Group [NHBPEP], 2000). Hypertensive disorders are classified into four categories by NHBPEP:

■ **Preeclampsia and eclampsia syndrome:** Preeclampsia is a systemic disease with hypertension accompanied by proteinuria after the 20th week of gestation. Ten percent of all first pregnancies are affected by preeclampsia–eclampsia (Gibson, Carson, & Letterie, 2007). **Eclampsia** is the onset of convulsions or seizures that cannot be attributed to other causes in a woman with preeclampsia.

■ **Preeclampsia superimposed on chronic hypertension:** Hypertensive women who develop new-onset proteinuria; proteinuria before the 20th week of gestation; or sudden increase in proteinuria or BP or platelet count <100,00/μL in women with hypertension and proteinuria before 20 weeks' gestation. Almost 25% of women with chronic hypertension develop preeclampsia (Cunningham et al., 2010; Gibson, Carson, & Letterie, 2007).

■ **Gestational hypertension:** Systolic BP ≥ 140/90 for the first time after 20 weeks, without proteinuria. Almost 50% of women with gestational hypertension develop preeclampsia syndrome. When the blood pressure increases appreciably, it can be a danger to the mother and the fetus. In the United States, gestational hypertension, formerly termed pregnancy-induced hypertension, develops in 5%–6% of all pregnancies (Gibson, Carson, & Letterie, 2007). Final diagnosis is made postpartum.

■ **Chronic hypertension:** Hypertension (BP ≥ 140/90) before conception or before the 20th week of gestation, or hypertension first diagnosed after 20 weeks' gestation that persists after 12 weeks postpartum; may put the woman at high risk for developing preeclampsia (ACOG, 2012).

Evidence-Based Practice: Cochrane Review: Antenatal Day Care Units versus Hospital Admission for Women with Complicated Pregnancy

Cowswell, T., Middleton, P., & Weeks, A. (2009) Antenatal day care units versus hospital admission for women with complicated pregnancy. *Cochrane Database of Systematic Reviews* 2009, Issue 4. Art. No.: CD001803. DOI: 10.1002/14651858.CD001803.pub2.

The use of antenatal day care units is widely recognized internationally as an alternative for inpatient care for women with pregnancy complications. Antenatal day care units allow women with pregnancy complications to spend part or most of a day at an outpatient setting cared for by nurses and midwives with physician and perinatologist consults receiving complication-based antenatal testing and assessments and interventions. Antenatal day care units have been widely used as an alternative to inpatient care for women with pregnancy complications including mild and moderate hypertension, and preterm premature rupture of the membranes. The objective of this review is to compare day care units with routine care or hospital admission for women with pregnancy complications in terms of maternal and perinatal outcomes, length of hospital stay, acceptability, and costs to women and health services providers. Randomized trials comparing antenatal day care with inpatient hospitalization for women with pregnancy complications were reviewed. Three trials with a total of 504 women were included.

Main Results

The findings were that women receiving day care had to make more visits to the hospital as outpatients but were less likely to stay in the hospital overnight. Care in day units did not seem to affect other outcomes for mothers and babies or increase or reduce interventions in labor; although women in one trial were less likely to have their labors induced if they received day care. Two studies provided evidence that women preferred day care to hospital admission, and no women expressed a preference for more inpatient care; most women in both groups felt they had received good care and were satisfied with it. Outcomes including mode of birth were similar for women in both groups, and there were no significant differences in infant birth weight.

Summary

Randomized trials to date have been too small to assess the effect of day care units on important clinical outcomes. There was, however, some evidence that women preferred day care to hospital admission. These findings may suggest a strategy to reduce hospitalizations for complications during pregnancy in the United States that extends beyond brief antenatal testing appointments done in the United States.

Preeclampsia

Preeclampsia is a hypertensive, multisystem disorder of pregnancy whose etiology remains unknown. Preeclampsia is best described as a pregnancy-specific syndrome of reduced organ perfusion secondary to vasospasm and endothelial activation (Cunningham et al., 2010).

Although management is evidence-based, preventative measures/screening tools are lacking, treatment remains symptomatic, and delivery remains the only cure. Preeclampsia is a disease of pregnancy that ranges from mild to severe and is hypertension accompanied by underlying systemic pathology that can have severe maternal and fetal impact.

- The incidence of preeclampsia complicating pregnancy is 4% (Martin et al., 2009).
- Despite extensive research, there is no consensus as to the cause of preeclampsia.
- The only cure for preeclampsia–eclampsia is delivery of the neonate and placenta.

The criteria for diagnosis of preeclampsia and preeclampsia superimposed on chronic hypertension are presented in Critical Component: Criteria for Diagnosis of Preeclampsia–Eclampsia and Preeclampsia Superimposed on Chronic Hypertension.

Pathophysiology of Preeclampsia

To understand the pathophysiological mechanisms of preeclampsia, it is important to review the normal physiological changes of pregnancy. Normal pregnancy is a vasodilated state in which peripheral vascular resistance decreases 25%. Within the first weeks, the woman's blood pressure falls, largely due to a general relaxation of muscles within the blood vessels. Diastolic blood pressure drops 10 mm Hg at midpregnancy and gradually returns to pre-pregnant levels at term. There is a 50% rise in total blood volume by the end of the second trimester, and cardiac output increases 30%–50%. Increased renal blood flow leads to an increased glomerular filtration rate. Because preeclampsia is a syndrome of reduced organ perfusion secondary to vasospasm and endothelial activation, the physiological changes that predispose women to preeclampsia also have an effect on other organs/systems such as the hepatic system, renal system, coagulation system, central nervous system, eyes, fluid and electrolytes, and pulmonary system (**Fig. 7-7**).

- In preeclampsia there is an increase in microvascular fat deposition within the liver, which is proposed as one cause of epigastric pain. Liver damage may be mild or may progress to HELLP syndrome (**H**emolysis, **E**levated **L**iver enzymes, and **L**ow **P**latelets). Hepatic involvement can lead to periportal hemorrhagic necrosis in the liver that can cause a subcapsular hematoma, which can result in right upper quadrant pain or epigastric pain and may signal worsening preeclampsia (NHBPEP, 2000).
- In 70% of preeclamptic patients, glomerular endothelial damage, fibrin deposition, and resulting ischemia reduce renal plasma flow and glomerular filtration rate (NHBPEP, 2000). Protein is excreted in the urine. Uric acid, creatinine, and calcium clearance are decreased and oliguria develops as the condition worsens. Oliguria is a sign of severe preeclampsia and kidney damage.
- The coagulation system is activated in preeclampsia and thrombocytopenia occurs, possibly due to increased platelet aggregation and deposition at sites of endothelial damage, activating the clotting cascade. A platelet count below 100,000 cells/mm³ is an indication of severe preeclampsia (NHBPEP, 2000).
- Endothelial damage to the brain results in fibrin deposition, edema, and cerebral hemorrhage, which may lead to hyperreflexia and severe headaches and can progress to eclampsia (NHBPEP, 2000).
- Retinal arterial spasms may cause blurring or double vision, photophobia, or scotoma (NHBPEP, 2000).
- The leakage of serum protein into extracellular spaces and into urine, by way of damaged capillary walls,

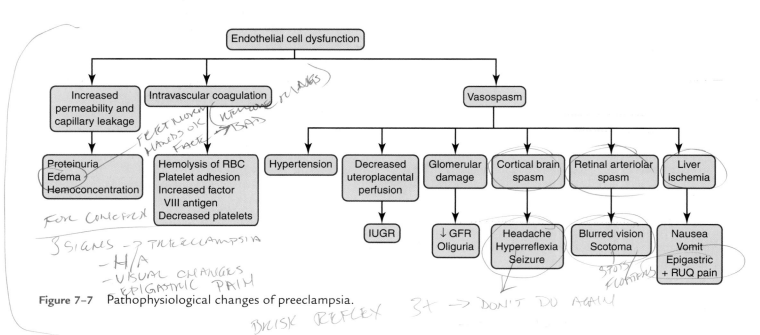

Figure 7-7 Pathophysiological changes of preeclampsia.

results in decreased serum albumin and tissue edema (NHBPEP, 2000).

■ Pulmonary edema is most commonly caused by volume overload related to left ventricular failure as the result of extremely high vascular resistance (Gilbert, 2007).

CRITICAL COMPONENT

Criteria for Diagnosis of Preeclampsia–Eclampsia and Preeclampsia Superimposed on Chronic Hypertension

Preeclampsia–Eclampsia

■ Diagnosed after the 20th week of pregnancy.
■ Blood pressure is >140 mm Hg systolic or >90 mm Hg diastolic with proteinuria (measurement of 3.0 g [300 mg/dL] or more of protein in a 24-hour urine collection period).
■ If proteinuria is absent, the diagnosis is suspected if headache, visual changes, abdominal pain, or laboratory abnormalities, specifically low platelets or elevated levels of liver enzymes, are noted along with hypertension.
■ Eclampsia describes grand mal seizure in a preeclamptic woman.

Edema occurs in many normal pregnant women and therefore is no longer considered a clinical marker for preeclampsia.

Preeclampsia Superimposed on Chronic Hypertension

■ New-onset proteinuria or an abrupt increase in proteinuria
■ Increase in blood pressure that previously had been under control
■ Changes in laboratory values, specifically platelet count <100,000 cells/mm³ and abnormal alanine transaminase (ALT) or aspartate aminotransferase (AST)

Because of poorer prognosis and difficulty in differentiating preeclampsia from an exacerbation of chronic hypertension, over diagnosis of preeclampsia is acceptable.

(Report of the National High Blood Pressure Education Program Working Group on High Blood Pressure in Pregnancy, 2000)

Risk Factors for Preeclampsia/Eclampsia

■ Nulliparity
■ Age younger than 19 or older than 35 years
■ Obesity
■ Multiple gestation
■ Family history of preeclampsia
■ Preexisting hypertension or renal disease
■ Previous preeclampsia or eclampsia
■ Diabetes mellitus

Risks for the Woman

■ Cerebral edema/hemorrhage/stroke
■ Disseminated intravascular coagulation (DIC)
■ Pulmonary edema
■ Congestive heart failure
■ Hepatic failure
■ Renal failure
■ Abruptio placenta

Risks for the Fetus and Newborn

■ Prematurity delivery may be indicated preterm related to deterioration of maternal status.
■ Intrauterine growth restriction (IUGR) related to decrease uteroplacental perfusion
■ Low birth weight
■ Fetal intolerance to labor because of decrease placental perfusion
■ Stillbirth

Assessment Findings

Accurate assessment is essential so that early recognition of worsening disease will allow for timely intervention that may improve maternal and neonatal outcome.

■ Elevated blood pressure: Hypertension with systolic pressure 140 mm Hg or greater and diastolic pressure 90 mm Hg or greater.
■ Proteinuria is 1+ or greater.
■ Lab values may indicate elevations in liver function tests, diminished kidney function, and altered coagulopathies.

Medical Management

Once diagnosed, the woman and fetus should be monitored weekly for indications of worsening condition, as preeclampsia can be a progressive disease (see Critical Component: Comparison of Assessment Findings between Mild and Severe Preeclampsia). Women can also present with abrupt onset of the disease. Indications of worsening of the disease from mild to severe and severe preeclampsia are treated with hospitalization and evaluation. Antihypertensive drugs are used to control elevated blood pressure, but because the only cure for preeclampsia is delivery, delivery is indicated in severe preeclampsia, even before term to protect the woman and fetus from severe sequelae. Care in labor and delivery includes use of magnesium sulfate to prevent seizures.

The primary goal in preeclampsia and preeclampsia superimposed on chronic hypertension is to control the woman's blood pressure and to prevent seizure activity and cerebral hemorrhage. Medical management includes:

■ Magnesium sulfate, a central nervous system depressant, has been proven to help reduce seizure activity without documentation of long-term adverse effects to woman and fetus (see Medication: Intravenous Administration of Magnesium Sulfate).
■ Antihypertensive medications are used to control blood pressure (**Box 7-3**).
■ Outpatient management for women with mild preeclampsia is an option if the woman can adhere to activity restriction, frequent office visits, and antenatal testing, and can monitor blood pressure (see Evidence-Based Practice: Cochrane Review: Antenatal Day Care Units versus Hospital Admission for Women with Complicated Pregnancy).
■ Delivery of the fetus and placenta is the only "cure" for preeclampsia. There are little data to suggest that any therapy alters the underlying pathophysiology. Therefore, all

BOX 7–3   ANTIHYPERTENSIVE MEDICATIONS

First-Line Drugs of Choice

Hydralazine (Apresoline, Neopreol) vasodilator: IV administration is used in severe preeclampsia; however, caution should be used to prevent rapid decreases in blood pressure. Rapid reduction in maternal blood pressure can decrease uteroplacental perfusion and decrease oxygen to fetus.

Methyldopa (Aldomet): Exact mechanism is unknown; may work on CNS. May take a few days for onset, so this drug is not a first choice in an acute situation. Research shows no long-term effects on fetus.

Labetalol (beta blocker): Slows the heart rate and decreases systemic vascular resistance. There is no significant research as to long-term effects on fetus.

Second-Line Drug

Nifedapine: Calcium channel blocker (Procardia) controls hypertension rapidly, increases cardiac index, and increases urinary output.

Sources: Deglin & Vallerand (2007); Gregg (2004); Sibai (2003).

---

other interventions are designed to safeguard the mother while allowing time for fetal maturity. Although delivery cures preeclampsia, its effect is not immediate and women remain at risk of continuing problems, including eclampsia, as long as five days postpartum (Peters & Flack, 2004).

CRITICAL COMPONENT

Comparison of Assessment Findings between Mild and Severe Preeclampsia

Abnormality	Mild	Severe
Systolic blood pressure	140–160 mm Hg	>160 mm Hg
Diastolic blood pressure	<100 mm Hg	110 mm Hg or higher
Proteinuria	Trace to 1+	Persistent 2+ or more
Headache	Absent	Present
Visual disturbances	Absent	Present
Upper abdominal pain	Absent	Present
Oliguria	Absent	Present
Seizure (eclampsia)	Absent	May be present
Serum creatinine	Normal	Elevated
Thrombocytopenia	Absent	Present
Liver enzyme elevation	Minimal	Marked
Fetal growth restriction	Absent	Obvious
Pulmonary edema	Absent	May be present

Mild preeclampsia may progress rapidly to severe preeclampsia.

Nursing Actions

- ■ Accurate assessment is essential in that early recognition of worsening disease allows for timely intervention and may improve maternal and neonatal outcome.
- ■ Blood pressure should be measured with the woman seated and her arm at heart level, using an appropriate sized cuff (**Fig. 7-8**). Placing the woman in a left lateral recumbent position is no longer recommended to evaluate blood pressure as it gives an inaccurately low blood pressure reading (Cunningham et al., 2005; NHBPEP, 2000).
- ■ Administer antihypertensive as per orders (generally for blood pressure >160/110 mm Hg) (see Box 7-3).
- ■ Administer magnesium sulfate as per orders (see Critical Component: Care of the Woman on Magnesium Sulfate).
- ■ Assess for CNS changes including headache, visual changes, deep tendon reflexes (DTRs), and clonus (**Box 7-4** and **Fig. 7-9**).
- ■ Auscultate lung sounds for clarity and monitor the respiratory rate.
- ■ Assess for signs and symptoms of pulmonary edema such as:
  - ■ *Shortness of breath, chest tightness or discomfort, cough, oxygen saturation less than 95%, increased respiratory and heart rates*

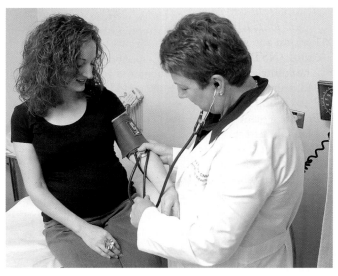

Figure 7–8   Take the woman's blood pressure while she is seated and with her arm at heart level.

BOX 7–4   ASSESSMENT OF DEEP TENDON REFLEXES

PHYSICAL ASSESSMENT	GRADE
None elicited	0
Sluggish or dull	1
Active, normal	2
Brisk	3
Brisk with transient or sustained clonus	4

(see Fig. 7-9)

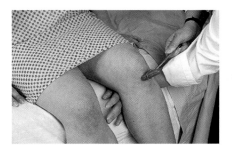

Figure 7–9 Assessing DTRs.

■ *Changes in behavior such as apprehension, anxiety, or restlessness*

■ Assess for epigastric pain or right upper quadrant pain indicating liver involvement.

■ Assess weight daily and assess for edema to assess for fluid retention.

■ Check urine for proteinuria (may include 24-hour urine collection) and specific gravity.

■ Evaluate laboratory values including:
  ■ *Elevations in serum creatinine (72 mg/dL)*
  ■ *Hematocrit levels (>35)*
  ■ *Low platelet count (100,000/mm³)*
  ■ *Elevated liver enzymes (AST >41 units/L, ALT >30 units/L)*

■ Perform antenatal fetal testing and fetal heart rate monitoring (NST and BPP).

■ Check intake of adequate calories and protein.

■ Maintain accurate I&O to evaluate kidney function. Total fluid intake may be restricted to 2,000 mL/24 hr.

■ Provide a quiet environment to decrease CNS stimulation.

■ Maintain bed rest in the lateral recumbent position.

■ Provide information to the woman and her family. Education is key in helping with the understanding of the disease process and the plan of care.

■ Report deterioration in maternal or fetal status to provider.

Medication

Intravenous Administration of Magnesium Sulfate

Continuous intravenous administration:

■ Loading dose: 4–6 g diluted in 100 mL of IV fluid administered over 15–20 minutes

■ Continuous infusion: 2 g/hr in 100 mL of IV fluid for maintenance

■ Laboratory evaluation: Measure serum magnesium level at 4–6 hours, after onset of treatment. Dosage should be adjusted to maintain a therapeutic level of 4–7 mEq/L.

■ Duration: Intravenous infusion should continue for 24 hours post-delivery.

■ **The antidote for magnesium toxicity is calcium gluconate or calcium chloride 5–10 mEq given IV slowly over 5–10 minutes.**

(Magpie Trial Collaborative Group, 2002; Sibai, 2003)

CRITICAL COMPONENT

Care of the Woman on Magnesium Sulfate

Potential Side Effects	Nursing Actions
Maternal: Nausea Flushing Diaphoresis Blurred vision Lethargy Hypocalcemia Depressed reflexes Respiratory depression-arrest Cardiac dysrhythmias Decreased platelet aggregation Circulatory collapse	Assess vital signs before beginning infusion and every 5–15 minutes during loading dose, then every 30–60 minutes until the patient stabilizes. Frequency is then determined by the patient status. Assess DTRs every 2 hours. Monitor strict intake and output. Patients with oliguria or renal disease are at risk for toxic levels of magnesium. Monitor serum magnesium levels (therapeutic level is 5–7 mg/dL). Monitor for signs and symptoms of magnesium toxicity:

■ Decreased reflexes could be a sign of pending respiratory depression.
■ Loss of DTRs
■ Respiratory depression: respiratory rate <14 breaths/min
■ Oliguria, urine output <30 mL/hr
■ Shortness of breath or respiratory rate <24
■ Chest pain
■ EKG changes
■ If toxicity is suspected, discontinue the infusion and notify the health care provider. Respiration difficulty and cardiac arrest can occur with magnesium levels above 12 mEq/L.
■ Keep calcium gluconate immediately available (1g IV).

Maintain seizure precautions and keep resuscitation equipment nearby. Patients receiving IV labetalol for blood pressure control should have cardiac monitoring. Maintain continuous fetal heart rate monitoring |
| **Fetal/neonatal:** Fetal heart rate decreased Variability Respiratory depression Hypotonia Decreased suck reflex Signs and symptoms of magnesium toxicity | Monitor FHR. Alert the neonatal team before delivery of use of magnesium sulfate in labor. |

(Mattson & Smith, 2011; Simpson, 2008)

Eclampsia

Eclampsia is the occurrence of seizure activity in the presence of preeclampsia (Gilbert, 2007). Eclampsia can occur ante-, intra-, or postpartum; about 50% of cases occur antepartum.

Eclampsia is thought to be triggered by one or more of the following:

■ Cerebral vasospasm
■ Cerebral hemorrhage
■ Cerebral ischemia
■ Cerebral edema

Warning signs of potential eclampsia include:

■ Severe persistent headaches
■ Epigastric pain
■ Nausea and vomiting
■ Hyperreflexia with clonus
■ Restlessness

Care during a seizure includes:

■ Remaining with the patient.
■ Calling for help.
■ Providing for patient safety by assessing airway and breathing.
    ■ *Lower the head of the bed and turn the woman's head to one side.*
    ■ *Anticipate the need for suctioning to decrease the risk of aspiration.*
■ Aspiration is the leading cause of maternal mortality (Poole, 2014).
■ Preventing maternal injury.
    ■ *If possible, a padded tongue blade should be inserted to prevent tongue injury (a tongue blade is still recommended by guidelines but not typically used in clinical practice).*
    ■ *Keep side rails up and padded if possible.*
■ Recording the time, length, and type of seizure activity.
■ Notifying the physician.

After the seizure, the following is done:

■ Rapidly assess maternal and fetal status.
■ Assess airway; suction if needed.
■ Administer supplemental oxygen: 10 L/min via mask.
■ Ensure IV access.
■ Administer magnesium sulfate per orders.
■ Provide a quiet environment.

HELLP Syndrome

HELLP syndrome (**H**emolysis, **E**levated **L**iver enzymes, and **L**ow **P**latelets) is the acronym used to designate the variant changes in laboratory values that can occur as a complication of severe preeclampsia (see Critical Component: Laboratory Values Indicative of HELLP Syndrome).

■ Hemolysis is a result of red blood cell destruction as the cells travel through constricted vessels.
■ Elevated liver enzymes result from decreased blood flow and damage to the liver.
■ Low platelets result from platelets aggregating at the site of damaged vascular endothelium causing platelet consumption and thrombocytopenia (Cunningham et al., 2010; Sibai, 2004).

Women with severe preeclampsia have an increased risk (7%–24%) of developing HELLP syndrome. HELLP may develop in women who do not present with the cardinal signs of severe preeclampsia. HELLP may appear at any time during the pregnancy in 70% of cases, and the immediate postpartum period accounts for 30% of cases (Queenan, Hobins, & Spong, 2005). The only definitive treatment is delivery. However, some women may experience worsening HELLP syndrome over the first 48-hour postpartum period. Women with only some of the laboratory changes are diagnosed with partial HELLP syndrome.

CRITICAL COMPONENT

Laboratory Values Indicative of HELLP Syndrome	
Platelets	<100,000/mm³
Liver enzymes (AST, ALT)	Elevated AST: >70 units/L Elevated ALT: >50 units/L
Bilirubin (indirect)	Elevated: >1.2 mg/dL
LDH	Elevated: >600 units/L

(Mattson & Smith, 2011).

Risks for the Woman

■ Abruptio placenta
■ Renal failure
■ Liver hematoma and possible rupture
■ Death

Risks for the Fetus and Newborn

■ Preterm birth
■ Death

Assessment Findings

■ The woman may present with a complaint of general malaise, nausea, and right upper gastric pain.
■ The woman may have unexplained bruising, mucosal bleeding, petechiae, and bleeding from injection and IV sites.
■ Assessment findings are related to alternations in laboratory tests associated with changes in liver function and platelets (see Critical Component: Laboratory Values Indicative of HELLP Syndrome).

Medical Management

The only definitive cure for HELLP syndrome is immediate delivery of the fetus and placenta. Resolution of disease is generally in 48 hours postpartum. Medical management may include replacement of platelets and is the same as those for the women with severe preeclampsia (Poole, 2014).

Nursing Actions

■ Perform a thorough assessment of the woman related to the diagnosis of preeclampsia.
■ Evaluate laboratory tests.
■ Notify the physician immediately if HELLP syndrome is suspected or lab values deteriorate.

- Administer platelets as per orders.
- Assessment and management are the same for the women diagnosed with HELLP syndrome as for the women with severe preeclampsia.
- Provide the woman and the family with information regarding HELLP and its treatment.
- Provide emotional support to the woman and her family, as the woman and family are at risk for increased levels of anxiety related to diagnosis (Mattson & Smith, 2011).

PLACENTAL ABNORMALITIES AND HEMORRHAGIC COMPLICATIONS

Major blood loss during pregnancy is a significant contributor to both maternal and fetal morbidity and mortality. Up to 1,000 mL/min of maternal blood flows through the placenta at term. Hemorrhage predisposes a woman to hypovolemia, anemia, infection, and premature birth. Significant maternal blood loss can result in decreased perfusion and oxygen to the fetus, resulting in progressive deterioration of fetal status and even death (Burke-Sosa, 2014). Placental abnormalities and hemorrhagic complications of pregnancy are presented in this section. The major causes of antepartum hemorrhage are placenta previa and placental abruption. The basic principles of immediate care of women with either type of antepartum hemorrhage include: assessment of maternal and fetal condition; prompt maternal resuscitation if this is required; and consideration of early delivery if there is evidence of fetal distress and if the baby is of sufficient maturity to be potentially capable of survival. Up to 15% of maternal cardiac output up to 1000 mL/min flows through the placental bed at term; unresolved bleeding can result in maternal exsanguination in 8 to 10 minutes (Burke-Sosa, 2014).

CRITICAL COMPONENT

Vaginal Bleeding

A sterile vaginal exam is contraindicated in **all** pregnant women with extensive vaginal bleeding until the source of bleeding is identified. If a vaginal exam is performed with a placenta previa torrential, vaginal bleeding could occur related to dislodging of the placenta from maternal tissues. Maternal blood loss results in decreased oxygen-carrying capacity, which directly impacts oxygen delivery to maternal organs and placental blood flow, thus decreasing oxygen to the fetus. Therefore, the management of placenta previa is dependent on maternal and fetal status.

Placenta Previa

The incidence of placenta previa is 1 in 300 deliveries (Cunningham et al., 2010). **Placenta previa** occurs when the placenta attaches to the lower uterine segment of the uterus, near or over the internal cervical os instead of in the body or fundus of the uterus. The cause is unknown (Gilbert, 2010). Hemorrhage is especially likely to occur during the third trimester with development of the lower uterine segment, and when uterine contractions dilate the cervix, thereby applying shearing forces to the placental attachment to the lower segment, or when separation is provoked by vaginal examination (Neilson, 2003). Placenta previa is most often diagnosed before the onset of bleeding when ultrasound is performed for other indications (Burke-Sosa, 2014).

There are four classifications of placenta previa (**Fig. 7-10**; Cunningham et al., 2010): *[handwritten: BEFORE VAG EXAM]*

- **Total placenta previa:** The placenta completely covers the internal cervical os.
- **Partial placenta previa:** The placenta partially covers the internal cervical os.
- **Marginal placenta previa:** The edge of the placenta is at the margin of the internal cervical os.
- **Low-lying placenta:** The placenta is implanted in the lower uterine segment in close proximity to the internal cervical os. *[handwritten: NOT PREVIA]*

Risk Factors for Placenta Previa

- Endometrial scarring
  - *Previous placenta previa*
  - *Prior cesarean delivery*
  - *Abortion*
  - *Multiparity*
- Impeded endometrial vascularization
  - *Advanced maternal age (>35 years)*
  - *Diabetes or hypertension*
  - *Cigarette smoking*
  - *Uterine anomalies/fibroids/endometritis*

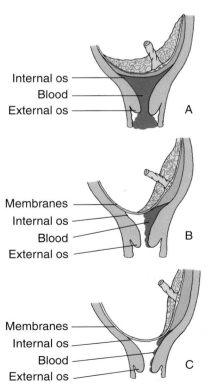

Figure 7–10   Classification of placenta previa. *A.* Total. *B.* Partial. *C.* Marginal/low-lying.

■ Increased placental mass
  ■ *Large placenta*
  ■ *Multiple gestation*

Risks for the Woman

■ Hemorrhagic and hypovolemic shock related to excessive blood loss
■ Because of the large volume of maternal blood flow to the uteroplacental unit at term, unresolved bleeding can result in maternal exsanguinations in 10 minutes.
■ Anemia
■ Potential Rh sensitization as Rh-negative women can become sensitized during any antepartum bleeding episode.

Risks for the Fetus and Newborn

■ Disruption of uteroplacental blood flow can result in progressive deterioration of fetal status, and the degree of fetal compromise is related to the volume of maternal blood loss (Burke-Sosa, 2014).
■ Blood loss, hypoxia, anoxia, and death (<10%) related to maternal hemorrhage may occur.
■ Fetal anemia may develop due to maternal blood loss.
■ Neonatal morbidity and mortality is related primarily to prematurity.

Assessment Findings

■ The classic presentation of a placenta previa is painless hemorrhage and fetal malposition.
■ Bleeding usually occurs near the end of the second trimester or in the third trimester of pregnancy, and initial bleeding episodes may be slight.
■ The first episode of bleeding is rarely life threatening or a cause of hypovolemic shock.
■ Ultrasound confirms placental location at the cervix.
■ A vaginal exam is contraindicated (see Critical Component: Vaginal Bleeding).

Emergency Medical Management

■ Cesarean delivery is necessary when either maternal or fetal status is compromised as a result of extensive hemorrhage.
■ Cesarean birth is necessary in practically all women with placenta previa because the placenta is at the cervix, and labor and cervical dilation results in placental hemorrhage (Cunningham et al., 2010).
■ Vaginal delivery may be attempted with a low-lying placenta if one can proceed with an emergency cesarean birth if needed.
■ Placenta previa may be associated with placenta accreta, placenta increta, or placenta percreta (see Chapter 10).
■ Blood is transfused as needed.

Medical Management After Stabilization

When the maternal and fetal status is stable and bleeding is minimal (<250 mL), prolonging pregnancy and delaying delivery may be possible. This expectant management or conservative management is performed when the fetus is premature to allow for fetal lungs to mature. This typically includes close observation and hospitalization. If the woman and fetus remain stable and bleeding stops, discharge home may be considered with maternal bed rest, antenatal surveillance, and close proximity to the hospital. A Cochrane Review of clinical trials revealed there was little evidence of any clear advantage or disadvantage to a policy of home versus hospital care (Neilson, 2003).

Nursing Actions

Nursing actions are related to maternal fetal status and the amount of vaginal bleeding and include:

■ Perform the initial assessment:
  ■ *Evaluation of color, character, and amount of vaginal bleeding*
  ■ *Arrangement for ultrasound to determine placental location*
  ■ *Determination of fetal well-being, gestational age, and fetal lung maturity*
  ■ *Assessment of vital signs for increased pulse and respiratory rate and falling blood pressure every 5–15 minutes if active bleeding. The woman can have up to a 40% maternal blood loss before exhibiting hemorrhagic hemodynamic changes in the blood pressure and pulse.*
■ Notify the physician of any of the following:
  ■ *Onset or increase in vaginal bleeding*
  ■ *Blood pressure less than 90/60 mm Hg; pulse less than 60 or more than 120 bpm*
  ■ *Respirations less than 14 or more than 26 breaths/min*
  ■ *Temperature greater than 100.4°F (38°C)*
  ■ *Urine output less than 30 mL/hr*
  ■ *Saturated oxygen less than 95%*
  ■ *Decreased level of consciousness*
  ■ *Onset or increase in uterine activity*
  ■ *Category II or III FHR pattern*
■ Assess abdominal pain, uterine tenderness, irritability, and contractions.
■ Initiate bed rest with bathroom privileges.
■ Maintain IV access with large-bore IV in case blood replacement therapy is needed.
■ Ensure availability of hold clot and blood components.
■ Assess FHR and UCs and facilitate antenatal testing as ordered.
■ Give corticosteroids to accelerate fetal lung maturity, if indicated.
■ Monitor lab values including CBC, platelets, and clotting studies.
■ See Critical Component: Nursing Activities to Promote Adaptation to Pregnancy Complications.
■ Inform the patient and family of maternal and fetal status.
■ Reassure the patient and her family.
■ Anticipate a cesarean birth if patient is unstable.
■ If undelivered and mother is RH negative, administer RhoGAM.

Placental Abruption

Placental abruption, also referred to **as abruptio placentae,** is the premature separation of a normally implanted placenta. Placental abruption is initiated by hemorrhage into the decidual basalis. A hematoma forms that leads to destruction of the placenta adjacent to it. In some instances spiral arterioles that nourish the decidua and supply blood to the placenta rupture. Bleeding into the decidua basalis results in hemorrhage and placental separation (**Fig. 7-11** and **Table 7-3**). The separation may be partial or total and can be classified as grade 1 (mild), 2 (moderate), or 3 (severe) (Gilbert, 2007). Bleeding with placental abruption is almost always maternal. This is a uniquely dangerous condition for the woman and fetus because of its potentially serious

complications. The reported frequency is 1 in 200 deliveries (Cunningham, 2010).

Maternal and fetal status determines the management of the pregnancy. The signs and symptoms of abruption can vary considerably and are:

- Severe sudden onset of intense abdominal pain
- Uterine contractions

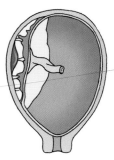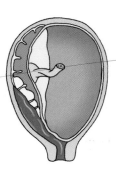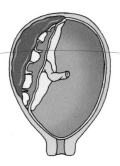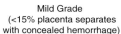

Mild Grade
(<15% placenta separates
with concealed hemorrhage)

Moderate Grade 2
(up to 50% placenta separates
with apparent hemorrhage)

Severe Grade 3
(>50% placenta separates
with concealed hemorrhage)

Figure 7–11   Three grades of abruptio placentae.

TABLE 7–3   CLASSIFICATIONS OF MANAGEMENT OF PLACENTAL ABRUPTION (BRUPTIO PLACENTAE)

	MILD: GRADE 1	MODERATE: GRADE 2	SEVERE: GRADE 3
DEFINITION	Less than one-sixth of placenta separates prematurely.	From one-sixth to one-half of placenta separates prematurely.	More than one-half of placenta separates prematurely.
SIGNS AND SYMPTOMS	Total blood loss <500 mL Dark vaginal bleeding (mild to moderate) Vague lower abdominal or back discomfort No uterine tenderness No uterine irritability	Total blood loss 1,000–1,500 mL 15%–30% of total blood volume Dark vaginal bleeding (mild to severe) Gradual or abrupt onset of abdominal pain Uterine tenderness present Uterine tone increased	Total blood loss >1,500 mL More than 30% of total blood volume Dark vaginal bleeding (moderate to severe) Usually abrupt onset of uterine pain described as tearing, knifelike, and continuous Uterus board-like (hard)
MATERNAL EFFECTS	Vital signs normal	Mild shock Normal maternal blood pressure Maternal tachycardia Narrowed pulse pressure Orthostatic hypotension Tachypnea	Moderate-to-profound shock common Decreased maternal blood pressure Maternal tachycardia significant Severe orthostatic hypotension Significant tachypnea
MATERNAL COMPLICATIONS	Normal fibrinogen of 450 mg/dL	Early signs of DIC common Fibrinogen 150–300 mg/dL	DIC usually develops unless condition is treated immediately. Fibrinogen <150 mg/dL
FETAL/NEONATAL COMPLICATIONS	Normal FHR pattern	FHR shows signs of fetal compromise.	FHR shows signs of fetal compromise and death can occur.

Source: Gilbert (2011).

■ Uterine tenderness
■ Dark vaginal non-clotting bleeding may or may not be present
■ If separation is in the center of the placenta, then blood may be trapped between the placenta and decidua, concealing the hemorrhage. A concealed hemorrhage occurs in about 10% of abruptions. This results in uterine tenderness and abdominal pain.
■ If the separation occurs at the edge of the placenta, then the blood usually escapes externally.
■ Signs of hypovolemia
■ Abnormal fetal heart rate

The fetal response to abruptio placenta depends on the volume of blood loss and the extent of uteroplacental insufficiency. Management depends on maternal and fetal status and gestational age. The cause of abruptio placenta is unknown but is associated with risk factors.

Risk Factors
■ Previous abruption increases risk up to 15%
■ Hypertensive disorders of pregnancy
■ Abdominal trauma (IMPROPER SEATBELT USE, IPV)
■ Cocaine, methamphetamine use, and/or cigarette smoking
■ Preterm premature rupture of membranes
■ Thrombophilia
■ Uterine anomalies/fibroids

Risks for the Woman
■ Hemorrhagic shock
■ Disseminated intravascular coagulation (DIC) of the release of thromboplastin into the maternal venous system triggering DIC
■ Hypoxic damage to organs such as kidneys and liver
■ Postpartum hemorrhage

Risks for the Fetus and Newborn
■ Preterm birth
■ Hypoxia, anoxia, neurological injury, and fetal death related to hemorrhage
■ Intrauterine growth restriction
■ Neonatal death (15%)

Assessment Findings
■ Maternal assessment findings include (see Table 7-3):
  ■ *Hypovolemic shock; hypotension; oliguria; thready pulse; shallow/irregular respirations; pallor; cold, clammy skin; and anxiety*
  ■ *Vaginal bleeding (but can be concealed hemorrhage)*
  ■ *Severe abdominal pain*
  ■ *Uterine contractions/tenderness/hypertonus/increasing uterine distention*
  ■ *Nausea and vomiting*
  ■ *Decreased renal output*
  ■ *Remember, during pregnancy signs of shock are usually not until 25%–30% of maternal blood loss has occurred.*
  ■ *Kleihauer–Betke test in maternal blood may be positive and indicate the presence of fetal red blood cells.*

■ Fetal assessment findings include (see Table 7-3):
  ■ *Tachycardia*
  ■ *Bradycardia*
  ■ *Category II or II FHR patterns including: loss or variability of FHR, late decelerations, decreasing baseline*

Emergency Medical Management
If abruption results in unstable or deteriorating maternal or fetal status, delivery by cesarean is indicated. Treatment includes:

■ Monitoring maternal volume status
■ Restoring blood loss
■ Monitor fetal status
■ Monitoring coagulation status
■ Correcting coagulation defects
■ Expediting delivery

Medical Management After Stabilization
If the maternal status is stable and the fetus is immature, then expectant management would include:

■ Hospitalization
■ Close monitoring of maternal and fetal status including:
  ■ *FHR*
  ■ *Maternal bleeding*
  ■ *Uterine activity*
  ■ *Abdominal pain*
  ■ *Vaginal bleeding*
  ■ *Maternal laboratory and coagulation studies*
■ Corticosteroids may be given to accelerate fetal lung maturity.
■ Tocolysis may be considered.

Nursing Actions
■ Monitor vaginal bleeding (can be concealed hemorrhage).
■ Assess abdominal pain.
■ Palpate the uterus for contractions/tenderness/hypertonus/increasing uterine distension.
■ Manage nausea and vomiting.
■ Assess for decreased renal output.
■ Monitor maternal cardiovascular status for hypotension and tachycardia.
■ Maintain IV access with a large-bore needle.
■ Administer oxygen at 8–10 L/min by mask.
■ Assess FHR for baseline changes, variability, and periodic changes indicative of an abnormal FHR.
■ Monitor lab values including CBC and clotting studies.
■ Provide emotional support to the woman and her family.
■ Provide information to the woman and her family regarding treatment plan and status of their infant.
■ Monitor lab values including CBC, platelets, and clotting studies.
■ Monitor ultrasound results and umbilical flow Doppler study trends.

- See Critical Component: Nursing Activities to Promote Adaptation to Pregnancy Complications.
- Inform the patient and family of maternal and fetal status.
- Reassure the patient and her family.
- Anticipate a cesarean birth if patient is unstable.
- If undelivered and mother is RH negative, administer RhoGAM.

Placenta Accreta

Placenta accreta is an abnormality of implantation defined by degree of invasion into the uterine wall of trophoblast of placenta. Placenta accreta can be diagnosed by ultrasound prenatally but typically is diagnosed after delivery when the placenta is retained. If the placenta does not separate readily, rapid surgical intervention is needed. Up to 90% of women lose more than 3,000 mL of blood operatively as a result of placenta accreta. A more comprehensive discussion of placenta accreta is in Chapter 10.

- **Placenta accreta:** Invasion of the trophoblast is beyond the normal boundary (80% of cases).
- **Placenta increta:** Invasion of the trophoblast extends into uterine myometrium (15% of cases).
- **Placenta percreta:** Invasion of the trophoblast extends into the uterine musculature and can adhere to other pelvic organs (5% of cases).

Abortion

Abortion is the spontaneous or elective termination of pregnancy before 20 weeks' gestation. Abortions are referred to as induced, elective, therapeutic, and spontaneous. **Induced abortion** is the medical or surgical termination of pregnancy before fetal viability. **Elective abortion** is termination of pregnancy before fetal viability at the request of the woman but not for reasons of impaired health of the mother or fetal disease. Termination of pregnancy is done transcervically through dilation of the cervix, then evacuation of the uterus mechanically by curettage, scraping of the contents, or vacuum. Legally induced abortions have an extremely low complication rate. Early medical abortion with medications such as mifepristone and misoprostol can be highly effective. **Therapeutic abortion** is termination of pregnancy for serious maternal medical indications or serious fetal anomalies. This section focuses on spontaneous abortion as it is associated with hemorrhage.

Spontaneous abortion (SAB) is abortion occurring without medical or mechanical means, also called **miscarriage.** Hemorrhage in the decidua basilis followed by necrosis of the tissue usually accompanies abortion. Approximately 10%–30% of pregnancies end in spontaneous abortion. The majority (80%) occur in the first 12 weeks of gestation and are termed early abortion, and more than half of those are a result of chromosomal abnormalities (Cunningham et al., 2010). Early spontaneous abortions typically are related to an abnormality of the zygote, embryo, fetus, or at times the placenta. Late spontaneous abortions are between 12 and 20 weeks' gestation.

Risk Factors for Spontaneous Abortion

- Increased parity
- Increased maternal and paternal age
- Endocrine abnormalities such as diabetes or luteal phase defects
- Drug use or environmental toxins
- Immunological factors such as autoimmune diseases
- Infections
- Systemic disorders
- Genetic factors
- Uterine or cervical abnormalities

Assessment Findings for Spontaneous Abortion

- Clinical manifestations and categories are listed in **Table 7-4**.
- Uterine bleeding first then cramping abdominal pain in a few hours to several days later
- Ultrasound confirms diagnosis.

Medical Management for Spontaneous Abortion

Medical management depends on classification and signs and symptoms and is presented in Table 7-4.

Nursing Actions Related to Care after Spontaneous Abortion

- Monitor vital signs per protocol and PRN.
- Monitor bleeding.
- Review labs.
- Give RhoGAM if indicated.
- Follow agency guidelines and facilitate and support the family's decisions about disposition of the products of conception.
- Assess significance of loss to woman and family (Gilbert, 2011).
  - *Acknowledge feeling of sadness, distress, or relief toward pregnancy loss.*
  - *Give parents' choices and opportunities for decision making.*
  - *Provide family with information on miscarriage, pregnancy loss, and support groups.*
- Provide psychological support appropriate to family's response.
- Discharge teaching related to self-care and warning signs including:
  - *Teach pericare.*
  - *Pelvic rest includes no tampons, douching, or sexual intercourse for several weeks.*
  - *Teach patient to monitor for excessive bleeding and signs and symptoms of infection such as fever and uterine tenderness or foul-smelling discharge.*
  - *Teach about diet high in iron and protein for tissue repair and red blood cell replacement.*
  - *Review plan for follow-up with care provider.*

Ectopic Pregnancy

An **ectopic pregnancy** develops as a result of the blastocyst implanting somewhere other than the endometrial lining of the uterus (**Fig. 7-12**). The embryo or fetus in an ectopic pregnancy is absent or stunted, and this is a nonviable pregnancy.

TABLE 7–4 CLASSIFICATION AND MANAGEMENT OF SPONTANEOUS ABORTIONS/MISCARRIAGE			
CLASSIFICATION	**DEFINITION**	**MANIFESTATIONS**	**MEDICAL MANAGEMENT**
THREATENED ABORTION	Approximately half of these pregnancies will abort. Continuation of pregnancy is in doubt.	Vaginal bleeding or spotting which may be associated with mild abdominal cramps in first half of pregnancy. Cervix closed Uterus soft, nontender, and enlarged appropriate to gestational age	There are no effective therapies for threatened abortion. Bed rest may be suggested.
INEVITABLE ABORTION	Termination of pregnancy is in progress	Cervix dilated Gross rupture of membranes Vaginal bleeding Mild-to-painful uterine contractions	If bleeding, ROM, pain, or fever, termination with D&C
INCOMPLETE ABORTION	Fragments of products of conception are expelled and part is retained in uterus.	Profuse bleeding because retained tissue parts interfere with myometrial contractions	D&C to evacuate uterus of products of conception
COMPLETE ABORTION	Products of conception are totally expelled from uterus	Minimal vaginal bleeding	No intervention if minimal bleeding
MISSED ABORTION	Embryo or fetus dies during first 20 weeks of gestation but is retained in uterus for 4 weeks or more afterward.	Amenorrhea or intermittent vaginal bleeding, spotting, or brownish discharge No uterine growth No fetal movement felt Regression of breast changes	Evacuation of products of conception based on weeks of gestation
SEPTIC ABORTION	Condition in which products of conception become infected during abortion process	Foul-smelling vaginal discharge	Evacuation of products of conception based on weeks of gestation; IV antibiotics
RECURRENT SPONTANEOUS ABORTION	Condition in which three or more successive pregnancies at less than 20 weeks have ended in spontaneous abortion		Treatment dependent on cause of spontaneous abortion

Sources: Cunningham et al. (2010); Gilbert (2011).

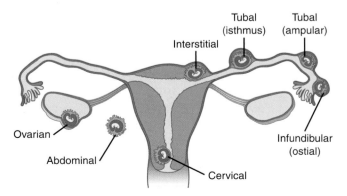

Figure 7–12 Sites for ectopic pregnancy.

The vast majority of ectopic pregnancies occur in the fallopian tube (95%), but the fertilized ovum can also implant in the ovary, cervix, or abdominal cavity (5%). Because the vast majority of ectopic pregnancies are tubal, the focus of this section is on tubal ectopic pregnancy. In a tubal pregnancy, the tube lacks a submucosal layer, and the fertilized ovum burrows through the epithelium of the tubal wall, tapping into the blood vessels; however, the tubal environment cannot support the rapidly proliferating trophoblast.

The incidence of tubal pregnancy is increasing and not always reported, but accounts for up to 10% of maternal mortality (Cunningham et al., 2010). Hemorrhage is the leading cause of death in women. Women with tubal pregnancy have diverse clinical symptoms that largely depend on whether there is a rupture.

Risk Factors for Ectopic Pregnancy (in order of risk)

- Prior tubal damage
  - *Tubal corrective surgery*
  - *Tubal sterilization*
  - *Previous ectopic pregnancies*
- Assisted reproduction
- Pelvic inflammatory disease
- Smoking
- Abdominal adhesions

Risks for the Woman

- Hemorrhage related to rupture of fallopian tube
- Decreased fertility related to removal of fallopian tube

Assessment Findings

Assessment Findings before Tubal Rupture

Most women now present prior to tubal rupture, and with advances in diagnosis and imaging the outcomes have dramatically improved. Common findings are:

- Pelvic or abdominal pain (95%)
- Abnormal bleeding (60%–80%)
- Abdominal and pelvic tenderness is uncommon.
- Uterine changes are minimal.
- Vital signs are stable prior to rupture.

Assessment Findings After Tubal Rupture

- Severe lower abdominal pain
- Pelvic pain described as sharp, stabbing, or tearing
- Vertigo or syncope
- Vital signs become unstable, indicating hypovolemia if hemorrhage is significant.
- Pain in neck or shoulder with peritoneal hemorrhage because of diaphragmatic irritation.

Medical Management

- Diagnosis generally is made with clinical signs, physical symptoms, serial human chorionic gonadotropin (hCG) levels, transvaginal ultrasonography, serum progesterone levels.
- Early diagnosis allows for surgical or medical management of unruptured ectopic pregnancy.
- Laparoscopy is preferred surgical method for hemodynamically stable women. Surgical management depends on the location and cause of the ectopic pregnancy, and extent of tissue involvement.
- Non-surgical medical management of ectopic pregnancy may be indicated in an unruptured and hemodynamically stable woman (ACOG, 2008). Methotrexate, a folic acid antagonist and type of chemotherapy agent, will cause dissolution of the ectopic mass.

Nursing Actions

- Ensure stabilization of cardiovascular status.
- Offer explanations and reassurance related to the plan of care.

- Assess response to diagnosis related to anxiety, fear, guilt.
- Provide support related to the pregnancy loss.
- Explain plan for follow-up care, which is determined by treatment plan, surgical or medical.
- Give RhoGAM if indicated.
- Assess significance of loss to woman and family (Gilbert, 2011):
  - *Acknowledge feeling of sadness, distress, or relief toward pregnancy loss.*
  - *Give parents' choices and opportunities for decision making.*
  - *Provide family with information on pregnancy loss and support groups.*
- Provide psychological support appropriate to family's response.
- Discharge teaching related to self-care and warning signs including:
  - *Teach patient to monitor for severe abdominal pain, excessive bleeding, and signs and symptoms of infection such as fever.*
  - *Teach about diet high in iron if woman experiences a high estimated blood loss (EBL).*
  - *Review plan for follow-up with care provider.*
  - *Teach patient appropriate pain management.*
  - *Teach patient signs and symptoms that need to be reported, such as severe abdominal pain, fever, bleeding.*
- Special considerations for teaching women treated with methotrexate (ACOG, 2008):
  - *Because methotrexate affects rapidly dividing tissues, gastrointestinal side effects, such as nausea, vomiting, and stomatitis, are the most common. Therefore, women treated with methotrexate should be advised not to use alcohol and nonsteroidal anti-inflammatory drugs (NSAIDs).*
  - *It is not unusual for women treated with methotrexate to experience abdominal pain 2–3 days after administration, presumably from the cytotoxic effect of the drug on the trophoblast tissue, causing tubal abortion.*

Gestational Trophoblastic Disease

The term **gestational trophoblastic disease** refers to a spectrum of placental related tumors. Gestational trophoblastic disease is categorized into molar and nonmolar tumors. Nonmolar tumors are grouped as gestational trophoblastic neoplasia or malignant gestational trophoblastic disease (ACOG, 2004). As an example, one of the nonmalignant tumors will be described.

A **hydatiform mole** is a benign proliferating growth of the trophoblast in which the chorionic villi develop into edematous, cystic, vascular transparent vesicles that hang in grape-like clusters without a viable fetus (**Fig. 7-13**). Hydatiform mole develops in 1 to 2 of 1,000 pregnancies in the United States (Cunningham et al., 2010). This is a nonviable pregnancy. In a normal pregnancy, the trophoblast cells develop into the placenta. The trophoblast cells have chorionic villi that form the endometrium. With a hydatiform mole pregnancy, there is a proliferation of the placenta and trophoblastic cells, which absorbs fluid from the maternal blood. Fluid accumulates into the chorionic villi and vesicles form

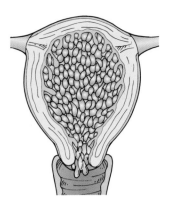

Figure 7-13 Hydatidiform mole.

out of the chorionic villi. The erythroblastic tissue of the complete hydatiform mole never develops into a fetus. The erythroblastic tissue of a partial hydatiform mole may include some fetal tissue, but this is always abnormal and never matures.

Risk Factors

■ Maternal age younger than 15 or older than 45 years
■ Previous molar pregnancy

Risks for the Woman

■ Increased risk of choriocarcinoma

Assessment Findings

■ Amenorrhea
■ Nausea and vomiting
■ Abnormal uterine bleeding ranges from spotting to profuse hemorrhage
■ Enlarged uterus
■ Abdominal cramping and expulsion of vesicles

Diagnosis of Medical Management

■ Diagnosis of molar pregnancy is much earlier than before because the routine use of ultrasound in early pregnancy detects the molar pregnancy earlier.
■ hCG and transvaginal ultrasound

Medical Management

■ Immediate evacuation of mole with aspiration/suction D&C
■ Follow-up of hCG levels for at least 6 months to detect trophoblastic neoplasia. After hCG levels fall to normal for 6 months, pregnancy can be considered.

Nursing Actions for Post Evacuation of Mole

■ Monitor for signs and symptoms of hemorrhage such as abnormal VS, abdominal pain, vaginal bleeding.
■ Assess uterus.
■ Offer explanations and reassurance related to the plan of care.
■ Offer emotional support related to pregnancy loss.
■ Assess response to diagnosis and treatment plan related to anxiety, fear, guilt.

■ Provide support related to the pregnancy loss.
■ Explain plan for follow-up care related to serial hCG.
■ Give Rhogam if indicated.
■ Assess significance of loss to woman and family (Gilbert, 2011).
    ■ *Acknowledge feeling of sadness, distress, or relief toward pregnancy loss.*
    ■ *Give parents' choices and opportunities for decision making.*
    ■ *Provide family with information on pregnancy loss and support groups.*
■ Provide psychological support appropriate to family's response.
■ Discharge teaching related to self-care and warning signs including:
    ■ *Teach patient to monitor for severe abdominal pain, excessive bleeding, and signs and symptoms of infection such as fever.*
    ■ *Review plan for follow-up with care provider.*
    ■ *Teach patient appropriate pain management.*
■ Emphasize importance of medical follow-up with regular HCG levels because of the risk of malignant trophoblastic disease and choriocarcinoma.
■ Prophylactic chemotherapy is not routinely recommended (ACOG, 2004).

INFECTIONS

Infection is a common complication of pregnancy. The impact of infection on pregnancy is dependent on the infectious organism involved. Some infectious agents, such as Trichomonas, are easily treated and affect only the mother. Other infections, such as rubella, can actively infect the fetus during pregnancy. Infections can be acquired by the fetus transplacentally, such as HIV; may ascend the birth canal; or can be acquired though contact at the time of a vaginal birth, such as herpes. In the following section, sexually transmitted diseases and TORCH infections are reviewed, highlighting maternal and fetal effects, treatment, and nursing implications.

Human Immunodeficiency Virus (HIV/AIDS)

The **human immunodeficiency virus (HIV)** organism is a retrovirus of the lentivirus family that has an affinity for the T-lymphocytes, macrophages, and monocytes. HIV/AIDS is a virus passed from one person to another through blood and sexual contact. The cases of HIV/AIDS among female adults and adolescents >13 years of age increased from 7% in 1985 to 27% in 2007 (Gilbert, 2011). According to the Centers for Disease Control, among female adults and adolescents diagnosed with HIV/AIDS in 2007, 83% of 10,977 HIV/AIDS cases were attributed to high-risk heterosexual contact, 16% to injection drug use, and 1% to other risk factors.

Transmission of HIV/AIDS is by exposure to blood or blood products or by-products. Transmission of HIV perinatally happens through transplacental, intrapartal, and breast milk exposure. Before the use of antiviral therapy in pregnancy, the risk of infection for a neonate to an HIV seropositive mother was approximately 25%, ranging from 13%–39%. However, today most pregnant women are on regular anti-retroviral drug regimen, decreasing their HIV viral load to undetectable. As a result, the rate of maternal-child transmission has decreased to less than 2% (ACOG, 2007).

Factors Associated with Increased Perinatal Transmission

- Mother with AIDS
- Preterm delivery
- Decreased maternal CD4 count
- High maternal viral load
- Chorioamnionitis
- Blood exposure due to episiotomy, vaginal laceration, and forceps delivery

Risks to Fetus and Newborn

- Risk of transmission is 20%–25% without the use of anti-retroviral drugs but can be as low as 2% with appropriate antepartal drug treatment.
- Preterm delivery
- Preterm PROM
- IUGR

Assessment Findings

- Physical findings include fever, fatigue, vomiting, diarrhea, weight loss, generalized lymphadenopathy, oral gingivitis, vaginitis, and opportunistic infection.

Medical Management

- Perform routine screening starting at first perinatal visit.
- Treatment of at least three antiretroviral drugs

Nursing Actions in Antepartal Period

- Provide education and counseling on plan of care.
- Provide education and counseling on potential consequences of pregnancy on HIV disease progress, risk for transmission, and consequences for neonate.
- Education to facilitate health promotion
  - *Adequate sleep*
  - *Adequate diet as protein deficiency can depress immunity; adequate zinc and vitamin A for cell growth*
  - *Avoidance of infection*
- Provide emotional support.
- If the woman is diagnosed with HIV during pregnancy, she needs extensive and ongoing education and counseling on plan of care and management.

Nursing Actions in Intrapartal Period

- Avoid using instruments during birth.
- Leave fetal membranes intact.
- Avoid fetal scalp electrode.
- Avoid episiotomy and assisted vaginal delivery.
- Provide and reinforce education.
- Provide emotional support.

Sexually Transmitted Infections

Sexually transmitted infections (STIs), sometimes referred to as **sexually transmitted diseases (STDs)** remain a major public health challenge in the United States. The Centers for Disease Control and Prevention (CDC, 2010) estimates that 19 million new infections occur every year, almost half of them among young people age 15–24 years. STIs affect women of every socioeconomic and educational level, age, race, and ethnicity.

In addition to the physical and psychological consequences, the costs of treating STIs are estimated at more than $17 billion annually (CDC, 2010). Women who are pregnant can become infected with the same STIs as women who are not pregnant. Pregnancy does not provide protection for the woman or the baby, and consequences of an STI can be serious in pregnancy, even life-threatening for the woman and her baby. Intrauterine or perinatal transmitted STIs can have severely debilitating effects on women, their partners, and their fetuses. All women should be screened for STIs during their first prenatal visit. **Table 7-5** shows the estimated number of women infected with specific STIs annually.

Risks for the Woman

- STIs can cause pelvic inflammatory disease (**Table 7-6**).
- Pelvic inflammatory disease (PID) can lead to infertility, chronic hepatitis, and cervical and other cancers.
- STIs during pregnancy can lead to PTL, PROM, and uterine infection.

Table 7-7 summarizes information on maternal effects and management of STIs (CDC, 2010).

Risks for the Fetus

- STIs can pass to the fetus by crossing the placenta; some can be transmitted to the baby during delivery as the baby passes through the birth canal (see Table 7-7).
- Harmful effects to babies include preterm birth, low birth weight, neonatal sepsis, and neurological damage.

TABLE 7–5 ESTIMATED INCIDENCES OF STIS IN PREGNANT WOMEN ANNUALLY	
STI	ESTIMATED NUMBER OF PREGNANT WOMEN
Bacterial vaginosis	1,080,000
Herpes simplex	880,000
Chlamydia	100,000
Trichomoniasis	124,000
Gonorrhea	13,200
Hepatitis B	16,000
HIV	6,400
Syphilis	<1,000
Source: Centers for Disease Control and Prevention (CDC) (2010).	

TABLE 7–6   PELVIC INFLAMMATORY DISEASE

PELVIC INFLAMMATORY DISEASE (PID)	Pelvic inflammatory disease is a general term that refers to an infection of the uterus, fallopian tubes, and other reproductive organs. It is a common and serious complication of STIs. Pregnant women with PID are at high risk for maternal morbidity and preterm delivery and should be hospitalized and treated with IV antibiotics.
INCIDENCE	An estimated more than 1 million women in the United States have an episode of acute PID.
CONSEQUENCES	Can lead to infertility, ectopic pregnancy, abscess formation, and chronic pelvic pain. Scar tissue in fallopian tubes increases the occurrence of ectopic pregnancies. 10%–15% of women with PID become infertile.
SIGNS AND SYMPTOMS OF PID	Signs and symptoms vary from none to severe including: Lower abdominal pain, fever, unusual vaginal discharge, painful urination, and irregular menstrual bleeding. Vague symptoms may go unrecognized.
TREATMENT	PID can be cured with antibiotics, but treatment does not reverse damage to reproductive organs.

Source: Centers for Disease Control and Prevention (CDC) (2010).

TABLE 7–7   SUMMARY OF FETAL AND MATERNAL EFFECTS AND MANAGEMENT OF STIS

INFECTION	MATERNAL EFFECTS	FETAL EFFECTS	MANAGEMENT	NURSING ISSUES
CHLAMYDIA *CHLAMYDIA TRACHOMATIS*	Three-fourths of women have no symptoms, so it is known as a "silent" disease; may have burning on urination or abnormal vaginal discharge.	Contact at delivery may cause conjunctivitis and/or premature birth. The efficacy of ophthalmia neonatorum prophylaxis is unclear.	Antibiotics Amoxicillin Azithromycin Erythromycin	Can lead to PID. Treat all infected partners. Retest in 3 weeks. *Pelvic Inflammatory Disease*
GONORRHEA *NEISSERIA GONORRHOEAE*	Most women have no symptoms but may have burning on urination, increased purulent yellow-green vaginal discharge, or bleeding between periods. Rectal infection can cause anal itching, discharge, and bleeding. Can lead to PID.	Contact at birth. Ophthalmia neonatorum may cause sepsis and/or blindness. To prevent gonococcal ophthalmia neonatorum, a prophylactic antibiotic ointment should be instilled into the eyes of all newborns.	Antibiotics Cephalosporin	Can lead to PID. Complete treatment.
GROUP B STREPTOCOCCUS *STREPTOCOCCUS AGALACTIAE* (GBS)	Women are typically asymptomatic carriers. Symptoms can include abnormal vaginal discharge, urinary tract infections, chorioamnionitis.	Transmission rates are low, 1%–2%, but infection can result in invasive GBS with permanent neurological sequelae.	If GBS-positive at 35–37 weeks of gestation or GBS status unknown, treat with antibiotics in labor to prevent neonatal transmission. Penicillin or ampicillin IV	GBS-positive women receive intrapartum antibiotic prophylaxis.

TABLE 7–7 SUMMARY OF FETAL AND MATERNAL EFFECTS AND MANAGEMENT OF STIS—cont'd

INFECTION	MATERNAL EFFECTS	FETAL EFFECTS	MANAGEMENT	NURSING ISSUES
HEPATITIS B (HBV)	50% asymptomatic May have low-grade fever, anorexia, nausea and vomiting, fatigue, rashes. Chronic infection can lead to cirrhosis of the liver and liver cancer.	90% of infected infants have chronic infection Cirrhosis of the liver Liver cancer	No specific treatment	HBsAg-positive pregnant women should be reported to the state or local health department for timely and appropriate prophylaxis for their infants. Immunoprophylaxis of all newborns born to HBsAg-positive women. HBIG to neonate at delivery and hepatitis B vaccination series initiated.
HEPATITIS CRNA VIRUS (HCV)	80% of persons infected have no symptoms. Can lead to chronic liver disease, cirrhosis, and liver cancer.	Exposure transplacentally. Estimated 2%–7% transmission rate. Little research on treatment of children.	Ribavirin and interferon, but are contraindicated in pregnancy.	Breastfeeding is not contraindicated.
HUMAN PAPILLO-MAVIRUS (HPV) Thirty or more types infect the genital area.	The majority of HPV infections are asymptomatic but can cause genital warts. Genital warts are flat, papular, or pedunculated growths on the genital mucosa.	Route of transmission unclear. Can cause respiratory papillomatosis.	Warts may be removed during pregnancy. Treatment reduces but does not eliminate HPV infection.	The presence of genital warts is not an indication for cesarean delivery.
SYPHILIS*TREPONEMA PALLIDUM*	Ulcer or chancre, then maculopapular rash advancing to CNS and multiorgan damage.	Transplacental transmission. Congenital syphilis may cause preterm birth, physical deformity, neurological complications, stillbirth, and/or neonatal death.	Penicillin	
TRICHOMONAS *TRICHOMONAS VAGINALIS*	Malodorous yellow-green vaginal discharge and vulvar irritation. Can lead to premature rupture of membrane and preterm labor.	Preterm delivery and low birth weight. Respiratory and genital infection.	Metronidazole	
CANDIDIASIS *CANDIDA ALBICANS**	Results from a disturbance in vaginal flora. Pruritus, vaginal soreness, dyspareunia, abnormal vaginal discharge with a yeasty odor.		Topical azole therapies	

Continued

TABLE 7–7   SUMMARY OF FETAL AND MATERNAL EFFECTS AND MANAGEMENT OF STIS—cont'd

INFECTION	MATERNAL EFFECTS	FETAL EFFECTS	MANAGEMENT	NURSING ISSUES
BACTERIAL VAGINOSIS†	50% of women are asymptomatic. A fishy odor and/or vaginal discharge. Can result in preterm labor and/or premature rupture of membranes.	Premature rupture of membranes, chorioamnionitis and/or preterm birth	Metronidazole or clindamycin	
HUMAN IMMUNODE-FICIENCY VIRUS (HIV/AIDS)	May be asymptomatic for years. HIV weakens the immune system. It may manifest as mononucleosis-like symptoms such as fever, fatigue, sore throat, and lymphadenopathy.	Early antiretroviral treatment has been shown to be effective in reducing maternal–fetal transmissions. Placental transmission but <2% transmission with maternal treatment with antiretroviral medications. 15%–25% transmission to fetus without maternal treatment. Antibody screening is not reliable during infancy because of maternally produced IgG antibodies to HIV are present up to 18 months.	Antiviral	Cesarean birth may be considered. Breastfeeding is contraindicated. Case management follow-up for both the woman and her baby.

Source: CDC (2010).
*Not an STI.
† A polymicrobial clinical syndrome

Assessment Findings

■ Many STIs in women are "silent" without signs and symptoms, making routine screening for STIs during the first prenatal visit an important part of routine prenatal care.

■ Physical findings include low-grade temperature, poor personal hygiene, genital warts, purulent urethral or cervical discharge, friable cervix, genital lesions, tender uterus, pain on motion of cervix, inguinal adenopathy, and rash on palms and soles of feet.

■ Positive STI cultures and test results

Medical Management (see Table 7-7)

■ Provide routine screening of STIs and HIV at first prenatal visit.

■ Treat bacterial STIs with antibiotics.

■ Prescribe antiviral medications for viral STIs to reduce symptoms.

Nursing Actions (see Table 7-7)

■ Provide information on STIs.

■ Provide emotional support.

■ Instruct the woman on correct administration of medications and other treatments and importance of completing treatment.

■ Instruct the patient on the warning signs of complication (fever, increased pain, bleeding).

■ Provide information on the importance of abstaining from intercourse until the patient and her partner are free of infection.

■ Provide the partner with treatment as indicated.

TORCH Infections

TORCH is an acronym that stands for Toxoplasmosis, Other (hepatitis B), Rubella, and Cytomegalovirus and Herpes simplex virus. TORCH infections are unique in their pathogenesis and have potentially devastating effects on the developing fetus (**Table 7-8**). Each disease is teratogenic to the developing fetus.

Risk Factors

The risk status for these infections varies based on route of transmission. Some are sexually transmitted diseases, such as

TABLE 7–8 TORCH INFECTIONS

INFECTION	MATERNAL EFFECTS	FETAL EFFECTS	PREVENTION AND MANAGEMENT	NURSING ISSUES
TOXOPLASMOSIS *TOXOPLASMA GONDII* Single-celled protozoan parasite. Transplacental transmission	Most infections are asymptomatic but may cause fatigue, muscle pains, pnuemonitis, myocarditis, and lymphadenopathy.	Severity varies with gestational age and congenital infection. Can lead to spontaneous abortion, low birth weight, hepatosplenomegaly, icterous, anemia, chorioretinitis, and/or neurological disease. Incidence of congenital infection is low.	Avoid eating raw meat and contact with cat feces. Treatment with sulfadiazine or pyrimethamine after the first trimester	Teach women to avoid raw meat and cat feces. Almost 50% of adults have an antibody to this organism.
OTHER INFECTIONS **HEPATITIS B** Direct contact with blood or body fluid from infected person.	30%–50% of infected women are asymptomatic. Symptoms include low-grade fever, nausea, anorexia, jaundice, hepatomegaly, preterm labor, and preterm delivery.	Infants have a 90% chance of becoming chronically infected, HBV carrier, and a 25% risk of developing significant liver disease.	Infant receives HBIG and hepatitis vaccine at delivery.	Universal screening recommended in pregnancy. HBV can be given in pregnancy.
RUBELLA **(GERMAN MEASLES)** Nasopharyngeal secretions Transplacental	Erythematous maculopapular rash, lymph node enlargement, slight fever, headache, malaise	Overall risk of congenital rubella syndrome is 20% for primary maternal infection in the first trimester with 50% if the woman is infected in the first 4 weeks of gestation. Anomalies include deafness, eye defects, CNS anomalies, and severe cardiac malformations.	Primary approach to rubella infection is immunization. If the woman is pregnant and not immune, she should not receive the vaccine until the postpartum period.	If the woman is not immune, she should not receive the vaccine until the postpartum period and be counseled to not become pregnant for 3 months.
CYTOMEGALOVIRUS **(CMV)** Virus of herpes group Transmitted by droplet contact and transplacentally	Most infections are asymptomatic, but 15% of adults may have mononucleosis-like syndrome.	Infection to fetus is most likely with primary maternal infection and timing of infection with first- and second-trimester exposure. May result in low birth weight, IUGR, hearing impairment microcephaly, and CNS abnormalities.	No treatment is available.	
HERPES SIMPLEX **VIRUS (HSV)** Chronic lifelong viral infection Contact at delivery and ascending infection	Painful genital lesions. Lesions may be on external or internal genitalia.	Transmission rate of 30%–50% among women who acquire genital herpes near time of delivery and is low (<1%) among women with recurrent genital herpes. Mortality of 50%–60% if neonatal exposure to active primary lesion is related to neurological complications of massive infection sepsis and neurological complications.	No cure available. Acyclovir to suppress outbreak of lesions.	★Most common viral STI. Protect the neonate from exposure with cesarean delivery if active lesion.

Source: Queenan, Hobbins, & Spong (2005).

herpes; others have various routes of transmission to woman (CDC, 2010).

Risk for the Woman

■ Depends on the infectious agent (CDC, 2010; see Table 7-8)

Risks for the Fetus

■ The usual route of transmission to the fetus is transplacentally (see Table 7-8).
■ Infections acquired in utero can result in intrauterine growth restriction, prematurity, chronic postnatal infection, and even death.

Assessment Findings

■ Maternal assessment findings vary with the organism (see Table 7-8).

Medical Management

■ Medical management varies based on the organism, trimester of exposure, and clinical evidence of neonatal sequelae (see Table 7-8).

Nursing Actions

■ Nursing considerations vary with the organism (see Table 7-8).
■ Provide emotional support.
■ Instruct woman on treatment plan.

TRAUMA DURING PREGNANCY

Trauma is the leading cause of maternal death during pregnancy and is more likely to cause maternal death than any other complication of pregnancy. The most common cause of maternal death by trauma is abdominal injury (resulting in hemorrhagic shock) and head injury. Injury to the pregnant woman can result from blunt or penetrating trauma. The most common cause of blunt injury is motor vehicle accidents. The most common cause of penetrating trauma is from gunshot wounds. The mechanisms of maternal and fetal injury, gestational age of the fetus, and secondary complications determine the maternal-fetal response to trauma. Maternal outcome in trauma corresponds to the severity of the injury. Fetal outcome depends on injury and maternal physiological response (Van Otterloo, 2011). It is essential to keep in mind that at term, 15% of maternal cardiac output, that is, 750 mL to 1000 mL/min, flow through the placental bed; unresolved bleeding can lead to maternal exsanguination in 8 to 10 minutes (Burke-Sosa, 2014).

Pregnancy causes both anatomic and physiological changes that impact the woman's response to traumatic injury. For example, increased plasma volume by 50% and increased red blood cell volume of 30% can mask hemorrhage. Any condition that results in maternal hypotension, such as hemorrhage or hypovolemia, results in vasoconstriction of the uterine arteries and shunting of blood to vital organs. The shunting of blood from the uteroplacental unit maintains maternal blood pressure at the expense of perfusion to the fetus. The pregnant woman has decreased oxygen reserves and decreased blood buffering capacity, which leaves the pregnant trauma patient vulnerable to hypoxemia and less able to compensate when acidemia occurs (Ruth & Miller, 2013). Two catastrophic events can occur during pregnancy after blunt trauma to the abdomen:

■ Placental abruption
■ Uterine rupture

Extensive discussion of management and care during trauma in pregnancy is beyond the scope of this chapter, but key elements of stabilization of the woman and the fetus and assessments are briefly reviewed. Treatment priorities for injured pregnant women typically are directed as they would be for non-pregnant women. Some important considerations related to pregnancy are presented in the following section.

Assessment Findings

Assessment findings are based on injury. Initial maternal evaluation is the systematic evaluation performed according to the standard Advanced Trauma Life Support (ATLS) protocols. Initial maternal evaluation and resuscitation takes precedence over fetal evaluation. Early recognition of maternal compromise and rapid resuscitation reduces maternal mortality, which in turn reduces fetal mortality.

■ Physiological changes in pregnancy might delay the usual vital sign changes of hypovolemia; blood loss of up to 1,500 mL can occur without a change in maternal vital sign changes.
■ Uterine contractions more frequently than every 10 minutes may be an indication of placental abruption (Cunningham et al., 2010).
■ Fetal well-being reflects maternal and fetal status, and conversely fetal heart rate changes may indicate maternal deterioration such as hypoxia.

Medical Management

Treatment priorities and medical management for the pregnant trauma patient are the same as for the non-pregnant woman in the initial evaluation. Admission and continuous fetal monitoring for 24 to 48 hours after stabilization, in particular for abdominal injuries because of the increased incidence of placental abruption, is recommended.

Nursing Actions

■ Treatment priorities for injured pregnant women typically are directed as they would be for non-pregnant women.
■ Initial actions in trauma care are focused on maternal stabilization.

PREGESTATIONAL COMPLICATIONS

Women who enter pregnancy with a preexisting disease or chronic medical condition are at increased risk for complication and are considered high-risk. These high-risk pregnancies require extensive surveillance and collaboration of multiple disciplines to achieve an optimal pregnancy outcome. Women often experience fear and anxiety for their health and that of the fetus regarding the impact of the chronic disease on the pregnancy outcome. Any preexisting medical disease can complicate the pregnancy or be exacerbated during pregnancy. Increasing numbers of women with chronic diseases are achieving pregnancy. Nursing care is focused on decreasing complications and providing support and education to patients and families to facilitate their participation in their health care during pregnancy.

Women and their families should participate in decision-making and the plan of care to optimize outcomes for both the woman and the fetus. Maternal safety is the prime consideration in all pregnancies. The major preexisting medical complications that impact pregnancy are discussed in this chapter, although all of the possible preexisting medical conditions impacting pregnancy are beyond the scope of this chapter. When caring for women who have preexisting diseases, textbooks on high-risk pregnancy management and perinatal journals are the best sources of information. (See Quality and Safety Education for Nurses (QSEN) Patient Centered Care.)

Quality and Safety Education for Nurses (QSEN) Patient–Centered Care

Recognize the patient or designee as the source of control and full partner in providing compassionate and coordinated care based on respect for the patient's preferences, values, and needs.

Women experiencing pregnancy complications are vulnerable in very special ways physiologically, psychologically, emotionally, and spiritually. Nurses are in a unique position to explore a woman's needs and advocate for the woman's participation in management of pregnancy complications. Some suggestions to foster respect for a woman's preferences, values, and needs include:

- Elicit patient values, preferences, and expressed needs as part of clinical interview, implementation of care plan, and evaluation of care.
- Communicate patient values, preferences, and expressed needs to other members of the health care team.
- Value the patient's expertise with her own health and symptoms.
- Respect patient and family preferences for degree of active engagement in care process.

Cardiovascular Disorders

Pregnancy complicated by cardiovascular disease is potentially dangerous to maternal and fetal well-being. The incidence of cardiac disease among pregnant women ranges from 0.5%–4% and varies in form and severity (Gilbert, 2011; Gaddipati & Troiano, 2013). **Cardiac disease** during pregnancy may be categorized as congenital, acquired, or ischemic. The spectrum and severity of heart disease observed in reproductive-age women is changing. Today, congenital heart disease accounts for more than half of cardiac disease in pregnancy,

and ischemic heart disease is on the rise as a result of obesity, hypertension, diabetes, and delayed childbearing (Arafeh, 2014). Some of the normal cardiac changes during pregnancy can exacerbate cardiac disease during pregnancy, including:

- Increase in total blood volume 30%–50%
- Increase in cardiac output that peaks at 28 to 32 weeks of gestation
- Plasma volume expansion by 45%
- Increase in RBC by 20%
- Increased cardiac output by 40%
- Increased heart rate by 15%
- Heart slightly enlarges and displaces upward and to the left anatomically.
- The weight of the gravid uterus can lie on the inferior vena cava, causing compression and hypotension and decreasing cardiac output.
- Increased estrogen leads to vasodilatation, which lowers peripheral resistance and increases cardiac output.
- Autonomic nervous system influences are more prominent on blood pressure.

Marked hemodynamic changes in pregnancy can have a profound effect on the pregnant woman with cardiac disease and may result in exceeding the functional capacity of the diseased heart (Cunningham et al., 2010; Arafeh, 2014; Mattson & Smith, 2004), resulting in:

- Pulmonary hypertension
- Pulmonary edema
- Congestive heart failure
- Maternal or fetal death

Extensive discussion of specific cardiac disorders and their management is beyond the scope of this text. Reference to texts that deal with management of high-risk pregnancy particularly during labor and delivery is indicated when caring for women with underlying heart disease, but general principles are presented. The management of cardiac disease is related to the cardiac disorder that is present and the impact it has on cardiac function responsible for specific symptoms.

Risks for the Woman

- Maternal mortality with cardiac disorders ranges from 1%–50% based on cardiac disorder.
- Maternal effects include severe pulmonary edema, systemic emboli, and congestive heart failure.

Risks for the Fetus and Newborn

- Fetal effects are a result of decreased systemic circulation and/or decreased oxygenation.
- If maternal circulation is compromised because of decreased cardiac function, uterine blood flow is reduced, which can result in intrauterine growth restriction. Fetal oxygenation is impaired when maternal oxygenation is impaired.
- Fetal hypoxia can result in permanent CNS damage depending on length and severity of decreased oxygenation.
- Neonatal death secondary to maternal cardiac disease ranges from 3%–50%.

Assessment Findings

- Diagnosis of cardiac disease is based on symptoms and diagnostic tests, which may include ECG, echocardiogram, and lab tests.
- The usual signs of deteriorating cardiac function include:
  - *Dyspnea, severe enough to limit usual activity*
  - *Progressive orthopnea*
  - *Paroxysmal nocturnal dyspnea*
  - *Syncope during or after exertion*
  - *Palpitations*
  - *Chest pain with or without activity*
  - *Fatigue*
  - *Cyanosis*
  - *Thromboembolitic changes*
  - *Fluid retention*

Medical Management

- Medical management varies based on cardiac disease and should include collaboration between obstetricians, maternal fetal medicine specialists, cardiologists, anesthesiologists, and other specialists as needed.
- Discuss with the woman estimations of maternal and fetal mortality, potential chronic morbidity, and interventions to minimize risk during pregnancy and delivery.
- Obtain laboratory test to evaluate renal function and profusion (electrolytes, serum creatinine, proteins, and uric acid).
- Invasive hemodynamic monitoring using pulmonary artery catheters, peripheral arterial catheters, or central venous pressure monitors may be necessary.
- Drug therapy is dependent on cardiac lesion.
- Vaginal delivery is recommended for most patients with cardiac disease.
- Preterm delivery may be indicated for deteriorating maternal or fetal status.

Nursing Actions

- Nursing measures are directed toward prevention of complications (Gilbert, 2011).
- Review the woman's history related to cardiovascular disorder, including previous therapies or surgery, current medications, and current functional classification of cardiac disease.
- Conduct a cardiovascular assessment (Gaddipati & Troiano, 2013) that includes:
  - *Auscultation of heart, lungs, and breath sounds*
  - *LOC, BP, HR, capillary refill check*
  - *Evaluation of respiratory rate and rhythm*
  - *Evaluation of cardiac rate and rhythm*
  - *Body weight and weight gain*
  - *Assessment of skin color, temperature, and turgor*
  - *Identification of pathological edema*
- Additional noninvasive assessment may include:
  - *O_2 saturation via pulse oximeter*
  - *Arrhythmia assessment with 12-lead EKG*
  - *Electrocardiogram*
  - *Urinary output*
  - *Electronic fetal monitoring*
- Review laboratory results related to renal function and perfusion.
  - *Electrolytes, blood urea nitrogen (BUN), serum creatinine, proteins, uric acid*
- Determine the patient's and family's understanding of the effect of her cardiac disease on her pregnancy.
- Provide information to the woman and her family regarding status of woman and fetus and plan of care.
  - *Antepartal testing including NSTs, BPPs, and ultrasounds*
  - *New medications may include anticoagulation therapy; therefore, women need to learn to give self-injections.*
- Provide emotional support to the woman and her family.
- Refer patient to high-risk pregnancy support groups.
- Facilitate home health and other referrals PRN.

Hematological Disorders

Pregnancy results in intravascular volume expansion, with the increase in plasma volume larger than the rise in erythrocyte volume, resulting in hemodilution of pregnancy that results in a drop in the hemoglobin and hematocrit. During pregnancy there is an increased potential for thrombosis resulting from increased levels of coagulation factors and decreased fibrinolysis, venous dilation, and obstruction of the venous system by the gravid uterus. Thromboembolyic diseases occurring most frequently in pregnancy include deep vein thrombosis and pulmonary embolism; both are addressed in Chapter 7.

Iron-Deficiency Anemia

Anemia complicates 15%–60% of all pregnancies (Yancy, 2011), and 75% of those anemias are a result of iron deficiency related to a diet low in iron content and insufficient iron stores. Pregnancy results in an intravascular volume expansion with the increase in plasma volume larger than the rise in RBCs, resulting in the hemodilution of pregnancy; the net result is a physiological drop in hemoglobin and hematocrit values. Iron deficiency anemia during pregnancy is the consequence primarily of expansion of plasma volume without normal expansion of maternal hemoglobin mass (Cunningham et al., 2010). **Anemia** is present if the hemoglobin drops below 11 g/dL in the first and third trimesters and below 10 g/dL in the second trimester (Yancy, 2011). Discussion of acquired and inherited anemias and hemoglobinopathies are beyond the scope of this chapter.

Risk Factors

- History of poor nutritional status or eating disorder
- Close spacing of pregnancies
- Multiple gestation
- Excessive bleeding
- Adolescence

Risks for the Woman

- Fatigue
- Reduced tolerance to activity

Risks for the Newborn

- Preterm birth
- Intrauterine growth restriction

Assessment Findings

- Pallor
- Fatigue, weakness, and malaise
- Reduced exercise tolerance and dyspnea
- Anorexia and/or pica
- Edema
- Hemoglobin below 10–11 g/dL
- Hematocrit below 30%

Medical Management

- Iron supplementation
  - *Supplement with 325 mg tid ferrous sulfate.*

Nursing Actions

- Refer the woman to a dietitian for nutritional counseling and reinforce dietary interventions.
- Advise that taking iron supplementation at bedtime and on an empty stomach may increase absorption and decrease gastrointestinal upset.
- Discuss strategies to deal with constipation PRN.
- Assess fatigue and develop interventions and a plan of care to deal with fatigue.

Pulmonary Disorders

Normal physiological changes of pregnancy can cause a woman with a history of compromised respiratory function to decompensate. Pulmonary disease has become more prevalent in women of childbearing age. Pulmonary diseases, such as pneumonia or tocolytic induced pulmonary edema, can develop during pregnancy whereas other conditions such as asthma preexist. It is important to remember that some of the normal respiratory changes during pregnancy can exacerbate respiratory disease during pregnancy. Alteration in the immune system and mechanical and anatomical changes have a cumulative effect to decrease tolerance to hypoxia and acute changes in pulmonary function (McMurtry-Baird & Kennedy, 2014; Gilbert, 2011). These include:

- Increased progesterone during pregnancy results in maternal hyperventilation and increased tidal volume.
- Changes in configuration of the thorax with advancing pregnancy decrease residual capacity and volume while oxygen consumption increases.
- Increased estrogen levels result in mucosal edema, hypersecretion, and capillary congestion.
- Respiratory physiology in normal pregnancy tends toward respiratory alkalosis.

Respiratory emergencies, such as pulmonary embolism and amniotic fluid embolism (anaphylactoid syndrome), are discussed in other sections of the chapter. Asthma is presented as an exemplar of the impact of pregnancy on a preexisting pulmonary disorder.

Asthma

Asthma is the most common form of lung disease that can impact pregnancy and complicates about 8% of pregnancies. **Asthma** is an irrevocable syndrome characterized by varying levels of airway obstruction, bronchial hyperresponsiveness, and bronchial edema.

Diagnosis and management goals of asthma during pregnancy are the same as for nonpregnant women. People with asthma have airways that are hyperresponsive to allergens, viruses, air pollutants, exercise, and cold air. This hyperresponsiveness is manifested by bronchospasm, mucosal edema, and mucus plugging the airways. Goals of therapy include:

- Protection of the pulmonary system from irritants
- Prevention of pulmonary and inflammatory response to allergen exposure
- Relief of bronchospasm
- Resolution of airway inflammation to reduce airway hyper-responsiveness
- Improve pulmonary function

Risks for the Woman

- Pregnancy has varying effects on asthma, with about one-third of pregnant women becoming worse, one-third improving, and one-third remaining the same (Gilbert, 2011).
- If symptoms worsen, they tend to do so between 17–24 weeks' gestation (Gilbert, 2011).
- With aggressive management of asthma, pregnancy outcomes can be the same as for nonasthmatic pregnant women.
- Uncontrolled asthma increases the risk of preeclampsia, hypertension, and hyperemesis gravidarum.

Risks for the Fetus and Newborn

- Hypoxia to the fetus is a major complication.
- Preterm birth
- Low birth weight

Assessment Findings

- Signs and symptoms of asthma:
  - *Cough (productive or nonproductive)*
  - *Wheezing*
  - *Tightness in chest*
  - *Shortness of breath*
  - *Increased respiratory rate (>20 breaths/min)*
- Signs and symptoms of hypoxia:
  - *Cyanosis*
  - *Lethargy*
  - *Agitation or confusion*
  - *Intercostal retractions*
  - *Respiratory rate >30 breaths/min*

Medical Management

Asthma should be aggressively treated during pregnancy, as the benefits of asthma control far outweigh the risks of medication use. During pregnancy, monthly evaluation of pulmonary function and asthma history are conducted. Serial ultrasound for fetal growth and antepartal fetal testing is done for moderately or severely asthmatic women.

- Medications commonly used for asthma management are considered safe during pregnancy and include bronchodilators, anti-inflammatory agents such as inhaled steroids, oral corticosteroids, allergy injections, and antihistamines.

Nursing Actions

- Take a detailed history and assessment of respiratory status, including pulmonary function and blood gases.
- Assess for signs and symptoms including cough, wheezing, chest tightness, and sputum production.
- Care for women with acute asthma exacerbations includes:
  - *Oxygen administration to maintain PaO$_2$ greater than 95%*
  - *Ongoing maternal pulse oximeter*
  - *Baseline arterial blood gases as per orders*
  - *Baseline pulmonary function tests performed to gather baseline data as per orders*
  - *Beta-agonist inhalation therapy as ordered*
- Monitor maternal oxygen saturation (should be at 95% to oxygenate the fetus).
- Assess fetal well-being and for signs of fetal hypoxia.
- Evaluate pulmonary function test results and laboratory tests (i.e., arterial blood gases).
- Explain the plan of care and goals.
- Teach the woman to avoid allergens and triggers.
- Teach the woman to monitor pulmonary function daily and her normal parameters.
- Teach the woman the role of medications, correct use of medications, and adverse effects of medications.
- Teach the woman to recognize signs and symptoms of worsening asthma and provide a treatment plan to manage exacerbations appropriately.
- Discuss warning signs and symptoms to report to the provider, such as dyspnea, shortness of breath, chest tightness, or exacerbations of signs and symptoms beyond the woman's baseline asthma status.

Gastrointestinal Disorders

Cholelithiasis, presence of gallstones in the gallbladder, occurs in approximately 8% of pregnancies (Gilbert, 2011). Decreased muscle tone allows gallbladder distension and thickening of the bile and prolongs emptying time during pregnancy, increasing the risk of cholelithiasis.

Assessment Findings

Colicky abdominal pain presents in the right upper quadrant; anorexia, nausea, and vomiting; the woman may have a fever. Gallstones are present on an ultrasound scan.

Medical Management

Cholelithiasis is typically treated with conservative management such as IV fluids, bowel rest, nasogastric suctioning, diet, and antibiotics. Increasingly, it is managed by surgical intervention with laparoscopic cholecystectomies (Cunningham et al., 2010).

If gallbladder disease is nonacute, surgical intervention may be delayed until the postpartum period.

Nursing Actions

- Manage pain, administering pain medication as needed.
- Manage nausea and vomiting, minimizing environmental factors that cause nausea and vomiting such as odors.
- Administer antiemetics as needed.
- Provide comfort measures based on symptoms.
- Explain procedures and plan of care including dietary restrictions.

Venous Thromboembolic Disease

Venous thromboembolic disease has two components: deep vein thrombosis (DVT) and pulmonary embolism (PE) (Gilbert, 2011). Pregnancy is a hypercoagulable state with increased fibrin generation, increased coagulation factors, and decreased fibrinolytic activity. Venous stasis in the lower extremities, increased blood volume, and compression of the inferior vena cava and pelvic veins with advancing gestation all combine to increase risk five times over non-pregnant women (Krivak & Zorn, 2007). About half of the cases of venous thromboembolism during pregnancy are associated with a common risk factor for thrombophilia. Acquired and/or inherited thrombophilia are associated with severe preeclampsia, abruption, intrauterine growth restriction (IUGR), intrauterine fetal demise (IUFD), preterm birth, and recurrent miscarriage (Simpson & Creehan, 2008). Thrombophilia can be an inheritable hypercoagulable condition caused by mutations in clotting mechanisms. The most common acquired thrombophilia during pregnancy is antiphospholipid antibody syndrome (APLA). These antibodies are a result of antigenic changes in endothelial and platelet membranes which promote thrombosis. Other risk factors for venous thrombosis during pregnancy include:

- Bed rest
- Obesity
- Severe varicose vein
- Dehydration
- Trauma
- History of thrombosis
- Medical conditions such as diabetes, heart disease, renal disease or serious infections

Assessment Findings

- Classic signs of DVT are dependant edema, unilateral leg pain, erythema, low-grade fever, and positive Homan's sign (i.e., pain with dorsiflexion of foot).
- A PE may present with shortness of breath, tachypnea, tachycardia, dyspnea, pleural chest pain, fever, and anxiety.

Medical Management

Objective tests for DVT include Doppler ultrasound, magnetic resonance venography, and pulsed Doppler study. Chest X-ray, CT, and electrocardiography are used to diagnose PE. Treatment goals include prevention of further clot propagation, prevention of PE, and prevention of further venous thromboembolism (Krivak & Zorn, 2007).

■ Anticoagulation therapy is required for women experiencing a DVT during pregnancy with heparin.
■ Treatment of PE is to stabilize a woman with a life-threatening PE and transfer to ICU. Thromboembolitic therapy and catheter or surgical embolectomy may be done.

Nursing Actions

■ Manage pain, administering pain medication as needed.
■ Teach woman how to administer heparin SQ to her abdomen.
■ Instruct woman to report side effects such as bleeding gums, nosebleeds, easy bruising, or excessive trauma at injection sites.

Maternal Obesity

Maternal obesity has long been recognized as a risk factor in pregnancy. There is a well-established risk factor for the development of preeclampsia, gestational and type 2 diabetes, and thrombosis (ACOG, 2013; Ramachenderan, Bradford, & McLean, 2008). Many of the systemic physiological alterations that occur during pregnancy may be altered when the pregnant woman is obese (Ramachenderan, Bradford, & McLean, 2008). For example:

■ The typical increase in cardiac output associated with pregnancy is compounded when a woman is obese and is influenced by the degree and duration of obesity. Cardiac output increases by 30–50 mL/min for every 100 g of fat deposited. Blood volume is increased as well. A degree of cardiac hypertrophy is normal during pregnancy, but obesity exaggerates the hypertrophy and contributes to myocardial dilation.
■ Although obese women can experience more frequent episodes of obstructive sleep apnea (OSA) than women with normal BMI, pregnancy may exert a protective effect on OSA occurrence.
■ Pregnant women are more prone to gastric reflux, given associated hormonal and anatomic changes. The incidence of hiatus hernia is greater in obese patients, and abdominal pressure and intragastric volume are increased in the obese patient.
■ Pregnancy is a hypercoagulable state, and obesity further increases the risk of thrombosis by promoting venous stasis, increasing blood viscosity, and promoting activation of the coagulation cascade.
■ A large panniculus, that is, a thick layer of adipose tissue in the abdominal area, sometimes called a fatty apron, may contribute to uterine compression and exaggerate the vena cava syndrome to which pregnant women are susceptible.

Assessment Findings

■ BMI of ≥30

Medical Management

■ Provide specific information on maternal risks of obesity in pregnancy.
■ Provide specific information on the increased risk for an infant with a neural tube defect and for a stillborn infant.
■ These risks require heightened and ongoing evaluation of the pregnant woman and fetus.

Nursing Actions

■ Reinforce information on maternal and fetal risks associated with obesity.
■ Provide teaching on signs and symptoms of preeclampsia, diabetes, sleep apnea, and vena cava syndrome.
■ Ensure woman understands plan of care for increased and ongoing evaluation of pregnancy.
■ Because pregnancy presents an ideal time during which to initiate simple healthy behaviors, such as walking and proper diet that can be maintained after birth, offer suggestions and encouragement for lifestyle changes.
■ Provide referrals to dietitian for nutritional counseling and reinforce guidelines for diet and weight gain.
■ Use caution when shifting the panniculus to assess for fetal heart sounds or when providing personal hygiene, as the redistributed weight may alter maternal hemodynamics and increase the risk of vena cava compression.
■ Encouraging the woman to sleep in a sitting position may help, as effects of obesity on the respiratory system are decreased in this position.
■ Making appropriate environmental changes to accommodate the larger patient, such as assuring that patient beds, examining tables, and chairs can support at least 400 pounds.

SUBSTANCE ABUSE

Alcohol, cigarette, and illicit drug use during pregnancy can cause poor pregnancy outcomes and early childhood behavioral and development problems. Recent reports show that alcohol use among pregnant women in the first trimester was 19.0%, for those in the second trimester 7.8%, and for the third trimester 6.2%. There were similar patterns for past-month binge alcohol use, cigarette use, and marijuana use (Substance Abuse and Mental Health Services Administration, Office of Applied Studies, 2009). The findings in this report suggest that many U.S. women, particularly those in the third trimester, are getting the message and abstaining from substance use. Still, a sizeable proportion of women in the first trimester of pregnancy were past-month users of alcohol, cigarettes, or marijuana, and one in seven women used cigarettes in the second or third trimester. In addition, many women are resuming use of these substances after childbirth, and that resumption appears to be rapid given the higher rates for mothers of infants under 3 months old compared with pregnant women in the second or third trimesters. Effective interventions for women to further reduce substance use during pregnancy and to prevent postpartum resumption of use could improve the overall health and well-being of mothers and infants.

Many pregnant women who use illicit drugs also use alcohol and tobacco, and it may be difficult to determine which complications are associated with which substance. Risks of specific complications vary based on substance used; however, general risks resulting from substance abuse for both the woman and fetus/newborn are presented. Pregnant women using illicit substances often fear legal consequences and may avoid seeking prenatal care. A nonjudgmental and factual approach with attention toward reducing risks offers the best approach for these complex pregnancies. Chemically dependent pregnant women may engage in other risky behaviors. A holistic, comprehensive approach to care that deals not only with the prenatal aspects of care, but also with the complex social and psychological contributing factors, is needed.

Smoking/Tobacco Use

Smoking during pregnancy increases the risk of premature delivery, low-birth-weight infants, and stillbirth. Pregnant women were more likely to have smoked cigarettes during their first trimester (22.9%) than during their second (14.3 %) or third (15.3 %) trimesters (Substance Abuse and Mental Health Services Administration, 2007). The same report cites studies suggesting that women who stop smoking by the first trimester give birth to infants with weight and body measurements comparable with those of infants of nonsmokers (US DHHS, 2008). The physiological effects of smoking are a result of transient intrauterine hypoxemia. The more the woman smokes, the greater the risk (March of Dimes, 2008a). Cigarette smoke contains many chemicals, in particular nicotine and carbon monoxide, that cause adverse pregnancy outcomes, particularly low birth weight and prematurity.

■ Nicotine reduces uterine blood flow.
■ Carbon monoxide binds to hemoglobin, reducing the oxygen-carrying capacity of the blood (Creasy, Resnik, & Iams, 2004).

Alcohol

Alcohol use during pregnancy can cause physical and mental birth defects, preterm births, and miscarriages. Because a safe level of alcohol intake during pregnancy cannot be determined, both the U.S. Surgeon General and the March of Dimes Foundation recommend that pregnant women not consume any alcohol. White women were more likely than Hispanic women to have drunk alcohol in the past month regardless of their pregnancy status. Generally, higher education status and higher family income were associated with higher rates of alcohol use among all women of childbearing age regardless of their pregnancy status. Among women aged 18–44, those with a college education were nearly twice as likely as their counterparts with less than a high school education to have used alcohol in the past month in each pregnancy status category. Similarly, women age 15–44 with annual family incomes of $75,000 or higher had the highest rates of alcohol use in the prior month compared with those with lower family incomes in all three pregnancy status

categories (Substance Abuse and Mental Health Services Administration, 2008). Other data from the CDC reports 12.2% of pregnant women (about 1 in 8) drink during pregnancy, and 1.9% of pregnant women (about 1 in 50) reported binge drinking in the past 30 days.

Pregnant women age 15-17 years may be in particular need of alcohol prevention services tailored for their age group because nearly 16% of them used alcohol in the past month. Pregnant women in this age group consumed an average of 24 drinks in the past month (i.e., they drank on an average of six days during the past month and an average of about four drinks on the days that they drank).

Alcohol is the most common teratogen (Gilbert, 2007). When a pregnant woman drinks, alcohol passes swiftly to the fetus through the placenta. Because alcohol is processed more slowly in the fetus's liver, the alcohol level can be even higher and can remain elevated longer. Drinking alcohol during pregnancy can result in a wide range of physical and mental birth defects. The term "fetal alcohol spectrum disorder" (FASD) is used to describe the many problems associated with alcohol exposure prior to birth.

Alcohol consumed during pregnancy increases the risk of alcohol-related birth defects, including growth deficiencies, facial abnormalities, central nervous system impairment, behavioral disorders, and impaired intellectual development (Bertrand, Floyd, Weber, O'Connor, Riley, Johnson, & Cohen, 2004). Each year in the United States up to 40,000 infants are born with FASDs (March of Dimes, 2008b). Chapter 17 provides additional information on FASDs. The consensus is that no level of drinking alcohol is considered safe in pregnancy.

Illicit Drugs

An average of 5.2% of pregnant women use illicit drugs such as marijuana, cocaine, amphetamines, heroin, and Ecstasy (US DHHS, 2008). The effect of the drug on placental function and fetal development depends on its nature. For example, cocaine causes vasoconstriction that can impact the placenta and uterus, resulting in abruption of the placenta or preterm birth (Foley, 2002; March of Dimes, 2006c). Women who use illicit drugs are counseled to stop, except for heroin users, for whom methadone treatment is recommended to prevent stillbirth.

Cocaine

Cocaine abuse and addiction is a complex problem which involves physiological changes in the brain as well as changes in psychosocial and environmental factors. Biologically, cocaine blocks the reuptake of catecholamines at the nerve terminal, which results in an increase in circulating catecholamines in the blood and leads to vasoconstriction. Cardiovascular and neurological complications such as hypertension, tachycardia, uterine contractions, myocardial infarction, dysrhythmias, subarachnoid hemorrhage, thrombocytopenia, seizures and even sudden death have been described among patients who abuse cocaine. Acute use of cocaine during the third trimester can result in preterm labor, a greater incidence of PROM, abruptio placentae, precipitous delivery, increased risk for meconium staining, and premature and low-birth-weight infants (Moran, 2011).

Heroin

Heroin abuse during pregnancy is linked to adverse consequences to both mother and fetus. It is believed that the hazards of heroin to the fetus are directly related to the physiological dependence effect on the fetus and the maternal lifestyle associated with heroin use. The primary effects of heroin include analgesia, sedation, feeling of well-being, and euphoria. Women who use heroin during pregnancy typically do not seek early prenatal care for fear of detection of heroin use and are at an increased risk to exposure to serious infections such as STDs, hepatitis, and HIV. The neonatal effects of prenatal heroin exposure include withdrawal symptoms, increased incidence of meconium aspiration at birth, increased incidence of sepsis, IUGR, and neurodevelopmental behavioral problems (Moran, 2011).

Marijuana

Marijuana use causes tachycardia and low blood pressure, which can result in orthostatic hypotension. Research has shown the neonates born to mothers who used marijuana during pregnancy can have an altered response to visual stimuli, increased tremilousness, and even a high-pitched cry which may indicate a problem with neurological development (Moran, 2011).

Risks for the Woman Using Substances during Pregnancy

- Preterm labor
- PPROM
- Poor weight gain and nutritional status
- Placental abnormalities (placenta previa, abruptio placentae)

Risks for the Fetus and Newborn

- Effects of maternal substance use on the neonate are detailed in Chapter 17.
- Stillbirth
- Low birth weight
- Preterm birth
- Intrauterine growth restriction
- Neonatal withdrawal syndrome (symptoms are dependent on drug used during pregnancy) (See Chapter 17)
- Sudden infant death syndrome (SIDS)

Assessment Findings in Women Using Substances during Pregnancy

A variety of screening tools have been proposed, and screening for smoking, alcohol use, and illicit drugs is recommended to start at the first prenatal visit. Universal screening of all pregnant women is recommended in a supportive and nonjudgmental manner (Gilbert, 2007). One simple screening tool includes asking the following four questions for a yes or no response, described as Ewing's 4 P's (Taylor, Zaichkin, & Bailey, 2002).

- Have you ever used alcohol or drugs during this **pregnancy?**
- Have you had a problem with drugs or alcohol in the **past?**
- Does your **partner** have a problem with drugs or alcohol?
- Do you consider one of your **parents** to have a problem with drugs or alcohol?

A yes answer to any of these questions should trigger further evaluation of habits.

Medical Management (Creasy, Resnik, & Iams, 2004)

- Screen for substance use in pregnancy with all pregnant women (American College of Obstetricians and Gynecologists, 2008).
- Refer to multispecialty clinics.
- Refer to drug treatment programs.
- Screen for domestic violence.
- Conduct frequent urine toxicology tests.
- Use targeted ultrasound to rule out congenital anomalies.
- Provide patient education.
- Conduct antepartal testing.

Nursing Actions for the Woman Using Substances during Pregnancy

- Women are more receptive to treatment and lifestyle changes during pregnancy; therefore, pregnancy may be a window of opportunity for chemically dependent women to enter treatment. To facilitate this, nurses must be armed with knowledge and information necessary to screen and identify women who abuse substances during pregnancy.
- Provide health education about the risks to the fetus of substance use during pregnancy and facilitate early diagnosis and appropriate intervention and referral.
- Laws governing drug screening during pregnancy vary from state to state. Nurses need to be aware of laws and local guidelines for toxicology screening of pregnant women and treatment options and availability of programs, as many treatment programs will not accept pregnant women.
- Counsel women who test positive for drug or alcohol use and those who smoke during pregnancy to stop and supply referrals to assist with cessation and refer to local treatment centers for pregnant women (**Box 7-5**).
- Maintain a nonjudgmental and nonpunitive attitude (Selleck & Redding, 1998); remember addiction is a disease.
- It has been proposed that government policies can be viewed as either "facilitative" or "adversarial" (Bornstein, 2003). Facilitative policies improve women's access to prenatal care, food, shelter, and treatment.
- Adversarial policies propose that women who fail to seek treatment are liable to criminal prosecution and may diminish utilization of prenatal care.
- Because of the substantial costs and repercussions of drug use during pregnancy for newborns, women, and society, it is essential to devise methods of intervention that decrease this risky behavior.
- Pregnant women aged 15–17 may be in particular need of alcohol prevention services tailored for their age group because of the high rates of alcohol use in pregnancy.

BOX 7–5   REFERRALS FOR INFORMATION AND SUPPORT ON QUITTING SUBSTANCE USE DURING PREGNANCY

Alcoholics Anonymous
    www.aa.org
Narcotics Anonymous
    www.na.org
Smoking Cessation
    www.ahrg.gov/consumer/tobacco/quits.htm
    www.helppregnantsmokersquit.com
    www.cancer.org
    www.smokefreefamilies.org
    www.marchofdimes.org

Many women who need substance abuse treatment may not receive it due to lack of money or child care, fear of losing custody of their children, or other barriers. For successful recovery, women often need a continuum of care for an extended period of time, including:

- Comprehensive inpatient or outpatient treatment for alcohol and other drugs
- Case management
- Counseling and other mental health treatment
- Medical and prenatal care
- Child care
- Transportation
- Follow-up pediatric and early intervention services for children
- Services that respond to women's needs regarding reproductive health, sexuality, relationships, and victimization
- Other support services, such as housing, education and job training, financial support services, parenting education, legal services, and aftercare.

A study of women who continued to use alcohol or drugs after learning they were pregnant found that they were more frequent users than spontaneous quitters, more likely to smoke cigarettes, and had more psychosocial stressors (Harrison & Sidebottom, 2009). Achieving higher rates of cessation may require approaches that simultaneously address substance use and impediments to quitting. Research shows that residential substance abuse treatment designed specifically for pregnant women and women with children can have substantial benefits in terms of recovery, pregnancy outcomes, parenting skills, and women's ability to maintain or regain custody of their children.

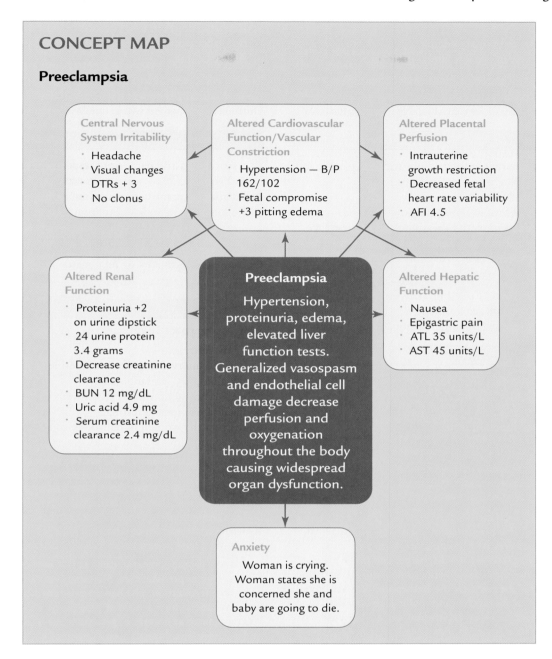

CONCEPT MAP

Preeclampsia

Central Nervous System Irritability
- Headache
- Visual changes
- DTRs + 3
- No clonus

Altered Cardiovascular Function/Vascular Constriction
- Hypertension — B/P 162/102
- Fetal compromise
- +3 pitting edema

Altered Placental Perfusion
- Intrauterine growth restriction
- Decreased fetal heart rate variability
- AFI 4.5

Altered Renal Function
- Proteinuria +2 on urine dipstick
- 24 urine protein 3.4 grams
- Decrease creatinine clearance
- BUN 12 mg/dL
- Uric acid 4.9 mg
- Serum creatinine clearance 2.4 mg/dL

Preeclampsia
Hypertension, proteinuria, edema, elevated liver function tests. Generalized vasospasm and endothelial cell damage decrease perfusion and oxygenation throughout the body causing widespread organ dysfunction.

Altered Hepatic Function
- Nausea
- Epigastric pain
- ATL 35 units/L
- AST 45 units/L

Anxiety
Woman is crying. Woman states she is concerned she and baby are going to die.

Problem No. 1: Central Nervous System Irritability
Goal: Prevent seizures and cerebral edema
Outcome: Patient will remain seizure free and not develop neurological sequelae.

Nursing Actions

1. Monitor CNS changes including headache, dizziness, blurred vision, and scotoma.
2. Maintain seizure precautions.
3. If treated with magnesium sulfate, see Critical Component: Care of the Woman on Magnesium Sulfate.
4. Restrict fluids to total of 125 mL/hr or as ordered.
5. Monitor I&O.
6. Assess DTRs.
7. Maintain bed rest in the lateral position.
8. Provide an environment that is conducive to decreased stimulation, such as low lights, decreased noise, and uninterrupted rest periods.
9. Teach the patient relaxation techniques.

Problem No. 2: Altered Cardiovascular Function/Vasoconstriction
Goal: Normal blood pressure
Outcome: Blood pressure within acceptable limits, below 140/90 mm Hg

Nursing Actions

1. Monitor BP every hour or more frequently if elevated.
2. Administer antihypertensive medication as ordered related to hypertensive parameters.

5. An appropriate gestational age to do glucose screening is:
   A. 22 weeks of gestation
   B. 26 weeks of gestation
   C. 30 weeks of gestation
   D. 34 weeks of gestation

6. Smoking during pregnancy increases the risk of:
   A. Low birth weight and prematurity
   B. Neonatal lung disease
   C. Preeclampsia

7. The goal of magnesium sulfate therapy in treating preeclampsia is to:
   A. Reduce blood pressure
   B. Delay delivery
   C. Prevent seizures
   D. Increase placental perfusion

8. Hypoglycemia is defined as a blood glucose below:
   A. 60 mg/dL
   B. 70 mg/dL
   C. 80 mg/dL
   D. 90 mg/dL

9. Management of women with pregestational diabetes should begin:
   A. Before conception
   B. At the end of the first trimester
   C. At the end of 20 weeks
   D. Before the onset of labor

10. An oxygen saturation below _____ is an abnormal finding for a pregnant woman.
    A. 90%
    B. 92%
    C. 95%
    D. 97%

11. The likelihood of dizygotic twinning is affected by:
    A. Advancing maternal age
    B. Use of assisted reproductive technology
    C. Maternal nutritional status

12. Women are more receptive to treatment and lifestyle changes during pregnancy, so pregnancy may be a window of opportunity for chemically dependent women to enter treatment.
    A. True
    B. False

References

American College of Obstetricians and Gynecologists. (2013). ACOG Committee opinion no. 549. Washington, DC; Author.

American College of Obstetricians and Gynecologists. (2008). ACOG Committee opinion no. 42. At risk drinking and illicit drug use: Ethical issues in Obstetric and gynecological practice. *Obstetrics & Gynecology, 112,* 449–60.

American College of Obstetricians and Gynecologists (2004). Diagnosis and treatment of gestational trophoblastic disease. Washington (DC): American College of Obstetricians and Gynecologists (ACOG); 2004 (ACOG practice bulletin; no. 53).

American College of Obstetricians and Gynecologists (2010). Committee opinion no. 445. Magnesium sulfate before antepartal preterm birth for neuroprotection. Washington DC: 669–671.

American College of Obstetricians and Gynecologists (2012). Chronic hypertension in pregnancy. Practice bulletin no. 125. Washington DC: Author.

American College of Obstetricians and Gynecologists. Medical management of ectopic pregnancy. Washington (DC): American College of Obstetricians and Gynecologists; 2008 (ACOG practice bulletin; no. 94).

American College of Obstetricians and Gynecologists. 2012. Management of preterm labor. Washington (DC): American College of Obstetricians and Gynecologists; 2003 May. 9 p. (ACOG practice bulletin; no. 127).

American College of Obstetricians and Gynecologists. (2004). Nausea and vomiting of pregnancy. Washington (DC): American College of Obstetricians and Gynecologists; 2004 (ACOG practice bulletin; no. 52).

American College of Obstetricians and Gynecologists. 2008. Use of progesterone to prevent preterm birth. Washington (DC): American College of Obstetricians and Gynecologists; 2008 (ACOG practice bulletin; no. 112), 963–5.

American College of Obstetricians and Gynecologists. (2007). Premature rupture of membranes. Washington (DC): American College of Obstetricians and Gynecologists; (ACOG practice bulletin; no. 80).

American College of Obstetricians and Gynecologists. (2011). Screening and Diagnosis of Gestational Diabetes Mellitus ACOG Committee opinion. Number 504. 118: 751–3.

Alwan, N., Tuffnell, D. J., & West, J. (2009). Treatments for gestational diabetes. *Cochrane Database of Systematic Reviews* 2009, Issue 3. Art. No.: CD003395. DOI: 10.1002/14651858.CD003395.pub2.

American Diabetes Association. (2006). Diagnosis and classification of diabetes mellitus. *Diabetes Care, 29,* S43–S48.

American Diabetes Association (ADA). (2004). Gestational diabetes mellitus. *Diabetes Care, 27,* S88–90.

Arafeh, J. (2014). Cardiac disease in pregnancy. Simpson, K. & Creehan, P. Perinatal nursing, 4th ed. Philadelphia: Lippincott, Williams & Wilkins.

Berhman, R., & Stith Butler, A. (Eds.). (2007). Preterm Birth: Causes, Consequences, and Prevention. Committee on Understanding Premature Birth and Assuring Healthy Outcomes Institute of Medicine of the Academies. Washington: The National Academies Press.

Berkman, N., Thorp, J., Lohr, K., Cary, T., Hartman, K., Gavin, N., Hasselblad, V., & Inicula, A. (2003). Tocolytic treatment for the management of preterm labor: A review of the evidence. *American Journal of Obstetrics and Gynecology, 188*(6), 1648–1659.

Bertrand, J., Floyd, R. L., Weber, M. K., O'Connor, M., Riley, E. P., Johnson, K. A., Cohen, D. E., National Task Force on FAS/FAE. (2004). Fetal Alcohol Syndrome: Guidelines for Referral and Diagnosis. Atlanta, GA: Centers for Disease Control and Prevention.

Bornstein, B. (2003). Pregnancy, drug testing, and the Fourth Amendment: Legal and behavioral implications: Pregnancy and reproduction issues. *The Journal of Family Psychology, 17,* 220–228.

Bowers, N. (2014). Multiple gestation. In Simpson, K. & Creehan, P. Perinatal nursing, 4th ed. Philadelphia: Lippincott, Williams & Wilkins.

Burke-Sosa, M.E. (2014). Bleeding in pregnancy. In Simpson, K. & Creehan, P. Perinatal nursing, 4th ed. Philadelphia: Lippincott, Williams & Wilkins.

Centers for Disease Control and Prevention (CDC). (2004a). Pelvic Inflammatory Disease-CDC Fact Sheet, May 2004. Retrieved from www.cdc.gov/std/PID/STDFact-PID.htm

Centers for Disease Control and Prevention (CDC). (2004b). STDs & Pregnancy- CDC Fact Sheet, May, 2004. Retrieved from www.cdc.gov/std/STDFact-STDs & Pregnancy.htm Centers for Disease Control and Prevention (CDC). (2005). Sexually

Transmitted Disease Surveillance, 2004. Atlanta: U.S. Department of Health and Human Service, September 2005.

Centers for Disease Control and Prevention (CDC). (2006). Sexually Transmitted Diseases Treatment Guidelines 2006. *MMRW* 2006:55 (no. RR-11).

Creasy, R., Resnik, R., & Iams, J. (Eds.). (2004). *Maternal-fetal medicine* (5th ed.). Philadelphia: W. B. Saunders.

Crowther, C., McKinlay, C., Middleton, P., & Harding, J. (2011). Repeat doses of prenatal corticosteroids for women at risk of preterm birth for improving neonatal health outcomes. *Cochrane Database of Systematic Reviews, (6)*.

Cunningham, E. G., Leveno, K. J., Bloom, S. L., Hauth, J. C., Rouse, D. J., & Spong, C. Y. (2010). *Williams Obstetrics* (23rd ed.). New York: McGraw-Hill.

Daley, J. (2014). Diabetes in pregnancy. In Simpson, K. & Creehan, P. Perinatal nursing, 4th ed. Philadelphia: Lippincott, Williams & Wilkins.

Gilbert, E. (2011). Labor and Delivery at Risk. In Mattson, S., & Smith J. (Ed.), Core Curriculum for Maternal-Newborn Nursing, Fourth Edition. St Louis, Elsevier Saunders pages 624-629.

Gilbert, E., (2011). *Manual of high risk pregnancy and delivery.*, 5th ed. St. Louis, C. V. Mosby.

Deglin, J., & Vallerand, A. (2009). *Davis's drug guide for nurses* (11th ed.). Philadelphia: F.A. Davis.

Durham, R. (1998). Strategies women engage in when managing preterm labor at home. *Journal of Perinatology, 18*, 61–64.

Doyle, L. W., Crowther, C. A., Middleton, P., Marret, S., Rouse, D. (2009). Magnesium sulphate for women at risk of preterm birth for neuroprotection of the fetus. *Cochrane Database of Systematic Reviews* 2009, Issue 1. Art. No.: CD004661. DOI: 10.1002/14651858.CD004661.pub3.

Eunice Kennedy Shriver National Institute of Child Health and Human Development, NIH, DHHS. (2008). Prematurity Research at the NIH (NA). Washington, DC: U.S. Government Printing Office.

Foley, E. (2002). Drug screening and criminal prosecution of pregnant women. *Journal of Obstetric and Gynecologic and Neonatal Nursing, 31*(2), 133–137.

Freda, M., Patterson, E., & Wieczorek, R. (2004). Preterm labor: Prevention and nursing management. In *Continuing education for registered nurses and certified nurse midwives* (3rd ed.). White Plains, NY: March of Dimes.

Gaddipati, S., & Troiano, N. (2013). Cardiac Disorders in Pregnancy. In Troiano, N., Harvey, C., & Chez, B. (Eds.). High Risk & Critical Care Obstetrics, 3rd ed., Association of Women's Health Obstetrics and Neonatal Nursing. Philadelphia: Wolters Kluwer/Lippincott Williams & Wilkins.

Gibson, P., Carson, M., & Letterie, G. (2007). Hypertension and pregnancy. emedicine specialties from WEBMD, December 13, 2007.

Goldstein, R. (2007). Management of Preterm Labor. In Queenan, J. (Ed.) High Risk Pregnancy. The American College of Obstetricians and Gynecologists.

Gregg, A. (2004). Hypertension in pregnancy. *Obstetrics and Gynecology Clinics of North America, 31*, 223–241.

Grey, B. (2006). A ticking uterus. *Lifelines, 10*, 380–389.

Griffith, J., & Conway, D. (2004). Care diabetes in pregnancy. *Obstetrics and Gynecology Clinics of North America, 31*, 243–256.

Harrison, P., & Sidebottom, A. (2009). Alcohol and Drug Use Before and During Pregnancy: An Examination of Use Patterns and Predictors of Cessation. *Maternal Child Health Journal 13*, 386–394.

Hodnett, E. (2010). Support during pregnancy for women at increased risk of low birthweight babies. *Cochrane Database of Systematic Reviews, (6)*.

Hoffert Gilmartin, A., Ural, S., & Repke, J. (2008). Gestational Diabetes Mellitus Review. *Obstetrics & Gynecology 1*(3),129–134.

Iams, J. (2007). Predication and Early Detection of Preterm Labor. In Queenan, J. (Ed.), High Risk Pregnancy. The American College of Obstetricians and Gynecologists.

Institute of Medicine. (2007). Preterm Birth: Causes, Consequences, and Prevention. National Academy Press, Washington, D.C. Published and unpublished analyses.

Kendrick, J. (2004). *Diabetes in pregnancy* (3rd ed.). White Plains, NY: March of Dimes Nursing Module.

Krivak, T., & Zorn, K. (2007). Venous Thromboembolism in Obstetric and Gynecology. In Queenan, J. (Ed.), High Risk Pregnancy. The American College of Obstetricians and Gynecologists.

Kröner, C., Turnbull, D., & Wilkinson, C. (2001). Antenatal day care units versus hospital admission for women with complicated pregnancy. *Cochrane Database of Systematic Reviews* 2001, Issue 4. Art. No.: CD001803. DOI:10.1002/14651858.CD001803.

Magpie Trial Collaborative Group. (2002). Do women with preeclampsia, and their babies, benefit from magnesium sulphate? The Magpie Trial: A randomized placebo-controlled trial. *The Lancet, 359*, 1877–1890.

Maloni, J. A. (1993). Bedrest during pregnancy: Implications for nursing. *Journal of Obstetric, Gynecologic, and Neonatal Nursing, 23*, 422–426.

Maloni, J. A. (1998). Antepartum bedrest: Case studies, research I nursing care. Washington, DC: Association of Women's Health, Obstetric and Neonatal Nurses.

March of Dimes. (2006a). Compendium on preterm birth: Epidemiology and biology of preterm birth. Produced in cooperation with American Academy of Pediatrics, The American College of Obstetricians and Gynecologists & Association of Women's Health, Obstetric and Neonatal Nurses.

March of Dimes. (2006b). Compendium on preterm birth: Employing systems-based practice for patient care. Produced in cooperation with American Academy of Pediatrics, The American College of Obstetricians and Gynecologists & Association of Women's Health, Obstetric and Neonatal Nurses.

March of Dimes. (2006c). Illicit drug use during pregnancy. Retrieved from www.marchofdimes.com/printableArticles/14332_1169.asp

March of Dimes. (2008a). Smoking during pregnancy. Retrieved from www.marchofdimes.com/printableArticles/14332_1171.asp

March of Dimes. (2008b). Drinking alcohol during pregnancy. Retrieved from www.marchofdimes.com/printableArticle/14332_1170.asp

March of Dimes. (2011). *Healthy Babies are Worth the Wait: Preventing Preterm Births through Community-Based Interventions: Implementation Manual.*

March of Dimes. (2012). PERINATAL DATA SNAPSHOTS: United States: Maternal and Infant Health Overview. Retrieved from ww.marchofdimes.com

Martin, J., Hamilton, B. Osterman, M. (2012) Three decades of twin births in the United States, 1980–2009. NCHS Data Brief USDHHS Washington, DC: Author.

Martin, J., Hamilton, B., Ventura, S., Osterman, M., Kirmeyer, S., Mathews, T., Wilson, E. (2011). Birth: Final data for 2009. *National Vital Statistic Reports, 57, 1*. Hyattville, MD: National Center for Health Statistics.

Matthews, A., Dowswell, T., Haas, D. M., Doyle, M., & O'Mathúna, D. P. 2010. Interventions for nausea and vomiting in early pregnancy. *Cochrane Database of Systematic Reviews*, Issue 9. Art. No.: CD007575. DOI: 10.1002/14651858.CD007575.pub2.

Mattson, S., & Smith, J. E. (Eds.). (2011). *Core curriculum for maternal-newborn nursing* (4th ed.). St. Louis, MO: Elsevier Saunders.

McMurtry-Baird, S., & Kennedy, B. (2014). Pulmonary complications in pregnancy. In Simpson, K. & Creehan, P. Perinatal nursing, 4th ed. Philadelphia: Lippincott, Williams & Wilkins.

Moran, B. (2011). Substance Abuse in Pregnancy. In Mattson, S., & Smith, J. E. (Eds.), *Core curriculum for maternal-newborn nursing* (4th ed.). St. Louis, MO: Elsevier Saunders.

Meis, P. (2007). 17 alpha Hydroxyprogesterone Caproate for the Prevention of Preterm Delivery. In Queenan, J. (Ed.), High Risk Pregnancy, The American College of Obstetricians and Gynecologists.

Meis, P. J., Klebanoff, M., Thom, E., Dombrowski, M.P., Sibai, B., Moawad, A.H., Spong, C.Y., Hauth, J.C., Miodovnik, M., Varner, M.W., Leveno, K.J., Caritis, S.N., Iams, J.D., Wapner, R.J., Conway, D., O'Sullivan, M.J., Carpenter, M., Mercer, B., Ramin, S.M., Thorp, J.M., Peaceman, A.M., & Gabbe, S. (2003). National Institute of Child Health and Human Development Maternal-Fetal Medicine Units Network. Prevention of recurrent preterm delivery by 17 alpha-hydryoxyprogesterone caproate. *New England Journal of Medicine, 348*(24), 2379–85.

Mignini, L. E., Villar, J., & Khalid, K. S. (2006). Mapping the theories of preeclampsia: The need for systematic reviews of mechanisms of the disease. *American Journal of Obstetrics and Gynecology, 194,* 317–321.

Morin, K., & Reilly, L. (2007). Caring for obese pregnant women. *JOGNN: Journal of Obstetric, Gynecologic & Neonatal Nursing, 36*(5), 482–489.

Nanda, K., Cook, L. A. A., Gallo, M. F., & Grimes, D. A. (2002). Terbutaline pump maintenance therapy after threatened preterm labor for preventing preterm birth. *Cochrane Database of Systematic Reviews* 2002, Issue 4. Art. No.: CD003933. DOI: 10.1002/14651858.CD003933.

National High Blood Pressure Education Program Working Group (NHBPEP). (2000). Working group report on high blood pressure in pregnancy (NHBPEP Publication No. 00-3029). Washington, DC: National Heart Lung and Blood Institute.

Neilson, J. P. (2003). Interventions for suspected placenta previa. *Cochrane Database of Systematic Reviews* 2003, Issue 2. Art. No.:CD001998. DOI: 10.1002/14651858.CD001998.

Owen, J., & Harger, J. (2007). Cerclage and Cervical Incompetency. In Queenan, J. (Ed.), High Risk Pregnancy. The American College of Obstetricians and Gynecologists.

Perkins, J. M., Dunn, J. P., & Jagasia, S. M. (2007). Perspectives in gestational diabetes mellitus: A review of screening, diagnosis, and treatment. *Clinical Diabetes, 25,* 57–62.

PeriStats. (2008). National Center for Health Statistics, final natality data. Retrieved from www.marchofdimes.com/peristats

Peters, R., & Flack, J. (2004). Hypertensive disorders of pregnancy. *Journal of Obstetric, Gynecologic, and Neonatal Nursing, 33,* 209–219.

Poole, J. (2014). Hypertension disorders in pregnancy. In Simpson, K. & Creehan, P. Perinatal nursing, 4th ed. Philadelphia: Lippincott, Williams & Wilkins.

Queenan, J., Hobbins, J., & Spong, C. (2005). *Protocols in high risk pregnancies.* Malden, MA: Blackwell.

Ramachenderan, J., Bradford, J., & McLean, M. (2008). Maternal obesity and pregnancy complications: a review. *Australian & New Zealand Journal of Obstetrics & Gynaecology, 48*(3), 228–235.

Reedy, N. (2014). Preterm labor and birth. In Simpson, K. & Creehan, P. Perinatal nursing, 4th ed. Philadelphia: Lippincott, Williams & Wilkins.

Roberts, D., & Dalziel, S. (2007). Antenatal corticosteroid maturation for women at risk for preterm birth (Cochrane Review). *Cochrane Database of Systematic Reviews* 2006, Issue 3. Art. No.: CD004454. DOI: 10.1002/14651858.CD004454.pub2.

Selleck, C. S., & Redding, B. A. (1998). Knowledge and attitude of registered nurses toward perinatal substance abuse [Clinical Studies]. *Journal of Obstetric and Gynecologic and Neonatal Nursing, 27,* 70–77.

Shah, P., & Shah, J. (2010). Maternal Exposure to Domestic Violence and Pregnancy and Birth Outcomes: A Systematic Review and Meta-Analyses. *Journal of Women's Health (15409996), 19*(11), 2017–2031. doi:10.1089/jwh.2010.2051

Shah, P., Zao, J., & Ali, S. (2011). Maternal Marital Status and Birth Outcomes: A Systematic Review and Meta-Analyses. *Maternal & Child Health Journal, 15*(7), 1097–1109. doi:10.1007/s10995-010-0654-z

Simpson, L. L. (2012). Maternal cardiac disease: update for the clinician. *Obstetrics and Gynecology, 119,* 345–59.

Sibai, B. (2003). Diagnosis and management of gestational hypertension and preeclampsia [An expert's view]. *Obstetrics & Gynecology, 102,* 181–192.

Sibai, B. (2004). Diagnosis, controversies, and management of the syndrome of Hemolysis, Elevated Liver Enzymes, and Low Platelet Count [High Risk Pregnancy Series: An expert's view]. *Obstetrics & Gynecology, 103,* 981–991.

Sosa, C., Althabe, F., Belizán, J., & Bergel, E. (2007). Bed rest in singleton pregnancies for preventing preterm birth (Cochrane Review). In: The Cochrane Library Issue 2, 2007. *Cochrane Database of Systematic Reviews* 2004, Issue 1. Art. No.: CD003581. DOI: 10.1002/14651858.CD003581.pub2.

Taylor, P., Zaichkin, J., & Bailey, D. (2002). Substance abuse during pregnancy: guidelines for screening. Olympia, WA, 2002, Maternal and Child Health. Retrieved from http://doh.wa.gov

U.S. Department of Health and Human Services, Substance Abuse and Mental Health Administration. (2008). Results from the 2007 National Survey on Drug Use and Health: National Findings, Office of Applied Studies, DHHS, publication no. SMA 08-4343. Rockville, MD: Author.

Substance Abuse and Mental Health Services Administration, Office of Applied Studies. (May 21, 2009). The NSDUH Report: Substance Use among Women During Pregnancy and Following Childbirth. Rockville, MD: Author.

Berhman, R., & Stith Butler, A. (Eds.). (2007). Preterm Birth: Causes, Consequences, and Prevention. Committee on Understanding Premature Birth and Assuring Healthy Outcomes Institute of Medicine of the Academies. Washington: The National Academies Press.

Substance Abuse and Mental Health Services Administration, Office of Applied Studies. (2007). The NSDUH report: Cigarette use among pregnant women and recent mothers. Rockville, MD: Author.

U.S. Department of Health and Human Services. (2004). The health consequences of smoking: A report of the Surgeon General. Atlanta, GA: Centers for Disease Control and Prevention, National Center for Chronic Disease Prevention and Health Promotion, Office on Smoking and Health. (Accessed July 5, 2012).

Substance Abuse and Mental Health Services Administration, Office of Applied Studies. (2008). The NSDUH Report: Alcohol Use among Pregnant Women and Recent Mothers: 2002 to 2007. Rockville, MD: Author.

U.S. Department of Health and Human Services. (2007).Preventing FASD: Healthy Women and Health Babies DHHS Publication No. (SMA) 07–4253.www.fasdcenter.samhsa.gov/links/links.aspx

Van Otterloo L. R. (2011). Trauma in Pregnancy. In Mattson, S., & Smith, J. E. (Eds.), *Core curriculum for maternal-newborn nursing* (4th ed.). St. Louis, MO: Elsevier Saunders. Pages 535-555.

Yancy, M. (2011). Other Medical Complications. In Mattson, S., & Smith, J. (Eds). (2011). Core Curriculum for Maternal-Newborn Nursing, Fourth Edition. AWHONN Saunders Elsevier. Pages 587-623.

Intrapartum Assessment and Interventions

EXPECTED STUDENT OUTCOMES

On completion of this chapter, the student will be able to:

☐ Define key terms.
☐ Describe the four stages of labor and the related nursing and medical care.
☐ Demonstrate understanding of supportive care of the laboring woman.
☐ Identify the five Ps of labor.
☐ Describe the mechanism of spontaneous vaginal delivery and related nursing care.

Nursing Diagnoses

▪ Deficient knowledge of labor process
▪ Pain related to the labor and delivery process
▪ Fear related to unknowns of labor; threat of potential harm to self or fetus
▪ Risk of ineffective maternal/fetal perfusion related to perfusion in labor
▪ Risk of infection related to vaginal exams after rupture of membranes

Nursing Outcomes

▪ The woman will understand the process and interventions related to labor.
▪ The woman will have decreased pain.
▪ The woman will have decreased fear during labor.
▪ The woman's vital signs and fetal heart rate remain stable.
▪ The woman will be free of infection.

INTRODUCTION

The **intrapartum period** begins with the onset of regular uterine contractions (UCs) and lasts until the expulsion of the placenta. The process by which this normally occurs is called **labor**. **Childbirth** is the period from the conclusion of the pregnancy to the start of extrauterine life of the infant. This chapter discusses the intrapartum/childbirth process, including the factors affecting labor and delivery, progression of labor and delivery, and the nursing care involved.

LABOR TRIGGERS

The question of when and how labor begins has been studied for years. The exact cause of the onset of labor is not completely understood, although there are several theories. Generally it is proposed that labor is triggered by both maternal and fetal factors (**Fig. 8-1**) (Mattson & Smith, 2011; Simpson & O'Brien-Abel, 2013).

Maternal Factors

▪ Uterine muscles are stretched to the threshold point, leading to release of prostaglandins that stimulate contractions.

Don't have time to read this chapter? Want to reinforce your reading? Need to review for a test?
Listen to this chapter on *DavisPlus*.

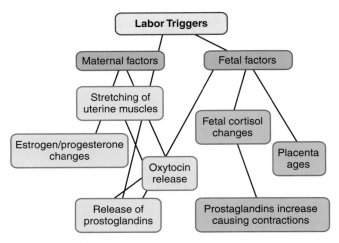

Figure 8–1 Labor triggers.

- Increased pressure on the cervix stimulates the nerve plexus, causing release of oxytocin by the maternal pituitary gland, which then stimulates contractions.
- Estrogen increases, stimulating the uterine response.
- Progesterone, which has a quieting effect on the uterus, is withdrawn, allowing estrogen to stimulate contractions.
- Oxytocin stimulates myometrial contractions. Oxytocin and prostaglandin work together to inhibit calcium binding in muscle cells, raising intracellular calcium levels and activating contractions.
- The oxytocin level surges from stretching of the cervix.

Fetal Factors

- As the placenta ages it begins to deteriorate, triggering initiation of contractions.
- Prostaglandin synthesis by the fetal membranes and the decidua stimulates contractions.
- Fetal cortisol, produced by fetal adrenal glands, rises and acts on the placenta to reduce progesterone that quiets the uterus, and increases prostaglandin that stimulates the uterus to contract.

THE PROCESS OF LABOR

Signs of Impending Labor

A few weeks before labor, changes occur that indicate the woman's body is preparing for the onset of labor. These changes are also referred to as **premonitory signs** of labor. These signs are:

- **Lightening** refers to the descent of the fetus into the true pelvis that occurs approximately 2 weeks before term in first-time pregnancies. The woman may feel she can breathe more easily but may experience urinary frequency from increased bladder pressure. In subsequent pregnancies, this may not occur until labor begins.
- **Braxton-Hicks** contractions: These are irregular UCs that do not result in cervical change and are associated with false labor. These contractions begin to coordinate

the many muscle layers of the uterus to perform when true labor begins.

- Cervical changes: The cervix becomes soft (ripens) and may become partially effaced and begin to dilate.
- Surge in energy: Some women may experience a burst of energy or feel the need to put everything in order; sometimes referred to as **nesting**.
- Gastrointestinal changes: Less commonly, some women may experience a 1- to 3-pound weight loss and some experience diarrhea, nausea, or indigestion preceding labor.
- Backache: The woman may experience low backache and sacroiliac discomfort due in part to the relaxation of the pelvic joints.
- Bloody show: The woman may experience a brownish or blood-tinged cervical mucus discharge referred to as **bloody show**.

FACTORS AFFECTING LABOR

Labor is defined by UCs that bring about effacement and dilation of the cervix. Factors that have been traditionally identified as the essential components in the outcome of labor and delivery include the "4 Ps":

- Powers (the contractions)
- Passage (the pelvis and birth canal)
- Passenger (the fetus)
- Psyche (the response of the woman)

In more recent times a fifth "P" has been added:

- Position (maternal postures and physical positions to facilitate labor)

Powers

Powers refer to the involuntary UCs of labor and the voluntary pushing or bearing down powers that combine to propel and deliver the fetus and placenta from the uterus (see Chapter 9 for assessment of UCs).

Uterine Contractions

- The uterine muscle, known as the myometrium, contracts and shortens during the first stage of labor.
- The uterus is divided into two segments known as the upper segment and the lower segment.
  - *The upper segment composes two-thirds of the uterus and contracts to push the fetus down.*
- The lower segment composes the lower third of the uterus and the cervix and is less active, allowing the cervix to become thinner and pulled upward.
- Uterine contractions are responsible for the dilation (opening) and effacement (thinning) of the cervix in the first stage of labor.
- Uterine contractions are rhythmic and intermittent.
- Each contraction has a **resting phase** or uterine relaxation period that allows the woman and uterine muscle a pause for rest. This pause allows blood flow to the uterus and placenta that was temporarily reduced during the contraction

phase. It is during this pause that much of the fetal exchange of oxygen, nutrients, and waste products occurs in the placenta. With every contraction, 500 mL of blood leaves the utero–placental unit and moves back into maternal circulation.

- Uterine contractions are described in the following ways (**Fig. 8-2**):
    - *Frequency: Time from beginning of one contraction to the beginning of another. It is recorded in minutes (e.g., occurring every 3–4 minutes).*
    - *Duration: Time from the beginning of a contraction to the end of the contraction. It is recorded in seconds (e.g., each contraction lasts 45–50 seconds).*
    - *Intensity: Strength of the contraction. It is evaluated with palpation using the fingertips on maternal abdomen and is described as:*
        - Mild: The uterine wall is easily indented during contraction.
        - Moderate: The uterine wall is resistant to indentation during a contraction.
        - Strong: The uterine wall cannot be indented during a contraction.
- There are three phases of a contraction (see Fig. 8-2):
    - *Increment phase: Ascending or buildup of the contraction that begins in the fundus and spreads throughout the uterus; the longest part of the contraction.*
    - *Acme phase: Peak of intensity but the shortest part of the contraction*
    - *Decrement phase: Descending or relaxation of the uterine muscle*
- Contractions facilitate cervical changes (**Fig. 8-3A, B, C**).
    - *Dilation and effacement occurs during the first stage of labor when UCs push the presenting part of the fetus toward the cervix, causing it to open and thin out as the musculofibrous tissue of the cervix is drawn upwards (see Fig. 8-3B).*

- *Dilation is the enlargement or opening of the cervical os.*
    - The cervix dilates from closed (or <1 cm diameter) to 10 cm diameter (see **Fig. 8-3C**).
    - When the cervix reaches 10 cm dilation, it is considered fully or completely dilated and can no longer be palpated on vaginal examination.
- *Effacement is the shortening and thinning of the cervix (Fig. 8-3A, B, C).*
    - Before the onset of labor the cervix is 2 to 3 cm long and approximately 1 cm thick (Fig. 8-3A).
    - The degree of effacement is measured in percentage and goes from 0% to 100%.
- *Effacement often precedes dilation in a first-time pregnancy. Effacement and dilation progression of the cervix occurs together in subsequent pregnancies.*

Bearing-down powers occur once the cervix is fully dilated (10 cm), and the woman feels the urge to push; she will involuntarily bear down. The urge to push is triggered by the Ferguson reflex, activated when the presenting part stretches the pelvic floor muscles. Stretch receptors are activated, releasing oxytocin, stimulating contractions (Simpson & O'Brien-Abel, 2013). The bearing-down powers are enhanced when the woman contracts her abdominal muscles and pushes.

Passage

The **passage** includes the bony pelvis and the soft tissues of the cervix, pelvic floor, vagina, and introitus (external opening to the vagina). Although all of these anatomical areas play a role in the birth of the fetus, it is the maternal pelvis that is the greatest determinate in the vaginal delivery of the fetus. The assessment of the size and shape of the pelvis is important. Assessment of the pelvis is performed manually through palpation with a vaginal exam by the care provider during pregnancy.

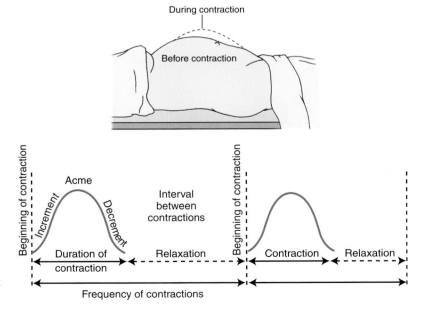

Figure 8–2 Phases, frequency, and duration of a contraction.

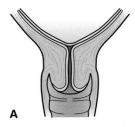

Figure 8–3A Cervical effacement and dilation. A. Cervix prior to labor is closed and not effaced.

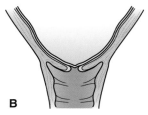

Figure 8–3B Cervix in latent phase of labor is effaced and starting to dilate.

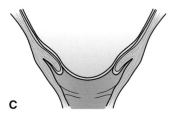

Figure 8–3C Cervix in labor is effaced and dilating.

Pelvis

- ■ Types of bony pelvis (**Fig. 8-4**):
  - ■ *Gynecoid (most common type and found in about 50% of women)*
  - ■ *Android*
  - ■ *Anthropoid*
  - ■ *Platypelloid (least common type and found in about 3% of women)*
- ■ The anatomical structure of the pelvis includes the ileum, the ischium, pubis, sacrum, and coccyx (**Fig. 8-5A**).
- ■ The bony pelvis is divided into (**Fig. 8-5B**):
  - ■ *False pelvis, which is the shallow upper section of the pelvis.*
  - ■ *True pelvis, which is the lower part of the pelvis and consists of three planes, the inlet, the midpelvis, and the outlet. The measurement of these three planes defines the obstetric capacity of the pelvis.*
- ■ The pelvic joints include the symphysis pubis, the right and the left sacroiliac joints, and the sacrococcygeal joints.
- ■ The actions of the hormones estrogen and relaxin during pregnancy soften cartilage and increase elasticity of the ligaments, thus allowing room for the fetal head.
- ■ **Station** refers to the relationship of the ischial spines to the presenting part of the fetus and assists in assessing for fetal descent during labor (**Fig. 8-6**). Station 0 is the narrowest diameter the fetus must pass through during a vaginal birth.

Soft Tissue

- ■ The soft tissue of the cervix effaces and dilates, allowing the descending fetus into the vagina.
- ■ The soft tissue of the pelvic floor muscles helps the fetus in an anterior rotation as it passes through the birth canal.
- ■ The soft tissue of the vagina expands to allow passage of the fetus.

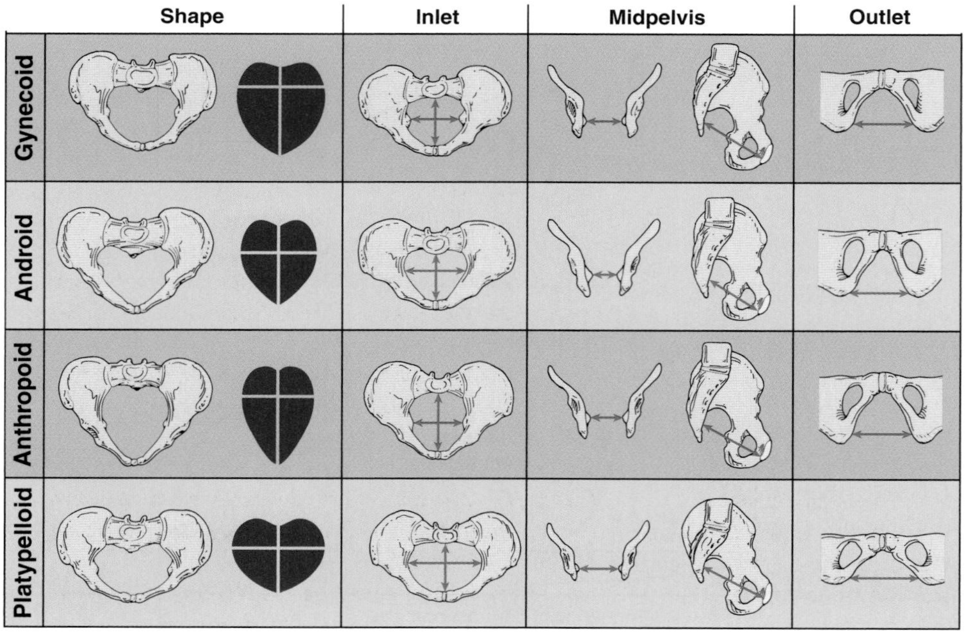

	Shape		Inlet	Midpelvis		Outlet
Gynecoid						
Android						
Anthropoid						
Platypelloid						

Figure 8–4 Pelvic types: gynecoid, android, anthropoid, and platypeloid.

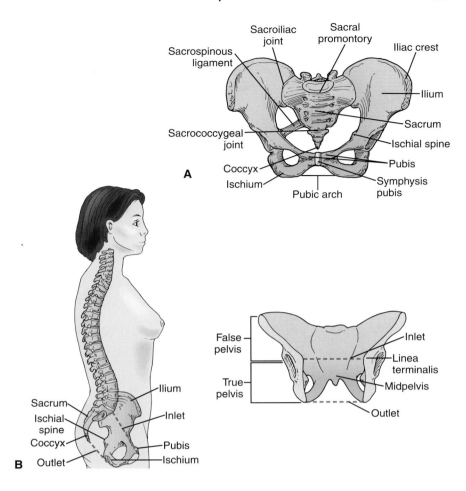

Figure 8–5 Pelvic structures. A. Anatomical structures of pelvis. B. Pelvic planes.

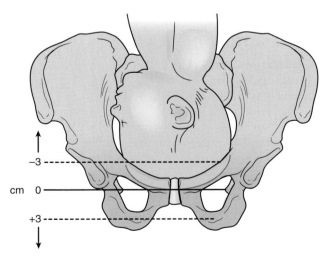

Figure 8–6 Station of presenting part: Fetal head in relation to ischial spines.

Passenger

The **passenger** is the fetus. It is the fetus and its relationship to the passageway that is the major factor in the birthing process. The relationship between the fetus and the passageway includes fetal skull, fetal attitude, fetal lie, fetal presentation, fetal position, and fetal size. At the onset of labor, the position

of the fetus with respect to the birth canal is critical (Cunningham et al., 2010). In general, in the United States, when a fetus is in a position other than cephalic (head first), a cesarean delivery is considered. Size of the fetus alone is less significant in the birthing process than the relationship among fetal size, position, and pelvic dimensions (Mattson & Smith, 2011).

Fetal Skull

■ The fetal head usually accounts for the largest portion of the fetus to come through the birth canal.

■ Bones and membranous spaces help the skull to mold during labor and birth.

■ **Molding** is the ability of the fetal head to change shape to accommodate/fit through the maternal pelvis (**Fig. 8-7**).

■ The fetal skull is composed of two parietal bones, two temporal bones, the frontal bone, and the occipital bone (**Fig. 8-8 A**).

■ *The **biparietal diameter (BPD)**, 9.25 cm, is the largest transverse measurement and an important indicator of head size (see **Fig. 8-8 B**).*

■ *The membranous space between the bones (sutures) and the fontanels (intersections of these sutures) allows the skull bones to overlap and mold to fit through the birth canal (see Fig. 8-8A and B).*

■ *Sutures are used to identify the positioning of the fetal head during a vaginal exam. By identifying the anterior*

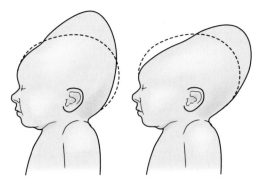

Figure 8–7   Molding of fetal head.

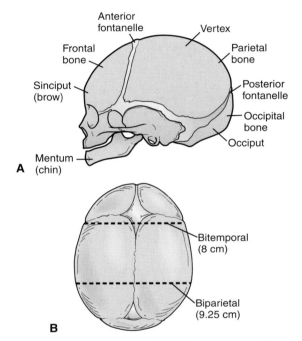

Figure 8–8   Bones of the fetal skull. A. Bones of fetal skull (side view) B. Diameter of fetal skull

fontanel in relationship to the woman's pelvis, the examiner can determine the position of the head and the degree of rotation that has occurred.

Fetal Attitude or Posture

Fetal attitude or posture is the relationship of fetal parts to one another. This is noted by the flexion or extension of the fetal joints (**Fig. 8-9**).

■ At term, the fetus's back becomes convex and the head flexed such that the chin is against the chest. This results in a rounded appearance with the chin flexed forward on the chest, arms crossed over the thorax, the thighs flexed on the abdomen, and the legs flexed at the knees.

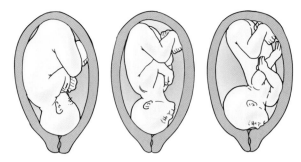

Figure 8–9   Fetal attitude or posture (flexed).

■ With proper fetal attitude, the head is in complete flexion in a vertex presentation and passes more easily through the true pelvis.

Fetal Lie

Fetal lie refers to the long axis (spine) of the fetus in relationship to the long axis (spine) of the woman.

■ The two primary lies are longitudinal and transverse (**Fig. 8-10**).
   ■ *In the longitudinal lie, the long axes of the fetus and the mother are parallel (most common).*
   ■ *In the transverse lie, the long axis of the fetus is perpendicular to the long axis of the mother.*
■ A fetus cannot be delivered vaginally in the transverse lie.

Presentation

Fetal presentation is determined by the part or pole of the fetus that first enters the pelvic inlet. There are three main presentations (**Fig. 8-11**):

■ Cephalic (head first) (Fig. 8-11A)
■ Breech (pelvis first) (Fig. 8-11B)
■ Shoulder (shoulder first) (Fig. 8-11C)

Presenting Part

The **presenting part** is the specific fetal structure lying nearest to the cervix. It is determined by the attitude or posture of the fetus.

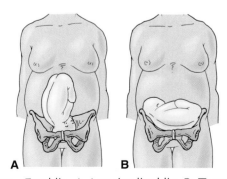

Figure 8–10   Fetal lie. A. Longitudinal lie. B. Transverse lie.

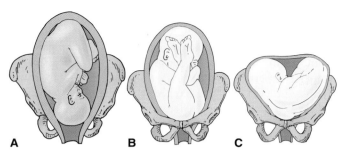

Figure 8–11 Fetal presentation. A. Cephalic. B. Breech. C. Shoulder.

Each presenting part has an identified denominator or reference point that is used to describe the fetal position in the pelvis.

■ Cephalic presentations: The presenting part is the head (**Fig. 8-12**).
  ■ *This accounts for 95% of all births (Mattson & Smith, 2011).*
  ■ *The degree of flexion or extension of the head and neck further classifies cephalic presentations.*
    ■ Vertex presentation indicates that the head is sharply flexed and the chin is touching the thorax. The denominator is the occiput (Fig. 8-12A).

■ Frontum or brow presentation indicates partial extension of the neck with the brow as the presenting part. The denominator is the frontum (Fig. 8-12B).
■ Face presentation indicates that the neck is sharply extended and the back of the head (occiput) is arching to the fetal back. The denominator is the mentum-chin (Fig. 8-12C).

■ Breech presentations: The presenting part is the buttock and/or feet (**Fig. 8-13**).
  ■ *Breech presentations are further classified into: see new suggested pictures*
    ■ **Complete** breech: Complete flexion of the thighs and the legs extending over the anterior surfaces of the body (see Fig. 8-13A)
    ■ **Frank** breech: Complete flexion of thighs and legs (see Fig. 8-13B)
    ■ **Footling breech**: Extension of one or both thighs and legs so that one or both feet are presenting (see Fig. 8-13C)

■ Transverse presentation: The presenting part is usually the shoulder (see Fig. 8-9C).
  ■ *This usually is associated with a transverse lie.*
■ Compound presentation: The fetus assumes a unique posture usually with the arm or hand presenting alongside the presenting part.

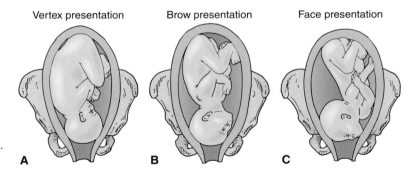

Vertex presentation   Brow presentation   Face presentation

Figure 8–12 Cephalic presentation, A. Vertex. B. Brow. C. Face.

A   B   C

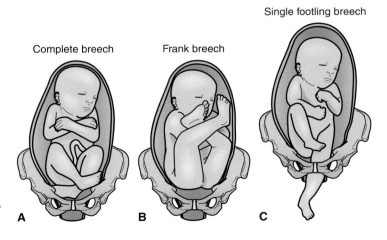

Single footling breech

Complete breech   Frank breech

Figure 8–13 Breech presentation. A. Complete. B. Frank. C. Footling.

A   B   C

Fetal Position

The **fetal position** is the relation of the denominator or reference point to the maternal pelvis (see **Fig. 8-14**).

- There are six positions for each presentation: right anterior, right transverse, right posterior, left anterior, left transverse, and left posterior.
- The occiput is the specific fetal structure for a cephalic presentation (see Fig. 8-11A).
- The sacrum is the specific fetal structure for a breech presentation (see Fig. 8-11B).
- The acromion is the specific fetal structure for a shoulder presentation (see Fig. 8-11C).
- The mentum is the specific fetal structure for the face presentation (see Fig. 8-12C).
- Position is designated by a three-letter abbreviation (Fig. 8-14):
  - *First letter: Designates location of presenting part to the left (L) or right (R) of the woman's pelvis (Fig. 8-14).*
  - *Second letter: Designates the specific fetal part presenting: occiput (O), sacrum (S), mentum (M), and shoulder (A) (Fig. 8-14).*
  - *Third letter: Designates the relationship of the presenting fetal part to the woman's pelvis such as anterior (A), posterior (P), or transverse (T) (Fig. 8-14).*

Psyche

Nursing care of the woman during the intrapartum period addresses not only the physical aspect of care but also the psychosocial aspect to result in woman's wellness and satisfaction. Preparation of childbirth, both physically and mentally, helps the woman manage labor. This preparation promotes in the woman a sense of security and safety. A woman's experience and satisfaction during the labor and birthing process can be enhanced when there is a coordination of collaborative goals between the woman and health care personnel in the plan of care (Perla, 2002). This is a critical part that influences her self-esteem, self-confidence, her relationship to others, and a general view she holds of life.

Factors that influence the woman's coping mechanism include her culture, expectations, a strong support system, and type of support during labor.

- Culture
  - *Culture influences the woman's reaction to labor expectations and how she interacts with others. Cultural influences may be most apparent in the newly immigrated woman. The nurse needs to be culturally aware and sensitive to the needs and practices of the individual.*
  - *Nurses need to integrate the woman's cultural and religious values, beliefs, and practices to provide a mutually acceptable plan of care. When the woman feels that the plan of care is one she is actively involved in and integrates her cultural and/or religious values, beliefs, and practices with the decision making, her feeling of safety and control are further facilitated (Cultural Awareness: Culture and Birth Traditions).*

Cultural Awareness: Culture and Birth Traditions

Giving birth is a pivotal life event, and the meaning of birth and parenthood is culturally defined (Moore, Moos, & Callister, 2010). Culture influences all aspects of a woman's response to labor and impacts factors such as:

- Who is with the woman in labor, their role, and who participates in decision making
- Preferences for use of pharmacological and non-pharmacological pain management in labor
- Who they want to care for them in relation to gender and modesty
- How they respond to labor, so the nurse needs to help women formulate their concerns, priorities, and decisions.

Behaviors in birth are complex and personal. It is important for nurses to have a general understanding of birth practices of the groups with which they work (Bar-Yam, 1994). Some strategies for providing culturally sensitive care are presented in Chapter 5 and in the Critical Component: Strategies for Nurses: Improving Culturally Responsive Care in Labor & Birth. By identifying the patient's beliefs and being sensitive to her experiences of the health care system, nurses can provide individualized care to her and her support system and provide information when there are differences encountered.

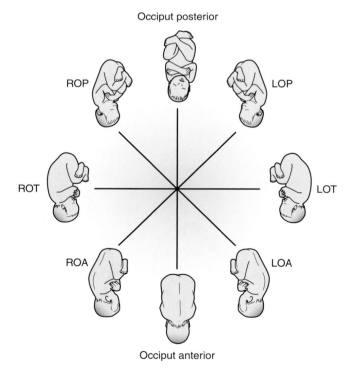

Figure 8–14 Variety of fetal positions with vertex presentation.

CRITICAL COMPONENT

Strategies for Nurses: Improving Culturally Responsive Care in Labor & Birth

- Learn the traditions of the cultural groups you care for and the specific preferences of each woman and her family.
- Recognize there are sub-cultures within cultures.
- Listen to the woman and her support persons and help them find meaningful and acceptable support activities.
- Identify who the client calls "family."
- Use the beliefs, values, customs, and expectations of the woman to shape her plan of care for labor and birth.
- Include notes on cultural preferences and family strengths and resources as part of all intake and ongoing assessments, and nursing care plans.
- Instead of focusing on technology, look beyond the routine and appreciate the needs of all women.
- Develop linguistic skills related to your client population.
- Learn to use nonverbal communication in an appropriate way.
- Learn about the communication patterns of various cultures.
- Recognize and acknowledge your own belief system while maintaining an open attitude.
- Examine the biases and assumptions you hold about different cultures.
- Avoid preconceptions and cultural stereotyping.
- Recognize all care is given within the context of many cultures.
- Advocate for organizational change that is flexible to cultural variations.

(Adapted from Simpson & O'Brien-Abel, 2013; Amidi-Nouri, 2011; Moore, Moos, & Callister, 2010.)

- Expectations
  - *Expectations for the birth experience are related to how childbirth is viewed by the woman (e.g., as a natural process or as a stressful or threatening experience). The nurse should review the woman's expectations to help alleviate fear and to help set realistic goals.*
    - Unrealistic expectations can cause an increase in maternal anxiety.
  - *Past experience and complications of pregnancy, labor, and birth strongly influence women's expectations of labor and response to labor.*
    - Women who have experienced a negative previous birthing experience are at risk for increased anxiety; women who experienced a positive previous birthing experience have lower anxiety levels.
    - Women that are recent immigrants may have had very different birth experiences in other countries, and that influences their expectations, hopes, and fears.
  - *Current pregnancy experience with difficulty conceiving, an unplanned pregnancy, or a high-risk pregnancy may increase a woman's anxiety and fears.*
- Support system
  - *The woman's perception of being able to maintain control during labor and delivery is an important contributing factor to a positive and favorable evaluation of childbirth.*

This includes control of pain perception, control over emotions and actions, and being able to influence decisions while being an active participant (Mackey, 1995).

- *Studies have shown that with a support person, be it a family member, friend, doula, or professional such as a nurse, the patient experiences a decrease in anxiety and has a feeling of being in more control. This results in a decrease in interventions, a significantly lower level of pain, and an enhanced overall maternal satisfaction (Hodnett, Gates, Hofmeyr, & Sakala, 2007).*
- *Nursing care of women in labor should incorporate the following types of support and interventions:*
  - Emotional support, including continuous presence, reassurance, and praise
  - Information about labor progress and advice regarding coping techniques
  - Comfort measures (e.g., comforting touch, massage, warm baths/showers, promoting adequate fluid intake and output)
  - Advocacy, including assisting the woman in articulating her wishes to others

Evidence-Based Practice: Supportive Care for Adolescents in Labor

Adolescents have a very different view of labor & birth as they struggle with self-identity and self-esteem. It can pose a challenge for providers and nurses to work with adolescents to promote a positive birthing experience. Nurses need to have an understanding of adolescent development, expectations, and needs to provide a positive birthing experience. According to Sauls (2010), four themes became apparent based on feedback of over 180 adolescents in three tertiary centers during their postpartum interviews:

- Respectful nurse caring: during interactions be kind, friendly, and make her feel welcome. Include her in decision making, informing her of her options related to her care.
- Assistance with pain control: Assist her with pain management options with explanations of both pharmacological and non-pharmacological. Assess often her ability to manage her pain.
- Nursing support of the adolescent's support person: Pay attention to her support person's emotional and physical needs. Encourage them as they work through labor, including them in explanations and plan of care discussions.
- Childbirth guidance: Orient her and her support system to hospital facilities and to the birthing process, anticipating questions and explaining procedures. Answer questions truthfully and in a manner that is appropriate for the age group.

Sauls, D. J. (2010). Promoting a Positive Childbirth Experience for Adolescents. *Journal of Obstetric, Gynecologic, and Neonatal Nursing, 39,* 703–712.

- Labor support
  - *Since the middle of the 20th century, a majority of women have given birth in a hospital rather than at home, even in poorer, less developed countries. Access to continuous care and support during labor has become the exception rather*

than the routine in the hospital setting. Concerns about the consequent dehumanization of women's birth experiences have resulted in demands for a return to continuous, one-to-one support by women for women during labor **(Fig. 8-15)** *(Evidence-Based Practice: Continuous Labor Support for Women During Childbirth).*

■ *Two complementary theoretical explanations have been offered for the effects of labor support on childbirth outcomes (Hodnett, Gates, Hofmeyr, & Sakala, 2007). Both explanations hypothesize that labor support enhances labor physiology and woman's feelings of control and competence.*

■ *First theory: During labor women may be uniquely vulnerable to unfamiliar environmental influences; current obstetric care frequently subjects women to institutional routines, high rates of intervention, unfamiliar personnel, and lack of privacy.*

■ These conditions may have an adverse effect on the progress of labor and on the development of feelings of competence and confidence; this may in turn impair adjustment to parenthood and establishment of breast-feeding, and increase the risk of depression.

■ This response may, to some extent, be buffered by the provision of support and companionship during labor.

■ *Second theory describes two pathways: enhanced passage of the fetus through the pelvis and soft tissues, and decreased stress response (Hodnett, 2002).*

■ Enhanced fetopelvic relationships may be accomplished by encouraging mobility and effective use of gravity, supporting women to assume their preferred positions and recommending specific positions for specific situations.

■ Studies of the relationships among fear and anxiety, the stress response, and pregnancy complications have shown that anxiety during labor is associated with high levels of the stress hormone epinephrine in the blood, which may lead to abnormal fetal heart rate (FHR) patterns in labor, decreased uterine contractility, a longer active labor phase with regular well-established contractions, and low Apgar scores (Lederman, 1986).

■ Emotional support, information and advice, comfort measures, and advocacy may reduce anxiety and fear and associated adverse effects during labor.

■ *Anxiety (a sense of uneasiness in response to a vague unspecific threat) can interfere with labor and increase nausea and crying, as well as interfering with the ability to focus.*

■ *Fear (a painful, uneasy feeling in response to an identifiable threat) can be fear related to the unknown, fear of injury to self and fetus, or fear of pain. Fear can decrease UCs and enhance the perception of pain. Procedures and an unfamiliar environment can result in a sense of loss of control and feeling of helplessness. Women in labor can feel abandoned (Mattson & Smith, 2011).*

■ *Nurses can help and support women to be actively involved in their own care by allowing time for discussion, listening to worries and concerns, and offering information to help women gain increased self-determination in the context of care (Nordgren & Fridlund, 2001).*

Position

Discussion of the influence on labor often includes a fifth "P," referred to as maternal position during labor and birth. The woman's position has an effect on both the anatomical and physiological adaptations to labor **(Fig. 8-16)**.

■ During the first stage of labor, an upright position (walking, sitting, kneeling, or squatting) and/or a lateral position is encouraged **(Fig. 8-17A)**.

■ *These positions are used to decrease the compression of the maternal descending aorta and ascending vena cava that could result in a compromised cardiac output. Compression of these vessels can lead to supine hypotension, resulting in decreased placental perfusion.*

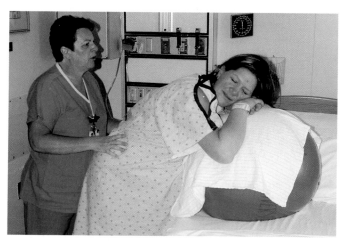

Figure 8–15 Woman receiving labor support from her nurse.

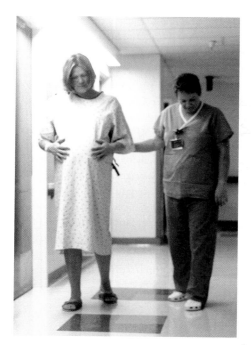

Figure 8–16 Woman walking in labor with her nurse.

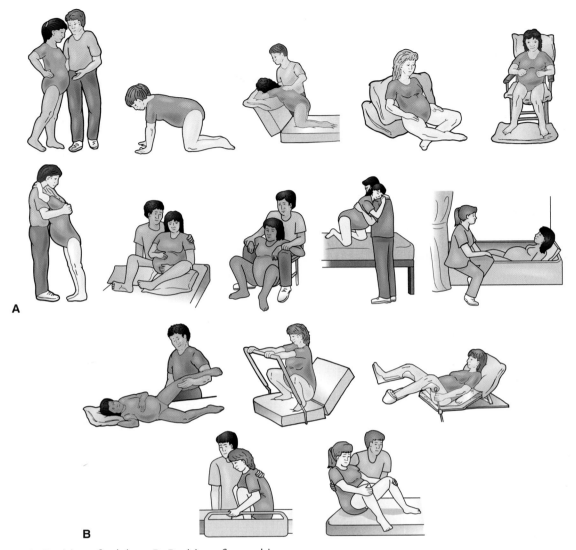

Figure 8–17 A. Positions for labor. B. Positions for pushing.

■ *The upright position has shown benefits of aiding in the descent of the infant and more effective contractions that result in shorter labor (Gupta, Hofmeyr, & Smyth, 2004).*
■ *Frequent position changes are associated with a reduction of fatigue, an increase of comfort, and improved circulation to both mother and fetus.*
■ During the second stage of labor, the upright position has been shown to increase the pelvic outlet and better aligns the fetus with the pelvic inlet (Fig. 8-17B) (Simkin & Ancheta, 2000).
■ The position most used in births in the United States is the lithotomy position, which allows for provider visualization and control during the delivery process.

ONSET OF LABOR

As the woman comes closer to term pregnancy, the uterus becomes more sensitive to oxytocin and the contractions increase in frequency and intensity. This can be an anxious time for the woman and family in trying to determine if she needs to proceed to the birthing center. An understanding of true versus false labor can help to alleviate some of these fears.

True Labor Versus False Labor

True labor contractions occur at regular intervals and increase in frequency, duration, and intensity (**Fig. 8-18**).

■ True labor contractions bring about changes in cervical effacement and dilation.
■ False labor is irregular contractions with little or no cervical changes.

Assessment of Rupture of the Membranes (ROM)

Spontaneous rupture of the membranes (SROM) may occur before the onset of labor but typically occurs during labor. Once the membranes have ruptured, the protective barrier to infection is lost, and ideally the woman should deliver within 24 hours to reduce the risk of infection to herself and her fetus.

Evidence-Based Practice: Continuous Support for Women During Childbirth

Hodnett, E., Gates, S., Hofmeyr, G., & Sakala, C. (2007). Continuous support for women during childbirth. *Cochrane Database of Systematic Reviews* 2007, Issue 3, Art. No. CD003766. DOI: 10.1002/1465185.CD003766.pbb2.

In recent decades in hospitals worldwide, continuous support during labor has become the exception rather than the routine. Concerns about the consequent dehumanization of women's birth experiences have led to calls for a return to continuous support by women for women during labor.

Objective of Systematic Review

Primary: To assess the effects, on women and their babies, of continuous, one-to-one intrapartum support compared with the usual care. Secondary: To determine whether the effects of continuous support are influenced by (1) routine practices and policies in the birth environment that may affect a woman's autonomy, freedom of movement, and ability to cope with labor; (2) whether the caregiver is a member of the staff of the institution; and (3) whether the continuous support begins early or later in labor.

Selection Criteria

All published and unpublished randomized controlled trials comparing continuous support during labor with usual care.

Main Results

Sixteen trials involving 13,391 women met inclusion criteria and provided usable outcome data. Primary comparison: women who had continuous intrapartum support were likely to have a slightly shorter labor, and were more likely to have a spontaneous vaginal birth and less likely to have intrapartum analgesia or to report dissatisfaction with their childbirth experiences. Subgroup analyses: In general, continuous intrapartum support was associated with greater benefits when the provider was not a member of the hospital staff, or when it began early in labor and in settings in which epidural analgesia was not routinely available.

Summary

Continuous support in labor increased the chance of a spontaneous vaginal birth, had no identified adverse effects, and women were more satisfied.

Supportive care during labor may involve emotional support, comfort measures, information, and advocacy. These may enhance normal labor processes as well as women's feelings of control and competence, and thus reduce the need for obstetric intervention. The review of studies included 16 trials from 11 countries, involving more than 13,000 women in a wide range of settings and circumstances. Women who received continuous labor support were more likely to give birth "spontaneously," i.e., give birth with neither cesarean birth nor vacuum nor forceps. In addition, women were less likely to use pain medications, were more likely to be satisfied, and had slightly shorter labors.

Common elements of this care include emotional support (continuous presence, reassurance, and praise); information about labor progress; advice regarding coping techniques and comfort measures (comforting touch, massage, warm baths/showers, promoting adequate fluid intake and output); and advocacy (helping the woman articulate her wishes to others).

A systematic review examining factors associated with women's satisfaction with the childbirth experience suggests that continuous support can make a substantial contribution to this satisfaction. When women evaluate their experience, four factors predominate: the amount of support from caregivers, the quality of relationships with caregivers, being involved with decision-making, and having high expectations or having experiences that exceed expectations (Hodnett, 2002).

Authors' Conclusions and Implications for Practice

Continuous support during labor should be the norm, rather than the exception. All women should be allowed and encouraged to have support people with them continuously during labor. In general, continuous support from a caregiver during labor appears to confer the greatest benefits when the provider is not an employee of the institution, when epidural analgesia is not routinely used, and when support begins in early labor.

Every effort should be made to ensure that women's birth environments are empowering, are not stressful, afford privacy, communicate respect, and are not characterized by routine interventions that add risk without clear benefit.

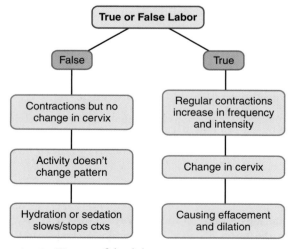

Figure 8–18   True vs. false labor.

Assessing the Status of Membranes

Different techniques may be used to confirm ROM:

■ *A speculum exam may be done to assess for fluid in the vaginal vault (pooling)*
■ *Nitrazine paper: The paper turns blue when in contact with amniotic fluid. Can be dipped in the vaginal fluid or fluid-soaked Q-tip can be rolled over the paper (**Fig. 8-19A**).*
■ *Ferning: During a sterile speculum exam a sample of fluid in the upper vaginal area is obtained.he fluid is placed on a slide and assessed for "ferning pattern" under a microscope (See **Fig. 8-19B**).*

A ferning pattern confirms ROM.

Use of AmniSure testing kit. The AmniSure ROM Test is a rapid, non-invasive immunoassay that aids clinicians with the diagnosis of ROM in pregnant women with signs and symptoms suggestive of the condition. According to published data it is ~99% accurate.

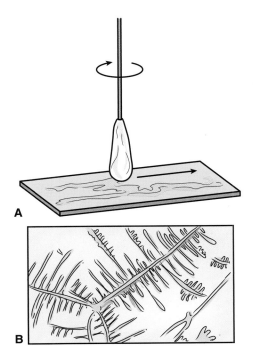

Figure 8–19 Assessment of rupture of membranes A. Placing fluid on nitrizine paper with Q-tip. B. Ferning pattern of dried amniotic fluid seen under microscope.

Nursing Actions

■ Assess the FHR.
   ■ *There is an increase risk of umbilical cord prolapse with ROM.*
   ■ *There is a higher risk of umbilical cord prolapse when the presenting part is not engaged.*
■ Assess the amniotic fluid for color, amount, and odor.
   ■ *Normal amniotic fluid is clear or cloudy with a normal odor that is similar to that of ocean water or the loam of a forest floor.*
   ■ *Fluid can be meconium stained and this needs to be reported to the care provider, as this may be an indication of fetal compromise in utero.*
■ Document the date and time of SROM, characteristic of fluid, and FHR.

Guidelines for Going to the Birthing Facility

■ By law, all pregnant women have access to medical care regardless of their ability to pay (**Box 8-1**).
■ Ongoing communication with your pregnancy care provider will help assure a smooth transition from pregnancy to labor management. By discussing when to go to the birthing facility before labor happens, women will have less anxiety and be more prepared for when labor begins. When to go to the birthing facility depends greatly on the past history of pregnancies, location of the birth center, and risk status of the pregnancy.

BOX 8–1 EMERGENCY MEDICAL TREATMENT AND ACTIVE LABOR ACT

The Emergency Medical Treatment and Active Labor Act (EMTALA) is a federal regulation that was enacted to ensure treatment for a woman seeking care in an emergency or if she thinks she is in labor, regardless of her ability to pay. Nurses who work in the labor and delivery unit(s) of the hospital need to be familiar with EMTALA regulations (Angelini & Mahlmeister, 2005). In general, the criteria for admission to the hospital for labor are cervical dilation to 3–4 cm and/or ruptured membranes (Cunningham et al., 2010).

■ A general rule of thumb for first-time pregnancy with no risk factor is to wait until contractions are 5 minutes apart, lasting 60 seconds, and are regular.
■ The woman should go to the birthing center when:
   ■ *The membrane ruptures, or "bag of waters" break.*
   ■ *The woman is experiencing intense pain.*
   ■ *There is an increase of bloody show.*

MECHANISM OF LABOR

The postponed changes in the presenting part required to navigate the birth canal constitute the mechanism of labor. These mechanisms are cardinal movements of labor (**Fig. 8-20**).

■ Engagement: When the greatest diameter of the fetal head passes through the pelvic inlet; can occur late in pregnancy or early in labor (see Fig. 8-20A)
■ Descent: Movement of the fetus through the birth canal during the first and second stages of labor (see Fig. 8-20A)
■ Flexion: When the chin of the fetus moves toward the fetal chest; occurs when the descending head meets resistance from maternal tissues; results in the smallest fetal diameter to the maternal pelvic dimensions; normally occurs early in labor (see Fig. 8-20A)
■ Internal rotation: When the rotation of the fetal head aligns the long axis of the fetal head with the long axis of the maternal pelvis; occurs mainly during the second stage of labor (see Fig. 8-20B)
■ Extension: Facilitated by resistance of the pelvic floor that causes the presenting part to pivot beneath the pubic symphysis and the head to be delivered; occurs during the second stage of labor (see Fig. 8-20C)
■ External rotation: During this movement, the sagittal suture moves to a transverse diameter and the shoulders align in the anteroposterior diameter. The sagittal suture maintains alignment with the fetal trunk as the trunk navigates through the pelvis (see Fig. 8-20D).
■ Expulsion: The shoulders and remainder of the body are delivered (see Fig. 8-20E).

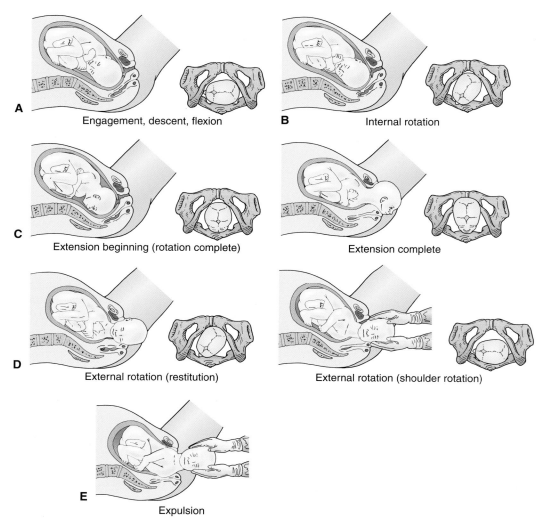

A Engagement, descent, flexion

B Internal rotation

C Extension beginning (rotation complete)

D External rotation (restitution)

Extension complete

External rotation (shoulder rotation)

E Expulsion

Figure 8–20 Cardinal movements of labor. A. Engagement, descent, and flexion. B. Internal rotation. C. Extension. D. External rotation. E. Expulsion.

STAGES OF LABOR AND CHILDBIRTH

Labor or parturition is the process in which the fetus, placenta, and membranes are expelled through the uterus. The care of women and families during labor and delivery requires astute and ongoing assessments of the bio-psycho–social adaptation of the woman and fetus. Because childbirth is a natural process, care should move forward on a continuum from noninvasive to least invasive intervention and from non-pharmacological to pharmacological interventions according to the desires of the woman and assessment of health care providers based on individual clinical situations (Simpson & O'Brien-Abel, 2013). See Critical Component: Care Practices That Support and Promote Normal Physiologic Birth.

In the United States in 2010, 98.8% of all births were delivered in hospitals. Among the 1.2% of out-of-hospital births,

---

CRITICAL COMPONENT

Care Practices That Support and Promote Normal Physiologic Birth

The World Health Organization and Lamaze International identified six birth practices that support and promote normal physiologic birth. They include:

1. Labor Begins on Its Own
2. Freedom of Movement throughout Labor
3. Continuous Labor Support
4. NO Routine Interventions
5. Spontaneous Pushing in Non-supine Positions
6. NO Separation of Mother and Baby

Romano, A., & Lothian, J. (2008). Promoting, Protecting & Supporting Normal Birth: A look at the Evidence. *Journal of Obstetrics, Gynecologic & Neonatal Nursing, 37,* 94–105.

67.0% were in a residence (home) and 28.0% were in a freestanding birthing center. Doctors of medicine (M.D.s) attended the vast majority (86.3%) of hospitals births in 2010, followed by certified nurse midwives (CNMs) (7.6%), and Doctors of Osteopathy (D.O.s) (5.7%) (Martin, Hamilton, Ventura, Osterman, Wilson, & Mathews, 2012). Because most babies are delivered in the hospital by physicians, nurses in the intrapartal setting have a key role in providing comprehensive and individualized care for women and their families. To provide this care, nurses must understand the process of labor, birth, and postpartum. By understanding the stages and phases of labor, the nurse can facilitate, assist, and provide care for the woman, the fetus, and her support system (see Concept Map and **Figure 8-21**).

Labor and birth is divided into four stages (**Table 8-1**):

■ **The first stage** begins with onset of labor and ends with complete cervical dilation.
■ **The second stage** begins with complete dilation of cervix and ends with delivery of baby.
■ **The third stage** begins after delivery of baby and ends with delivery of placenta.
■ **The fourth stage** begins after delivery of the placenta and is completed 4 hours later; it is the immediate postpartum period.

First Stage

The first stage of labor is defined as the progression of cervical changes. This stage is divided into three phases: latent phase, active phase, and transition. Characteristics of the first stage of labor are:

■ It begins with onset of true labor and ends with complete cervical dilation (10 cm) and complete effacement (100%).
■ Stage 1 is longest stage, typically lasting 12 hours for primigravidas and 8 hours for multigravidas.
■ There are normally tremendous variations in lengths of labor (Cunningham et al., 2010).

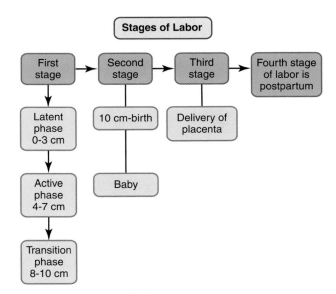

Figure 8–21   Stages of labor.

■ The bag of waters or fetal membranes usually ruptures during this stage.
■ The woman's cardiac output increases.
■ The woman's pulse may increase.
■ Gastrointestinal motility decreases, which leads to increase in gastric emptying time (Mattson & Smith, 2011).
■ The woman experiences pain associated with UCs that result in the dilation and effacement of the cervix.
■ The first stage has three phases: the latent, active, and transition phases (see Table 8-1).

Assessment

Assessment during all phases of the first stage of labor includes:

■ Maternal vital signs
■ The woman's response to labor and pain
■ FHR and UCs
■ Cervical changes
■ Fetal position and descent in the pelvis

Nursing Actions

Nursing actions during all phases of the first stage of labor are related to:

■ Diet and hydration
  ■ *Typically once admitted to the hospital, medical orders limit oral intake to clear liquids*
  ■ *The WHO recommends women dictate their oral intake of carbohydrates to decrease maternal ketosis. (Sharts-Hopko, 2010)*
■ Activity and rest
  ■ *Encouraging frequent position changes and upright positions assists labor progression, facilitates fetal descent, and decreases pain perception.*
■ Elimination
  ■ *Frequent emptying of bowel and bladder assists in comfort of the mother, provides more pelvic room as baby descends, and decreases pressure and injury to the urethra and bowel.*
■ Comfort
  ■ *Providing comfort measures and therapies facilitates labor progress, decreases pain perception, and supports maternal coping mechanisms to manage the labor process. See Critical Component: Non-pharmacologic Strategies for Nurses and Comfort Measures in Labor.*
■ Support and family involvement
  ■ *Shown to provide emotional and physical support to the laboring mother, decreasing stress and possibly facilitates labor progress. See Critical Component: Non-pharmacologic Strategies for Nurses and Comfort Measures in Labor.*
■ Education
  ■ *Providing education and information about labor, procedures, and hospital policies will decrease maternal and family anxiety and fear. Empowers the women to make informed decisions.*
■ Safety
  ■ *Providing a safe friendly environment will enhances the birthing experience.*
■ Documentation of labor admission and progression (**Figs. 8-22** and **8-23**)

(Text continues on page 205)

TABLE 8–1 STAGES AND PHASES OF LABOR

STAGES OF LABOR	1st			2nd	3rd	4th
Phases	Latent	Active	Transition	Expulsive	Placenta	Immediate Postpartum
Length	Primip: average 9 hours up to 19 hours Multip: average 6 hours up to 14 hours	Primip: average 5 hours or 0.5 cm/hr Multip: average 2–3 hours or 1.2 cm/hr	Primip: average 2 hours Multip: average 1–2 hours	Primip: average 1–2+ hours Multip: average less than 1 hour	1–20 minutes	First 2–4 hours after delivery
Cervix	Effacing; dilating to 4 cm	Effacing; dilating to 7 cm	Effacing; dilating to 10 cm	Fully dilated and effaced	Closing	Closing
Uterine Contractions	Frequency: 5–15 min Duration: 10–30 sec Intensity: mild	Frequency: 3–5 min Duration: 30–45 sec Intensity: mod/strong	Frequency: 1–2 min Duration: 40–60 sec Intensity: strong	Frequency: 1–2 min Duration: 50–90 sec Intensity: less painful, expulsive	Less painful contractions	Cramping
Show	None or some	Increasing	Heavy	Heavy		
Membranes	Usually intact	Intact or ruptured	Usually ruptured	Ruptured		
Station	Primip: 0 Multip: −2–0	Primip: 0 – + 2 Multip: 0 – + 2	Primip: 0 – + 2 Multip: 0 – + 2	Primip: progress to + 4 Multip: progress to + 4		
Biological Response	Cramps, backache Excited, anxious, happy, relief, curious, quiet or talkative, needs information and reassurance	May become restless, have labored respiration and tendency to hyperventilate Increasing fears, increasing anxieties, serious, feels threatened May be more serious and inwardly focused	Leg cramps, nausea, vomiting, hiccups, belches, perspiration on forehead and upper lip, a pulling or stretching sensation deep in pelvis Panic, emotional, irritable response to external environment stimuli	Intra-abdominal pressure is exerted (bearing down), urge to push, perineum bulges and flattens, perineal burning and stretching Desires to sleep between contractions, amnesic between contractions	Uterus rises and becomes globular shape, gush or flood as placenta separates, umbilical cord lengthens, cramping May want to sleep, proud, happy, relief, may or may not display emotions	Postpartum chills, hunger, thirst, drowsy, moderate to heavy lochia, usually painless uterine contractions
Personal System	Thoughts centered on self, labor, and baby	Needs human presence	Becomes limited, losing control, thoughts are on self, uncooperative, amnesic between contractions, dependent	Slow to react, focus on delivery	Relieved	

Maternal Biological System	1. B/P, pulse, resp. temp q 1–2 hour 2. Begin Friedman graph 3. Assess cervical changes by SVE 4. Assess FHR and UC's 30 minutes or per protocol 5. Ascertain presence of bloody show and ROM 6. Encourage relaxation 7. Clear liquids or intake per protocol 8. Encourage void q 2 hours 9. Position of comfort	1. B/P, pulse, resp. temp q 1–2 hour 2. Friedman graph 3. Assess cervical changes by SVE PRN 4. Assess FHR and UCs q 15–30 minutes or per protocol 5. Assess vaginal secretions and for ROM 6. Relaxing environment 7. Clear liquids or intake per protocol 8. Encourage void q 2 hours 9. Side or semi-Fowlers position 10. Wet washcloth, mouth care, perineal care, clean dry linen	1. B/P, pulse, resp. temp. q 1 hour 2. Friedman graph 3. SVE to assess cervix, fetal position 4. Assess FHR and UCs q 15 minutes or per protocol 5. Assess vaginal secretions and for ROM 6. Relaxing environment 7. Clear liquids or intake per protocol 8. Check bladder distention 9. Encourage slow breathing 10. Relieve muscle leg cramps 11. Multip—prepare for delivery at 8 cm	1. B/P, pulse, resp. q 1 hour 2. SVE to assess position, station and progress 3. Assess FHR & UC q 5–15 min or per protocol 4. Assess patients readiness and urge to push 5. Prepare primip for delivery at 10 cm 6. Assist in comfortable position for pushing, encourage upright positions 7. Use squatting bars and birthing balls 8. Teach and utilize open glottis pushing 9. Support and facilitate patient's spontaneous pushing efforts 10. Encourage to rest between contractions 11. Ice chips or intake per protocol	1. B/P, pulse, resp. q 15 minutes 2. Assess for bleeding 3. Assess for placental detachment 4. Encourage relaxation 5. Ice chips or intake per protocol	1. VS q 15 min × 1 hour the q 30 minutes 2. Assess fundus, lochia q 15 minutes × 1 hour, then 30 minutes 3. Inspect perineum q 15 min × 1 hour, then q 30 minutes 4. Check for bladder distention 5. Position of comfort 6. Diet and fluid as tolerated
Pain	1. Initiate non-pharmacological pain management strategies 2. Assist in diversional activities 3. Encourage control breathing 4. Position changes and ambulation 5. Use non-pharmacological pain management strategies	1. Relaxation and controlled breathing 2. Back rub 3. Pharmacological pain management 4. Position changes and ambulation 5. Use non-pharmacological pain management strategies	1. Relaxation and controlled breathing 2. Palpate contractions lightly 3. Pharmacological pain management 4. Position changes 5. Use non-pharmacological pain management strategies	1. Support leg, chest, arms, and back 2. Positioning 3. Pharmacological pain management 4. Relaxation breathing between contractions 5. Assist with breathing and pushing 6. Use nonpharmacological pain management strategies	1. Relaxation breathing 2. Positioning 3. Use non-pharmacological pain management strategies	1. Positioning 2. Analgesics 3. Use non-pharmacological pain management strategies

Continued

TABLE 8–1   STAGES AND PHASES OF LABOR—cont'd

STAGES OF LABOR

Phases	1st			2nd	3rd	4th
	Latent	Active	Transition	Expulsive	Placenta	Immediate Postpartum
Fetal Biological System	1. Assess FHR q 30 minutes or per protocol 2. Leopold's maneuver for fetal position 3. SVE exam of patient 4. Position patient off of back	1. Assess FHR q 15–30 minutes or per protocol 2. Position patient off of back	1. Assess FHR q 15 minutes or per protocol 2. Position patient off of back	1. Assess FHR after each contraction 2. Observe perineum for crowning	1. Assess condition of newborn at birth 2. Apgar scores 1 min and 5 minutes 3. Maintain airway 4. Maintain body heat 5. Facilitate early contact with parents 6. Baby I.D.	1. V.S. q 15 minutes × 1 hr, then q 30 minutes 2. Facilitate contact with parents 3. Initiate breast feeding 4. Give routine meds 5. Maintain thermoregulation 6. Initial assessment
Social System	1. Patient's identification of support person(s) 2. Assist support person(s) in his/her role 3. Include support person(s) in patient teaching and care 4. Encourage support person(s) to remain with patient	1. Assist support person(s) with comfort measures and positions of comfort for patient 2. Assist support person in relaxation breathing exercises 3. Encourage support person(s) to remain with patient 4. Assist support person in focusing on patient labor	1. Assist support person with relaxation breathing 2. Assist support person identifying changes and tension and keeping patient relaxed 3. Reassurance	1. Prepare support person(s) for delivery—scrubs, mask, cap, shoe covers 2. Assist support person(s) with relaxations breathing 3. Assist support person in supporting patient during contractions and pushing	1. Reassurance 2. Praise 3. Early contact with baby 4. Explain procedures	1. Support person(s) to remain with patient and baby 2. Explain procedures, education

Labor and Delivery Admission Record

PT. NAME: _____   **AGE:** _____   **CARE PROVIDER:** _____

ADMIT DATE/TIME: _____

EDC	LMP	Weeks of Gestation	Gravida	Para	Term	Preterm	Spontaneous Abortion	Elective Abortion	Living	Stillborn	C-Section	VBAC

T	P	R	BP	Height	Weight	Pre-Pregnant weight	Weight Gain	How Admitted		Accompanied By	

Date/Time Care Provider Notified	Date/Time Seen By Care Provider	Reason for Admission

		Nutritional screen:	Describe Last Solid Intake (Include Date/Time):

Onset of Labor   **Contraction Frequency (Min)**

Dilatation (cm)   **Effacement (%)**   **Station**

Contraction Duration (Sec)   **Contraction Quality**
None   Mild   Moderate   Strong

Pelvic Exam By:

Pain Level Assessment: *Pain scale 0–10*

Admission Membranes: Intact   Ruptured   Bulging   Unknown

Fern: N/A   Negative   Positive   Equivocal

AROM/SROM (Date/Time):

Amniotic Fluid:
Amount: None   N/A   Copious   Large   Moderate   Small   Scant
Color: N/A   Clear   Bloody   Meconium   Heavy   Light   Particulate
Odor: None   N/A   Normal   Foul
Amniotic Fluid Comments:

Vaginal Bleeding: None   Normal   Frank bleeding

Describe Vaginal Bleeding:

Mental Status: Alert   Anxious   Confused

Feeding Preference: Breast   Bottle   Breast/bottle   Undecided

Support Person: None   Husband   Partner   Other

Support Person(s) Name:

Anesthesia Plans: None Local Epidural Spinal General Pudendal Paracervical

Anesthesia Plans Other:

Anesthesia Class: Yes   No   Yes, Previous Pregnancy

Attended Prenatal Class: Yes   No   Yes, Previous Pregnancy

Labor Teaching Initiated: Yes   No   N/A
  Fetal Well-being   Yes   No   N/A
  Labor Progress   Yes   No   N/A
  Pain Relief Measures   Yes   No   N/A
  Other

Nutritional screen:
[ ] N/A
[ ] History of Diabetes/Gestational Diabetes
[ ] History of Eating Disorder
[ ] Multiple Pregnancy
[ ] Special Diet/Vegetarian Diet
[ ] Pt. is 18 Years Old or Younger
[ ] Failure to Gain at Least 1/2 lb. per Wks. of Gestation
[ ] Food Allergies
[ ] Other _____

Describe Last Solid Intake (Include Date/Time):

Describe Last Fluid Intake (Include Date/Time):

In-Pt. Dietary Referral Entered in Computer: Yes No N/A   **In-Pt. Dietary Referral Entered in Computer:** Yes No N/A

Medication Allergy: Yes   No
Medication Allergy Detail:

Food Allergies: Yes   No
Food Allergy detail:

Latex Allergy: Yes   No
Describe Latex Reaction:

Allergy Sticker on Chart: Yes N/A   **Allergy Band on Patient:** Yes N/A

Prenatal Vitamins This Pregnancy: Yes   No   **Anticoagulants This Pregnancy:** Describe: Yes   No

For current prescription/over the counter medications taken during pregnancy see Home Medication Order Sheet.

Prescription/over the counter medications previously taken during pregnancy:

Addressograph

(continued on next page)

Labor and Delivery Admission Record (continued)

PT. NAME: _____

GBS Yes Negative Results Results: Positive Date: Tested: No Unknown	**Drug Use:** Denies Yes *If Yes, Describe:* **Drug Use Comments:**

GBS
Tested: Yes / No
Results: Negative / Positive / Unknown
Results Date:

Blood Type/Rh: | Rhogam | **This Pregnancy:** N/A Yes No No Record

Rubella: Immune Non-immune Unknown **HBsAg:** Negative Positive Unknown **RPR:** Non-Reactive Reactive Unknown

Hemoglobin = _____ g/dl Initials: _____ **HIV:** Non-Reactive Reactive
Reference Range: 11–14 g/dl (pregnancy)

Heart Disease: Yes No   Hypertension: Yes No

MVP: Yes No   Diabetes: Yes No

Asthma: Yes No   DVT: Yes No

Blood Transfusion: Yes No
Blood Transfusion Reason/Yr:

Sexually Denies Chlamydia Syphilis Gonorrhea
Transmitted HIV HPV/Genital Warts Herpes
Diseases: Other _____

Exposure to Infectious Denies Measles Mumps HIV/AIDS
Disease This Pregnancy: Chicken Pox TB Hepatitis
Other _____

Cervical Denies D & C LEEP Cervical biopsy
Procedures: Laser Cryo/Cautery
Other _____

History of Major
Illness or Surgery:

Patient History Detail:

Past Pregnancy None PIH Cystitis Pyelitis Preterm Labor
Complications: Preterm Birth Anemia Rh Sensitization
Positive GBS Other _____
Comments:

Complications None PIH Cystitis Preterm Labor
Current Anemia Rh sensitization
Pregnancy: Placental abnormalities
Comments: Other _____

Fetal Assessments None Non-Stress Test OCT
Done This Pregnancy: CVS BPP US Amnio

Previous Labor Durations:

Sibling History:

Family N/A Adopted Heart Disease HTN Diabetes Cancer
History: Bleeding Disorder Other _____
Family History Comments:

Smoke Denies <5 per day 5–10 per day
Use/Frequency: >10 per day >20 per day

Alcohol Use: Denies Occasional 3–5 Drinks/Week 6 or More Drinks/Week

Drug Use: Denies Yes *If Yes, Describe:*
Drug Use Comments:

Contact Lenses: Yes No Soft Lenses Hard Lenses Lenses In Lenses Out

Glasses: Yes No **Dentures:** Yes No

Body Piercing: Yes No **Body piercing Location/Removed:**

Support System After Birth: Family Friends Community None
If None, Social Service Referral Entered In Computer: Yes No N/A

History of Abuse: Denies Emotional Physical Sexual Other _____ *If Other, Describe*
Social Service Referral Entered in Computer: Yes No N/A

Special Needs: None Spiritual Cultural Emotional Other _____
Hearing/vision impaired: Yes No *If Other, Describe*

Social Service Referral Entered in Computer: Yes No N/A
Pastoral Service Referral Entered in Computer: Yes No N/A

Interpreter needed? Yes No Primary language: _____

Psychosocial Comments:

Room Orientation: EFM Bed Phone Call Light Visitors Computer

Does the Patient Have an Advance Directive?

Yes — **If Yes, is Copy in Chart?** Yes / No — **If No Copy on Chart, Remind Pt. to Have Family Member Bring Copy AND Send Advance Directive Referral to Pastoral Services** — **Referral Entered in Computer:** Yes / No

No — **If No, Does Pt. Want Additional Information or Assistance?** Yes / No — **If Yes, Was Referral Sent to Pastoral Care?** Yes / No — **Referral Entered in Computer:** Yes / No

Disposition of Valuables: Sent Home Kept with Pt. Valuables in Security Office Pt. Encouraged to Take Valuables Home Other _____
Valuables Comments:

Pt. Wants Other Physician or Family Notified: Yes No

Other Physician/Family Notified:

Morse Fall Scale Score:
[ ] < 45, low fall risk; initiate appropriate interventions
[ ] > 50, high fall risk; initiate appropriate interventions
[ ] ≥ 4 medications associated with increased fall risk;
    high fall risk; initiate appropriate interventions

Initiate Care Plan if:
[ ] Anticipated physiological fall risk
[ ] Unanticipated physiological fall risk
[ ] Accidental fall risk

Immunization History
Vaccines: Influenza Yes No Date ____
Pneumonia Yes No Date ____
Tetanus Yes No Date ____
PPD Yes No Date ____

Nursing Assessment Summary: _____

Requests cord blood banking: Y N
Cord blood banking type: ☐ NA
☐ St. Louis Cord Blood Bank
☐ Private cord blood bank

Addressograph

Figure 8–22 Labor and delivery admission sheet.

		DATE:				KEY
		TIME:				**Variability**
Cervix	Dilation					Ab = Absent (undetectable)
	Effacement					Min = Minimal (>0 out ≤5 bpm)
	Station					Mod = Moderate (6–25 bpm)
Fetal Heart	Baseline Rate					Mar = Marked (>25 bpm)
	Variability					**Accelerations**
	Accelerations					+ = Present and appropriate for gestational age
	Decelerations					∅ = Absent
	STIM/pH					**Decelerations**
	Monitor Mode					E = Early
Uterine Activity	Frequency					L = Late
	Duration					V = Variable
	Intensity					P = Prolonged
	Resting Tone					**Stim/pH**
	Monitor Mode					+ = Acceleration in response to stimulation
	Oxytocin milliunits/min					∅ = No response to stimulation
	Pain					Record number for scalp pH
	Coping					**Monitor mode**
	Maternal Position					A = Auscultation/Palpation
	O2/LPM/Mask					E = External u/s or toco
	IV					FSE - Fetal spiral electrode
	Nurse Initials					IUPC = Intrauterine pressure catheter

Patient Name: Physician/CNM:

KEY (continued)
Frequency of uterine activity
∅ = None
Irreg = Irregular
Intensity of uterine activity
M = Mild
Mod = Moderate
Str = Strong
By IUPC = mm Hg
Resting tone
R = Relaxed
By IUCP = mm Hg
Coping
W = Well
S = Support provided
For pain use 0–10 scale
Maternal position
A = Ambulatory
U = Upright
SF = Semi-Fowler's
RL = Right lateral
LL = Left lateral
MS = Modified Sims'

Narrative notes:

Figure 8–23   Labor documentation.

Latent Phase

The **latent phase,** is the early and slower part of labor with an average length of 9 hours for primiparous and 5 hours for multiparous women. Women in this phase are usually both excited and apprehensive about the start of labor. They are talkative and able to relax with the contractions. Many women choose to stay home during this phase, although some women are admitted to the birth center during this time. Indications for admittance to the birth center are if there is cervical change/ROM or fetal intolerance of labor. Most can go back home to a more relaxed setting at this stage and return to the birth center when labor progresses. Awaiting admission until active labor decreases the need for medical interventions, and facilitates fetal descent and labor support of the family to the patient.

Characteristics of this phase are:

■ Cervical dilation from 0 to 3 cm with effacement from 0 to 40%.
■ Contractions occur every 5–10 minutes, lasting 30–45 seconds, and mild intensity. Women often describe them as feeling like strong menstrual cramps.

Medical Interventions

■ Order laboratory tests, which may include complete blood count (CBC), urinalysis, and possible drug screening.
■ Order IV or saline lock.
■ Order intermittent fetal monitoring or continuous fetal and uterine monitoring.

CRITICAL COMPONENT

Nonpharmacological Strategies for Nurses and Comfort Measures in Labor

Labor support is a repertoire of techniques used to help women with the process of childbirth (Wood & Carr, 2003). Providing support and comfort is one of the primary activities of nurses and includes:

Emotional Support

- Sustaining physical presence, eye contact
- Verbal encouragement, reassurance, and praise
- Listening to woman and family
- Distraction

Physical Support

- Comfort measures such as ice chips, fluids, food, and pain medications
- Hygiene including mouth care, pericare, and changing soiled linens
- Assistance with position changes and ambulation
- Reassuring touch, massage
- Application of heat and cold
- Hydrotherapy in shower and tub. Hydrotherapy is safe and effective as a complementary pain management therapy (Stark & Miller, 2009).

- Calm environment (dim lighting, quiet, music, minimize interruptions)

Informational Support

- Provide information on the progress of labor.
- Explain all procedures.
- Communicate in lay language so the woman and her family understand.
- Offer advice
- Use interpreters as needed.

Advocacy

- Support decisions made by the woman and her family.
- Ensure respect for the woman's decisions.
- Manage the environment, which includes visitors.
- Translate the woman's wishes to others

Support of the Partner and Family

- Offer support and praise.
- Role model therapeutic behaviors.
- Assist the partner with food and rest.
- Provide breaks if desired or needed.

(Wood & Carr, 2003; Burke, 2013)

Nursing Actions (see Clinical Pathway and Concept Map)

- Admit to the labor unit and orient the woman, her partner, and family to the labor room.
- The review of the prenatal record will give information from pregnancy onset to the present. The prenatal record should include: all lab tests and ultrasounds (for estimated date of delivery (EDD) and placental location) as well as any prior obstetrical history (pregnancy, births, abortions, and living children) should be included. A review of allergies and medications, trends in vital signs and weight gain, chronic conditions, or pregnancy-related complications will also be a part of the record. Biochemical and infectious disease laboratory test results; for example, Group B streptococcus (GBS) status, are also included
- Complete labor and delivery admission record (Fig. 8-22).
- Review childbirth plan and discuss the woman's expectations.
  - *Woman may present with a birth plan: Some providers and childbirth educators encourage the family to think about how they "see" the labor and birth process. It is a wish list that allows the woman to express her wishes and preferences and communicate with care providers during her prenatal appointments. This discussion should include hospital policies and medical interventions. Review this plan with the woman during the admission process and clarify what you can and cannot*

  provide. This will facilitate open communication and show respect for her expectations.
- Teach and reinforce relaxation and breathing techniques.
  - *Support what they have been practicing or teach techniques as needed to decrease pain and anxiety.*
- Obtain laboratory tests as per orders.
  - *Provides information on patient status and health.*
- Start IV or insert saline lock, if ordered.
  - *Provides access for fluids and or medications if needed.*
- Review the woman's report of onset of labor.
- Assess and record the following (see Fig. 8-22 and Clinical Pathway and Concept Map):
  - *Maternal vital signs*
  - *FHR*
  - *Uterine contractions*
  - *Cervical dilation and effacement; and fetal presentation, position, and station by performing a sterile vaginal examination (SVE)* (**Fig. 8-24**, see **Box 8-2**).
  - *Status of membranes*
  - *Amniotic fluid for color, amount, consistency, and odor*
  - *Vaginal bleeding or bloody show for amount and characteristics of vaginal discharge*
  - *Fetal position with Leopold maneuver* (**Fig. 8-25**, see **Box 8-3**)
  - *Deep tendon reflexes*
  - *Signs of edema*
  - *Heart and lung sounds*

■ *Emotional status*
■ *Pain and discomfort*
■ Review laboratory results, note blood Rh status hematocrit and hemoglobin and dipstick urine for glucose and protein.
■ Review GBS status, if GBS positive intrapartum IV antibiotic prophylaxis is given.
  ■ *Group B streptococci (GBS), also known as Streptococcus agalactiae, is an important cause of perinatal morbidity and mortality. Between 10% and 30% of pregnant women are colonized with GBS in the vagina or rectum. Implementation of national guidelines for intrapartum antibiotic prophylaxis since the 1990s has resulted in an approximate 80% reduction in the incidence of early-onset neonatal sepsis due to GBS. Vertical transmission of GBS during labor or delivery may result in invasive infection in the newborn during the first week of life. Penicillin remains the drug of choice, with ampicillin as an alternative (American college of Obstetrics & Gynecology, 2011).*
■ Intrapartum GBS prophylaxis (CDC, 2010) is indicated:
  ■ *Previous infant with invasive GBS disease*
  ■ *GBS bacteria during and trimester of current pregnancy*
  ■ *Positive GBS vaginal-rectal screening culture in late gestation during current pregnancy*
  ■ *Unknown GBS status at onset of labor with <37 weeks gestation, or ROM >18 hours, or temperature > 100.4°F or >38.0°C or intrapartum NAAT positive for GBS*
■ Document allergies, history of illness, and last food intake.
■ Encourage fluid intake; food may or may not be restricted.
■ Provide comfort measures (see Critical Component: Non-pharmacologic Strategies for Nurses and Comfort Measures in Labor).
■ Encourage the woman to walk as much as possible by:
  ■ *Explaining the importance of walking in facilitating labor progression and fetal descent and rotation and in making UCs more efficient*
  ■ *Walking with the woman, which can provide a comforting and reassuring presence and distraction*
■ Assess cultural needs and incorporate beliefs in the nursing care and delivery plan.
■ Establish a therapeutic relationship through active listening and providing labor support (**Box 8-4**).
■ Incorporate understanding of the couple's maturity level, educational level, and previous experience into nursing care.
■ Review the labor plan with the woman and her partner.
■ Inquire about concerns and questions the woman and/or her partner have concerning the labor and birth process.
■ Provide clear explanations and updates on progress.
  ■ *Above noted nursing actions will provide information to the nurse to facilitate teaching moments, decrease patient anxiety, and support the plan of care.*

QSEN

Teamwork and Collaboration: Leading Health Care Organizations Issue Recommendations for Quality Patient Care in Labor and Delivery

Although the infant mortality rate in the United States declined in 2010, the U.S. rate remains higher than most European nations. In addition, U.S. health care providers have seen an increase in pregnancy complications. These trends, along with the recognition that collaboration among physicians, midwives, and nurses is essential to positive health outcomes, prompted professional organizations from the nation's leading obstetrics, family medicine, and pediatric organizations to develop joint recommendations. The "Call to Action" includes recommendations for health care providers and administrators:

■ Ensure that patient-centered care and patient safety are organizational priorities that guide decisions for policies and practices.
■ Foster a culture of openness by promoting the active communication of good outcomes and opportunities for improvement.
■ Develop forums to facilitate communication and track issues of concern.
■ Provide resources for clinicians to be trained in the principles of teamwork, safety, and shared decision-making.
■ Develop methods to systematically track and evaluate care processes and outcomes.
■ Facilitate cross-departmental sharing of resources and expertise.
■ Ensure that quality obstetric care is a priority that guides individual and team decisions.
■ Identify and communicate safety concerns, and work together to mitigate potential safety risks.
■ Disseminate and use the best available evidence, including individual and hospital-level data, to guide practice patterns.

The joint call to action underscores the collective belief among health care providers that ongoing collaboration is a key element to improving health care outcomes. By providing interprofessional collaboration and care management for families in labor, the overall experience can promote optimal patient care, satisfaction, and maternal and fetal outcomes (AWHONN, 2011).

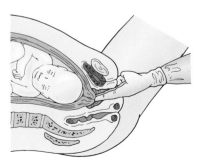

Figure 8–24 Sterile vaginal exam.

BOX 8–2 STERILE VAGINAL EXAM

Intrapartal Sterile Vaginal Exam

To perform a vaginal exam, the labia are separated with a sterile gloved hand. Fingers are lubricated with a water-soluble lubricant. The first and second fingers are inserted into the introitus; the cervix is located and the following parameters are assessed (Fig. 8-24):

■ Cervical dilation: This measurement estimates the dilation of the cervical opening by sweeping the examining finger from the margin of the cervical opening on one side to that on the other.
■ Cervical effacement: This measurement estimates the shortening of the cervix from 2 cm to paper thin measured by palpation of cervical length with the fingertips. The degree of cervical effacement is expressed in terms of the length of the cervical canal compared to that of an unaffected cervix. When it is reduced by one-half (1 cm), it is 50% effaced. When the cervix is thinned out completely, it is 100% effaced.
■ Position of cervix: Relationship of the cervical os to the fetal head and is characterized as posterior, midposition, or anterior.
■ Station: Level of the presenting part in the birth canal in relationship to the ischial spines. Station is 0 when the presenting part is at the ischial spines or engaged in the pelvis.
■ Presentation: Cephalic (head first), breech (pelvis first), shoulder (shoulder first)
■ Fetal position: Locate presenting part and specific fetal structure to determine fetal position in relation to the maternal pelvis.

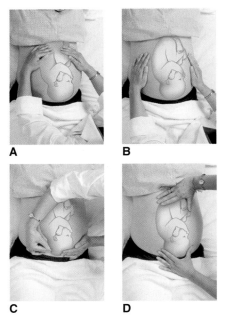

A **B**

C **D**

Figure 8-25 Leopold's maneuver.

BOX 8–3 LEOPOLD'S MANEUVERS

The purpose of Leopold's maneuvers is to inspect and palpate the maternal abdomen to determine fetal position, station, and size (Fig. 8-25).

■ The first maneuver is to determine what part of the fetus is located in the fundus of the uterus.
■ The second maneuver is to determine location of the fetal back.
■ The third maneuver is to determine the presenting part.
■ The fourth maneuver is to determine the location of the cephalic prominence.

Mattson & Smith (2004).

BOX 8–4 STANDARD OF PRACTICE. AWHONN PRACTICE STATEMENT: PROFESSIONAL NURSING SUPPORT OF LABORING WOMEN

Association for Women's Health, Obstetric and Neonatal Nurses (AWHONN) maintains that continuously available labor support by a professional registered nurse is a critical component to achieve improved birth outcomes. AWHONN views labor care and labor support as powerful nursing functions, and believes it is incumbent on health care facilities to provide an environment that encourages the unique patient–nurse relationship during childbirth. Only the registered nurse combines adequate formal nursing education and clinical patient management skills with experience in providing physical, psychological, and sociocultural care to laboring women. The registered nurse facilitates the childbirth process in collaboration with the laboring woman. The nurse's expertise and therapeutic presence influence patient and family satisfaction with the labor and delivery experience. Evidence supports women who are provided with continuously available support during labor experience improved labor and delivery outcomes compared with those who labor without a skilled support person. The support provided by the professional registered nurse should include:

■ Assessment and management of the physiological and psychological processes of labor
■ Provision of emotional support and physical comfort measures
■ Evaluation of fetal well-being during labor
■ Instruction regarding the labor process
■ Patient advocacy and collaboration among members of the health care team
■ Role modeling to facilitate family participation during labor and birth
■ Direct collaboration with other members of the health care team to coordinate patient care

AWHONN (2000a).

Active Phase

The **active phase** (dilation to 7 cm) of labor averages 3–6 hours in length. It is typically shorter for multigravidas (Table 8-1). Women in this phase may have decreased energy and experience fatigue. They become more serious and turn attention to internal sensations. As labor progresses, most women turn inward. Characteristics of this phase are:

■ The cervix dilates, on average, 0.5 cm/hr for primiparous women and 1.5 cm/hr for multiparous women. Current evidence suggests that the slowest dilation rate for primiparous women in early active labor is 0.5cm/hr. (Neal et al., 2010).

- Cervical dilation progresses *from* 4 cm–7 cm with effacement of 40%–80%.
- Fetal descent continues.
- Contractions become more intense, occurring every 2–5 minutes with duration of 45–60 seconds.
- Discomfort increases, and this is typically the time the woman comes to the birth center or hospital if she has not done so already.

Medical Interventions

- Rupture membranes if not previously ruptured if indicated.
- Evaluate fetal status by fetal monitoring as indicated, either intermittent or continuous.
- Perform internal monitoring with application of internal fetal electrode and/or uterine transducer, if necessary.
- Pain assessment: order pain medication or epidural anesthesia.
- Evaluate progression in labor.

Nursing Actions (see Clinical Pathway and Concept Map)

- Monitor FHR and contractions every 15–30 minutes.
- Monitor maternal vital signs every 2 hours; every 1 hour if ROM.
- Perform intrapartal vaginal exam as needed to assess cervical changes and fetal descent (Box 8-2).
- Assess pain (location and degree).
- Administer analgesia as per orders and desire of woman.
- Evaluate effectiveness of epidural or other pain medication.
- Monitor intake and output (I&O), hydration status, and for nausea and vomiting.
- Offer oral fluids as per orders (ice chips, popsicles, carbohydrate liquids, and water). Encourage the woman to listen to her body in regard to hydration and nausea and allow her to decide when she has had enough intake.
- Offer clear explanations and updates of progress.
- Promote comfort measures (see Critical Component: Non-pharmacologic Strategies for Nurses and Comfort Measures in Labor).
- Assist with elimination (bladder distension can hinder fetal descent).
- Encourage breathing and relaxation methods (see Box 8-4).
  - *Review and reinforce relaxation techniques.*
  - *Maintain eye contact and physical proximity to the woman.*
  - *Develop a rhythm and breathing style to deal with each contraction.*
  - *Use a direct and gentle voice and have a calm and confident manner.*
  - *Use touch of massage if acceptable to the woman.*
- Interdisciplinary collaboration management of labor assists in communicating the woman's progress and status with other care providers.
- Incorporate the support person in care of patient by:
  - *Role modeling supportive behaviors*
  - *Offering support and praise*
  - *Assisting partner with food and rest*
  - *Providing breaks if desired or needed*

- Explain procedures before initiating, asking for permission from the patient.
- Assess the environment for adjustments to be made; typically decrease stimulation with dim lighting and decrease noise and interruptions.
- Provide reassurance, updates on progress, and positive reinforcement.

Transition Phase

The transition phase (dilation to 10 cm), is usually the most difficult but shortest of the first stages of labor (Table 8-1). In transition, women are easily discouraged and irritable, and may be overwhelmed and panicky. They often feel and act out of control. Characteristics of this phase are:

- Cervical dilation from 8–10 cm with complete (100%) effacement
- Intense contractions every 1–2 minutes lasting 60–90 seconds
- Exhaustion and increased difficulty concentrating
- Increase of bloody show
- Nausea and vomiting
- Backache: woman complains of back pressure, hand goes over hip, rubbing and pressing on area.
- Trembling
- Diaphoresis: especially upper lip and facial area
- Strong urge to bear down or push, more vocal with primal noises and facial expressions.

Medical Interventions

- Perform amniotomy (AROM) if not previously done.
- Assess fetal position and cervix.
- Prepare for delivery

Nursing Actions (see Clinical Pathway and concept Map)

- Assess FHR and UCs every 15 minutes.
- Provide calming support and reassurance, speaking slowly in low, soothing tone, giving short and clear directs such as: "You are in control;" "It is normal to feel so much pressure as the baby moves down;" "You are doing a great job working with your contractions."
  - *Woman who are given encouragement and empowered to follow their body will have less anxiety and fear of the process and will perform with more control and conviction.*
- Encourage the woman to breathe during contractions and rest between contractions by staying with patient and breathing with her (see Box 8-4). Assist with breathing and relaxation methods by demonstrating breathing through demonstration and reinforcement.
  - *Providing support and encouragement will assist in decreasing fear and anxiety.*
- Assess I&O and assist with toileting as needed.
  - *Bladder distension may hinder fetal descent, cause bladder trauma and discomfort.*
- Promote comfort measures (see Critical Component: Non-pharmacologic Strategies for Nurses and Comfort Measures in Labor).

- Attend to the hygiene needs of the woman, such as mopping her brow and face, providing pericare, and changing chux.
  - *Providing comfort and hygiene measures shows attention to and respect for the patient's personal needs.*
- Prepare the room and couple for delivery.
  - *Familiarize the woman and support people with usual routine and keep them informed of what to expect.*
  - *Open the delivery tray.*
  - *Turn on the infant radiant warmer.*
- Use brief explanations, as the woman's focus is narrowed.
- Remain in the room with the woman and family.
- Provide encouragement and reassurance to the woman and her support person(s).
  - *Keep them apprised of labor progress, such as changes in cervical dilation.*
  - *Compliment them on their effective breathing and relaxation techniques.*

Second Stage

The woman enters the **second stage** of labor when cervical dilation is complete (10 cm) (see Table 8-1). This stage ends with the birth of the baby (**Fig. 8-26**). Women in the second stage may have a burst of energy, be more focused, and may feel like they are able to actively participate in facilitating birth with active pushing efforts. Characteristics of this stage are:

- Typically lasts 50 minutes for primigravidas and 20 minutes for multigravidas, although a second stage of several hours is normal.
- Woman may feel an intense urge to push or bear down when the baby reaches the pelvic floor.
  - *Studies have shown that bearing down in the second stage is less tiring and more effective when begun after the woman has the urge to do so instead of beginning to push without an urge to (Roberts, 2002, 2003). In nulliparous women with epidurals, there was a 27% less pushing time for those who delayed their efforts until they felt the urge to push (Ferguson's reflex), which decreased maternal fatigue, provided increased maternal satisfaction in the birth experience, and allowed women to fully participate in postpartum activities (Gillesby et al., 2010).*
  - *Contractions are intense, occurring every 2 minutes and lasting 60–90 seconds in duration.*
  - *Bloody show increases.*
  - *The perineum flattens and the rectum and vagina bulge.*

Labor Position and Bearing Down

Variation in practice exists in positioning of women during the second stage of labor. Many women maintain a semirecumbent position, but there are benefits to a more upright position. Along with the timing of the bearing-down efforts, which include the spontaneous versus the directed pushing, the way a woman pushes has also been studied. Two types have been studied for the effects on the fetus: the closed-glottis (Valsalva maneuver) and the open-glottis pushing (see Evidence-Based Practice: Guideline of Nursing Management

of Second Stage of Labor). The results are that fetal hypoxia and acidosis have been associated with the prolonged breath holding (closed glottis) and forceful pushing efforts. No significant differences have been found in the duration of the second stage of labor with the timing and how a woman pushes (Mayberry et al., 2000).

Evidence-Based Practice: AWHONN Evidence-Based Clinical Practice Guideline: Nursing Management of Second Stage of Labor

Association of Women's Health, Obstetric and Neonatal Nurses (AWHONN) clinical practice recommendations for management of pushing include:

- Assess the woman's knowledge of pushing techniques, expectations for pushing, presence of Ferguson's reflex (urge to bear down), and readiness to push as well as the fetal presentation, position, and station.
- Encourage open glottis pushing for 4–6 seconds followed by a slight exhale, repeating this pattern for five or six pushes per contraction. Open glottis refers to spontaneous, involuntary bearing down accompanying the forces of the uterine contraction and is usually characterized by expiratory grunting or vocalizations. This spontaneous method usually involves five or six pushes of 4–6 seconds' duration with each contraction.
- Whenever possible, discourage the traditional practice of breath holding for 10 seconds with each contraction. Closed glottis pushing, also referred to as the Valsalva technique, involves a voluntary or directed strenuous bearing-down effort against a closed glottis for at least 10 seconds. This method usually involves two to three pushes of 10 seconds each during a contraction.
- Provide birthing aids such as birthing balls, squat bars, birthing stools, and cushions to support the woman and the pelvis.
- Evaluate the effectiveness of pushing efforts and descent of the presenting part.
- Support and facilitate the woman's spontaneous pushing efforts.
- Evaluate the effectiveness of upright or other positions on fetal descent, rotation, and maternal-fetal condition.
- Upright positioning for the second stage of labor refers to the patient's position sitting with the head of the bed at a 45-degree angle or greater, squatting, kneeling, or standing during the second stage of labor. Benefits of upright positioning include: pelvic diameter may be increased by 30%, shortened duration of second stage, pain may be decreased, and perineal trauma may be decreased.
- Ferguson's reflex is a physiological response of the woman, activated when the presenting part of the fetus is at least at +1 station; it is usually accompanied by spontaneous bearing-down efforts. Pushing efforts may be delayed until the Ferguson reflex is present.
- Delayed pushing is waiting for fetal descent and or initiation of Ferguson's reflex before pushing begins in the second stage of labor. Delayed pushing is also referred to as "laboring down," "passive pushing," and "rest and descend."
- Delayed pushing may also be appropriate for women with epidural anesthesia/analgesia who do not feel the urge to push.

AWHONN. (2000b). Evidence-Based Clinical Practice Guideline, Nursing Management of the Second Stage of Labor. Clinical Practice Recommendation. Washington, DC: Author.

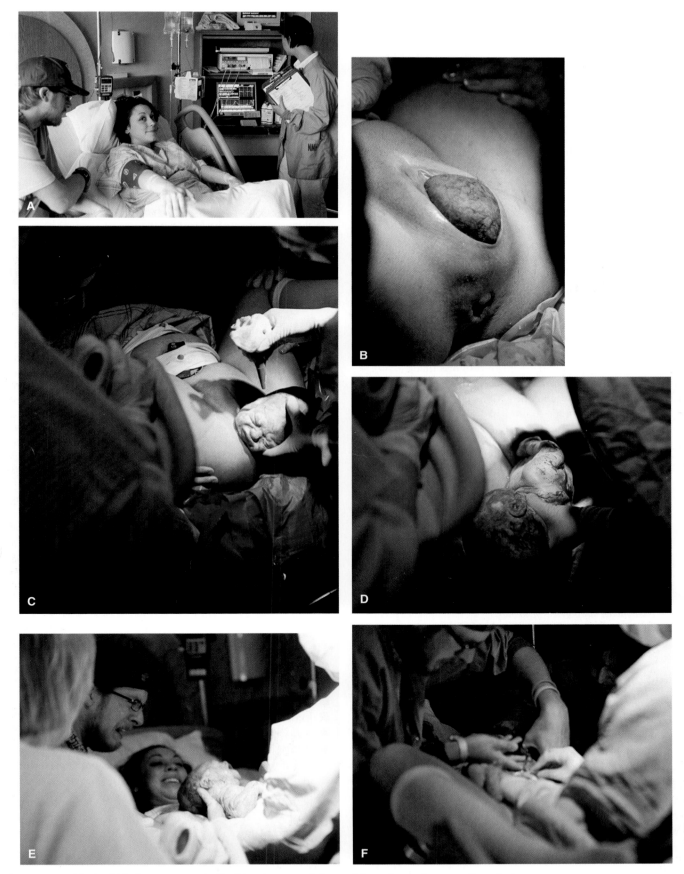

Figure 8–26 Vaginal birth sequence. A. Pushing in an upright position allows the use of gravity to promote fetal descent. B. Crowning. C. Birth of the head. D. Birth of the shoulders. E. The infant is shown to the new parents. F. The baby's father cuts the umbilical cord.

Medical Interventions

■ Prepare for delivery.
■ Provide reassurance to the woman while she pushes and brings baby down through the birth canal.
■ Perform episiotomy if necessary (**Box 8-5**).
■ Assist the woman in the birthing of her child.

Nursing Actions (see Clinical Pathway)

■ Instruct the woman to bear down with the urge to push (see Evidence-Based Practice guideline).
　■ *More progress is made and fewer traumas are noted to mother and fetus with spontaneous pushing efforts.*
■ Monitor for fetal response to pushing; check FHR every 5–15 minutes or after each contraction.
　■ *Assessing fetal heart rate response to pushing efforts*
■ Provide comfort measures.
■ Support and encourage woman's spontaneous pushing efforts.
■ Attend to perineal hygiene as needed, as the woman may pass stool with pushing.
　■ *Provides a cleaner pathway*
■ Give praise and encouragement of progress made.
　■ *Support and empowerment of woman's efforts*
■ Encourage rest between contractions by breathing with the patient and therapeutic touch.
　■ *Decreases fatigue and hypoxia in fetus by providing increased oxygenation*
■ Review and reinforce pushing technique by:
　■ *Maintaining eye contact.*
　■ *Developing a rhythm and pushing style to deal with each contraction that maximizes the woman's urge to push.*
　■ *Using direct, simple, and focused communication, avoiding unnecessary conversation.*
■ Advocate on the woman's behalf for her desires of the delivery plan.
■ Assist the support person and partner.
　■ *Role model supportive behaviors.*
　■ *Offer support, praise, and encouragement.*
　■ *Assist with food and rest and provide breaks.*

Third Stage

The **third stage** of labor begins immediately after the delivery of the fetus and involves separation and expulsion of the placenta and membranes (see Table 8-1). As the infant is born, the uterus spontaneously contracts around its diminishing contents. This sudden decrease in uterine size is accompanied by a decrease in the area of placental implantation. This results in the decidual layer separating from the uterine wall. Placental separation typically occurs within a few minutes after delivery. Once the placenta separates from the wall of the uterus, the uterus continues to contract until the placenta is expelled (**Fig. 8-29**). This process typically takes 5–30 minutes post-delivery of the baby and occurs

BOX 8–5　EPISIOTOMY AND LACERATIONS

Episiotomy is an incision in the perineum to provide more space for the presenting part at delivery (see **Fig. 8-27**). Routine use of episiotomy at delivery is no longer typical.

A median or midline episiotomy is at the midline and tends to heal more quickly with less discomfort.

A mediolateral episiotomy is cut at a 45-degree angle to the left or right and may be used for a large infant. It tends to heal more slowly, causes greater blood loss, and is more painful.

Lacerations are tears in the perineum that may occur at delivery (see **Fig. 8-28**):

Lacerations can occur in the cervix, vagina, and/or the perineum (Fig. 8-28A).

A first-degree laceration involves the perineal skin and vaginal mucous membrane (Fig. 8-28B).

A second-degree laceration involves skin, mucous membrane, and fascia of the perineal body (Fig. 8-28C).

A third-degree laceration involves skin, mucous membrane, and muscle of the perineal body and extends to the rectal sphincter (Fig. 8-28D).

A fourth-degree laceration extends into the rectal mucosa and exposes the lumen of the rectum (Fig. 8-28E).

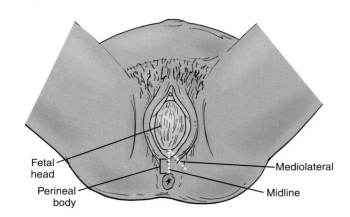

Figure 8–27　Episiotomy locations.

spontaneously. Signs that signify the impending delivery of the placenta include:

■ Upward rising of the uterus into a ball shape
■ Lengthening of the umbilical cord at the introitus
■ Sudden gush of blood from the vagina
■ Active management of placental delivery consists of the use of uterotonics, controlled cord traction, and uterine massage (Murray & Huelsmann, 2009).

Normal blood loss for a vaginal birth is approximately 500 mL. The placenta, membranes, and cord are examined by the care provider for completeness and anomalies. Uterotonics may be administered after the delivery of the placenta. See Medication: Uterotonics. These may be administered IV or IM.

Medication

Uterotonics

- **Oxytocin**—(Pitocin) Classification: hormone/oxytocic
  - Route/Dosage: IV (slow push or added to IV fluids) 1–20 milliunits. IM 10–20 milliunits.
  - Actions: Stimulates uterine smooth muscle that produces intermittent contractions. Has vasopressor and antidiuretic properties.
  - Indications: labor induction and augmentation. Control of PP (postpartum) bleeding after placental expulsion.
- **Mehtylergonovine**—(Methergine) Classification: oxytocic/ergot alkaloids
  - Route/Dosage: PO 200–400 mcg (0.4–0.6 mg) every 4–6 hours for 2–7 days. IM 200 mcg (0.2 mg) every 2–5 hours up to 5 doses. IV (for emergencies only) same dosage as IM.
  - Actions: Directly stimulates smooth and vascular smooth muscles causing sustaining uterine contractions.
  - Indications: Prevent or treat PP hemorrhage/uterine atony/subinvolution. Contraindicated in hypertensive patients.
- **Carboprost**—Tromethamine (Hemabate) Classification:Prostaglandin
  - Route/Dosage: IM 250 mcg injected into a large muscle or the uterus.
  - Actions: Contraction of uterine muscle
  - Indications: Uterine atony
- **Misoprostol**—(Cytotec) Classification: antiulcer/prostaglandins
  - Route/Dosage: PO/Rectally 200-1,000 mcg
  - Actions: Acts as a prostaglandin analogue causes uterine contractions.
  - Indications: To control PP hemorrhage. This medication is used off label and is not yet approved by the FDA for this use.

(Deglin, J., & Vallerand, A. (2009). Davis's Drug Guide for nurses, 11th ed. Philadelphia: F.A. Davis.)

Medical Interventions

- At delivery, the neonate is often placed skin-to-skin on mother's abdomen.
- Await delivery of the placenta.
- Inspect the placenta after delivery.
- Order pain medications and uterotonics if necessary.

Nursing Actions (see Clinical Pathway and Concept Map)

- Assess maternal vital signs every 15 minutes.
- Encourage the woman to breathe with contractions and relax between contractions.
- Encourage mother-baby interactions by providing immediate newborn contact, if the newborn is stable (see Critical Component: Newborn Family Attachment).
- Administer pain medications as per order.
- Complete documentation of the delivery (**Fig. 8-30**).
- Documentation of delivery includes labor summary, delivery summary for mother and baby, infant information, infant resuscitation, and documentation of personnel in attendance.
- Explain all forthcoming procedures.
- Stay with the woman and her family.

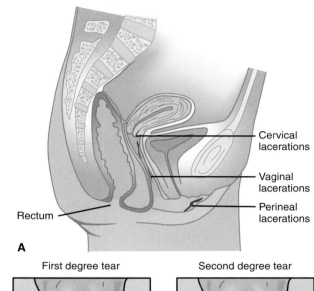

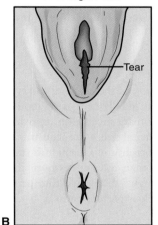

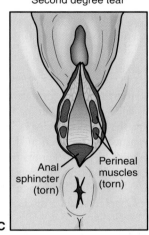

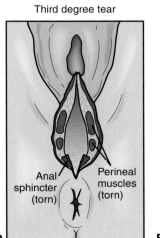

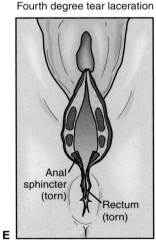

Figure 8–28 A. Potential locations of lacerations. B. First-degree tear. C. Second-degree tear. D. Third-degree tear. E. Fourth-degree tear

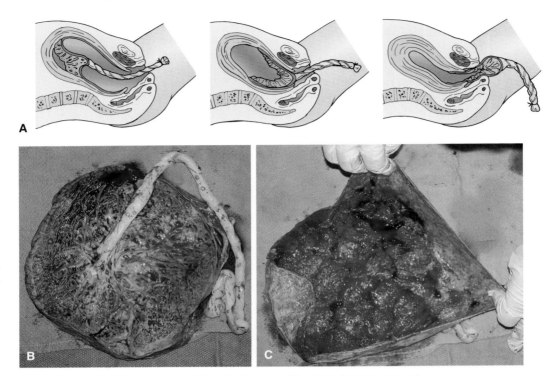

Figure 8–29   A. Delivery of the placenta. B. Delivered placenta (fetal side). C. Inside of placenta (maternal side).

Fourth Stage

The **fourth stage** begins after delivery of the placenta and typically ends within 4 hours or with the stabilization of the mother. After the placenta delivers, the primary mechanism by which hemostasis is achieved at the placental site is vasoconstriction produced by a well-contracted myometrium. During this stage, the nurse is caring for both the woman and her newborn child (see Table 8-1). This stage also begins the postpartum period (see Chapter 12 for a discussion of postpartum period).

Medical Interventions

■ Repair the episiotomy or laceration (see Box 8-5, Fig. 8-27, and Fig. 8-28).
■ Inspect the placenta.
■ Assess the fundus for firmness.
■ Order uterotonics.
■ Order pain medications, if necessary.

Nursing Actions (see Clinical Pathway and Concept Map)

■ Explain all procedures.
■ Assess the uterus for position, tone, and location, intervening with fundal massage as necessary.
■ Assess lochia for color, amount, and clots. May weigh initial blood loss on scale to estimate EBL (1 gm=1 cc)
■ Administer medications as per orders.
■ Assist the care provider with repair of lacerations and/or episiotomy.
■ Assess maternal vital signs every 15 minutes.
■ Monitor perineum for unusual swelling or hematoma formation.

■ Apply ice packs to the perineum.
■ Monitor for bladder distention.
   ■ *Assist the woman to the bathroom and measure void.*
■ Assess for return of full motor-sensory function if epidural or spinal anesthesia is used.
■ Assess pain and medicate as per orders.
■ Stay with the mother and family.
■ Offer congratulations and reassurance on a job well done to the woman and family.
■ Encourage mother-baby interaction by:
   ■ *Providing immediate newborn contact*
   ■ *Assisting with early breastfeeding, if desired*
   ■ *Pointing out the newborn's quiet, alert state*
■ Monitor newborn status, including temperature, heart and respiratory rates, skin color, adequacy of peripheral circulation, type of respiration, level of consciousness, and tone and activity every 30 minutes.
■ Provide an opportunity for the support person to interact with newborn (**Fig. 8-31**).

CRITICAL COMPONENT

Newborn Family Attachment

An important goal during the fourth stage is the newborn-family attachment. This is promoted by allowing early contact with the newborn and encouragement of eye contact and touch, and also by allowing time to hold the newborn. Positive maternal bonding behaviors include making eye contact, touching and talking to the baby, and other positive behaviors such as smiling and cuddling the newborn. This is often the best time to institute breastfeeding. The newborn may remain in the labor and delivery room with the family for all of the immediate recovery period.

Delivery/Newborn Record

LABOR SUMMARY

Time   Date

Regular contractions began: _____
Time of Oxytocin start: _____
BOW ruptured: _____
(best estimate) 4cm: _____
10cm: _____

Labor description:
- [ ] spontaneous   [ ] AROM for induction
- [ ] augmented, oxytocin   [ ] no labor
- [ ] induced, oxytocin

- [ ] Cervical ripening agent _____
- [ ] IUPC
- [ ] Amino infusion
  Previous C/S: [ ] No   VBAC   [ ] No
                [ ] Yes attempted: [ ] Yes

Analgesics: before delivery
drug   dose   time
_____   _____   _____
_____   _____   _____
_____   _____   _____

Steroids for lung maturity: Date _____ Time _____ Date _____ Time _____
Antibiotic started: (prior to birth): [ ] <4 hrs [ ] ≥4 hrs [ ] >24 hrs
  Why: [ ] GBS ⊕ Pending / Preterm   # Doses before birth _____
       [ ] Cardiac prophylaxis
       [ ] Fever / Chorioamnionitis
       [ ] Other: _____
Peak maternal temp [ ] <99.5   [ ] 99.5–101.9   [ ] ≥102

Amniotic fluid rupture:
- [ ] Spontaneous
- [ ] Artificial

Color:
- [ ] Clear
- [ ] Light mec. (stain)
- [ ] Medium mec.
- [ ] Thick mec.
- [ ] Cloudy
- [ ] Bloody

Fetal monitoring in labor:
- [ ] Auscultation only
- [ ] External monitor
- [ ] Internal monitor
- [ ] Both
- [ ] IFM site

Labor analgesia:
- [ ] none   [ ] epidural
- [ ] narcotic   [ ] both
- [ ] _____ cervical dil @ epid

DELIVERY SUMMARY

Baby [____] **of a** [____] **gestation**
  Birth Order   Plurality

                    Time   Date
DELIVERY: _____   _____
PLACENTA: _____   _____
C/S start time: _____
Uterine incis. time: _____
C/S finish time: _____

INFANT   (circle)   Boy   Girl

Weight _____ lb _____ gm
Length _____ in _____ cm
Head circ _____ in _____ cm

Delivery Outcomes: **Feeding:**
- [ ] live birth admitted for regular care   [ ] Breast
- [ ] live birth admitted to trans. nursery   [ ] Bottle
- [ ] live birth admitted to NICU
- [ ] neonatal death in delivery room   Gest. Age @
- [ ] fetal death before admission   Delivery
- [ ] fetal death after admission   _____

I.D. BAND #: [_____]
Bands Checked by:
_____ RN   _____ RN

Cord Blood to Lab: [ ] Yes   [ ] No
Cord Gases Sent: [ ] Yes   [ ] No
Specimen to Lab: [ ] Type _____
Culture to Lab: [ ] Type _____

GROUP B STREP SCREEN

Universal Risk Factors
- [ ] Previous GBS infected infant
- [ ] ⊕ urine cx for GBS in current pregnancy

Culture Based
- [ ] negative
- [ ] positive
- [ ] not available

Risk Based (Intrapartum)
- [ ] No risk factors
- [ ] < 37 weeks
- [ ] ROM ≥ 18 hours
- [ ] Maternal temp ≥ 100.4

APGAR SCORE

	1 min	5 min
Heart Rate		
Respiratory Effort		
Muscle Tone		
Reflex Irritability		
Color		
TOTAL		

Cord around neck X [____]

Umbilical Vessel Number: [____]

- [ ] Voided in DR
- [ ] Stool in DR

RESUSCITATION

Respirations: [ ] Spontaneous
              [ ] Delayed _____ min

Check ALL that apply: [ ] Narcan Given
- [ ] suction   Time: _____
- [ ] oxygen   Dose: _____
- [ ] mask vent   Route: _____
- [ ] intubation for   By whom: _____
      resuscitation   **For Meconium Babies:**
- [ ] chest compression   [ ] Not intubated
- [ ] medications   [ ] Intubated – ∅ Below Cords
- [ ] volume   [ ] Intubated – Meconium noted

Note: _____
_____
_____
_____
_____

DELIVERY–MOTHER

Method of Delivery:
- [ ] Vertex, Vaginal
- [ ] Breech, Vaginal
- [ ] Cesarean Section
- [ ] Vacuum
- [ ] Forceps

Episiotomy/Laceration:
- [ ] None
- [ ] Median
- [ ] Mediolateral
- [ ] Laceration
- [ ] Repaired

PLACENTA:
- [ ] Spontaneous
- [ ] Assist
- [ ] Manual
Abnormalities:

Medications at Delivery:
drug   dose   time
Pitocin IV IM _____ units _____ _____
_____   _____   _____
_____   _____   _____

PEDIATRICIAN:

Newborn attended by _____ RN/MD
[ ] Newborn admitted time: _____ am/pm
MR # _____   Pat # _____
Pediatrician notified of delivery: K # _____
  Name _____ MD
  Date _____ Time _____ am/pm
  Via _____ by _____

DELIVERING PHYSICIAN/CNM:	APN/NICU STAFF AT DELIVERY:	ANESTHESIOLOGIST:
ASSIST MD/CNM:	OB/RN AT DELIVERY:	RN SIGNATURE DATE/TIME:

Patient's Data/Addressograph

Figure 8–30 Documentation of delivery.

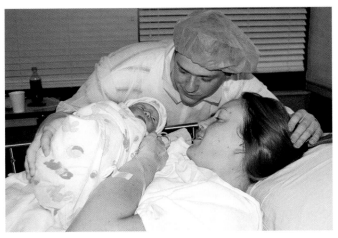

Courtesy of Chapman family

Figure 8–31   Newly delivered baby in the delivery room with family.

THE NEWBORN

Newborn transition and initial care typically occur in the labor and delivery room. Initial assessments can be safely done with the infant skin-to-skin on the mother's abdomen after delivery, if the infant is stable. Apgar scores should be obtained at 1 minute and 5 minutes after birth. If the 5-minute Apgar score is less than 7, additional scores should be assigned every 5 minutes up to 20 minutes. Temperature, heart and respiratory rates, skin color, adequacy of peripheral circulation, type of respiration, level of consciousness, tone, and activity should be monitored and recorded at least every 30 minutes until the newborn's condition has remained stable for at least 2 hours.

The **Apgar score** is a rapid assessment of five physiological signs that indicate the physiological status of the newborn and includes (**Table 8-2**):

■ Heart rate based on auscultation
■ Respiratory rate based on observed movement of chest
■ Muscle tone based on degree of flexion and movement of extremities
■ Reflex irritability based on response to tactile stimulation
■ Color based on observation

Each component is given a score of 0, 1, or 2. An Apgar score of:

0–3 indicates severe distress
4–6 indicates moderate difficulty with transition to extrauterine life
7–10 indicates stable status.

The Apgar score is not used to determine the need for resuscitation, nor is it predictive of long-term neurological outcome of the neonate (American Academy of Pediatrics [AAP] and American College of Obstetrics and Gynecology [ACOG], 2006). Rather it is a rapid, objective, convenient shorthand for reporting the status of the newborn and the response to resuscitation immediately after birth.

At every delivery, there should be one person who is solely responsible for assessment of the neonate response to the birth and who has the capacity to initiate resuscitation of the neonate if needed. Only 1% of neonates need extensive resuscitation at birth (AAP & AHA, 2011). The initial steps of resuscitation are to provide warmth by placing the baby under a radiant heat source, positioning the head in a "sniffing" position to open the airway, clearing the airway if necessary with a bulb syringe or suction catheter, drying the baby, and stimulating breathing. Further discussion of neonatal resuscitation is beyond the scope of this book except to mention optimal management of oxygen during neonatal resuscitation becomes particularly important because of the evidence that either insufficient or excessive oxygenation can be harmful to the newborn infant. More recent guidelines recommend use of a pulse oximeter to provide a continuous assessment of the pulse without interruption of other resuscitation measures. Once positive pressure ventilation or supplementary oxygen administration is begun, assessment should consist of simultaneous evaluation of three vital characteristics: heart rate, respirations, and the state of oxygenation, the latter optimally determined by a pulse oximeter. The most sensitive indicator of a successful response to each step is an increase in heart rate (Kattwinkel, Perlman, Aziz, Colby, Fairchild, Gallagher, Hazinski, Halamek, Kumar, Little, McGowan, Nightengale, Ramirez, Ringer, Simon, Weiner, Wyckoff, & Zaichkin, 2010). The sequence/algorithm for neonatal resuscitation is presented in **Figure 8-32**.

TABLE 8–2   NEONATAL APGAR SCORE

Sign	SCORE		
	0	1	2
RESPIRATORY EFFORT	Absent	Slow, irregular	Good cry
HEART RATE	Absent	Slow, below 100 bpm	Above 100 bpm
MUSCLE TONE	Flaccid	Some flexion of extremities	Active motion
REFLEX ACTIVITY	None	Grimace	Vigorous cry
COLOR	Pale, blue	Body pink, blue extremities	Completely pink

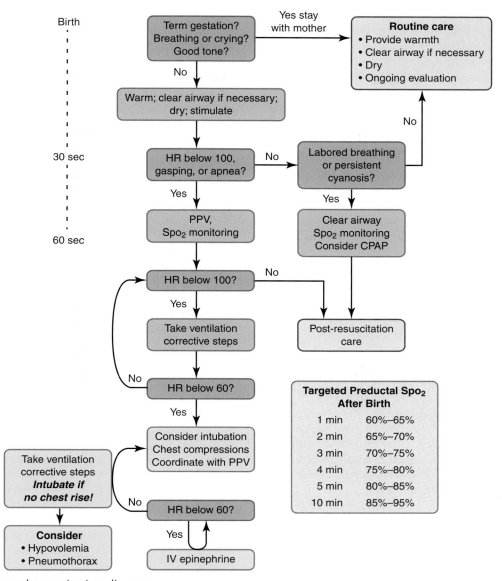

Figure 8–32 Neonatal resuscitation diagram.

Overview of neonatal resuscitation flow diagram:

Newly born infants who do not require resuscitation can generally be identified by a rapid assessment of the following 3 characteristics:

    Term gestation?
    Crying or breathing?
    Good muscle tone?

If the answer to all 3 of these questions is "yes," the baby does not need resuscitation and should not be separated from the mother. The baby should be dried, placed skin-to-skin with the mother, and covered with dry linen to maintain temperature. Observation of breathing, activity, and color should be ongoing.

The initial steps of resuscitation are to provide warmth by placing the baby under a radiant heat source, positioning the head in a "sniffing" position to open the airway, clearing the airway if necessary with a bulb syringe or suction catheter, drying the baby, and stimulating breathing.

If the answer to any of the above assessment questions is "no," the infant should receive one or more of the following 4 categories of action in sequence:

A. **Airway** Initial steps in stabilization (provide warmth, clear airway if necessary, dry, stimulate)

B. **Breathing** Ventilation

C. **Circulation** Chest compressions

D. **Drug** Administration of epinephrine and/or volume expansion

Kattwinkel J, Perlman JM, Aziz K, Colby C, Fairchild K, Gallagher J, Hazinski MF, Halamek LP, Kwmar P, Little G, McGowan JE, Nightengale B, Ramirez MM, Ringer S, Simon WM, Weiner GM, Wyckoff M, Zaichkin J; American Heart Association (2010) Neonatal resuscitation: 2010 American Heart Association Guidelines for Cardiopulmonary Resuscitation and Emergency Cardiovascular Care. *Pediatrics.* 126(5):e 1400-13. Epub 2010 Oct 18.

A comprehensive discussion of the newborn's transition to extrauterine life, physical assessment, and routine procedures are presented in Chapter 15.

One of the first procedures after birth is newborn identification. Perinatal nurses must be meticulous when recording the identification band number, and birth and newborn information, and applying identification bands to mothers and newborns. Institutional policies for newborn identification and newborn safety may vary.

Routinely three medications are administered to newborns:

■ Erythromycin ointment is administered to the eyes as prophylaxis to prevent gonococcal and *Chlamydia* infections.
■ Vitamin K is administered via intramuscular injection to prevent hemorrhagic disease caused by vitamin K deficiency.
■ Hepatitis B virus vaccine is recommended for all newborns (American Academy of Pediatrics Committee on Infected Diseases, 2009).

Newborn care is discussed in Chapter 15.

MANAGEMENT OF PAIN AND DISCOMFORT DURING LABOR AND DELIVERY

Pain in childbirth is a universal experience and considered a normal occurrence. Most pain in labor results from normal physiologic events (Burke 2014). Pain associated with labor has been described as one of the most intensely painful experiences possible. Labor pain differs from other conditions in which pain is experienced in several ways.

Understanding the cause and characteristics of pain in the labor and delivery setting helps the nurse develop a plan of care for the woman in each stage of the labor process. Labor pain is acute pain and presents in many ways. During the first stages of labor pain is caused by uterine muscle hypoxia, accumulation of lactic acid in the muscles, lower uterine and cervical stretching, traction on pelvic organs, and pressure on the bony pelvis. During the second stage, pain is due to pelvic muscle distention and pressure on the perineum, cervix, urethra, and rectum. Back pain during labor is thought to be caused by pressure of the fetal occiput on the maternal spine and pelvis.

Factors influencing pain response include both the physical and psychosocial:

■ Rate of cervical dilation and strength of contractions
■ Size and position of fetus impacts length of labor.
■ Sleep deprivation and exhaustion from long labor increases pain perception.
■ Culture of the woman influences her response to labor and pain. Pain behaviors are culturally bound (see Cultural Awareness: Culture and Birth Traditions).
■ The woman's labor support system can affect her anxiety level and perception of pain.

■ Previous birth experiences may increase or decrease anxiety.
■ Childbirth preparation may decrease anxiety and decrease pain.
■ The woman's expectations influence her satisfaction with her birth experience (Evidence-Based Practice: Maternal Satisfaction).

Pain in childbirth is transmitted from the periphery of the body along nerve pathways to the brain. This pain is attributable to:

■ Uterine contractions resulting in uterine pain from a decrease in blood supply to the uterus
■ Increased pressure and stretching of the pelvic structures resulting in the pulling and expansion of ligaments, muscle, and peritoneum
■ Cervical dilation and stretching resulting in the stimulation of the nerve ganglia.

Evidence-Based Practice: Maternal Satisfaction

Florence, D., & Palmer, D. (2003). Therapeutic choices for the discomforts of labor. *Journal of Perinatal & Neonatal Nursing, 17*(4), 238.

Hodnett, E. (2002). Pain and women's satisfaction with the experience of childbirth: A systematic review. *American Journal of Obstetrics and Gynecology, 186*(5), S160–S172.

Research has shown that maternal satisfaction post-birth is influenced by the degree of pain endured but is far more influenced by whether the actual birth event met the woman's personal expectations (Hodnett, 2002). Satisfaction with the labor experience is based on variables that include cultural influence, previous experiences, communication from family and providers, and prenatal education (Florence & Palmer, 2003).

Gate Control Theory of Pain

The use of the gate control theory of pain can be applied to the process of labor and birth (**Fig. 8-33**). This theory states that sensation of pain is transmitted from the periphery of the body along ascending nerve pathways to the brain. Because of the limited number of sensations that can travel along these pathways at any given time, an alternate activity can replace travel of the pain sensation, thus closing the gate control at the spinal cord and reducing pain impulses traveling to the brain. Based on this premise, the application of pressure to certain areas of the body, the cutaneous stimulation such as effleurage (gentle stroking of the abdomen), or the use of heat or cold can have a direct effect on closing the gate, which then limits the transmission of pain. A similar gating mechanism can be found in the descending nerve fibers from the hypothalamus and cerebral cortex. Strategies such as breathing, focusing, and visual and auditory stimulation may affect whether pain impulses reach the level of conscious awareness.

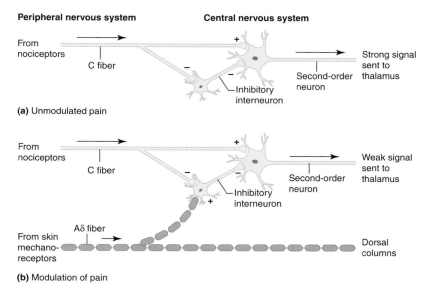

Figure 8–33   Gate control theory of pain modulation. (a). Normally C-fibers carrying slow pain signals block inhibitory interneurons and transmit their signals across the synapse unimpeded. (b). A-delta fibers carrying pleasurable signals from touch excite inhibitory interneurons, which then block the transmission of slow pain signals (+ equals transmission, − equals no transmission).

Non-pharmacological Management of Labor Discomfort

Non-pharmacological management of labor discomfort includes preparation by the woman for childbirth, cutaneous stimulation, thermal stimulation, mental stimulation, and the presence of a support person(s). It is essential that nurses have a repertoire of strategies to manage discomfort and pain during labor (see Critical Component: Non-pharmacologic Strategies for Nurses and Comfort Measures in Labor). A willingness to try a variety of strategies, adapt those that are effective, and modify and abandon those that are not effective are important aspects of care. Usually no one strategy works for very long in labor, making flexibility and adaptability key qualities for labor nurses.

- Childbirth preparation methods: Education and explanation of birth process is offered through classes to the woman and her support person before the delivery time. In these classes, the woman and her partner learn about pregnancy, the labor process, the painful aspects of labor, and methods to help relieve the discomforts of pregnancy and childbirth.
- Relaxation and breathing techniques: Varied breathing patterns that promote relaxation and avoidance of pushing before complete cervical dilation. Most childbirth preparation methods teach some form of relaxation and breathing techniques (**Fig. 8-34**). Most women are taught to take a deep breath at the beginning of the contraction to signal the onset of the contraction and then to breathe slowly during the contraction. As labor pain increases, the woman may need to breathe in a more rapid and shallow manner. On occasion, a woman will experience hyperventilation from this type of breathing. Symptoms are related to respiratory alkalosis and include tingling of the fingers or circumoral numbness, light-headedness, or dizziness. This undesirable side effect can be eliminated by having the woman breathe into a bag or cupped hands. This

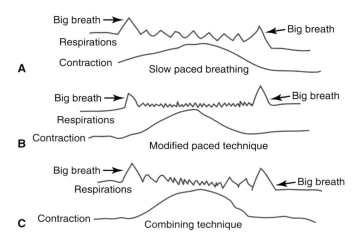

Figure 8-34   Space breathing technique graph. A. Slow-paced breathing is with big breath at beginning and end of contraction; the typical rate is fewer than 10 breaths per minute B. Modified paced breathing is with a big breath at the beginning and end of the contraction and rapid shallow breaths that are comfortable for the woman at a rate of about twice normal respirations. C. Combining technique. Big breath at the beginning and end of the contraction with more rapid and shallow breathing at the peak of the contraction.

causes her to rebreathe carbon dioxide and reverses the respiratory alkalosis. Discuss with the woman and her support team how they plan on managing labor. This will stimulate conversation, facilitate a plan of care to assist them in pain management, and give an opportunity to teach and or support them as needed.

- **Effleurage** is cutaneous stimulation done by lightly stroking the abdomen in rhythm with breathing during contractions. Another form of cutaneous stimulation is back massage and/or counter pressure to the sacral area by another.

Counter pressure is exerted to the sacral area with the heel of the hand or fist to relieve the sensation of intense pain in the back caused by internal pressure of the fetal head. This increased internal pressure by the fetal head is often associated with the posterior position of the fetus during labor. As labor advances, women may not want to be touched.

■ Thermal stimulation: Application of warmth or cold, such as use of warm showers or ice packs. The use of hydrotherapy via whirlpools, warm baths, or showers is very effective and promotes relaxation and comfort. This may reduce the woman's anxiety and promote well-being, causing a reduction in catecholamine production, which interferes with uterine contractility. Application of cold may release musculoskeletal pain, and the numbing effect of cold may decrease the sensation of pain.

■ Mental stimulation: Focal points, imagery, and music help the woman to concentrate on something outside her body. This helps her to focus away from the pain. With imagery, the woman is encouraged to bring into her mind a picture of a relaxing scene.

■ Support person(s): Significant other(s) and/or a doula provide emotional support and physical comfort and aids in a beneficial form of care. Research has shown that support early in labor significantly relieves pain, improves outcomes, decreases interventions and complication rates, and thus enhances overall maternal satisfaction (Simkin & O'Hara, 2002). A doula can also be used as a support for women during pregnancy through postpartum. Doulas are unique in that they are trained to provide support, promote comfort, and instill confidence to the laboring woman. Doulas are trained through many organizations and are paid by the family that hires them. Doulas do not perform clinical tasks and do not have direct communication responsibility to care providers (Burke, 2014). Some studies have shown that women who used a doula had shorter labors, less use of analgesia, fewer instrument deliveries, and decreased C-sections (Hodnett et al., 2003).

Complementary Therapy

Many therapies have been used to promote relaxation and decrease the perception of pain while providing a complement to decrease the use of pharmacological interventions (Zwelling, Johnson, & Allen, 2006).

■ Aromatherapy: Use of essential oils: can be inhaled (such as by vaporizers) or used in a carrier oil or lotion to be used with massage to promote relaxation and decrease the perception of pain. A few drops placed in a bath can be an adjunct to hydrotherapy. Lavender and jasmine oils promote relaxation and decrease pain perception, while peppermint may decrease feelings of nausea.

■ Massage: Multiple studies have shown massage to decrease pain and promote relaxation, which in turn promotes labor progress. A quiet, soothing voice along with encouraging the woman to image a safe place assists in relaxation. This used in conjunction with aromatherapy has proven to enhance relaxation in laboring women, allowing for the women to have better control of their labor.

■ Birthing ball: This ball (65-cm) came out of physical therapy programs but has been used successfully in the labor suite. It facilitates an upright position, opens the pelvis, and allows the woman to roll or bounce as she deems necessary to manage her contractions and pain.

■ Hydrotherapy: The use of water has been used in many areas of medicine for many years to promote relaxation and pain control. The use of a shower or large tub is ideal for releasing endorphins, decreasing muscle tension, and promoting circulation. The use of hydrotherapy with ruptured membranes (ROM) has shown no increase of infections. The many benefits of hydrotherapy include: less medication needs, less anesthesia, faster labors, facilitation of fetal positions (which decreases the number of instrumental deliveries), fewer episiotomies, decrease in blood pressure and edema, promotes diuresis and increased satisfaction in the birthing experience.

■ Music therapy: Music calms the spirit, and decreases stress and distress by diverting attention from the pain receptors and promoting relaxation.

All of these complementary therapies are being used in some form today either alone or in conjunction with each other, in all birthing venues, from home births to stand-alone birth centers to hospital suites. They can assist the woman and her support team by providing comfort, empowering the birth experience as the woman sees it, and promoting a safe non-invasive birth.

Most classes teach a variety of strategies to manage labor pain. Specific methods include:

■ Dick-Read method: Advocates birth without fear by education and environmental control and relaxation.

■ Lamaze: Promotes psychoprophylaxis with conditioning and breathing.

■ Bradley: This is husband-coached childbirth and support by working with and managing the pain rather than being distracted from it.

Pharmacological Management of Labor Discomfort

Pharmacological management of discomfort and pain in labor requires the nurse to assess the woman's preferences for pain management throughout labor. The decision to use pain medication in labor should be made by the woman in collaboration with her physician or midwife. The unique circumstances of every labor influence the experience and perception of pain (Burke, 2014).

■ Assessment of pain is an essential part of nursing care.
  ■ *Assessment of labor pain should include intensity, location, pattern, and degree of distress for the woman, as well as using pain scale with numerical self report using a scale of 1–10.*
■ The use of medication in the relief of pain during labor falls into two major categories:
  ■ *Analgesia (**Table 8-3**)*
  ■ *Anesthesia (**Table 8-4**)*
■ Basic principles when using analgesia include:
  ■ *Labor should be established.*

TABLE 8–3 ANALGESIC MEDICATIONS IN LABOR

MEDICATION	CLASS	SIDE EFFECTS	NURSE INTERVENTION
Meperidine (Demerol) 50–100 mg IM 25–50 mg IV Morphine 5 mg–10 mg IM 2 mg–5 mg IV	Opioid	CNS depression Neonatal respiratory depression	Avoid use when close to delivery time (about 1 hour).
Butorphanol (Stadol) 2 mg–4 mg IM 0.5 mg–2 mg IV Nalbuphine (Nubain) 10 mg IM or IV	Opioid agonist–antagonist	No respiratory depression in woman or neonate	Check maternal history for drug abuse. Do not give to drug dependent woman due to possible precipitation of sudden withdrawal response in woman and baby. Monitor effective response.
Sublimaze (Fentanyl) 50–100 mg IM 25–50 mg IM May be used in conjunction with regional anesthesia	Short acting opioid antagonist Crosses the placenta rapidly Synthetic opioid	FHR changes Hypotension Maternal/fetal/neonatal CNS depression Respiratory depression	Monitor for side effects such as sedation, nausea, vomiting, itching. Monitor respiratory rate and effort.

Faucher & Brucker (2000); Florence & Palmer (2003); Spratto & Woods (2006); Burke (2013).

TABLE 8–4 ANESTHESIA IN LABOR AND DELIVERY

TYPE OF ANESTHESIA	TIME GIVEN AND EFFECTS	ADVERSE EFFECTS	NURSING IMPLICATIONS
LOCAL: Anesthetic injected into perineum at episiotomy site	Second stage of labor, immediately before delivery Anesthetizes local tissue for episiotomy and repair	Risk of a hematoma Risk of infection	Monitor for: Return of sensation to area Increased swelling at site of injection
REGIONAL: **Pudendal Block:** Anesthetic injected in the pudendal nerve (close to the ischial spines) via needle guide known as "trumpet"	Second stage of labor, prior to time of delivery Anesthetizes vulva, lower vagina and part of perineum for episiotomy and use of low forceps	Risk of local anesthetic toxicity Risk of a hematoma Risk of infection	Monitor for: Return of sensation to area Increased swelling Signs and symptoms of infection Urinary retention
Epidural Block: Anesthetic injected in the epidural space: Located outside the dura mater between the dura and spinal canal via an epidural catheter	First stage and/or second stage of labor Can be used for both vaginal and cesarean births Has the potential of 100% blockage of pain Can be used with opioids such as Sublimaze to allow walking during first stage of labor and effective	Most common complication is hypotension Other side effects include nausea, vomiting, pruritis, respiratory depression, alterations in FHR	**Pre-anesthesia care** Obtain consent. Check lab values—especially for bleeding or clotting abnormalities, platelet count. IV fluid bolus with normal saline or lactated Ringer's. Ensure emergency equipment is available. Do time-out procedure verification

Continued

TABLE 8–4 ANESTHESIA IN LABOR AND DELIVERY—cont'd			
TYPE OF ANESTHESIA	**TIME GIVEN AND EFFECTS**	**ADVERSE EFFECTS**	**NURSING IMPLICATIONS**
	pushing in second stage of labor		**Post-procedure care.** Monitor maternal vital signs and FHR every 5 min initially and after every re-bolus then every 15 minutes and manage hypotension or alterations in FHR. Urinary retention is common and catheterization may be needed. Assess pain and level of sensation and motor loss. Position woman as needed (on side to prevent inferior vena cava syndrome) Assess for itching, nausea and vomiting, and headache and administer meds PRN. When catheter discontinued, note intact tip when removed.
Spinal Block: Anesthetic injected in the subarachnoid space	Second stage of labor or in use for cesarean section. Rapid acting with 100% blockage of sensation and motor functioning. Can last up to 3 hours.	Adverse effects are similar to the epidural with the addition of a spinal headache. A blood patch often provides relief.	Interventions are same as for epidural. Monitor site for leakage of spinal fluid or formation of hematoma. Observe for headache.
GENERAL ANESTHESIA: Use of IV injection and/or inhalation of anesthetic agents that render the woman unconscious.	Used mainly in emergency cesarean birth	Risk for fetal depression Risk for uterine relaxation Risk for maternal vomiting and aspiration	Obtain consent. Ensure woman is NPO. IV with large-bore needle. Place indwelling urinary catheter. Administer medications to decrease gastric acidity as ordered such as antacids: Bicitra or Proton pump inhibitor: Protonix. Place wedge to hip to prevent vena cava syndrome. Assist with supportive care of newborn.

AWHONN (2001a and b); Pitter & Preston (2001); Spratto & Woods (2006).

■ *Medication should provide relief to the woman with minimal risk to the baby.*
  ■ Neonatal depression may occur if medication is given within an hour before delivery.
  ■ Women with a history of drug abuse may have a lessened effect from pain medication and require higher doses.
■ Basic principles for anesthesia include:
  ■ *Local anesthesia is used at the time of delivery for episiotomy and repair.*
  ■ *Regional anesthesia is used during labor and at delivery.*
    ■ Regional anesthesia includes the pudendal block, epidural block, and spinal block.

■ *Regional or general anesthesia is used for cesarean deliveries. (Chapter 11 addresses care of cesarean birth women.)*

Parenteral Opioids

The use of opioids in labor is common. Advantages include availability, ease of administration, and cost. Depending on the dose, route of administration, and stage of labor parenteral analgesia does not illuminate pain but causes a blunting effect, leading to a decrease in sensation of pain and inducing somnolence (Burke 2013). Opioids cross the placenta and can cause neonatal respiratory depression.

Nitrous Oxide Analgesia

A new interest in self-administered nitrous oxide for labor analgesia has emerged in recent years in the United States. It has been used widely in Europe for decades, with favorable results (Stewart & Collins, 2012). A recent published review concludes nitrous oxide analgesia is safe for mothers, neonates, and those who care for women during childbirth (Rooks, 2011). In the context of obstetric analgesia, "nitrous oxide" usually refers to a half-and-half combination of oxygen and nitrous oxide gas, called by the trade name "Nitronox." It is self-administered by the laboring woman using a mouth tube or face mask, when she determines that she needs it, about a minute before she anticipates the onset of a strong contraction until the pain eases. Its use can be started and stopped at any point during labor, according to the needs and preferences of the woman. It takes effect in about 50 seconds after the first breath and the effect is transient—essentially gone when no longer needed. It is simple to administer and does not interfere with the release and function of endogenous oxytocin, and has no adverse effects on the normal physiology and progress of labor. This analgesia may be of help for women who want to have an unmedicated birth but may need help at some point during labor and want whatever method they use to be under their control (Rooks, 2007).

Epidural Anesthesia

Epidural anesthesia is one of the most common forms of pain relief during labor used in the United States. In a recent report 61 % of women who had a singleton birth in a vaginal delivery in 2008 received epidural or spinal anesthesia (Osterman & Martin, 2011). Epidural anesthesia involves the placement of a very small catheter and injection of local anesthesia and or analgesia between the fourth and fifth vertebrae into the epidural space. A **combined spinal epidural analgesia (CSE)** involves the injection of local anesthetic and/or analgesic into the subarachnoid space. Some patients may be able to ambulate with this type of anesthesia; hence it is referred to as a "walking epidural." Because of the widespread use of epidural anesthesia in labor, AWHONN has generated evidence-based practice guidelines for care of pregnant women receiving regional anesthesia/analgesia (AWHONN, 2011).

- Three of every five women undergoing labor in the United States use this method each year and the rate of epidural use in labor appears to be increaeseing (Osterman & Martin, 2011). Some research shows that epidural analgesia is associated with a lower rate of spontaneous vaginal delivery, a higher rate of instrumental (e.g., vacuum suction and/or forceps) vaginal delivery, longer labors, and increased incidence of intrapartum fevers and/or suspected sepsis (Buckley, 2005; Osterman & Martin, 2011). A review of the evidence has concluded that research about the effects of regional anesthesia/analgesia on the progress of labor may not be significant (AWHONN, 2011).
- Elevations in maternal temperature associated with regional anesthesia have been reported, but it is unclear whether they are a response to infection versus a response

to sympathetic blockade. They may be associated with decreased maternal hyperventilation, reduced perspiration, and altered thermoregulatory transmission.

- A wide variety of medications and dosing regimens are used for regional analgesia/anesthesia. Nurses are responsible for knowing general information about classification of these medications, their actions, potential side effects, and complications (AWHONN, 2011).

CRITICAL COMPONENT

Epidural Anesthesia

- Nurses monitor, but not manage, the care of women receiving epidural anesthesia.
- Catheter dosing of intermittent and continuous infusion of regional analgesia/anesthesia is outside the scope of registered nursing.
- Only qualified, licensed anesthesia providers should perform insertion, injection, and/or manage rate changes of a continuous infusion (AWHONN, 2011).
- Responsibilities of nurses caring for women receiving regional anesthesia/analgesia are assessment, monitoring, and interventions to minimize complications.
- After the stabilization of the patient after regional anesthesia, the nurse monitors the woman's vital signs, mobility, level of consciousness, and perception of pain, as well as fetal status.

Nursing Actions Before the Epidural

Nursing actions are based on AWHONN guidelines (2011):

- Assess woman's level of pain.
- Determine the woman's and her family's knowledge and concerns about epidural anesthesia.
- Provide information about options for anesthesia/analgesia.
- Notify obstetrical and anesthesia care providers when the woman requests epidural anesthesia.
- Assess and document baseline blood pressure, pulse, respiratory rate, and temperature.
- Assess FHR to confirm a normal FHR pattern; if indeterminate or abnormal, report to the physician or midwife.
- Encourage the patient to void before initiation of epidural anesthesia.
- If ordered, administer an IV bolus as ordered to decrease incidence of hypotension.
- Obtain platelet count, blood type, and screen.
- Conduct a pre-procedure verification process per facility policy.
- Conduct time out.

Nursing Actions During Administration of Epidural Anesthesia

- Assist the anesthesia provider, anesthesiologist, or nurse anesthetist (CRNA) with placement of the epidural, including placement of patient in the lateral position with head flexed toward chest, or sitting position with head flexed on chest, elbows on knees and feet supported on stool (AWHONN, 2011) (**Fig. 8-35** and **Fig. 8-36**).

Nursing Actions After Epidural Administration (AWHONN, 2011)

■ Monitor vital signs according to agency protocols generally every 5–15 minutes. Assess for hypotension and respiratory distress.
  ■ *Up to 40% of women may experience hypotension. Difficulty breathing may indicate the catheter is in the subarachnoid space.*
  ■ *Hypotension is defined as systolic blood pressure less than 100 mm Hg or a 20% decrease in blood pressure from pre-anesthesia levels. Notify the anesthesia provider if the patient becomes hypotensive.*
  ■ *Assess FHR every 5–15 minutes*
■ Facilitate lateral or upright positioning with uterine displacement.
  ■ *Helps to avoid supine hypotension.*
■ Assess for effectiveness of the epidural and the woman's pain levels and description of pain (see Critical Component: Epidural Anesthesia).
  ■ *Notify the anesthesia provider of inadequate pain relief.*
■ Assess for sedation if opioid medication is administered with local anesthesia.
  ■ *Drowsiness can occur in up to 50% of women who receive combination local/opioid analgesia.*
■ Assess the level of motor blockade according to agency criteria.
  ■ *If the patient receives an epidural that allows ambulation: Before ambulation, the nurse assesses somatosensory status, motor strength, and ability to ambulate.*
■ Monitor for pruritis.
  ■ *Up to 90% of women who receive opioids in epidurals have itching. Medicate as indicated.*
■ Monitor for nausea and vomiting.
  ■ *Up to 50% of women experience this and may be treated with antiemetics.*
■ Assess for post-procedural headache.
  ■ *Occurs in up to 3% of women related to leakage of spinal fluid with inadvertent puncture. If this occurs, it should be reported to the anesthesia provider.*
■ Assess the woman for urinary retention.
  ■ *This occurs in some women who receive epidural anesthesia because of decreased motor function. Catheterization is typically necessary.*
■ Assess the partner's or support person's response to epidural pain relief and answer questions (see Evidence-Based Practice: Expectant Fathers and Labor Epidurals).
■ Monitor uterine contractions as uterine activity may slow for up to 60 minutes after epidural placement. This may be a side effect of the neuroaxial block and usually no treatment is needed. Some providers will initiate oxytocin augmentation to stimulate contractions.
■ Monitor for signs and symptoms of intravascular injection including: This normally occurs during placement and is monitored by a test dose being given by the anesthesiologist.

■ *Maternal tachycardia or bradycardia*
■ *Hypertension*
■ *Dizziness*
■ *Tinnitus (ringing in the ears)*
■ *Metallic taste in the mouth*
■ *Loss of consciousness*

If intravascular injection occurs, the anesthesia care provider should be immediately notified and care includes administering oxygen, fluids, and medication as ordered. Initiating CPR may be necessary.

■ A higher level of anesthesia is necessary for a cesarean birth than for labor (**Fig. 8-37**).

Evidence-Based Practice: Expectant Fathers and Labor Epidurals

Chapman, L. (2000). Expectant fathers and labor epidurals. *Maternal Child Nursing, 25,* 133–138.

A qualitative research study using grounded theory methodology was conducted with the aim to describe and explain the expectant father's experience during labor and birth when epidural anesthesia/analgesia is used for labor pain management. Based on the research data a theory, "cruising through labor," was developed. The epidural labor process is different from nonepidural labor and is comprised of six phases:

■ Holding out
■ Surrendering
■ Waiting
■ Getting
■ Cruising
■ Pushing

Expectant fathers explained that before the epidural they felt like they were "losing" their partner as the increasing pain caused the woman to focus inward and away from interaction with those in the labor room. The expectant fathers explained that they felt a loss of connection with their partner and a loss of control. They felt that the pain of labor overtook their partner and was all-encompassing. The men further explained that they felt helpless, frustrated, and a sense of losing her to the pain of labor.

The men explained that the labor nurse played a significant role in supporting them during this time. The major supportive behaviors by the nurse were:

■ Remaining in the labor room
■ Explaining what was happening to their partner
■ Including the men in the care of their partner

Expectant fathers reported that once the epidural was administered and the woman experienced relief from labor pain, they saw a dramatic change in their partner's behavior. They often stated, "She's back," that she was comfortable and able to interact with those around her. One man stated, "She wasn't in pain. Her color was back. Her pain was gone. She wasn't throwing up. She was back. She was comfortable."

Men further explained that the effects of the epidural in decreasing the degree of labor pain allowed the men to shift their focus from labor pain management to enjoying the labor and birthing experience (**Fig. 8-38** and **Fig. 8-39**).

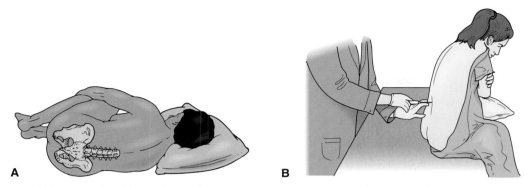

Figure 8–35 Lateral (A) and sitting (B) positions for placement of spinal and epidural block.

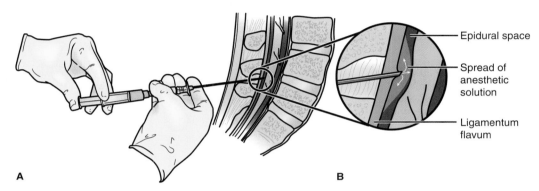

Epidural space

Spread of anesthetic solution

Ligamentum flavum

A

B

Figure 8–36 Technique for epidural block.

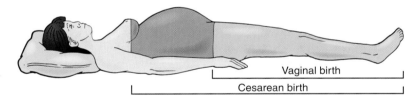

Vaginal birth

Cesarean birth

Figure 8–37 Levels of anesthesia necessary for vaginal and cesarean births.

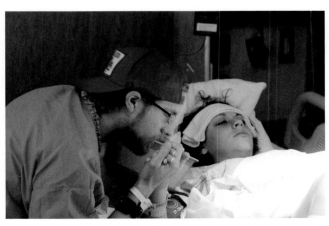

Figure 8–38 Partners experiencing labor together.

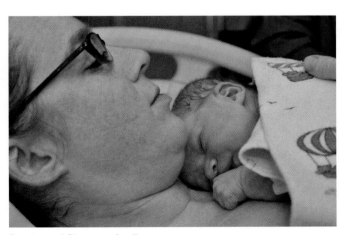

Courtesy of Chapman family

Figure 8-39 A new family.

Clinical Pathway for Intrapartal Maternal and Fetal Assessment

	Active Labor	Second Stage Labor (Active Pushing)	Third Stage of Labor (Delivery of Placenta)	Fourth Stage of Labor (Immediate Postpartum)
Maternal Vital Signs	P, R, BP every hour; temp every 2 hours unless ROM then every hour	P, R, BP every hour; temp every 2 hours unless ROM then every hour	P, R, BP every 15 minutes	P, R, BP every 15 minutes
FHR	Every 15–30 minutes*	Assessment every 5–15 minutes*	NA	Initiate neonatal transition care
Uterine Activity	Every 15–30 minutes**	Assessment every 5–15 minutes**	NA	NA Fundal and lochia checks every 15 minutes
Pain Status	Every 30 minutes and PRN	Assessment every 15 minutes	Assessment every 15 minutes	Assessment every 15 minutes
Response to Labor	Every 30 minutes and PRN	Assessment every 15 minutes	Assessment every 15 minutes	
Comfort Measures	Every 30 minutes and PRN	Assessment every 15 minutes and PRN	Assessment every 15 minutes and PRN	Assessment every 15 minutes and PRN
Maternal Position	Every 30 minutes and PRN	Change every 30 minutes and PRN		
Vaginal Exam/Fetal Station/Progress in Descent	As needed	As needed, at least every 30 minutes	NA	NA
Intake and Output	Every 8 hours	Assess bladder distension		Assess bladder distension

P, pulse; R, respirations, BP, blood pressure; FHR, fetal heart rate.
*FHR characteristics include baseline rate, variability, and presence or absence of accelerations and periodic or episodic decelerations.
**Uterine activity included contraction frequency, duration, intensity, and uterine resting tone.
Source: AWHONN (2008).

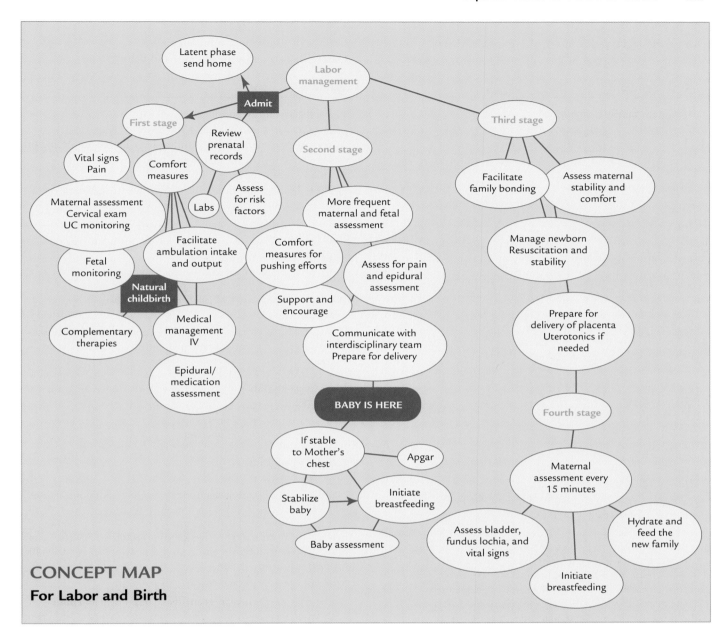

CONCEPT MAP
For Labor and Birth

First Stage of Labor
Goal: Safe delivery for mother and baby
Outcome: Safe delivery for mother and baby

Nursing Actions

1. Perform admission procedures and orient patient to setting.
2. Review prenatal records.
3. Assess FHR and uterine activity.
4. Assess maternal vital signs and pain.
5. Assist with ambutation and maternal position changes.
6. Provide comfort measures.
7. Discuss pain management options.
8. Administer pain meds PRN.
9. Monitor I&O and provide oral and/or IV hydration as indicated.
10. Provide ongoing assessment of labor progress.
11. Request an immediate bedside evaluation by a physician or CNM.

Second Stage of Labor
Goal: Safe delivery for mother and baby
Outcome: Safe delivery for mother and baby

Nursing Actions

1. Perform more frequent maternal and fetal assessment.
2. Review prenatal records.
3. Assess FHR and uterine activity.
4. Assess maternal vital signs and pain.
5. Encourage open glottis pushing efforts.
6. Provide comfort measures for pusing efforts.
7. Provide ongoing assessment and encouragement of labor progress.
8. Communicate with interdisciplinary team.
9. Prepare for delivery.

Third Stage of Labor
Goal: Safe delivery of placenta and transition for baby
Outcome: Safe delivery of placenta and transition for baby

Nursing Actions

1. Facilitate family bonding.
2. Assess maternal vital signs and pain.
3. Assess maternal stability.
4. Prepare for delivery of placenta and need for uterotonics.

Fourth Stage of Labor
Goal: Safe recovery of mom and baby
Outcome: Safe recovery of mom and baby

Nursing Actions

1. Facilitate family bonding.
2. Assess maternal vital signs and pain.
3. Assess maternal stability, fundus, lachia, bladder, perineum.
4. Provide comfort measures and pain meds.
5. Initiate breastfeeding.
6. Provide food and fluids for patient when stable.

TYING IT ALL TOGETHER

As the nurse, you admit Margarite Sanchez to the labor and delivery unit. She arrived in the triage unit at midnight in early labor. She presented with uterine contractions that were 5 minutes apart for 3 hours. Patient is a 28-year-old G3 P1 Hispanic woman. She is 39 weeks' gestation. José, her husband, has accompanied her to the unit. Two years ago, she had a normal spontaneous vaginal delivery NSVD after an 18-hour labor for a baby girl, Sonya, that was 7 lbs., 3 oz.

Margarite's cervix is now 4 cm/80%/0 station and fetal position is left occiput anterior (LOA).

Prenatal Labs
Blood type O+
RPR NR
GBS negative
Hgb
Hct
Hepatitis negative
Vital signs: Blood pressure 110/60; pulse 84 bpm; respiratory rate 18; temperature 98.6°F (37°C).

Began prenatal care at 10 weeks of gestation and received regular prenatal care. She gained 22 pounds during pregnancy, and her current weight is 164 lbs. She is 5 feet, 4 inches tall. She has no prior medical complications and has experienced a normal pregnancy. Her first pregnancy ended in miscarriage at 8 weeks' gestation. She has no allergies to food or medication. She does not have a birth plan and states, "I just hope for a normal delivery and a healthy baby."

Detail the aspects of your initial assessment.

EFM reveals a FHR pattern that is normal, category I, with a FHR baseline of 140s moderate variability with accelerations to 160s (20 seconds. She is uncomfortable with contractions and rates her pain at 5. She requests ambulation, as she feels more comfortable with walking.

At 0120 she has SROM for a large amount of clear amniotic fluid. FHR is baseline 130s with moderate variability, and accelerations and contractions are every 3 minutes and feel moderate to palpation. Her SVE reveals her cervix is 5 cm/90/0 station. She is very uncomfortable with contractions but does not want pain medication at this time. José appears anxious and at a loss for how to help his wife.

What are your immediate priorities in nursing care for Margarite and José Sanchez?
Discuss the rationale for the priorities.

What teaching would you include?
State nursing diagnosis, expected outcome, and interventions related to managing her labor pain.
What are appropriate interventions to manage her labor pain nonpharmacologically?

At 2 A.M. Margarite is increasingly uncomfortable with contractions and cries out that she can no longer take the pain. Her cervical exam is 6/100/0. She requests pain medication and is given a dose of Nubain at 0215 for pain relief in active labor. José asks how much longer the labor will be and when the baby will be born.

Detail the aspects of your ongoing assessment.
What are your current priorities in nursing care for Margarite Sanchez?
Discuss the rationale for the priorities.
Further teaching would include the following:
State nursing diagnosis, expected outcome, and interventions related to this problem.

At 0410 Margarite is very uncomfortable with contractions and cries out that she feels more pressure. She vomits a small amount of bile-colored fluid, and is perspiring and breathing hard with contractions. Her cervical exam is 8/90/0. She requests pain medication and is given a dose of Nubian at 0440 for pain relief in transition.

What are appropriate interventions?

At 0630 Margarite reports an urge to bear down and push with contractions, is very uncomfortable with contractions, and cries out that she feels more pressure. Her sterile vaginal exam (SVE) reveals she is 10 cm/100% and +1 station. She has a strong urge to push with contractions that are every 2 minutes and strong to palpation. The fetal heart rate is 130 with moderate variability, and the FHR drops to 90 bpm for 40 seconds with pushing efforts.

What are your immediate priorities in nursing care for Margarite Sanchez?
Discuss the rationale for the priorities.
What does the FHR indicate?
Teaching would include the following:
State nursing diagnosis, expected outcome, and interventions related to managing her labor pain.

Margarite continues to bear down, using open glottis pushing with contractions, and the fetal head is descending with contractions. The fetal heart rate is 130 with moderate variability and the FHR drops to 90 bpm for 40 seconds with pushing efforts. At 7:30 A.M. Margarite is increasingly unfocused with contractions and states, "I can't push...call my doctor to get the

TYING IT ALL TOGETHER—cont'd

baby out!" José is at her side, holding her hand and encouraging her pushing efforts.

What are your immediate priorities in nursing care for Margarite Sanchez? Discuss the rationale for the priorities.

At 0815 Margarite continues to bear down with contractions and the fetal head is descending with contractions. The FHR is 130 with moderate variability and the FHR drops to 90 bpm for 40 seconds with pushing efforts. Margarite is focused with contractions. The fetal head is starting to crown with pushing efforts.

What are your immediate priorities in nursing care for Margarite Sanchez?
Discuss the rationale for the priorities.

Her doctor comes into the labor and delivery room and she delivers a baby boy at 0839, with a second-degree perineal laceration. Her son weighs 3,800 g and 1- and 5-minute Apgar scores are 8 and 9.

Both Margarite and José begin to cry when their son is born, and José holds his son and hugs his wife. The placenta is delivered apparently intact at 0845. Both Margarite and her son are stable, and you initiate immediate postpartum and transition care for the mother and baby.

■ ■ ■ Review Questions ■ ■ ■

1. The primary reason for administering Nubain to a woman in active labor is to:
   A. Slow uterine contractions
   B. Relieve nausea and vomiting
   C. Relieve pain
   D. Promote dilation

2. Labor pain in active labor is primarily caused by:
   A. Cervical dilation
   B. Uterine contractions
   C. Fetal descent
   D. Perineal tearing

3. Passenger, as one of the 4 Ps of labor, refers to:
   A. The position of the mother
   B. The passage of the vagina
   C. The fetal descent in the pelvis
   D. The fetus

4. Nurses manage the care of patients receiving regional anesthesia.
   A. True
   B. False

5. Supportive activities in labor are:
   A. Interventions ordered by the care provider
   B. Techniques used to help women in labor
   C. Derived from adhering to the birth plan
   D. Pharmacological interventions

6. An involuntary urge to push is most likely a sign of:
   A. Malposition of the fetus
   B. Transition to active labor
   C. Low fetal station
   D. Imminent delivery

7. False labor is characterized by:
   A. Irregular uterine contractions and cervical change
   B. Back pain that radiates to the lower abdomen
   C. The presence of bloody show
   D. Irregular contractions with no cervical change

8. Women who have a support person with them in labor are more likely to:
   A. Have epidural anesthesia
   B. Have a precipitous labor
   C. Experience fewer birth complications
   D. Experience more interventions

9. A sterile vaginal exam reveals that the woman is 5 cm/80% effaced/0 station. Based on this exam the woman is:
   A. In the transition phase
   B. In the latent phase
   C. In the active phase

10. A common side effect of epidural anesthesia in labor includes:
    A. Maternal hypotension
    B. Maternal hypertension
    C. Variable decelerations in the FHR
    D. Hypertonic labor pattern

References

Akinsipe, D., Villaloos, L., & Ridley, R., (2012). A Systematic Review of Implementing an Elective Labor Induction Policy. *Journal of Obstetric, Gynecologic, and Neonatal Nursing 41*(4), 5–15.

American College of Obstetricians and Gynecologists (2011). Prevention of early-onset group B streptococcal disease in newborns. Committee Opinion No. 485. American College of Obstetricians and Gynecologists. Obstetrics & Gynecology 117.

American Academy of Pediatrics (AAP) and American College of Obstetrics and Gynecology (ACOG). (2006). The Apgar score. *Pediatrics 117*(4), 1444–1447.

American Academy of Pediatrics & American Heart Association, (2011). *Textbook of Neonatal Resuscitation* (6th ed.) Elk Grove Village, IL: Author.

American Academy of Pediatrics Committee on Infectious Diseases, (2009). 2009 Red Book. (28th ed.). Elk Grove Village, IL: Author.

Amidi-Nouri, A. (2011). Culturally Responsive Nursing Care. In A. Berman & S. Snyder, *Kozier & Erb's Fundamentals of Nursing* (9th ed.). San Francisco: Pearson.

Angelini, D., & Mahlmeister, L. (2005). Liability in triage: Management of EMTALA regulations and common obstetric risks. *Journal of Midwifery & Women's Health, 50*(6), 472–478.

Association of Women's Health, Obstetric and Neonatal Nurses (AWHONN). (2000a). *Professional nursing support of laboring women.* AWHONN Practice Statement. Washington, DC: Author.

Association of Women's Health, Obstetric and Neonatal Nurses (AWHONN). (2000b). *Nursing management of the second stage of labor.* Evidence-Based Clinical Practice Guideline. Washington, DC: Author.

Association of Women's Health, Obstetric and Neonatal Nurses (AWHONN). (2001a). *Role of the registered nurse in the care of the pregnant woman receiving analgesia/anesthesia by catheter techniques (epidural, intrathecal, spinal, PCEA catheters).* AWHONN Clinical Position Statement. Washington, DC: Author.

Association of Women's Health, Obstetric and Neonatal Nurses (AWHONN). (2011). *Nursing care of the woman receiving analgesia/anesthesia in labor.* Evidence-Based Clinical Practice Guideline. (2nd ed.). Washington, DC: Author.

Association of Women's Health, Obstetric, and Neonatal Nurses (AWHONN). (2008). *Fetal heart rate monitoring: Principles and practice* (4th ed.). Washington, DC: Author.

Bar-Yam, N. B. (1994). Learning about culture: A guide for birth practitioners. *International Journal of Childbirth, 9*(2), 8–10.

Buckley, L. (2005). Evidence-based care sheet: *Epidural analgesia in labor & childbirth.* Glendale, CA: Cinahl Information Systems, January 11, 2005.

Burke, C. (2013). Pain in labor: Nonpharmacologic and pharmacologic management. In AWHONN Perinatal Nursing. (4th ed.). Philadelphia: Lippincott.

Centers for Disease Control and Prevention (2010). Prevention of Perinatal Group B Streptococcal Disease. MMWR: 59.

Chapman, L. (2000). Expectant fathers and labor epidurals. *Maternal Child Nursing, 25,* 133–138.

Cunningham, F., Leveno, K., Bloom, S., Hauth, J., Rouse, D., & Spong, C. (2005). *Williams Obstetrics* (2nd ed.). New York: McGraw-Hill.

Deglin, J., & Vallerand, A. (2009). Davis's Drug Guide for nurses, 11th ed. Philadelphia: F.A. Davis.

Faucher, M., & Brucker, M. (2000). Intrapartum pain: Pharmacologic management [Clinical Issues: Pharmacology Update in Obstetric and Gynecologic Nursing]. *Journal of Obstetric, Gynecologic, and Neonatal Nursing, 29*(2), 169–180.

Florence, D., & Palmer, D. (2003). Therapeutic choices for the discomforts of labor. *Journal of Perinatal & Neonatal Nursing, 17*(4), 238.

Gillesby, E., Burns, S., Dempsey, A., Kirby, S., Mongensen, K., Naylor, et al. (2010). Comparison of Delayed versus Immediate Pushing During Second Stage of Labor for Nulliparous Women with Epidural Anesthesia. *Journal of Obstetric, Gynecologic, & Neonatal Nursing, 39*(6), 635–644.

Gupta, J., Holmeyr, G., & Smyth, R. (2006). Position in the second stage of labour for women without epidural anaesthesia. *Cochrane Database of Systematic Reviews* 2004, Issue 1. Art. No.: CD002006. DOI: 10.1002/14651858.CD002006.pub2.

Hodnett, E. (2002). Pain and women's satisfaction with the experience of childbirth: A systemic review. *American Journal of Obstetrics and Gynecology, 186*(5), S160–S172.

Hodnett, E., Gates, S., Hofmeyr, G., & Sakala, C. (2007). Continuous support for women during childbirth. *Cochrane Database of Systematic Reviews* 2007, Issue 3. Art. No.: D003766. DOI: 10.1002/14651858.CD003766.pub2.

Kattwinkel, J., Perlman, J. M., Aziz, K., Colby, C., Fairchild, K., Gallagher, J., Hazinski, M. F., Halamek, L. P., Kumar, P., Little, G., McGowan, J. E., Nightengale, B., Ramirez, M. M., Ringer, S., Simon, W. M., Weiner, G. M., Wyckoff, M., Zaichkin, J. American Heart Association Neonatal resuscitation: 2010 American Heart Association Guidelines for Cardiopulmonary Resuscitation and Emergency Cardiovascular Care. *Pediatrics.* 2010 Nov; 126(5):e1400-13. Epub 2010 Oct 18.

Kennedy, B., Ruth, D., & Martin, E. (2009). Intrapartum management modules: A perinatal Education program (4th ed.). Philadelphia: Wolters Kluwer/Lippincott Williams & Wilkins.

Lederman, R. (1986). Maternal anxiety in pregnancy: Relationship to health status. *Annual Review of Nursing Research, 2,* 27–61.

Mackey, C. (1995). Women's evaluation of their childbirth performance. *Maternal-Child Nursing Journal, 23*(2), 57–72.

Mandel, D., Pirko, C., Grant, K., Kauffman, T., Williams, L., & Schneider, J. (2010). A Collaborative Protocol on Oxytocin Administration: Bringing Nurses, Midwives & Physicians Together. *Nursing for Women's Health, 13*(6), 482–485.

Martin, J., Hamilton, B., Ventura, S., Osterman, M., Wilson, E., & Mathews, T. (2012). Births: Final Data for 2010. *National Vital Statistics Reports, 61*(1). Hyattsville, MD: National Center for Health Statistics.

Martin, J., Hamilton, B., Sutton, P., Ventura, S., Menacker, F., & Munson, M. (2005). Births: Final Data for 2003. *National Vital Statistics Reports, 54*(2). Hyattsville, MD: National Center for Health Statistics.

Mattson, S., & Smith, J. E. (2011). *Core curriculum for maternal-newborn nursing* (4th ed.). St. Louis, MO: Elsevier Saunders.

Mayberry, L., Wood, S., Strange, L., Lee, L., Heisler, D., & Neilsen-Smith, K. (2000). *Second-stage labor management: Promotion of evidence-based practice and a collaborative approach to patient care.* Washington, DC: Association of Women's Health, Obstetric and Neonatal Nurses.

Moore, M., Moos, M., & Callister, L. (2010). *Cultural Competence: An Essential   Journey for Perinatal Nurses.* White Plains NY: March of Dimes Foundation.

Murray, M. L., & Huelsmann, G. M. (2009). Labor & Delivery Nursing: A Guide to Evidence-Based Practice. New York: Springer Publishing Company.

Neal, J., Lowe, N., Patrick, T., Cabbage, L., & Corwin, E. (2010). What is the Slowest-Yet-Normal Cervical Dilation Rate among Nulliparous Women with Spontaneous Labor Onset? *Journal of Obstetric, Gynecologic, and Neonatal Nursing, 39*(4), 361–369.

Nordgren, S., & Fridlund, B. (2001). Patients' perceptions of self-determination as expressed in the context of care. *Journal of Advanced Nursing, 35*(1), 117–125.

Perla, L. (2002). Patient compliance and satisfaction with nursing care during delivery and recovery. *Journal Nursing Care Quality, 16*(2), 60–66.

Osterman MJK, Martin JA. (2011) Epidural and spinal anesthesia use during labor: 27-state reporting area, 2008. National vital statistics reports; vol 59 no 5. Hyattsville, MD: National Center for Health Statistics.

Pitter, C., & Preston, R. (2001). Modern pharmacologic methods in labor analgesia. *International Journal of Childbirth Education, 16*(2), 15–19.

Roberts, J. (2002). The 'push' for evidence: Management of the second stage. *Journal of Midwifery & Women's Health, 47*(1), 2–15.

Roberts, J. (2003). A new understanding of the second stage of labor: Implications for nursing care. *Journal of Obstetric, Gynecologic, and Neonatal Nursing, 32*(6), 794–801.

Romano, A., & Lothian, J. (2008). Promoting, Protecting & Supporting Normal Birth: A look at the Evidence. *Journal of Obstetrics, Gynecologic & Neonatal Nursing, 37*, 94-105.

Rooks, J. (2007). Guest editorial. Nitrous oxide for pain in labor—why not in the United States? *Birth: Issues In Perinatal Care, 34*(1), 3–5.

Rooks, J. P. (2011). Safety and Risks of Nitrous Oxide Labor Analgesia: A Review. *Journal of Midwifery & Women's Health, 56*(6), 557–565. DOI:10.1111/j.1542-2011.2011.00122.x.

Sauls, D. J. (2010). *Promoting a Positive Childbirth Experience for Adolescents. Journal of Obstetric, Gynecologic, and Neonatal Nursing,* 39, 703–712.

Sharts-Hopko, N., (2010). Oral Intake During Labor: A Review of the Evidence. *Maternal Child Nursing, July August 2010.*

Simkin, P., & Ancheta, R. (2000). *The labor progress handbook: Early intervention to prevent and treat dystocia.* Oxford: Blackwell Science.

Simkin, P., & O'Hara, M. (2002). Nonpharmacologic relief of pain during labor: Systemic reviews of five methods. *American Journal of Obstetrics & Gynecology, 186*(5), S131–S159.

Simpson, K., & O'Brien-Abel, N., (2013). *Labor and Birth, AWHONN. Perinatal Nursing.* (4th ed.). Philadelphia: Lippincott.

Spratto, G., & Woods, A. (2006). *2006 PDR nurse's drug handbook.* Clifton Park, NY: Delmar.

Stark, M., & Miller, M. (2009). Barriers to the use of hydrotherapy in labor. *JOGNN: Journal of Obstetric, Gynecologic & Neonatal Nursing, 38*(6), 667–675. DOI:10.1111/j.1552-6909.2009.01065.x.

Stewart, L., & Collins, M. (2012). Nitrous Oxide as Labor Analgesia. *Nursing For Women's Health, 16*(5), 398–409. DOI:10.1111/j.1751-486X.2012.01763.x.

Wood, S., & Carr, K. (2003). *The art and science of labor support.* White Plains, NY: March of Dimes.

Zwelling, E., Johnson, K., & Allen, J. (2006). How to Implement Complementary Therapies for laboring Women. *Maternal Child Nursing, 31*(6), 364–370.

Fetal Heart Rate Assessment

9

EXPECTED STUDENT OUTCOMES

On completion of this chapter, the student will be able to:
- ☐ Define terms used in electronic fetal monitoring (EFM).
- ☐ Identify the modes of fetal monitoring, auscultation, and EFM.
- ☐ Describe the components of fetal heart rate (FHR) patterns essential to interpretation of monitor strips.
- ☐ Articulate the physiology of FHR accelerations and decelerations.
- ☐ Distinguish between Category I, II, and III patterns and appropriate nursing actions based on these interpretations.

Nursing Diagnoses

- ☐ Knowledge deficit related to fetal monitoring
- ☐ Impaired fetal gas exchange related to:
  - ■ Umbilical cord compression
  - ■ Placental insufficiency
- ☐ Risk of fetal injury related to metabolic acidemia

Nursing Outcomes

- ☐ The pregnant woman and family will verbalize basic understanding of fetal monitoring.
- ☐ Nursing actions to decrease risk of fetal injury will be initiated if injury Category II or III patterns are present.

INTRODUCTION

This chapter is an introduction to basic electronic fetal monitoring (EFM) concepts. Fetal heart rate (FHR) assessment began almost 200 years ago when Europeans (Swiss surgeon Mayor in 1818 and nobleman Kergaradec in 1821) (Freeman et al., 2003) reported the presence of fetal heart sounds via auscultation (hearing sounds via ear-to-abdomen or stethoscope). It continues to be the primary method for intrapartum fetal surveillance despite concerns regarding its efficacy and ability to improve neonatal outcomes (Freeman, 2002; Tucker et al., 2009).

The goal of fetal monitoring is the interpretation and ongoing assessment of fetal oxygenation (Feinstein, Torgersen, & Atterbury, 2003). EFM is a technique for fetal assessment based on the fact that the FHR reflects fetal oxygenation (Lyndon, O'Brien-Abel, & Simpson, 2014). Current practice indicates that EFM is used for virtually all women during labor in the United States. EFM is essential in the assessment of maternal and fetal well-being in antepartal and intrapartal settings (Menihan & Kopel, 2008).

Nurses are expected to independently assess, interpret, and intervene related to interpretations of EFM patterns. Assessments and interactions with monitored women and their families are individualized and geared to providing information and explanation, and reducing anxiety. Clear and accurate communication with care providers and the perinatal team is essential for optimizing perinatal care (see Quality and Safety Education for Nurses (QSEN) Teamwork and Collaboration). Assessment of FHR in the intrapartal period is the focus of this chapter.

TERMINOLOGY RELATED TO FETAL ASSESSMENT

Definitions used in this chapter are from the National Institute of Child Health and Human Development (NICHD). Research Planning Workshop (1997) and the 2008 NICHD Workshop Report on Electronic Fetal Monitoring: Update on Definitions, Interpretations and Research Guidelines publications (Macones et al., 2008; ACOG Practice Bulletin, July 2010). There is a current movement to standardize language

Don't have time to read this chapter? Want to reinforce your reading? Need to review for a test? Listen to this chapter on DavisPlus.

233

for FHR interpretations because of variations in language used at present. It is critical for labor units to select one set of definitions for FHR patterns for all types of professional communications (Simpson, 2004a; AWHONN, 2009) (**Table 9-1** and **Box 9-1**). Clinicians should be familiar with these definitions and use them consistently in clinical practice.

QSEN Teamwork and Collaboration

The QSEN definition for teamwork and collaboration is to function effectively within nursing and inter-professional teams, fostering open communication, mutual respect, and shared decision-making to achieve quality patient care. Communication and collaboration are particularly essential related to EFM. Some suggestions to foster your development in this area related to EFM include:

■ Follow communication practices that minimize risks associated with EFM communication among providers.

■ Appreciate the importance of intra- and inter-professional collaboration to improve patient outcomes.
■ Integrate the contributions of others who play a role in helping patient and family achieve a healthy birth.
■ Respect the centrality of the patient/family as core members of any health care team.
■ Acknowledge your own potential to contribute to effective team functioning in this critical setting.

TABLE 9–1 TERMINOLOGY RELATED TO FETAL HEART RATE ASSESSMENT

TERMINOLOGY	DEFINITION
BASELINE FHR	Mean fetal heart rate (FHR) rounded to increments of 5 beats per minute (bpm) during a 10-minute window, excluding accelerations and decelerations.
BASELINE VARIABILITY	Fluctuations in the baseline FHR that are irregular in amplitude and frequency. The fluctuations are visually quantified as the amplitude of the peak to trough in bpm. It is determined in a 10-minute window, excluding accelerations and decelerations. It reflects the interaction between the fetal sympathetic and parasympathetic nervous system. • Absent: Amplitude range is undetectable • Minimal: Amplitude range is visually undetectable ≤5 bpm • Moderate: Amplitude from peak to trough 6 bpm to 25 bpm • Marked: Amplitude range >25 bpm
ACCELERATIONS	Visually apparent, abrupt increase in FHR above the baseline. The peak of the acceleration is ≥15 bpm over the baseline FHR for ≥15 seconds and >2 minutes. • Before 32 weeks' gestation acceleration is ≥10 beats over the baseline FHR for ≥10 seconds. **Prolonged accelerations** are ≥2 minutes, but ≤10 minutes.
DECELERATION	Transitory decrease in the FHR from the baseline. • **Early deceleration** is a visually apparent gradual decrease in FHR below the baseline. The nadir (lowest point) of the deceleration occurs at the same time as the peak of the UC. In most cases the onset, nadir, and recovery of the deceleration are coincident or mirror the contraction. • **Variable deceleration** is a visually apparent abrupt decrease in the FHR below baseline; the decrease in the FHR is ≥15 bpm lasting ≥15 seconds and <2 minutes in duration. • **Late deceleration** is a visually apparent gradual decrease of FHR below the baseline. Nadir (lowest point) of the deceleration occurs after the peak of the contraction. In most cases the onset, nadir, and recovery of the deceleration occurs after the respective onset, peak, and end of the UC. • **Prolonged deceleration** is a visually apparent abrupt decrease in FHR below baseline that is ≥15 bpm lasting ≥2 minutes but ≤10 minutes. • **Sinusoidal pattern** is defined as having a visually apparent smooth sine-like wave like undulating pattern in FHR baseline with a cycle frequency of 3–5/min that persists for ≥ 20 minutes.
TACHYCARDIA	Baseline FHR of >160 bpm lasting 10 minutes or longer.
BRADYCARDIA	Baseline FHR of <110 bpm lasting for 10 minutes or longer.
NORMAL FHR	FHR pattern that reflects a favorable physiological response to the maternal fetal environment.
ABNORMAL FHR	FHR pattern that reflects an unfavorable physiological response to the maternal fetal environment.

Sources: NICHD (2008); Lyndon & Ali (2009); ACOG (2010); Macones et al. (2008).

BOX 9-1 COMMON ABBREVIATIONS FOR ELECTRONIC FETAL MONITORING

bpm	beats per minute
ED	Early deceleration
EFM	Electronic fetal monitoring
FHR	Fetal heart rate
FSE	Fetal scalp electrode
IA	Intermittent auscultation
IUPC	Intrauterine pressure catheter
LD	Late deceleration
MVU	Montevideo units
PD	Prolonged deceleration
TOCO	Tocodynamometer
VAS	Vibroacoustic stimulation
UC	Uterine contractions
US	Ultrasound
VD	Variable deceleration
VE	Vaginal examination

MODES OR TYPES OF FETAL AND UTERINE MONITORING

Auscultation

Auscultation is use of the fetoscope or Doppler to hear the FHR by externally listening without the use of a paper recorder (Feinstein et al., 2008) (**Fig. 9-1**). Auscultation with a fetoscope allows the practitioner to hear the sounds associated with the opening and closing of ventricular valves via bone conduction. A Doppler, by contrast, uses ultrasound technology, using sound waves deflected from fetal heart movements (similar to that used on an electronic fetal monitor external ultrasound transducer). This ultrasound device then converts information into a sound that represents cardiac events.

Auscultation limits assessment data to FHR baseline, rhythm, and changes from baseline. Auscultation cannot detect certain types of decelerations and variability, which are enabled only by a combination of a paper recorder and ultrasound technology (part of electronic fetal monitoring).

Research evidence supports the use of intermittent auscultation (IA) as a method of fetal surveillance during labor for low-risk pregnancies (Lyndon & Ali, 2008; Feinstein, Sprague, & Trepanier, 2008). **Box 9-2** provides the Clinical Position Statement of the Association of Women's Health, Obstetric and Neonatal Nurses (AWHONN) with regard to fetal heart monitoring. In summary, fetoscope and Doppler obtain information differently but are both appropriate in some auscultation clinical situations.

Palpation of Contractions

When the uterus contracts, the musculature becomes firm and tense and can be palpated with the fingertips by the nurse. The frequency, duration, tone, and intensity of contractions can be assessed by palpation (AWHONN, 2009).

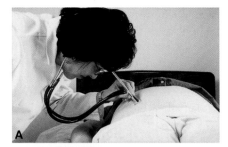
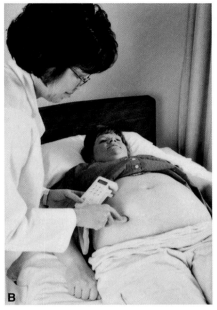

Figure 9–1 Auscultation of fetal heart rate. *A.* Fetoscope. *B.* Doppler ultrasound stethoscope.

BOX 9–2 AWHONN FETAL HEART MONITORING CLINICAL POSITION STATEMENT

The professional organization for perinatal nursing states: "AWHONN supports the assessment of the laboring woman and her fetus through the use of auscultation, palpation and/or electronic monitoring techniques...to assess and promote maternal and fetal well being." AWHONN "does not support the use of EFM as a substitute for appropriate professional nursing care and support of women in labor" (AWHONN, 2008, p. 1).

The policy statement recommends ongoing education in the interpretation of fetal assessment. The policy recommends that guidelines are developed in facilities specifying modes and frequency of fetal assessment as well as policies that address communication and collaboration essential to providing quality care and optimizing patient outcomes.

Source: AWHONN (2008).

This is a subjective assessment and can be biased by the fat distribution around the pregnant woman's uterus.

■ Palpation of uterine contractions is done by the nurse placing her fingertips on the fundus of the uterus and assessing the degree of tension as the contractions occur.

■ The intensity of contractions is measured at the peak of the contraction and is rated as:
  ■ *Mild or 1+ feels like the tip of the nose (easily indented)*
  ■ *Moderate or 2+ feels like the chin (can slightly indent)*
  ■ *Strong or 3+ feels like the forehead (cannot indent uterus)*
■ The resting tone is measured between contractions and listed as either soft or firm uterine tone.

External Electronic Fetal and Uterine Monitoring

External electronic fetal and uterine monitoring uses an ultrasound device to detect FHR and a pressure device to assess uterine activity (**Fig. 9-2** and **Box 9-3**), which is attached to a paper recorder.

■ The FHR is measured via an ultrasound transducer.
  ■ *External EFM detects FHR baseline, variability, accelerations, and decelerations.*
  ■ *Erratic FHR recordings or gaps on a paper recorder may be due to inadequate conduction of ultrasound signal displacement of the transducer (may be picking up maternal heart rate), fetal or maternal movement, inadequate ultrasound gel, or fetal arrhythmia (may need to auscultate to verify).*
■ Contractions are measured via a **tocodynamometer,** an external uterine monitor.
  ■ *The relative frequency and duration of uterine contractions (UCs), and relative resting tone, which is the tone of the uterus between contractions, can be measured by this method.*
  ■ *External uterine monitors cannot measure pressure/intensity.*
  ■ *Pressure/intensity of the contraction must be estimated by palpation of contractions.*
  ■ *Contractions not recording on a paper recorder may be due to transducer not on area of uterus palpated to be strongest area of contraction; resting tone not dialed to 15–20 mm Hg when uterus is relaxed.*

BOX 9–3 GUIDELINES FOR PLACEMENT OF AN EXTERNAL ELECTRONIC FETAL MONITOR

Explain the procedure to the woman and her family. For example:
  "The monitor records your baby's heart rate, uterine contractions, and tells us the baby's response to uterine contractions. We place two monitors on your abdomen and secure them with belts. You can move around in bed and we will adjust the monitors."

FHR
Use Leopold's maneuver to locate fetal back.

Apply ultrasound gel to FHR ultrasound transducer and place it on the woman's abdomen at the location of the fetus's back and move the transducer until clear signal and FHR is heard. Secure with monitor belt.

UCs
Place the uterine activity sensor (tocodynamometer) in the fundal area where the contraction feels strongest to palpation. Secure the monitor with a belt.

Internal Electronic Fetal and Uterine Monitoring

Internal electronic fetal monitoring uses a fetal scalp electrode (FSE)/internal scalp electrode (ISE) that is applied to the presenting part of the fetus to directly detect FHR. Internal electronic uterine monitoring involves an intrauterine pressure catheter (IUPC) placed in the uterine cavity to directly measure uterine contractions (**Fig. 9.3** and **Box 9-4**). Membranes must be ruptured for both methods (AWHONN, 2009).

The decision to insert an FSE is based on the need for continuous FHR tracing when troubleshooting methods do not alter quality of tracing. A nurse or care provider certified to attach this should be aware of relative contraindications to direct methods of monitoring. These include chorioamnionitis, active maternal genital herpes and human immunodeficiency

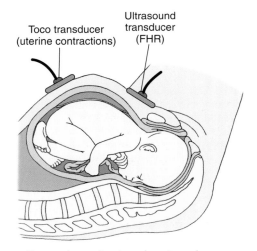

Figure 9–2 External monitoring showing placement of the ultrasound and tocodynamometer.

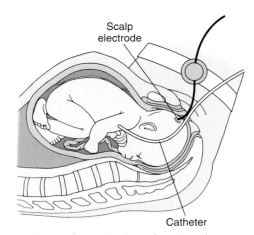

Figure 9–3 Internal monitoring, showing placement of the fetal scalp electrode and intrauterine pressure catheter.

BOX 9–4 GUIDELINES FOR PLACEMENT OF AN INTERNAL ELECTRONIC FETAL MONITOR

Explain the procedure to the woman and her family. For example:

"The internal fetal scalp electrode allows us to directly monitor your baby's heart rate. It is clipped on the baby's scalp with a vaginal exam and the monitor is attached to your leg. You can still move around and go to the bathroom."

"The intrauterine pressure catheter tells us exactly how strong your contractions are. It is a direct measurement of the pressure of your contractions. It is placed in your uterus with a vaginal exam."

FHR	UCs
Placement of the FSE requires skills and techniques of vaginal examination and EFM as well as risks, limitations, and contraindications (primarily preexisting infections such as herpes or HIV).	Placement of an IUPC is an invasive procedure where the nurse should have knowledge and understanding of indications and contraindications and risks of internal monitoring. For placement of the IUPC, the manufacturer directions are reviewed as there are several types of IUPC with different set-up guidelines. The IUPC and the guide tube are inserted in the vagina with a vaginal exam, and the catheter is advanced through the cervix into the uterus.
For placement of FSE, a vaginal exam is performed and the guide tube with the electrode is advanced and attached to the presenting part of the fetus.	

- *IUPC monitoring can detect actual frequency, duration, and strength of UCs and resting tone in mm Hg.*
- *Uterine contraction intensity is measured using an IUPC = Peak pressure minus the baseline pressure in mm Hg.*
- *Contraction intensity varies during labor, from 30 mm Hg in early spontaneous labor to 70 mm Hg in transition to 70–90 mm Hg in the second stage.*
- ***Peak pressure** is the maximum uterine pressure during a contraction measured with an IUPC. **Resting tone or baseline pressure** is the uterine pressure between contractions and should be about 5–25 mm Hg.*
- *The contraction and resting tone intensity is a combination of pressure from myometrial muscle contraction as well as intrauterine hydrostatic pressure (pressure exerted from amniotic fluid above the catheter). Therefore, positioning of the patient—measuring IUPC pressures in left, right, supine, and lateral—will prevent possible erroneous conclusions about induction or augmentation management (AWHONN, 2009).*
- *Uterine contractions may also be quantified via Montevideo units (MVUs) measured by the peak pressure for each contraction in a 10-minute period. ACOG has recommended at least 200 MVUs every 10 minutes for 2 hours as adequate uterine contraction intensity for normal progress of labor.*
- *An IUPC can be used to perform an amnioinfusion.*
- *The IUPC is inserted by the care provider. Some institutions may have protocols for nurses to insert IUPCs; nurses need to check hospital policy on IUPC insertion.*

virus (HIV), and conditions that preclude vaginal exams (placenta previa and undiagnosed vaginal bleeding).

IUPC monitoring is initiated based on the clinical need for additional uterine activity information. It may be used when external monitoring is inadequate due to maternal obesity or due to lack of progress in labor when quantitative analysis of uterine activity is needed for clinical decision making. In addition, an IUPC may be inserted to treat a worsening Category II tracing (e.g., recurrent variable decelerations with nadir greater than 60 mm Hg from baseline) via amnioinfusion. IUPCs provide an objective measure of the frequency and duration of contractions, as well as the intensity of contractions (as opposed to palpation, which is subjective) and resting tone both expressed in mm Hg.

- FHR is measured via an internal fetal spiral electrode (FSE).
  - *Internal EFM detects FHR baseline, variability, accelerations, decelerations, and limited information on some types of arrhythmias.*
  - *It is attached to the presenting part of the fetus by the nurse or care provider.*
- Contractions are measured via an **intrauterine pressure catheter (IUPC).**
  - *IUPC provides an objective measure of the pressure of contractions expressed as mm Hg.*

Telemetry

This is a type of continuous electronic fetal monitoring which involves connecting the patient to a radio frequency transmitter that allows the patient to walk and take a bath without having to be connected to the monitor. Nurses can oversee the fetal and uterine information as if the patient were connected directly to the monitor (Tucker et al., 2009). It can be used in all phases of labor.

Monitor Paper Used for the Electronic Fetal Monitor

Monitor paper is used for EFM (**Fig. 9-4**). Assuming that the paper speed is 3 cm per minute (standard for the United States), each dark vertical line represents 1 minute and each lighter vertical line represents 10 seconds.

The FHR is recorded on the top grid of the paper while uterine contractions are recorded on the lower grid. Some EFM systems allow for maternal pulse (obtained via a pulse oximeter attached to the laboring mother) also to be recorded on the paper in the top grid. Clinicians may need this additional information to distinguish between maternal and fetal heart rate. Both external and internal fetal monitors may inadvertently pick up maternal rate, which is especially critical if the fetus is not tolerating labor or actually dead (Murray, 2004).

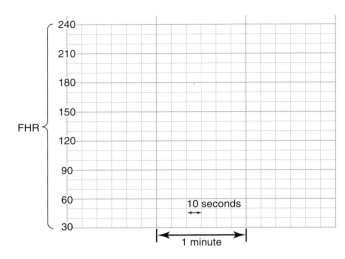

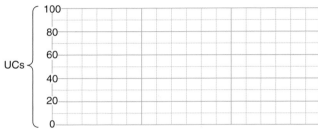

Figure 9–4 Monitor paper indicating timing on grid.

A WHONN STANDARDS FOR FREQUENCY OF ASSESSMENT OF FHR

Frequency of FHR assessment is based on assessment of risk status, stage of labor, and ongoing clinical assessment (AWHONN, 2008a; Lyndon & Ali, 2009) (**Box 9-5; Fig. 9-5**).

■ The frequency of assessment increases:
   ■ *When indeterminate Category II or abnormal Category III FHR characteristics are heard*
   ■ *Before and after rupture of membranes or administration of medication*
■ When indeterminate or abnormal characteristics are heard, electronic FHR monitoring is used to:
   ■ *Clarify pattern interpretation*
   ■ *Assess baseline variability*
   ■ *Further assess fetal status*
■ In the presence of risk factors, continuous EFM is recommended and the FHR should be evaluated:
   ■ *Every 15 minutes in the active phase*
   ■ *Every 5 minutes while pushing*
■ It is common practice for all women to have a baseline EFM tracing of at least 20 minutes at the time they are first evaluated in labor.
■ Routine continuous FHR monitoring remains controversial. Refer to Evidence-Based Practice: Continuous Electronic Heart Rate Monitoring for Fetal Assessment During Labor.

■ A decision tree for managing fetal assessment may be utilized (Fig. 9-5).

> ## Evidence-Based Practice: Electronic Fetal Heart Rate Monitoring for Fetal Assessment During Labor
>
> Alfirevic, Z. (2008). Continuous cardiotocography (CTG) as a form of electronic fetal monitoring (EFM) for fetal assessment during labour. *Cochrane Database of Systematic Reviews, (4).*
>
> A review was conducted to compare the efficacy and safety of routine continuous EFM of labor with intermittent auscultation using the results of published randomized controlled trials (RCTs). This review found 12 trials involving over 37,000 women. But most studies were not of high quality, and the review was dominated by one large, well-conducted trial of almost 13,000 women who received care from one person throughout labor in a hospital where the membranes either ruptured spontaneously or were artificially ruptured as early as possible and oxytocin stimulation of contractions was used in about a quarter of the women. There was no difference in the number of babies who died during or shortly after labor (about 1 in 300). Neonatal seizures in babies were rare (about 1 in 500 births), but they occurred significantly less often when continuous EFM was used to monitor fetal heart rate. There was no difference in the incidence of cerebral palsy, although other possible long-term effects have not been fully assessed and need further study. Continuous monitoring was associated with a significant increase in cesarean section and instrumental vaginal births. Both procedures are known to carry the risks associated with a surgical procedure, although the specific adverse outcomes have not been assessed in the included studies.
>
> Authors' Conclusions
>
> Continuous EFM during labor is associated with a reduction in neonatal seizures, but there are no significant differences in cerebral palsy, infant mortality, or other standard measures of neonatal well-being. However, continuous EFM was associated with an increase in cesarean sections and instrumental vaginal births. The authors believe the real challenge is how best to convey this uncertainty to women to enable them to make an informed choice without compromising the normality of labor.

INFLUENCES ON FETAL HEART RATE

An understanding of FHR physiology aids in the interpretation of FHR patterns. The FHR responds to multiple physiological factors. The following sections review the influences on the FHR.

Utero-Placental Unit

At term, about 10%–15% of maternal cardiac output (600–750 mL) perfuses the uterus per minute. Oxygenated blood from the mother is delivered to the intervillous space in the placenta via the uterine arteries. Maternal-fetal exchange of oxygen, carbon dioxide, nutrients, waste products, and water occurs in the intervillous space across the membranes that separate fetal and maternal circulations. Oxygen and carbon

BOX 9–5   AWHONN STANDARDS FOR FREQUENCY FOR FHR ASSESSMENT

Intermittent Auscultation (IA)

In the absence of risk factors, FHR should be auscultated:

- Every 1 hour in the latent phase of labor
- Every 5–30 minutes in the active and transition phase
- Every 5–15 minutes in the second stage

In the presence of risk factors (e.g., when there is thick meconium, the mother has a fever, or there is an obvious problem with the placenta, or when the fetus is not tolerating the stress of labor well as evidenced by late decelerations), continuous EFM is recommended.

Intermittent auscultation can only interpret Category I and Category II FHR characteristics as all Category III patterns include assessment of FHR variability not possible with intermittent auscultation (IA).

Intermittent Electronic Fetal Monitoring (EFM)

In the absence of risk factors, FHR should be evaluated:

- Every 30 minutes in the active phase of labor
- Every 5–15 minutes in the second stage, although typically in the second stage there is continuous EFM.

In the presence of risk factors, continuous EFM is recommended.

Source: Lyndon & Ali (2009).

---

dioxide diffuse across the membranes rapidly and efficiently (Menhan & Kopel, 2008).

- Effective transfer of oxygen and carbon dioxide between fetal and maternal blood streams is dependent on:
  - *Adequate uterine blood flow*

- *Sufficient placental area*
- *Unconstricted umbilical cord*
- Appropriate oxygenation to the fetus depends on:
  - *Adequate oxygenation of the mother*
  - *Adequate blood flow to the placenta*
  - *Adequate uteroplacental circulation*
  - *Adequate umbilical circulation*
  - *The fetus's own innate ability to initiate compensatory mechanisms to regulate the FHR*
- Additional factors in the fetal environment that influence fetal oxygenation include:
  - *Uteroplacental function*
  - *Uterine activity*
  - *Umbilical cord issues*
  - *Maternal physiological function*
- Having a basic understanding of the extrinsic influence on FHR, such as normal physiological changes in pregnancy, uterine and placental blood flow, and umbilical blood flow, improves the nurse's ability to assess FHR patterns (Lyndon & Ali, 2009)
- The influences related to labor are discussed in Chapter 10.

Autonomic Nervous System

Parasympathetic Nervous System

- Parasympathetic stimulation decreases the heart rate.
- The parasympathetic nervous system is primarily mediated by vagus nerve innervating sinoatrial (SA) and atrioventricular (AV) nodes in the heart.
- Vagus nerve stimulation slows FHR and helps maintain variability.
  - *Variability in FHR develops at 28–30 weeks of gestation.*

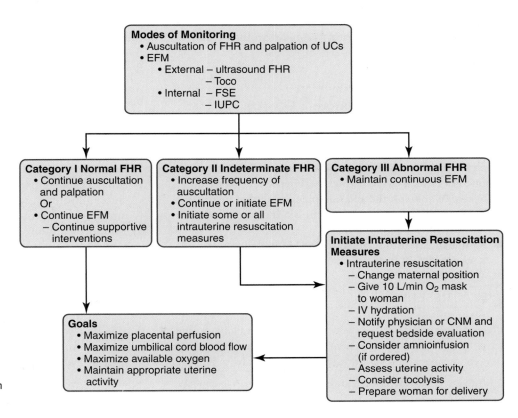

Figure 9–5   Decision-making in FHR assessment.

Sympathetic Nervous System

- Sympathetic nervous system (SNS) stimulation increases the FHR.
- Nerves are distributed widely in the fetal heart, and stimulation produces an increase in strength of fetal heart contraction.
- SNS is responsible for FHR variability.
- Action occurs through release of norepinephrine.
- Stimulation of SNS increases fetal heart rate.
- SNS may be stimulated during hypoxemia.

Baroreceptors

- Baroreceptors are stretch receptors in the aortic arch and the carotid arch which detect pressure changes.
- They provide a protective homeostatic mechanism for regulating heart rate by stimulating a vagal response and decreasing FHR, fetal blood pressure, and cardiac output.

Central Nervous System (CNS)

- CNS is the integrative center responsible for variations in FHR and baseline variability related to fetal activity.
- CNS regulates and coordinates autonomic activities.
- Mediates cardiac and vasomotor reflexes
- Responds to fetal movement

Chemoreceptors

- Chemoreceptors are located in the aortic arch and the central nervous system (CNS).
- They respond to changes in fetal O_2 and CO_2 and pH levels. Decreased O_2 and increased CO_2 cause peripheral chemoreceptors to stimulate the vagal nerve and slow the heart rate, and central chemoreceptors respond to an increased heart rate and an increased blood pressure.

Hormonal Regulation

- The fetus responds to a decrease in O_2 or uteroplacental blood flow by releasing hormones that maximize blood flow to vital organs such as the heart, brain, and adrenals.
- Epinephrine, norepinephrine, catecholamines, and vasopressin facilitate hemodynamic changes in response to changes in fetal oxygenation. Fetal hypoxia causes a release of epinephrine and norepinephrine that increases FHR and blood pressure. Vasopressin increases blood pressure in response to hypoxia.
- Renin–angiotensin secreted by the kidneys produces vasoconstriction in response to hypovolemia.

*F*ETAL RESERVES

Placental reserve describes the reserve oxygen available to the fetus to withstand the transient changes in blood flow and oxygen during labor (Lyndon & Ali, 2009). In a healthy maternal-fetal unit, the placenta provides oxygen and nutrients beyond the baseline needs of the fetus.

- When oxygen is decreased, blood flow is deferred to vital fetal organs to compensate.
- When placental reserves of oxygen are decreased or depleted, the fetus may not be able to adapt to or tolerate decreased oxygen that occurs during a labor contraction.
- Fetal adaptation to the stresses of labor occurs through homeostatic mechanisms.
  - *Prolonged or repeated hypoxemia may deplete reserves, resulting in decompensation.*
  - *Interpretation of FHR data requires the ability to differentiate three types of fetal responses:*
    - Nonhypoxic reflex responses such as FHR accelerations
    - Compensatory responses to hypoxemia, such as variable decelerations
    - Impending decompensation responses such as late decelerations (Lyndon & Ali, 2009)

Umbilical Cord Blood Acid-Base Analysis After Delivery

Umbilical cord blood acid-base acidosis analysis can be a useful objective way to quantify fetal acid base balance at birth. An understanding of respiratory and metabolic acidosis and acidemia and associated clinical applications is required to interpret the findings (AWHONN, 2009).

Although maternal and fetal components of oxygen transport are similar, there are features of oxygen transport that are unique to the fetus. Fetal oxygen transport is directly dependent on the maternal transport system. The fetus has lower oxygen tension (25%) than the adult (100%). Fetuses have higher oxygen affinity (due to different fetal hemoglobin) than adults. The amount of oxygen being transported to the fetus may be affected by the sufficiency of blood flow to the uterus and placenta, the integrity of the placenta, and the flow of blood through the umbilical cord.

Normally, the fetus is able to maintain normal aerobic metabolism even though there are transient decreases in blood flow to the uterus. However, when available oxygen in the intervillous space falls below 50% of normal levels, there is a sequential process that occurs:

1) Redistribution of blood to vital organs (heart, brain, and adrenal glands). In scenarios when oxygen is altered chronically, fetal growth will decelerate and lead to intrauterine growth retardation.
2) Fetal myocardium will change in oxygen consumption, leading to changes in FHR such as fetal heart variability.
3) Fetus will convert from aerobic to anaerobic metabolism.

In fetal heart muscle cells, normal cellular metabolism utilizes glucose and oxygen or aerobic metabolism. Carbon dioxide and water are the waste products that need to be taken away from the muscle cell by the fetal blood flow and increase of hydrogen ions in the tissue (acidosis).

When the fetus experiences hypoxia, the fetus may switch to anaerobic metabolism, which is non-oxygen dependent. The waste product produced during this process is lactic acid. Accumulation of this acid leads to cell death and eventually to acidemia (increase of hydrogen ions in the blood).

Shortly after birth, blood is drawn from the umbilical vein and one of the umbilical arteries. The umbilical vein represents oxygen supply available to the fetus, and the arterial blood best represents fetal usage of oxygen because it is the end point of fetal metabolism as blood returns to the placenta.

Respiratory acidosis occurs when an elevated PCO_2 level is present. An elevated PCO_2 is indicative that the fetus is still processing oxygen via aerobic metabolism. It can develop rapidly in the fetus during acute hypoxia but can also be corrected rapidly when carbon dioxide is allowed to diffuse. Base excess with acidemia, during anaerobic metabolism, can become elevated. With a normal PCO_2, it may reflect a prolonged hypoxic insult (Tucker et al., 2009).

The following box contains normal values for umbilical cord blood. Note that greater absolute values for base deficit or excess (bicarbonate concentration which increases to compensate for greater hydrogen ion concentration) are associated with acidemia. Also, acidemia is determined by the pH level. Our goal for a vigorous infant at birth is a pH of ≥ 7.1 and a base excess of ≥–12 (**Box 9-6**).

NICHD Criteria for Interpretation of FHR Patterns

A variety of systems and terminology have been used in the interpretation of FHR patterns. The FHR should be interpreted within the context of the overall clinical circumstances. Clinical conditions that impact FHR patterns include gestational age, prior results of fetal assessment, medications, maternal medical conditions, and fetal conditions. FHR patterns are dynamic and transient and require frequent assessment. A careful review of current evidence has resulted in a new recommendation for FHR interpretation in the intrapartum period from NICHD based on a three-tier category system (see Critical Component: Three-Tier FHR Interpretation System).

■ Category I FHR tracings are normal. They are strongly predictive of a well-oxygenated, nonacidotic fetus with a normal fetal acid-base balance. They may be followed in a routine manner and no action is required.

■ Category II FHR tracings are indeterminate. They are not predictive of abnormal fetal acid-base status, yet there is not adequate evidence to classify them as Category I or III. They require evaluation and continued surveillance and reevaluation in the context of the clinical circumstances.

■ Category III FHR tracings are abnormal. They are predictive of abnormal fetal acid-base status and require prompt evaluation. Depending on the clinical situation, efforts to resolve the underlying cause of the abnormal fetal heart rate pattern should be made expeditiously.

A more complex 5-tier system has also been proposed to standardize management of FHR (Parer & Ikeda, 2007) (see Critical Component: Five-Tier FHR Interpretation System).

BOX 9–6   UMBILICAL CORD BLOOD ACID BASE NORMAL

ARTERIAL CORD BLOOD MEASURES	NORMAL VALUES	TARGET VALUES
ph	7.20–7.3	≥7.10
PCO_2 (mm Hg)	49.9–50.3	<60
HCO_3 (mEg/L) Bicarbonate	22–24	>22
Base excess (mEg/L)	–2.7 to –4.3	>–12
PO_2 (mm Hg)	15–23	>20

Sources: Lyndon & Ali (2009); Cunningham et al. (2010).

CRITICAL COMPONENT

Three-Tier FHR Interpretation System

Category I Normal

FHR tracings include **all** of the following:

■ Baseline rate 110–160 bpm
■ Baseline variability moderate
■ Late or variable deceleration absent
■ Early decelerations absent or present
■ Accelerations absent or present

Category II Indeterminate

FHR tracings include all FHR tracings not categorized as Category I or III.
    They include **any** of the following:

■ Bradycardia not accompanied by absent variability
■ Tachycardia
■ Minimal baseline variability
■ Absent baseline variability not accompanied by recurrent decelerations
■ Marked baseline variability
■ Absence of induced accelerations after fetal stimulation
■ Recurrent variable decelerations with minimal or moderate variability
■ Prolonged decelerations ≥2 minutes but ≤10 minutes
■ Recurrent late decelerations with moderate variability
■ Variable decelerations with other characteristics such as slow return to baseline "overshoots" or "shoulders"

Category III Abnormal

FHR tracings that are **either**:

■ Absent variability with any of the following:
  ■ Recurrent late decelerations
  ■ Recurrent variable decelerations
  ■ Bradycardia
■ Sinusoidal pattern

(Macones et al., 2008; Lyndon & Ali, 2009)

CRITICAL COMPONENT

Five-Tier FHR Interpretation System

FHR 5-Tier System

FHR 5-tier is based on the five-color system developed by Drs. Parer and Ikeda. The intent of their system is to standardize management of different fetal heart rate (FHR) tracings. The system divides all FHR tracings into one of five categories: green (no acidemia, no intervention required), blue, yellow, orange, or red (evidence of actual or impending fetal asphyxia, rapid delivery recommended). Each color has assigned to it: (a) risk of acidemia, (b) risk of evolution to a more serious pattern, or (c) recommended action.

Category		Risk of Acidemia	Risk of Evolution	Action	Risk of Acidemia Related to Variability, Baseline Heart Rate and Recurrent Decelerations										
					Decelerations		Recurrent variables			Recurrent late			Prolonged		
I	Green	0	Very low	none			Mild	Moderate	Severe	Mild	Moderate	Severe	Mild	Moderate	Severe
IIA	Blue	0	Low	Inform M.D. Conservative measures	None	Early	All else	Last 30-60 sec and touch 70 BPM OR last > 60 sec and touch 80 BPM	Last 1-2 min and touch 70 BPM OR last > 2 min and touch 80 BPM	< 15 BPM below baseline	15-44 BPM below baseline	> 45 BPM below baseline	> 80 BPM	80 to 70 BPM	≤ 70 BPM
IIB	Yellow	0	Moderate	Increased surveillance Conservative measures											
IIC	Orange	Acceptably low	High	Prepare for possible urgent delivery											
III	Red	Unacceptably high	Not a consideration	Deliver											

Moderate variability (normal)

FHR
Tachycardia	
Normal	(110-160 BPM)
Mild bradycardia	(> 80 BPM)
Moderate bradycardia	(80 to 70 BPM)
Severe bradycardia	(≤ 70 BPM)

Minimal variability

FHR
Tachycardia	
Normal	(110-160 BPM)
Mild bradycardia	(> 80 BPM)
Moderate bradycardia	(80 to 70 BPM)
Severe bradycardia	(≤ 70 BPM)

Absent variability

FHR
Tachycardia	
Normal	(110-160 BPM)
Mild bradycardia	(> 80 BPM)
Moderate bradycardia	(80 to 70 BPM)
Severe bradycardia	(≤ 70 BPM)
Sinusoidal	
Marked variability	

REFERENCE: Parer JT, Ikeda T.A framework for standardized management of intrapartum fetal heart rate patterns. Am J Obstet Gynecol. 2007 Jul;197(1):26 e1-6 PMD: 17618744
Parer JT, Hamilton EF.Comparison of 5 experts and computer analysis in rule-based fetal heart rate interpretation. Am J Obstet Gynecol. 2010 Nov;203(5):451.e1-7. Epub 2010 July 15.PMD: 20633869
Coletta, J., Murphy, E., Rubeo, Z., et al. (2012). The 5-tier system of assessing fetal heart rate tracings is superior to the 3-tier system in identifying fetal academia. American Journal of Obstetrics and Gynecology; 206:226.e1-5.

The National Institute of Child Health and Human Development (NICHD) three-tier system of classifying FHR tracings has been criticized for having too wide a range of tracings in category II. Some researchers and clinicians believe that the five-tier color-coded system classifies EFM tracings more effectively. The five-tier system is being adopted by an increasing number of hospitals in the United States.

FHR AND CONTRACTION PATTERN INTERPRETATION

Three major areas are assessed when interpreting FHR pattern: FHR baseline, periodic and episodic changes, and uterine activity.

- Interpretation of FHR baseline includes:
  - *Baseline rate*
  - *Baseline variability*
- Interpretation of periodic and episodic changes includes:
  - *Accelerations*
  - *Decelerations (early, variable, late, and prolonged)*
- Interpretation of uterine activity includes:
  - *Frequency*
  - *Duration*
  - *Intensity*
  - *Resting tone*
  - *Relaxation time between UCs*

Baseline Fetal Heart Rate

Baseline FHR is the mean FHR rounded to increments of 5 beats per minute (BPM) during a 10-minute window excluding accelerations, decelerations, or marked variability (**Fig. 9-6**). There must be at least 2 minutes of identifiable baseline segments (not necessarily contiguous) in a 10-minute period or the baseline for that period is indeterminate.

Characteristics

- The normal range is 110–160 bpm.
- FHR baseline above 160 bpm for at least 10 minutes is tachycardia.
- FHR baseline below 110 bpm for at least 10 minutes is bradycardia.

Medical Management

- Assess the baseline over a 10-minute period.

Nursing Actions

- Assess the baseline over 10-minute period.

Fetal Tachycardia

Tachycardia is a FHR above 160 bpm that lasts for at least 10 minutes (**Fig. 9-7**).

- Tachycardia may be a sign of early fetal hypoxemia, especially with decreased variability and decelerations.
- If tachycardia persists above 200–220 bpm, fetal demise may occur.
- A number of causes of fetal tachycardia, such as maternal fever or exposure to medications such as terbutaline, do not reflect a risk of abnormal acid-base balance.

Characteristics

- Baseline FHR above 160 bpm that lasts for at least 10 minutes.

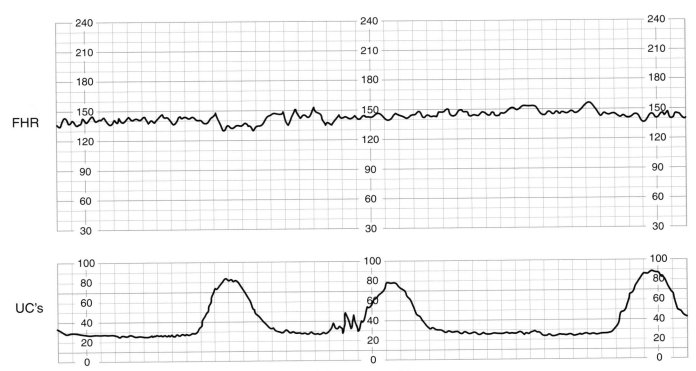

Figure 9–6 Normal fetal heart rate with moderate variability. *Top.* Fetal heart rate. *Bottom.* Contractions.

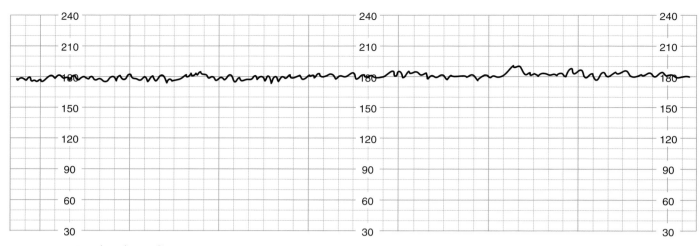

Figure 9–7 Fetal tachycardia.

■ It is often accompanied by a decreased or absent baseline variability due to the relationship to the increased parasympathetic and sympathetic tone.

Causes

Maternal related causes:

■ *Fever*
■ *Infection*
■ *Chorioamnionitis*
■ *Dehydration*
■ *Anxiety*
■ *Anemia*
■ *Medications such as betasympathomimetic, sympathomimetic, ketamine, atropine, phenothiazines, and epinephrine*
■ *Illicit drugs*

Fetal related causes:

■ *Infection or sepsis*
■ *Activity/stimulation*
■ *Compensatory effort following acute hypoxemia*
■ *Chronic hypoxemia*
■ *Fetal tachyarrhythmia*
■ *Cardiac abnormalities*
■ *Anemia*

Medical Management

■ Treat the underlying cause of tachycardia, such as antibiotics for infection or fluids for dehydration.
■ Consider delivery.

Nursing Actions

■ Assess maternal vital signs (particularly temperature and pulse), as maternal fever and tachycardia increase FHR.
■ Initiate interventions to decrease maternal temperature, if elevated.
  ■ *Give medications as ordered (i.e., antibiotics, antipyretics)*
  ■ *Use ice packs to decrease maternal fever.*

■ Assess hydration by checking skin turgor, mucous membranes, urine specific gravity, and intake and output.
  ■ *Hydrate the woman by oral intake and/or IV fluids.*
■ Reduce anxiety by explaining, reassuring, and encouraging.
■ Assess FHR variability and consider need for position change or oxygen to promote fetal oxygenation.
■ Decrease or discontinue oxytocin.
■ Notify the physician or midwife.

Fetal Bradycardia

Fetal bradycardia is a baseline FHR of less than 110 bpm.

■ A decreased FHR can lead to decreased cardiac output, which causes a decrease in umbilical blood flow that leads to decreased oxygen to the fetus, causing fetal hypoxia.
■ Unresolved bradycardia may result in fetal hypoxia and needs immediate intervention.
■ Sudden profound bradycardia (less than 80 bpm) is an obstetrical emergency.
■ Bradycardia may be tolerated by the fetus if the FHR remains above 90 bpm with variability.
■ Bradycardia with normal variability may be benign.
■ Bradycardia with loss of variability or late decelerations is associated with current or impending fetal hypoxia (NICHD, 1997).
■ Sudden, profound bradycardia is an obstetrical emergency.

Characteristics

■ FHR less than 110 bpm for more than 10 minutes (**Fig. 9-8**)

Causes

Maternal related:

■ *Supine position*
■ *Dehydration*
■ *Hypotension*

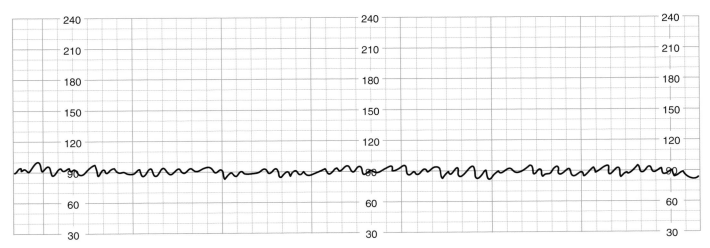

Figure 9–8 Fetal bradycardia.

- *Acute maternal cardiopulmonary compromise (cardiac arrest, seizures)*
- *Rupture of uterus or vasa previa*
- *Placental abruption*
- *Medications such as anesthetics and adrenergic receptors*

Fetal related:

- *Fetal response to hypoxia*
- *Umbilical cord occlusion*
- *Acute hypoxemia*
- *Late or profound hypoxemia*
- *Hypothermia*
- *Hypokalemia*
- *Chronic fetal head compression*
- *Fetal bradyarrythmias*

Medical Management

- Intervene related to the cause of bradycardia.
- Consider delivery.

Nursing Actions

- Confirm if EFM is monitoring FHR versus maternal HR.
- Assess fetal movement.
- Assess the fetal response to fetal scalp stimulation. This is done when FHR is between contractions and when it is definitely determined that baseline has changed.
- Perform a vaginal exam and assess for a prolapsed cord.
- Assess maternal vital signs (especially blood pressure).
- Assess hydration and hydrate prn to reduce UCs and promote fetal oxygenation.
- Depending on FHR variability and other FHR characteristics, consider:
  - *Maternal position change (left or right lateral) to promote fetal oxygenation*
  - *Discontinuing oxytocin to reduce UCs*
  - *Giving oxygen 10 L/min via nonbreather face mask to promote fetal oxygenation*

- *Modifying pushing to every other contraction or stop pushing until the FHR recovers to promote fetal oxygenation*
  - *Encourage open glottis pushing efforts*
  - *Discourage prolonged or sustained breath holding with pushing*
- *Support the woman and her family*
- *Notifying the physician or midwife*

Baseline Variability

Baseline variability refers to the fluctuations in the baseline FHR that are irregular in amplitude and frequency. Cycles portray the peak to trough (rise and fall) of the heart rate within its baseline range over a minute. It is the most important predictor of adequate fetal oxygenation and fetal reserve during labor (AWHONN, 2009). It is a reflection of an intact pathway from the cerebral cortex to the midbrain (medulla oblongata) to the vagus nerve and finally to the heart, and an interaction between the fetal sympathetic and parasympathetic nervous system. Accelerations and decelerations are excluded from the evaluation of baseline variability.

Characteristics

Variability is described as follows:

- **Absent:** Amplitude range is undetectable (**Fig. 9-9**)
- **Minimal:** Amplitude range undetectable ≤5 bpm range (**Fig. 9-10**)
- **Moderate:** Amplitude from peak to trough 6 bpm to 25 bpm (**Fig. 9-11**). Moderate variability predicts a well-oxygenated fetus with normal acid-base balance at the time.
- **Marked:** Amplitude range greater than 25 bpm (**Fig. 9-12**)

Minimal or absent variability can occur when the fetus is in a sleep, sedated by certain central nervous system depressants, such as opiates or magnesium sulfate, or a central

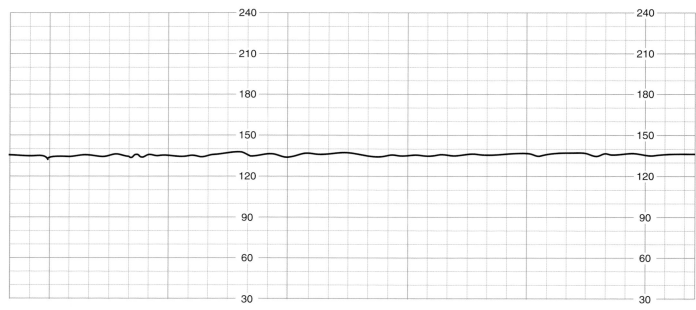

Figure 9-9   Absent variability (abnormal).

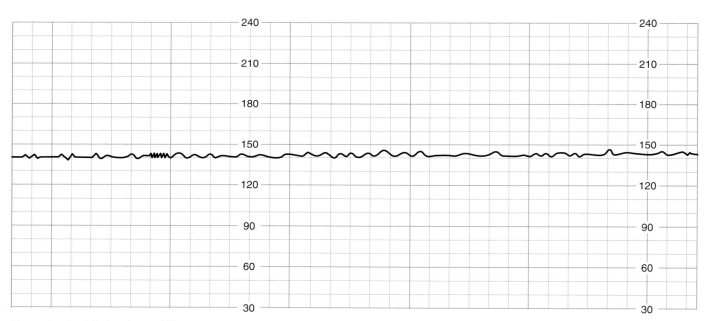

Figure 9-10   Minimal variability.

nervous system that has been previously injured. Minimal or absent variability can also be significant for presence of fetal hypoxia or acidosis especially if persisting over 60 minutes despite interventions as listed below.

Causes of Minimal or Absent Variability

■ Maternal-related:
  ■ *Supine hypotension*
  ■ *Cord compression*
  ■ *Uterine tachysystole*
  ■ *Drugs (prescription, illicit drugs, alcohol)*
■ Fetal-related:
  ■ *Fetal sleep*
  ■ *Prematurity*

Medical Management

■ Consider artificial rupture of membranes (AROM) and more invasive internal monitoring with fetal spiral electrode (FSE).
■ Manage cause of decreased variability.
■ Consider delivery.

Nursing Actions

■ Change the maternal position to promote fetal oxygenation.
■ Assess fetal response to fetal scalp stimulation or vibroacoustic stimulation (VAS).
■ Assess hydration. Give IV bolus to reduce uterine activity and promote uterine perfusion.

■ Discontinue oxytocin to reduce uterine activity.
■ Deliver oxygen to the woman at 10 L/min via non-breather face mask to promote fetal oxygenation.
■ Consider invasive monitoring such as internal FSE.
■ Support the woman and her family.
■ Notify the physician or midwife.

Periodic and Episodic Changes

Periodic changes are accelerations or decelerations in the FHR that are in relation to uterine contractions and persist over time. They include accelerations and four types of decelerations: early, variable, late, and prolonged.

Episodic changes are acceleration and deceleration patterns not associated with contractions. Accelerations are the most common episodic change.

Fetal Heart Rate Accelerations

The presence of FHR accelerations is predictive of adequate central fetal oxygenation and reflects the absence of fetal acidemia. They identify a well-oxygenated fetus and require no intervention. The absence of FHR accelerations, especially in the intrapartum period, however, does not reliably predict fetal acidemia.

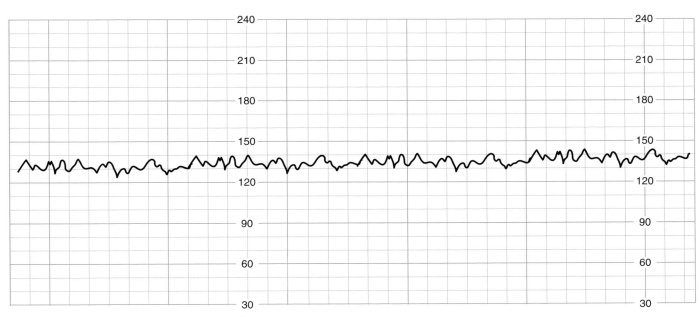

Figure 9–11 Moderate variability (normal).

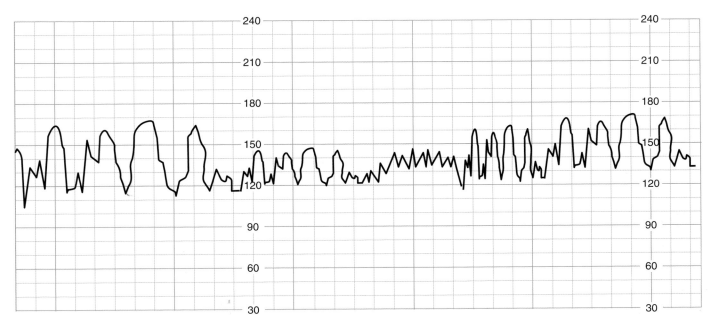

Figure 9–12 Marked variability.

Characteristics

FHR accelerations are the visually abrupt, transient increases (onset to peak <30 seconds) in the FHR above the baseline (**Fig. 9-13**).

■ They are 15 beats above the baseline and last from 15 seconds to less than 2 minutes.
■ Before 32 weeks' gestation, accelerations are defined as acceleration ≥10 bpm or greater over the baseline FHR for ≥10 seconds.
■ Prolonged accelerations are ≥2 minutes, but ≤10 minutes.

Causes

■ Sympathetic response to fetal movement
■ Transient umbilical vein compression

Medical Management

■ None

Nursing Actions

■ Record accelerations in the woman's labor documentation.

Fetal Heart Rate Decelerations

Fetal heart rate decelerations are transitory decreases in the FHR baseline. They are classified as early, variable, late, and prolonged decelerations.

■ They are classified according to their shape, timing, and duration in relationship to the contraction.
■ Decelerations are defined as **recurrent** when they occur with at least 50% of UCs over a 20-minute period
■ Decelerations are defined as **intermittent** when they occur with fewer than 50% of UCs over a 20-minute period.

Early Decelerations

Early decelerations are visually apparent, usually symmetrical, with a gradual decrease and return of FHR associated with a UC (**Fig. 9-14**).

■ They do not occur early or before the contraction starts; thus, this term is something of a misnomer.

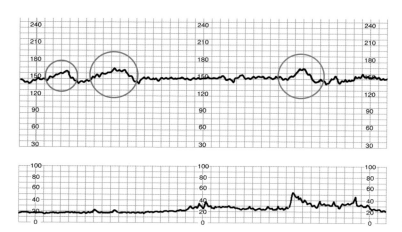

Figure 9–13 Fetal heart rate accelerations.

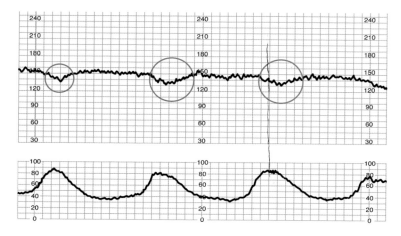

Figure 9–14 Early decelerations.

Characteristics

■ The **nadir** (the lowest point of the deceleration) occurs at the peak of the contraction.
■ Generally the onset, nadir, and the recovery mirror the contraction.

Causes

■ When a UC occurs, the fetal head is subjected to pressure that stimulates the vagal nerve.
■ Fetal head compression resulting in increased intracranial pressure, decreased transient cerebral blood flow, and corresponding decrease in Po_2 with stimulation of cerebral chemoreceptor (**Fig. 9-15**)

Medical Management

■ None

Nursing Actions

■ Early decelerations are benign and no intervention is needed.

Variable Decelerations

A **variable deceleration** is a visually apparent abrupt decrease in the FHR.

■ They are the most common decelerations seen in labor.
■ When variable decelerations persist over time, fetal tolerance is confirmed by the presence of variability or accelerations in the FHR (Lyndon & Ali, 2009).
■ An acceleration that precedes or follows the deceleration is a shoulder. It is a compensatory response to hypoxemia and is an increase in the FHR of 20 bpm for <20 seconds.

Characteristics

■ They can be periodic or episodic and may vary in duration, depth or nadir, and timing in relation to UCs (**Fig. 9-16**).
■ The decrease in FHR is ≥15 bpm lasting ≥15 seconds and <2 minutes in duration.
■ The shape can be a U, W, or V.
■ The depth of the deceleration is not related to fetal hypoxemia or acidosis.
■ They can mimic early or late decelerations.

CRITICAL COMPONENT

Intrauterine Resuscitation Interventions

Interventions for category II and III indeterminate or abnormal FHR patterns are referred to as **intrauterine resuscitation** (See Fig. 9-5). These interventions maximize uterine blood flow, umbilical circulation, and maternal fetal oxygenation (AWHONN, 2009; Lyndon & Ali, 2009; Simpson, 2004b; Lyndon, O'Brien-Abel, Simpson, 2014, Simpson & James, 2005). Interventions include:

■ Maternal positioning to minimize or correct cord compression and decrease frequency of UCs and improve uterine blood flow (either left or right)
■ Administration of IV bolus of fluid of at least 500 mL of lactated Ringer's to maximize maternal intravascular volume and improve uteroplacental perfusion
■ Correct maternal hypotension with positioning, hydration, and ephedrine prn
■ Administration of O_2 at 10 L/min via non-rebreather face mask to improve fetal oxygen status
■ Reduction of uterine activity if UCs are too frequent, as there may be insufficient time for blood to perfuse placenta.
  ■ Decrease or discontinue oxytocin.
  ■ Remove cervical ripening agent, if possible.
  ■ Terbutaline may be used to relax the uterus.
■ Amnioinfusion has been used to resolve variable FHR deceleration by correcting umbilical cord compression as a result of oligohydramnios in the first stage of labor.
  ■ Amnioinfusion is a procedure in which a saline solution at room temperature is introduced transcervically via an IUPC to correct the FHR decelerations associated with cord compression and/or decreased amniotic fluid.

■ Encourage physiologic pushing techniques, alter pushing efforts, or stop pushing, or pushing with every other or every third UC to provide time for fetus to recover when FHR is indeterminate or abnormal during the second stage.
■ Support the woman and her family to decrease anxiety or pain, and improve uterine blood flow and maximize oxygenation to fetus.
■ Obtain fetal acid-base status if possible with scalp or Vas or fetal scalp sampling if available.

Abnormal FHR patterns are associated with fetal acidemia.

■ Notify primary provider.
■ The presence of one of the abnormal patterns warrants immediate bedside evaluation by a physician who can initiate a cesarean birth.
■ Notify or activate OR, anesthesia, and pediatric teams as indicated.
■ Move patient to OR as indicated.

When a Category II or III FHR pattern is identified, initial assessment may also include:

■ Assess maternal vital signs, especially:
  ■ Maternal temperature for maternal fever and maternal blood pressure for hypotension
■ Assess uterine activity for uterine tachysystole.
■ Perform cervical exam to assess for:
  ■ Umbilical cord prolapse
  ■ Rapid cervical dilation
  ■ Rapid descent of fetal head

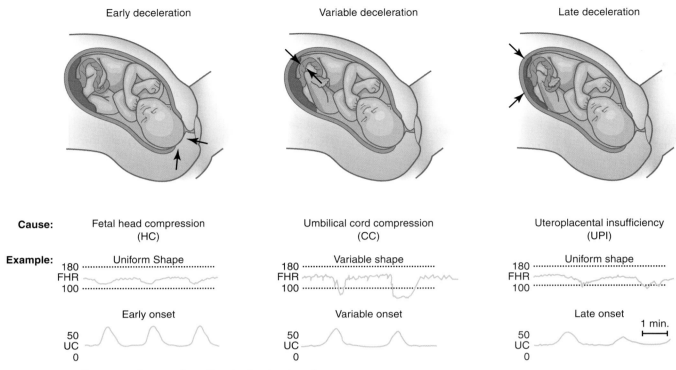

Early deceleration	Variable deceleration	Late deceleration

Cause: Fetal head compression (HC) | Umbilical cord compression (CC) | Uteroplacental insufficiency (UPI)

Example: Uniform Shape | Variable shape | Uniform shape

Early onset | Variable onset | Late onset

Figure 9-15   Causes and examples of periodic decelerations.

- An overshoot or rebound overshoot is a gradual smooth acceleration in FHR of 10–20 bpm for >60–90 seconds.
- Characteristics of normal variable decelerations include:
  - *Duration of <60 seconds*
  - *Rapid return to baseline*
  - *Accompanied by normal baseline and variability*
- Characteristics of indeterminate or abnormal variable decelerations include:
  - *Prolonged return to baseline*
  - *Persistence to less than 60 bpm and 60 seconds*
  - *Presence of overshoots tachycardia*
  - *Repetitive overshoots and absent variability*

Causes

- Umbilical cord occlusion
- Umbilical cord compression triggers a vagal response that slows the FHR, usually related to decreased cord perfusion.

- This results in initial compression of the umbilical vein (decreased PO_2 and chemoreceptor stimulation) and then compression of the more muscular umbilical arteries (fetal hypertension with resultant baroreceptors stimulation; remember that hypertension is often accompanied with a corresponding drop in heart rate) (see Fig. 9-15).
- Prolonged cord compression produces a decrease in PO_2 with direct myocardial depression, adrenal activation, and rebound tachycardia (note: rebound tachycardia does not always occur).
- Variable decelerations can also occur with sudden descent of the vertex late in active phase of labor (i.e., head compression).
- These appear different from early decelerations in that they are usually not repetitive nor smooth or regular in shape.

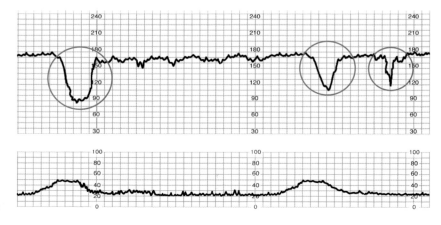

Figure 9-16   Variable decelerations.

Medical Management

■ Consider amnioinfusion (see Critical Component: Amnioinfusion).
■ Consider tocolytics.
■ Consider delivery.

Nursing Actions (see Critical Component: Intrauterine Resuscitation Interventions and Fig. 9-5)

■ Change the maternal position to promote fetal oxygenation.
■ Perform SVE to evaluate cord and labor progress and perform fetal scalp stimulation.
■ Perform amnioinfusion if ordered to alleviate umbilical cord compression by increasing volume of fluid in uterus and thereby correcting umbilical cord compression (see Critical Component: Amnioinfusion).
■ Administer O_2 at 10 L/min via non-rebreather face mask to improve fetal oxygen status.
■ Decrease or discontinue oxytocin.
■ Consider need for tocolytic to reduce UCs.
■ Consider more invasive monitoring with fetal spiral electrode (FSE).
■ Modify pushing.
■ Support the woman and her family to decrease anxiety or pain.
■ Notify the physician or midwife.
■ Plan for delivery and care of the neonate.

CRITICAL COMPONENT

Amnioinfusion

Amnioinfusion is a therapeutic option when there are recurrent variable decelerations as a result of decreased amniotic fluid. During amnioinfusion, room temperature normal saline is infused into the uterus transcervically via an intrauterine pressure catheter to increase intraamniotic fluid to cushion the umbilical cord and reduce cord compression.

Indications: Variable decelerations in first stage of labor
Contraindications: Vaginal bleeding, uterine anomalies, and active infection

Careful monitoring of maternal and fetal response is needed; documentation of fluid infused is also important to avoid iatrogenic polyhydramnios.

(Lyndon & Ali, 2009, Lyndon, O'Brien-Abel, & Simpson,2014)

Late Decelerations

Late deceleration is a visually apparent symmetrical gradual decrease of FHR associated with UCs.

■ Late decelerations can be a sign of fetal intolerance to labor.
■ Fetal tolerance of late decelerations is assessed by evaluating the baseline, presence of variability, and the presence of accelerations.

Characteristics

■ Onset is gradual with onset to nadir ≥30 seconds **(Fig. 9-17)**.
■ Nadir (lowest point) of the deceleration occurs after the peak of the contraction.
■ In most cases the onset, nadir, and recovery of the deceleration occurs after the respective onset, peak, and end of the UC.
■ Nadir decreases 10–20 bpm and rarely 30–40 bpm (Freeman, Garite, & Nageotte, 2003).

Causes

■ Reflect fetal response to transient or chronic uteroplacental insufficiency
■ Related to decreased availability of O_2 because of uteroplacental insufficiency (see Fig. 9-15)
■ Suppression of the fetal myocardium
■ Late decelerations are not completely understood.
  ■ *Usually related to placental insufficiency (in which case they are often accompanied by decreased or absent FHR variability)*
  ■ *Late decelerations with moderate variability reflect a compensatory response and are not associated with significant fetal acidemia.*
  ■ *Late decelerations with minimal or absent variability reflect hypoxia and represent a risk of significant fetal acidemia.*
  ■ *Can be related to aorto-caval compression or obstetrical anesthesia, in which case they are usually accompanied by moderate FHR variability and can be corrected by position change or improving maternal blood pressure. This latter type of late deceleration is sometimes referred to as a "reflex late deceleration."*
  ■ *Fetal hypoxia stimulates chemoreceptors when it is acute (i.e., recently occurring) and, if prolonged, results from direct myocardial depression.*
  ■ *Maternal related factors associated with decreased uteroplacental circulation include:*
    ■ Hypotension from regional anesthesia, supine positioning, or maternal hemorrhage
    ■ Maternal hypertension, gestational or chronic
    ■ Placental changes affecting gas exchange such as postmaturity or placental abnormalities
    ■ Decreased maternal hemoglobin or oxygen saturation from severe anemia or cardiopulmonary disease
    ■ Uterine tachysystole

Medical Management

■ Interventions are directed at causes of late decelerations.
■ Consider tocolytics.
■ Consider delivery.

Nursing Actions (see Critical Component: Intrauterine Resuscitation Interventions and Fig. 9-5)

■ The degree to which the deceleration is abnormal depends on the status and response of the fetus after the deceleration.
■ Change the maternal position to promote fetal oxygenation.

- Discontinue oxytocin (consider terbutaline) to reduce uterine activity.
- Assess hydration. Give an IV bolus to promote fetal oxygenation.
- Consider fetal scalp stimulation or VAS to assess fetal status.
- Administer O_2 at 10 L/min via non-rebreather face mask to improve fetal oxygen status.
- Consider more invasive monitoring with fetal spiral electrode (FSE).
- Support the woman and her family.
- Notify the physician or midwife.
- Plan for delivery and care of the neonate.

Prolonged Decelerations

Prolonged deceleration is a visually apparent abrupt decrease in FHR below baseline that is ≥15 bpm, lasting ≥2 minutes but <10 minutes (**Fig. 9-18**).

- Prolonged decelerations that are not recurrent and are preceded and followed by normal baseline and moderate variability are not associated with fetal hypoxemia.

Characteristics

- Episodic decelerations that last >2 minutes and <10 minutes
- May be abrupt or gradual

Causes

- May be any mechanism that causes a profound change in the fetal O_2
- Interruption of uteroplacental perfusion
  - *Tachysystole*
  - *Maternal hypotension*
  - *Abruptio placenta*
- Interruption of umbilical blood flow
  - *Cord compression*
  - *Cord prolapse*
- Vagal stimulation
  - *Profound head compression*
  - *Rapid fetal descent*

Medical Management

- Treat the cause of prolonged deceleration.
- Consider amnioinfusion.
- Consider tocolytics.
- Consider delivery.

Nursing Actions (see Critical Component: Intrauterine Resuscitation Interventions and see Fig. 9-5)

- Assess baseline variability preceding and following deceleration.
- Change the maternal position to improve fetal oxygenation.
- Discontinue oxytocin (consider terbutaline) to decrease the UCs.
- Administer O_2 at 10 L/min via non-rebreather face mask to improve fetal oxygen status.
- Assess hydration. Give an IV bolus to promote fetal oxygenation.
- Perform SVE to assess labor and cord, and perform scalp stimulation.
- Perform amnioinfusion, if ordered, to alleviate umbilical cord compression.
- Consider more invasive monitoring with fetal spiral electrode (FSE).
- Support the woman and her family.
- Notify the physician or midwife.
- Plan for delivery and care of the neonate.

Uterine Activity and Contraction Patterns

Uterine activity is an integral part of fetal monitoring interpretation. Interpretation of the FHR pattern is done in concurrence with uterine activity. Interpretation of uterine activity includes assessment of contractions' frequency, duration, and intensity, and uterine resting tone (**Fig. 9-19**). Uterine activity can be monitored by palpation or via an IUPC.

- **Frequency of contractions** is determined by counting number of contractions in a 10-minute period, counting from the start of one contraction to the start of the next contraction in minutes. It is recorded in

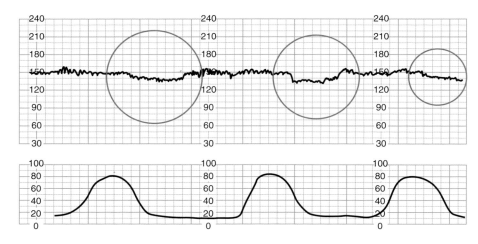

Figure 9–17 Late decelerations.

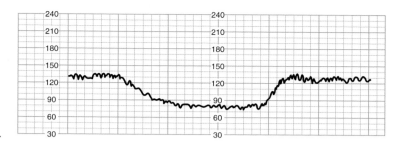

Figure 9-18 Prolonged deceleration.

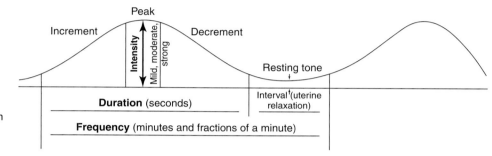

Figure 9-19 Example of contraction frequency, duration, intensity, and resting tone.

minutes (i.e., frequency of contractions is every 3 minutes).
- **Duration of contractions** is measured by counting from the beginning to the end of one contraction and measured in seconds. Because contractions often vary in their duration, this is often calculated for several contractions and expressed as a range.
- **Intensity** is strength of the contraction and measured by palpation, or internally by an IUPC in mm Hg.
- **Resting tone** is the pressure in the uterus between contractions. It is measured by an IUPC when internal fetal monitoring is used or by palpation when an external monitor is used. It is described as the number of mm Hg when the uterus is not contracting when an IUPC is being used and as "soft" if the uterus feels relaxed by palpation.
- **Normal:** 5 or fewer contractions in 10 minutes averaged over a 30-minute window
- **Tachysystole:** More than 5 contractions in 10 minutes over a 30-minute window

Tachysystole

Tachysystole, also referred to as **hyperstimulation,** is excessive uterine activity (**Fig. 9-20**).

- *Contraction patterns that may contribute to fetal hypoxia*
- *Tachysystole should be treated regardless of fetal response.*
- *Tachysystole can result in decreased uteroplacental blood flow and result in indeterminate or abnormal fetal heart rate patterns.*

Characteristics of Tachysystole

- More than 5 contractions in 10 minutes
- Contractions lasting 2 minutes or longer

- Contractions occurring within 1 minute of each other
- Increasing resting tone greater than 20–25 mm Hg, peak pressure greater than 80 mm Hg, or Montevideo units greater than 400

Causes

- Tachysystole can be spontaneous or stimulated labor.
- Most commonly, tachysystole can be caused by medications used for cervical ripening, induction, and augmentation of labor.

Medical Management

- Manage cause of tachysystole (e.g., discontinuing oxytocin, removing cervical ripening medication). See Chapter 10.

Nursing Actions

- Reducing uterine activity can be accomplished with a variety of interventions, such as the following (these practices are known as intrauterine resuscitation):
  - *Changing maternal position*
  - *Providing hydration*
  - *Using IV fluid bolus*
  - *Reducing maternal anxiety or pain*
  - *Administering a tocolytic (terbutaline)*
  - *Supporting woman and family*

SPECIAL MONITORING CIRCUMSTANCES

Monitoring the Preterm Fetus

As noted in Chapter 7, preterm labor can be defined as the onset of labor at less than 37 weeks' gestation. With the current preterm birth rate continuing to rise (Martin et al., 2010),

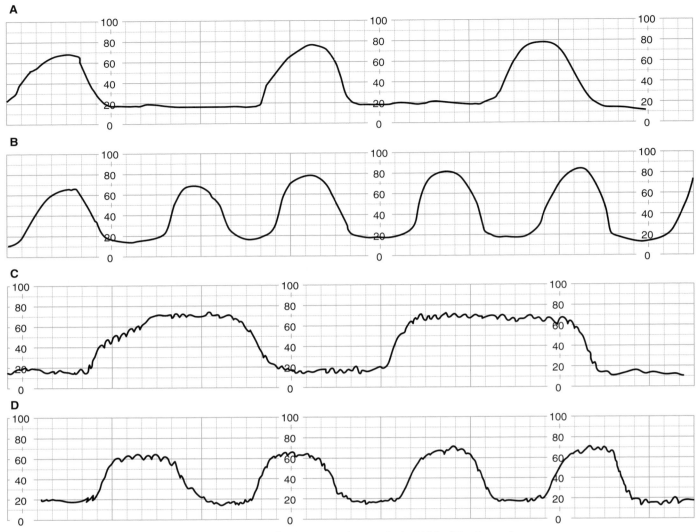

Figure 9-20 Examples of UC patterns. *A.* Normal UCs. *B.* Tachysystole (<5 UCs 10 minutes). *C.* Tachysystole (tetanic contraction verified by palpation). *D.* Tachysystole (inadequate interval of resting tone between UCs).

monitoring a preterm fetus during the antepartum and intrapartum period is a common occurrence in many obstetrical units. Two important points to remember when caring for the mother with a preterm fetus are:

■ Physiologic responses of the preterm fetus are dependent on the stage of development of the fetus.
■ Physiologic responses and tolerance to stress (maternal tachycardia and sepsis) in the preterm fetus can be different (more rapid deterioration) from those in the term fetus.

Characteristics include:

■ Higher baseline although still within normal FHR range
■ Accelerations may be of lower amplitude (see earlier section on accelerations)—accelerations of at least 10 bpm of baseline lasting 10 seconds are considered to be acceptable for fetus less than 32 weeks' gestation (Mascones et al., 2008). However, once the preterm fetus (sometimes as early by 24–26 weeks) demonstrates

accelerations of 15 beats per minute above baseline that last for 15 seconds, the fetus is generally held to that criteria in subsequent evaluations (Baird & Ruth, 2002).
■ Variability may be decreased, although specific parameters have not been quantified (Freeman, Garite, & Nageotte, 2003).
■ Variable decelerations may occur more frequently in the preterm fetus even in the absence of contractions (Druzin, Smith, Gabbe, & Reed, 2007). During labor, variable decelerations occur in approximately 70%–75% of preterm fetuses compared to 30%–50% in term fetuses (Freeman, Garite, & Nageotte, 2003).
■ Late and prolonged decelerations occur at the same frequency in preterm labor as in term labor. But conditions associated with late decelerations, such as IUGR, preeclampsia, and abruption, are more commonly present during preterm labor (Simpson, 2004).

■ Magnesium sulfate decreases FHR variability and acceleration amplitude in preterm infants.
■ Beta-sympathomimetics (e.g., terbutaline) are associated by tachycardia in both mother and fetus.

The preterm fetus is more likely to be subjected to hypoxia. These include conditions such as preeclampsia, abruption, and intrauterine infection that frequently are either the indication for, or a cause of, preterm delivery. The loss of variability in a preterm fetus is more predictive of acidosis and depressed Apgar scores at birth than for a term infant (Froen, Heazell, Tveit, Saaseted, Fretts, & Flenady, 2008).

It is therefore important to continually evaluate trends and continually assess the maternal and fetal condition when making clinical decisions regarding the antepartum and intrapartum management of the preterm fetus.

Monitoring the Woman with Multiple Gestation

Current monitors have the capability of monitoring twins (or higher multiples) at the same time due to the presence of two ultrasound transducers on the same monitor. The dual tracings distinguish each fetus by a thicker or darker tracing for one fetus and a thinner or lighter tracing for the other. To more clearly distinguish between the fetuses, their positions on the mother's abdomen can be documented as well as the transducers appropriately labeled. In identifying twins or higher multiples, the more advanced (lower in uterus) fetus is labeled as A, the next one B, and so on. Once the membranes are ruptured, it is recommended that the more advanced fetus is monitored by a scalp electrode, to distinguish it from the other fetus. Two monitors are required for higher multiples, with the third fetus on the second monitor which has an identical clock setting to the first one (Tucker et al., 2004).

At the time of birth, the first twin that is delivered may not necessarily be twin A, especially with cesarean sections. In that case, the medical chart should be written as first twin (B) and second twin (A) or vice versa.

Other Topics

Monitoring of fetal arrhythmias and sinusoidal pattern (a Category III or impending decompensation fetal response) is beyond the scope of this chapter. Resources are cited for more in-depth exploration and advanced concepts in fetal monitoring. Antenatal fetal surveillance and testing are discussed in Chapter 6.

DOCUMENTATION OF ELECTRONIC MONITORING INTERPRETATION—UTERINE ASSESSMENT

Documentation of fetal monitoring consists of the elements described in Critical Component: Assessment and Documentation of Electronic Fetal Monitoring and **Figure 9-21.**

CRITICAL COMPONENT

Assessment and Documentation of Electronic Fetal Monitoring

FHR	UC
External/ultrasound	External/tocodynamometry
■ FHR baseline ■ Baseline variability ■ Presence of accelerations ■ Periodic or episodic decelerations	■ Frequency ■ Duration ■ Palpate strength of UCs and resting tone
Internal/fetal scalp electrode	Internal/intrauterine pressure catheter
■ FHR baseline ■ Baseline variability ■ Presence of accelerations ■ Periodic or episodic decelerations ■ FHR dysrythmias	■ Frequency ■ Duration ■ Strength of uterine contractions and resting tone (in mm Hg)

Patient Name:		Physician/CNM:			
	DATE:				KEY
	TIME:				**Variability**
Cervix	Dilation				Ab = Absent (undetectable)
	Effacement				Min = Minimal (>0 out ≤5 bpm)
					Mod = Moderate (6–25 bpm)
	Station				Mar = Marked (>25 bpm)
Fetal Heart	Baseline Rate				**Accelerations**
					+ = Present and appropriate
	Variability				for gestational age
	Accelerations				Ø = Absent
					Decelerations
	Decelerations				E = Early
					L = Late
	STIM/pH				V = Variable
					P = Prolonged
	Monitor Mode				**Stim/pH**
					+ = Acceleration in response
Uterine Activity	Frequency				to stimulation
					Ø = No response to stimulation
	Duration				Record number for scalp pH
					Monitor mode
	Intensity				A = Auscultation/Palpation
					E = External u/s or toco
	Resting Tone				FSE - Fetal spiral electrode
					IUPC = Intrauterine pressure
	Monitor Mode				catheter
					P = Palpation
	Oxytocin milliunits/min				T = Telemetry
	Pain				**Frequency of uterine activity**
					Ø = None
	Coping				Irreg = Irregular
					Intensity of uterine activity
	Maternal Position				M = Mild
					Mod = Moderate
	O2/LPM/Mask				Str = Strong
					By IUPC = mm Hg
	IV				**Resting tone**
					R = Relaxed
	Nurse Initials				By IUCP = mm Hg
Narrative notes:					**Coping**
					W = Well
					S = Support provided
					For pain use 0–10 scale
					Maternal position
					A = Ambulatory
					U = Upright
					SF = Semi-Fowler's
					RL = Right lateral
					LL = Left lateral
					MS = Modified Sims'

Figure 9–21   Example of FHR documentation.

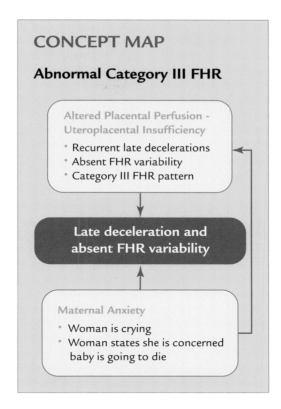

CONCEPT MAP

Abnormal Category III FHR

Altered Placental Perfusion - Uteroplacental Insufficiency
* Recurrent late decelerations
* Absent FHR variability
* Category III FHR pattern

Late deceleration and absent FHR variability

Maternal Anxiety
* Woman is crying
* Woman states she is concerned baby is going to die

Problem No. 1: Category III FHR
Goal: Improve placental perfusion. Fetus will become well perfused and oxygenated; cord gases indicate no respiratory or metabolic acidosis.
Outcome: Fetus will become well perfused and oxygenated; cord gases indicate no respiratory or metabolic acidosis.

Nursing Actions

1. Change maternal position (left, right, lateral, or hands and knees).
2. Administer 500 cc IV bolus of fluid.
3. Perform cervical exam to assess cord prolapse, rapid cervical dilation, or rapid descent of the fetal head.
4. Assess uterine activity for uterine tachysystole.
5. Assess maternal vital signs, especially temperature, for maternal fever, and blood pressure for hypotension.
6. Administer O_2 at 10 L/min via non-rebreather face mask to improve fetal oxygen status.
7. Consider discontinuing oxytocin if in use.
8. Consider use of terbutaline to stop UCs.
9. Alter pushing efforts, or stop pushing, or pushing with every other or every third UC to provide time for fetus to recover when FHR is Category III during second stage.
10. Request an immediate bedside evaluation by a physician or midwife.

Problem No. 2: Anxiety related to harm for fetus
Goal: Decreased anxiety
Outcome: Patient verbalizes that she feels less anxious.

Nursing Actions

1. Be calm and attentive in interactions with the patient and her family.
2. Explain all procedures and interventions.
3. Explain current fetal status.
4. Assist patient with breathing and relaxation techniques.
5. Encourage the patient and her family to verbalize their feelings regarding concern for the fetus.
6. Remain with the patient and her family.

■ ■ ■ Review Questions ■ ■ ■

1. Which of the following indicates a Category I fetal heart rate?
   A. Baseline rate of 170 bpm, decreased variability, no fetal heart rate decelerations
   B. Baseline rate of 150 bpm, moderate variability, accelerations to 170 bpm for 20 seconds
   C. Baseline rate of 150 bpm, decreased variability, no fetal heart rate decelerations
   D. Baseline rate of 130 bpm, average variability, decreases after uterine contractions

2. Potential causes of late decelerations include:
   A. Maternal fever
   B. Umbilical cord compression
   C. Uteroplacental insufficiency
   D. Fetal activity

3. The goal of maternal position changes for a prolonged deceleration is:
   A. Maximizing uterine blood flow
   B. Increasing uterine contractions
   C. Maximizing maternal oxygenation
   D. Increasing maternal movement

4. Increased information provided by assessment of uterine contractions with an intrauterine pressure catheter includes:
   A. Frequency, duration, intensity, and resting tone
   B. Frequency, duration, and intensity
   C. Intensity only
   D. Labor progress

5. Fetal heart rate should be assessed in a low-risk woman in active labor:
   A. Every 5 minutes
   B. Every 10 minutes
   C. Every 15 minutes
   D. Every 30 minutes

5. Fetal heart rate should be assessed in a low-risk woman in active phase of labor:
   A. Every 5 minutes
   B. Every 10 minutes
   C. Every 15 minutes
   D. Every 30 minutes

6. Variable decelerations are typically related to:
   A. Cord compression
   B. Head compression
   C. Uteroplacental insufficiency
   D. Uterine hyperstimulation due to hypovolemia

7. Nursing interventions related to late decelerations include all of the following except:
   A. Initiate pitocin induction
   B. Initiate IV bolus
   C. Change maternal position
   D. Initiate oxygen therapy

References

Alfirevic, Z. (2008). Continuous cardiotocography (CTG) as a form of electronic fetal monitoring (EFM) for fetal assessment during labour. *Cochrane Database of Systematic Reviews,* (4).

American College of Obstetrics and Gynecologists. (2010). *Management of Intrapartum Fetal Heart Rate Tracing, Practice Bulletin #116. Obstetrics and Gynecology,* 116(5), 1232–1240.

Association of Women's Health, Obstetric and Neonatal Nurses (AWHONN). (2009). *Fetal Heart Monitoring Principles and Practices, Fourth Edition.* Washington, DC.

Coletta, J., Murphy, E., Rubeo, Z., et al. (2012). The 5-tier system of assessing fetal heart rate tracings is superior to the 3-tier system in identifying fetal academia. *American Journal of Obstetrics and Gynecology;* 206:226.e1-5.

Cunningham, E. G., Leveno, K. J., Bloom, S. L., Hauth, J. C., Rouse, D. J., & Spong, C. Y. (2010). *Williams Obstetrics* (23rd ed.). New York: McGraw-Hill.

Feinstein, N., Sprague, A., & Trepanier, M. (2008). *Fetal heart rate auscultation* (2nd ed.) Washington, DC: Association of Women's Health, Obstetric and Neonatal Nurses.

Freeman, R. (2002). Problems with intrapartum fetal heart rate monitoring interpretation and patient management. *American College of Obstetricians and Gynecologists,* 100(4), 813–826.

Freeman, R., Garite, T., & Nageotte, M. (2003). *Fetal heart rate monitoring* (3rd ed.). Philadelphia: Lippincott Williams & Wilkins.

Lyndon, A. & Ali, L. U. (Eds.). (2009). *AWHONN's Fetal heart rate monitoring: Principles and practice* (4th Ed.). Dubuque, IA: Kendal/Hunt.

Lyndon, A., O'Brien-Abel, N., & Simpson, K. (2014) Fetal assessment during labor in Simpson, K., & Creehan, P., (2014). *Perinatal nursing* (4th ed.). Philadelphia: Lippincott Williams & Wilkins.

Macones, G., Hankins, G., Spong, C., Hauth, J., & Moore, T. (2008). The 2008 National Institute of Child Health and Human Development Workshop Report on Electronic Fetal Monitoring: Update on Definitions, Interpretation, and Research Guidelines. *Journal of Obstetric, Gynecologic and Neonatal Nurses,* 37, 510–515.

Martin, J. A., Hamilton, B. E., Sutton, P. D. (2010). *Are Preterm Births on Decline in the United States? Recent Data from the National Vital Statistics System,* Vital Statistics system NCHS Data Brief, No. 31. Hyattsville, MD: U.S. Department of Health and Human Services, DCD, National Center for Health Statistics.

Menihan, C., & Kopel, E. (2008). *Electronic Fetal Monitoring, Concepts and Applications, Second Edition.* Philadelphia: Lippincott Williams & Wilkins.

Murray, M. (2004). Maternal or Fetal Heart Rate? Avoiding Intrapartum Misidentification, *Journal of Obstetrical Gynecological and Neonatal Nursing,* 33(1), 93–103.

National Institute of Child Health and Human Development. (1997). Electronic fetal heart rate monitoring: Research guidelines for interpretation. *Journal of Obstetric Gynecology and Neonatal Nursing,* 26(6), 635–640.

National Institute of Child Health and Human Development Research Planning Workshop. (1997). Electronic fetal heart rate monitoring: Research guidelines for interpretation. *American Journal of Obstetrics and Gynecology,* 177(6), 1385–1390.

Parer, J. T., & Hamilton, E. F. (2010). Comparison of 5 experts and computer analysis in rule-based fetal heart rate interpretation. *American Journal of Obstetrics and Gynecology* 203(5): 451.e1-7.

Parer, J. T., & Ikeda, T. (2007). A framework for standardized management of intrapartum fetal heart rate patterns. *American Journal of Obstetrics and Gynecology,* 197:26.e1-26.e6.

Simpson, K. (2004a). Standardized language for electronic fetal heart rate monitoring. *American Journal of Maternal/Child Nursing,* 29(5), 336.

Simpson, K. (2004b). Fetal assessment in the adult intensive care unit. *Critical Care Nursing Clinics of North America, 16,* 233–242.

Simpson, K. (2009). *Cervical ripening and induction and augmentation of labor* (3rd ed., updated). Washington, DC: Association of Women's Health, Obstetric and Neonatal Nurses.

Simpson, K., & James, D. (2005). Efficacy of intrauterine resuscitation techniques in improving fetal oxygen status during labor. *American College of Obstetricians and Gynecologists, 105*(6), 1362–1368.

Tucker, S., Miller, S., & Miller, D. (2009). *Fetal Monitoring, A Multidisciplinary Approach, Sixth Edition.* St Louis: Mosby Inc.

High-Risk Labor and Birth

OBJECTIVES

Expected student outcomes:

- ☐ Define key terms.
- ☐ Describe the primary causes of dystocia and the related nursing and medical care.
- ☐ Demonstrate understanding of knowledge related to induction of labor and augmentation of labor and vaginal birth after cesarean birth.
- ☐ Identify potential complications of dystocia in labor and related medical and nursing care.
- ☐ Identify and manage high-risk pregnancy, labor, and delivery to promote healthy outcomes for the mother and infant.
- ☐ Describe the key obstetrical emergencies and the related medical and nursing care.

Nursing Diagnoses

- ■ Risk of maternal injury related to interventions implemented for dystocia
- ■ Risk of maternal injury related to obstetrical emergencies
- ■ Risk of fetal injury related to complications of labor and birth
- ■ Anxiety related to labor and birth complications.

Nursing Outcomes

- ■ The woman will understand the causes of dystocia and interventions to achieve a normal labor pattern.
- ■ The woman will give birth without maternal or fetal injury.
- ■ The woman will give birth to a healthy infant without complications.
- ■ The woman verbalizes understanding of the situation and plan of care and uses effective coping methods.

INTRODUCTION

Most pregnant women go into labor spontaneously and have a normal labor and spontaneous vaginal birth. However, interventions to initiate or accelerate labor and birth are increasingly common. This chapter presents problems encountered during labor and birth and interventions related to those complications. Nurses have a key role in identification of complications and implementing nursing actions in response to them to improve maternal and neonatal outcomes.

DYSTOCIA

Dystocia is abnormal labor that results from abnormalities of the power, the passenger, or the passage (American College of Obstetrics and Gynecology [ACOG], 2003). It is diagnosed when there is an alteration in the progress of labor related to cervical dilation and/or descent of the fetus.

Dystocia is the most common reason for primary cesarean sections (Queenan, Hobbins, & Spong, 2005). It is associated with the same factors that influence normal labor; the 4 Ps are discussed in Chapter 8:

- ■ **Powers** of labor (uterine contractions [UCs])
- ■ **Passenger** (fetal aspects/position)
- ■ **Passage** (pelvis)
- ■ **Psychological** response of the woman

Dysfunctional labor is abnormal UCs that prevent the normal progress of cervical dilation or descent of the fetus. Abnormal uterine activity typically has a hypertonic or hypotonic pattern. The American College of Obstetricians and Gynecologists (ACOG, 1995) currently suggests two practical classifications of abnormal labor in the active phase:

- ■ Protraction disorders: Slower than normal labor
- ■ Arrest disorders: Complete cessation of UCs

The primary issues impacting nursing care with regard to dystocia are related to uterine factors, which are described in

Don't have time to read this chapter? Want to reinforce your reading? Need to review for a test?
Listen to this chapter on *DavisPlus*.

this chapter. Other factors are presented in Chapter 8. Risk factors for dystocia include:

- Congenital uterine abnormalities such as bicorniate uterus (SEPTUM IMMIDDLE)
- Malpresentation of the fetus such as occiput posterior, or face presentation
- Cephalopelvic disproportion
- Tachysystole of the uterus with oxytocin
- Maternal fatigue and dehydration
- Administration of analgesia or anesthesia early in labor
- Extreme maternal fear or exhaustion, which can result in catecholamine release interfering with uterine contractility.

Hypertonic Uterine Dysfunction

Hypertonic uterine dysfunction is uncoordinated uterine activity. Contractions are frequent and painful but ineffective in promoting dilation and effacement. When this occurs in early labor it may be referred to as **prodromal labor.** Women who experience hypertonic uterine dysfunction are at risk for exhaustion related to the prolonged labor, and the fetus is at risk for fetal intolerance of labor and asphyxia related to decreased placental profusion.

Risk Factors

- Nulliparous woman are more subject to abnormal early labor. (FIRST PREGNANCY)

Assessment Findings

- Painful, frequent UCs with inadequate uterine relaxation between UCs with little cervical changes (**Fig. 10-1B**).
- May be Category II (indeterminate) or Category III (abnormal) fetal heart rate (FHR) related to prolonged labor and inadequate uterine relaxation

Medical Management

- Evaluate labor progress.
- Evaluate cause of labor dysfunction.
- Hydrate to improve uterine perfusion and coordination of UCs.
- Provide pain management to allow the woman to sleep and prevent exhaustion. (SLEEPING THE PATIENT)

Nursing Actions

- Promote rest to try to break the pattern of frequent but ineffective UCs. The pattern typically becomes effective when the woman sleeps for a period of several hours and awakens in a normal labor pattern of active labor. Methods used to promote uterine rest are:
  - *Administration of pain medication such as Demerol or morphine as per order to decrease labor contractions and allow the uterus to rest*
  - *Promotion of relaxation*
    - Warm shower or tub bath
    - Quiet environment
    - Minimal interruptions to allow for long period of sleep

- Hydrate the woman with IV or PO fluids if tolerated. Dehydration can result in dysfunctional labor.
- Assess FHR and UCs.
- Evaluate labor progress with a sterile vaginal exam (SVE).
- Inform the woman and family of the progress of labor and explain interventions.
- Inform the care provider of the woman's response and progress in labor.

Hypotonic Uterine Dysfunction   PALPATE FOR (MILD/MOD) FIRM CONTRACTIONS ACT PRESSURE INTRUUT CATH!

Hypotonic uterine dysfunction occurs when the pressure of the UC is insufficient (IUPC pressure <25 mm Hg) to promote cervical dilation and effacement (Gilbert & Harmon, 2003). Typically, the woman makes normal progress during the latent phase of labor, but during active labor the UCs become weaker and less effective for cervical changes and labor progress (see Fig. 10-1A). The woman is at risk for exhaustion and infection related to the prolonged labor, and the fetus is at risk for fetal intolerance of labor and asphyxia.

Risk Factors

- Multiparous women often have more problems in the active phase. (TYP W/ BABIES CLOSE TOGETHER)
- Extreme fear may result in catecholamine release, interfering with uterine contractility.

Assessment Findings   IN ACTIVE PHASE

- Decreased frequency, strength, and duration of UCs
- Little or no cervical change
  - *Less than 0.5 cm/hr progress in cervical dilation for a primiparous woman in active labor*
  - *Less than 1.0 cm/hr progress in cervical dilation for a multiparous woman in active labor*
- Increased fear and anxiety levels

Medical Management

- Evaluate labor progression.
- Determine the cause of the dysfunction.
- Consider obstetrical interventions:
  - *Augment labor with oxytocin. (ENHANCE)*
  - *Perform amniotomy.*
  - *Perform cesarean birth when other interventions have failed or when there are signs of fetal intolerance of labor.*

Nursing Actions

- Assess uterine activity.
- Assess maternal and fetal status.
- Stimulate uterine activity to achieve a normal labor pattern using the following methods:
  - *Ambulate and change the position of the woman to promote comfort and labor progress.*
  - *Hydrate with IV or PO as per orders as dehydration can result in dysfunctional labor.*
  - *Administer IV fluids to maximize maternal fluid volume, to correct maternal hypotension and improve placental perfusion.*
  - *Augment labor with oxytocin as per protocol.*

CONTINUOUS DILATION SLEEP NOS

- Evaluate labor progress with SVE.
- Inform the woman and the family of the progress of labor and explain interventions.
- Provide emotional support. Anxiety levels can increase due to prolonged labor; increased anxiety and fear can interfere with effective UCs.
- Maintain good aseptic technique to minimize the risk of infection if ROM. *D/T Labor ↑ Length*
  - *Minimize vaginal exams.* (only have to know)
  - *Maintain perineal cleanliness.*
- Inform the care provider of the woman's response and progress in labor.

Precipitous Labor

Precipitous labor is a labor that lasts fewer than 3 hours from onset of labor to birth. The current rate of precipitous labor for women is 2.4% (Martin et al., 2011). Women who experience a precipitous labor often have higher anxiety and pain levels related to the rapid and intense labor experience. Precipitous labor and/or birth places the woman at risk for postpartum hemorrhage related to uterine atony or lacerations. It places the fetus/neonate at risk for hypoxia and at risk for central nervous system (CNS) depression related to hypoxia from the rapid birth. (pressure on head)

Risk Factors

- Grand multiparity
- History of precipitous labor

Assessment Findings (long + strong)

- Hypertonic UCs (tetanic UCs) that are occurring every 2 minutes or more frequently, lasting greater than 60 seconds and strong (**Fig. 10-2**).
- Potential for Category II (indeterminate) or Category III (abnormal) FHR and nursing actions are based on FHR pattern (see Chapter 9). (FHR affected)
- Rapid cervical dilation such that labor is less than 3 hours.

Medical Management

- Prepare for and stand by for precipitous birth.

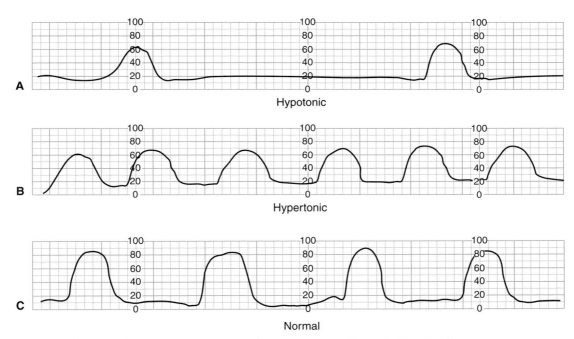

Figure 10–1   Hypertonic versus hypotonic versus normal uterine contractions. A. Hypotonic uterine contraction pattern. B. Hypertonic uterine contraction pattern. C. Normal uterine contraction pattern.

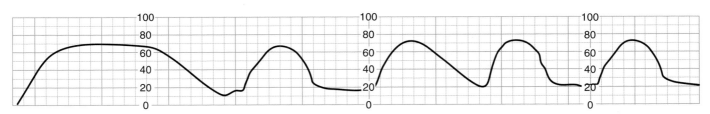

Figure 10–2   Tetanic uterine contractions.

Nursing Actions

- Remain in the room with the woman since birth is often very rapid with precipitous labor.
- Monitor FHR and UCs every 15 minutes.
- Assess labor progress and cervical change closely with sterile vaginal exams (SVEs).
  - *Assess the cervix if the woman states she feels pressure or feels like "the baby is coming!" It may be a sign of impending birth.*
- Support the woman and the family. This type of labor can be frightening, overwhelming, and painful.
- Anticipate potential maternal postpartum complications such as hemorrhage and lacerations.
- Anticipate potential neonatal complications such as hypoxia and CNS depression related to rapid birth.
- Prepare for delivery.

Inadequate Expulsive Forces

Inadequate expulsive forces occur in the second stage of labor when the woman is not able to push or bear down. It was previously thought that limiting the second stage to 2 hours was essential to decrease fetal morbidity and mortality. It is now known that waiting beyond 2 hours is safe for the fetus and the 2-hour time frame is no longer clinically valid.

- The fetus is at higher risk for asphyxia related to prolonged second stage of labor.
- The woman with a prolonged second stage, beyond 4 hours, is at risk for operative vaginal birth and perineal trauma.

Risk Factors

- Maternal exhaustion
- Epidural anesthesia because woman may not feel the urge to push

Assessment Findings

- Inadequate or ineffective pushing with little or no descent of the fetal head with expulsive pushing efforts
- Potential for Category II (indeterminate) or Category III (abnormal) FHR

Medical Management

- Evaluate the woman's progress, maternal-fetal status, and likelihood of vaginal birth.
- Augment with oxytocin.
- Assist birth with vacuum or forceps.
- Perform cesarean birth when other interventions are ineffective or signs of fetal intolerance to labor.

Nursing Actions

- Assess fetal descent.
- Evaluate fetal response to expulsive pushing.
- Facilitate the second stage of labor by doing the following:
  - *Coaching the woman in bearing-down efforts*
  - *Minimizing the Valsalva maneuver by using open glottis push strategies*
  - *Maintaining adequate pain relief for the woman with labor epidurals*
  - *Changing the maternal position to a more upright position to facilitate fetal descent*
  - *Supporting the woman's involuntary pushing efforts*

Fetal Dystocia

Fetal dystocia may be caused by excessive fetal size, malpresentation, multifetal pregnancy, or fetal anomalies. The fetus can move through the birth canal most effectively when the head is flexed and is presenting anterior to the woman's pelvis (occiput anterior position). This allows the smallest diameter of the fetal head to enter the maternal pelvis and the most flexible part of the fetal body, the back of the neck, to adapt to the curve of the birth canal. When the fetal position is other than flexed and vertex or the fetus is large in comparison to the maternal pelvis, labor may be difficult and vaginal birth a challenge. Complications of fetal dystocia are:

- Neonatal asphyxia related to prolonged labor
- Fetal injuries, such as bruising
- Maternal lacerations
- Cephalopelvic disproportion (CPD) (see Critical Component: Cephalopelvic Disproportion)

CRITICAL COMPONENT

Cephalopelvic Disproportion (CPD)

Cephalopelvic disproportion is a condition in which the size, shape, or position of the fetal head prevents it from passing through the lateral aspect of the maternal pelvis *or* when the maternal pelvis is of a size or shape that prevents the descent of the fetus through the pelvis. A diagnosis of CPD often necessitates a cesarean birth. CPD can rarely be diagnosed until labor has progressed for some time.

The success of any labor depends on the complex interrelationship of several factors:

- Fetal size, presentation, and position
- Size and shape of the maternal pelvis
- Quality of the UCs

Risk Factors

- Abnormal fetal presentation or position such as face, brow, or breech (**Table 10-1**)
- Fetal anomalies, such as hydrocephalus, and/or any other fetal anomaly that interferes with fetal descent through the birth canal
- Fetal macrosomia; birth weight greater than 4500 g

Assessment Findings

- FHR may be heard above the umbilicus versus in the lower uterine segment; this is a sign that the fetus may be in position other than vertex.
- The SVE reveals a buttocks or face when malpresentation is the cause of dystocia.
- The presenting part is not engaged in the maternal pelvis.
- There is no fetal descent through the pelvis.

TABLE 10–1   MALPRESENTATION OF THE FETUS

MALPRESENTATION	DESCRIPTION	IMPLICATIONS
OCCIPUT POSTERIOR	The occiput of the fetus is in the posterior portion of the pelvis rather than the anterior. As the fetus moves through the birth canal, the occiput bone presses on the woman's sacrum. Rotation of fetal head may occur during fetal descent.	Prolonged labor and prolonged second stage Severe back pain
FACE PRESENTATION	Fetal head is in extension rather than flexion as it enters the pelvis.	Labor and pushing may be prolonged. Cesarean delivery may be indicated. The neonate's face may have extensive bruising.
BROW PRESENTATION	Fetal head presents in a position midway between full flexion and extreme extension. This causes the largest diameter of the head to engage in the pelvis.	Prolonged second stage of labor.
SHOULDER PRESENTATION/COMPOUND PRESENTATION	Shoulder presentation: The fetal spine is vertical to the maternal pelvis. Compound presentation: One or more fetal extremities accompany the presenting part.	Higher risk of prolapsed cord. Cesarean delivery is typically indicated.

Continued

TABLE 10–1   MALPRESENTATION OF THE FETUS—cont'd

MALPRESENTATION	DESCRIPTION	IMPLICATIONS
BREECH PRESENTATIONS Frank breech 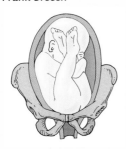 Complete breech 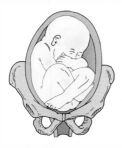 Footling breech (single) 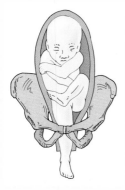 Footling breech (double) 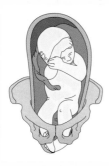	Frank breech: Thighs flexed alongside body, feet are close to the head Complete breech: One or both knees are flexed. Footling breech: Either one (single footling) or both (double footling) feet present before the buttocks.	Dysfunctional labor Fetal injury Increased risk of prolapsed cord Typically cesarean birth is indicated.

Medical Management

■ Confirm the fetal position with SVE and ultrasound.
■ Determine the type of obstetrical interventions, such as use of vacuum extractor, forceps, or need for cesarean birth.

Nursing Actions

■ Perform Leopold's maneuver as described in Chapter 8 to determine the fetal position.
■ Assess the location of the FHR.
■ Assess the fetal position with SVE.
■ Alert the care provider if there is any question regarding fetal presentation, position, or absence of fetal descent.

Pelvic Dystocia

Pelvic dystocia is related to the contraction of one or more of the three planes of the pelvis. During the prenatal period, the care provider determines the general pelvic size and configuration by vaginal examination. Pelvic measurements are not typically done. Descent and engagement of fetal head in labor indicate adequate pelvic inlet. The outcome of labor is dependent on the interrelationship of the size and shape of the pelvis, fetal size, presentation and position, and quality of the UCs (see Critical Component: Cephalopelvic Disproportion).

The three contractions of the pelvic planes are:

■ Inlet contraction occurs when the widest part of the pelvis is small.
■ Midpelvis contraction related to prominent ischial spines, convergent pelvic side walls, and a narrow sacrosciatic notch may result in arrest of descent of the vertex.
■ Outlet contraction can be estimated by measuring the transverse diameter of the pelvis. Normally, the antero-posterior diameter is 14 cm.

Risk Factors

■ Small pelvis
■ Abnormal pelvic shape

Assessment Findings

■ Delayed descent of fetal head

Medical Management

■ Evaluate the pelvis for contraction of one or more of the planes of the pelvis.
■ Evaluate the descent and engagement of the fetal head.

Nursing Actions

■ Perform SVE to evaluate the progress of labor and fetal descent into pelvis (i.e. check station).

Maternal Obesity

The World Health Organization and the National Institute of Health define obesity as a BMI of 30 or greater. Maternal obesity was recognized as a risk factor in pregnancy more than 50 years ago. A global epidemic of obesity is unfolding, resulting in new challenges for the management of obesity in up to 30% of pregnant women. The obstetric complications of maternal obesity are generally related to issues of maternal pre-pregnancy obesity rather than excessive weight gain during pregnancy (Catalano, 2007). Maternal obesity is a well-established risk factor for the development of preeclampsia, gestational diabetes, and thrombosis. The impact on pregnancy also translates to complications in labor, including labor induction, cesarean births, and failed vaginal birth after cesarean (Ramachenderan, Bradford, & McLean, 2008; Morin & Reilly, 2007). It is currently recommended that every perinatal department should have policies and practices specific to this patient population (Maher, 2014).

Risks at Delivery

■ Abnormal progress of labor
■ Fetal macrosomia
■ Shoulder dystocia
■ Higher rates of operative vaginal birth and cesarean birth
■ Performing epidural or spinal anesthesia on morbidly obese patients may be extremely problematic.
■ Not only do obese women experience higher rates of failed vaginal birth after cesarean (VBAC), but obese women who have a VBAC experience higher rates of infection.
■ Increased postoperative complications including wound infection, delayed wound healing, excessive blood loss, DVT, and endometritis (Catalano, 2007)

Assessment Findings

■ Delayed descent of fetal head
■ Abnormal labor progress

Nursing Actions

■ Anticipate impact of pregnancy complications listed above on labor and birth.
■ Assess for normal progress of labor.
■ Assure that patient beds, examining tables, and chairs can support patient's weight.
■ Facilitate patient positioning for administering epidural analgesia to obese women.

LABOR INTERVENTIONS

The majority of pregnant women go into labor spontaneously at term (37–42 weeks' gestation) and progress through the labor and birth experience without complications. Increasingly, the approach to labor has shifted from a natural process to one that should be "managed" by the woman, nurse, and care provider. Management of labor has resulted in an increase in labor interventions, including induction of labor (which may also include cervical ripening) and augmentation to speed up labor. This section reviews interventions to induce (initiate) and augment (strengthen) labor.

Labor interventions are medically indicated when either the condition or safety of the woman or fetus would be improved with birth. Because spontaneous labor is associated with fewer complications than induced labor, induction of labor without a medical indication is discouraged.

Despite risks to the woman and fetus (such as increased rates of cesarean birth), labor interventions such as elective induction are at an all-time high (see Critical Component: Elective Induction of Labor). Because of the potential risks associated with induction of labor, elective induction should be undertaken only after fully informing the woman of risks and benefits and establishing a gestational age of 39 weeks or greater. The nurse providing care for the woman during cervical ripening, induction, or augmentation of labor should be aware of the indications, actions, expected results, and potential risks of each agent. Before any agent is used, maternal status and fetal well-being should be established and cervical status should be assessed and documented (Simpson, 2009).

PATIENT EDUCATION

Healthy Mom&Baby, the consumer magazine from the Association of Women's Health, Obstetric and Neonatal Nurses (AWHONN), launched the "Go the Full 40" campaign in early 2012. This educational campaign is designed to help women understand the many reasons it's important for a mom to carry her baby to term. With 40 reasons, *Healthy Mom & Baby* is busting the myth that it's okay for babies to be born just a little early. In fact, babies need the benefit of a full-term pregnancy. Inducing labor before 40 weeks is associated with prematurity, cesarean surgery, hemorrhage, and infection. Babies born before 37 completed weeks of gestation are at risk for breathing problems, feeding issues, jaundice, low blood sugar, and problems stabilizing their own body temperature.

Labor Induction

Induction of labor is the deliberate stimulation of UCs before the onset of spontaneous labor to facilitate a vaginal delivery. According to the National Center for Health Statistics, the rate of induction of labor has increased significantly during the past 15 years from an induction rate of 9.5% in 1990 to 23.2% in 2009, more than a 100% increase (Martin et al., 2011). Data show that outcomes for newborns are greatly improved when gestation is longer than 39 weeks. Yet studies indicate that almost one-third of all babies delivered in the United States are electively delivered—most for convenience. This impacts short-term neonatal morbidity. New guidelines are being set by the Joint Commission to decrease elective inductions of labor prior to 39 weeks' gestation (Institute for Healthcare Improvement, 2010).

CRITICAL COMPONENT

Elective Induction of Labor

It is estimated that 25%–50% of inductions are elective or non-medical. Prior to elective induction, fetal maturity must be confirmed to be 39 weeks or greater by the following:

1. Ultrasound before 20 weeks' gestation confirms gestational age of 39 weeks or greater.
2. Fetal heart tones have been documented as present by Doppler for 30 weeks.
3. It has been 36 weeks since a positive serum or urine pregnancy test was confirmed.

(American College of Obstetricians and Gynecologists. (2009). Induction of Labor ACOG Practice Bulletin, No 107. Washington DC: ACOG.)

The nurse may face a dilemma when women are admitted for induction or cervical ripening without documented indications for the induction. It is the nurse's responsibility to ensure that the woman is fully informed by her provider before beginning a procedure (Simpson, 2009).

Induction of labor is a complex intervention that leads to a "cascade of interventions" that typically includes:

■ Intravenous (IV) fluids
■ Activity restriction or bed rest
■ More frequent or continuous electronic fetal monitoring
■ Increased pain medication use and epidural anesthesia
■ Amniotomy
■ Prolonged stay in the labor unit (Simpson, 2013; Simpson & Atterbury, 2003; Simpson & O'Brien-Abel, 2013)

A number of methods of induction of labor have been proposed as effective in initiating labor. When the decision has been made to induce labor, the next important question raised is how to induce labor. When deciding on the method of induction of labor, certain clinical factors are considered, including:

■ Parity
■ Status of membranes: Ruptured or intact
■ Status of the cervix: Favorable or unfavorable
■ History of previous cesarean births

All these factors or clinical situations are thought to be important to a provider in making the decision about which method of labor induction should be used. Labor induction is thought to be less successful when the cervix is unfavorable (not ripe). It is more successful in parous women than in nulliparous women. Little attention has been given to the combination of these factors, which may be important to women and clinicians when attempting to make informed decisions about induction of labor (Kelly, Alfirevic, Hofmeyr, Kavanagh, Neilson, & Thomas, 2009).

Oxytocin Induction

A pharmacological method for induction of labor is administration of oxytocin. Oxytocin is the most common induction agent used worldwide to initiate labor. It has been used alone, in combination with amniotomy, or after cervical ripening with other pharmacological or non-pharmacological methods. Before the introduction of prostaglandin agents, oxytocin was used as a cervical ripening agent as well.

■ Endogenous oxytocin is a peptide synthesized by the hypothalamus that is transported to the posterior lobe of the pituitary gland, where it is released in the maternal circulation in response to vaginal and cervical stretching. The release of oxytocin stimulates UCs.
■ Synthetic oxytocin is identical to endogenous oxytocin.
■ A uterine response occurs to oxytocin in 3–5 minutes, with a half-life of 10 minutes.
■ Considerable controversy exists related to dose and rate increase intervals when oxytocin is used for induction of labor.

There was a trend to use higher doses of oxytocin, termed "active management of labor" (**Box 10-1**). This dosing regimen

BOX 10–1   PRINCIPLES OF ACTIVE MANAGEMENT OF LABOR

The original research on active management of labor included only nulliparous women in spontaneous, active labor (O'Driscoll, Jackson, & Gallagher, 1970; O'Driscoll, Strange, & Minoque, 1973). The following is the summary of their findings:

True labor was defined as UCs with either bloody show, spontaneous rupture of membranes, or 100% cervical effacement.

Women received 1:1 labor care from the midwife or nurse.

Amniotomy was performed if membranes did not rupture spontaneously once labor was diagnosed.

If cervical dilation did not proceed at 1 cm/hour, oxytocin was administered at beginning at 6 mU/min and increasing by 6 mU/min every 15 minutes until adequate labor was established (maximum dose 40 mU/min).

The principles of active management have not been shown to decrease the cesarean birth rate in the United States.

---

is based on research conducted in the 1970s in Dublin, Ireland. However, current evidence supports lower dose infusions (Simpson, 2002), with research reporting more successful vaginal births, fewer operative vaginal deliveries, and less tachysystole and lower cesarean birth rates. Continued increases in oxytocin rates over a long period during induction can result in oxytocin receptor desensitization or down-regulation, making oxytocin less effective in producing normal UCs.

Indications

■ Post-term pregnancy
■ Pregnancy-induced hypertension
■ Preeclampsia/eclampsia
■ Maternal medical conditions (e.g., diabetes mellitus, renal disease, chronic pulmonary disease, cardiac disease, chronic hypertension)
■ Premature rupture of membranes (PROM)
■ Chorioamnionitis
■ Fetal stress or compromise, such as severe intrauterine growth restriction, oligohydramnios, or isoimmunization
■ Fetal demise
■ History of rapid labors/distance from the hospital
■ Psychosocial considerations

Contraindications

■ Any contraindications for vaginal birth
■ Previous vertical (classical) uterine scar or prior transfundal uterine scar
■ Placental abnormalities such as complete placenta previa or vasoprevia
■ Abnormal fetal position
■ Umbilical cord prolapse
■ Active genital herpes
■ Pelvic abnormalities

Risks Associated With Inductions

■ Tachysystole leading to Category II (indeterminate) or Category III (abnormal) FHR pattern is the primary

---

complication of oxytocin in labor (see Critical Component: Tachysystole).

■ Side effects of oxytocin use are primarily dose related; tachysystole and subsequent FHR decelerations are common side effects (ACOG, 1999) (see Critical Component: Administering Oxytocin in Labor).

■ Water intoxication can occur with high concentrations of oxytocin with large quantities of hypotonic solutions but usually only with prolonged administration with at least 40 mU/min.

Assessment Findings

■ The woman understands the indication for induction.
■ Assessment findings and prenatal records reflect an indication for induction.
■ If elective induction, confirmed gestational age of 39 or more weeks

Medical Management

■ Advise of indication for induction of labor and order induction of labor as per institutional protocol.
■ Be available to respond to complications.

CRITICAL COMPONENT

Tachysystole

Tachysystole, previously referred to as hyperstimulation, is excessive uterine activity and is the most concerning side effect of oxytocin because it can result in a progressive adverse effect on fetal status (Simpson & O'Brien-Abel, 2013) (**Fig. 10-3**). UCs cause an intermittent decrease in blood flow in the intervillous space where oxygen exchange occurs. The decreased intervillous blood flow associated with tachysystole leads to decreased oxygen to the fetus. Tachysystole can result in progressive deterioration in fetal status and hypoxemia that result in an abnormal fetal heart rate. Tachysystole may result in abruptio placenta or uterine rupture, which are rare complications (ACOG, 1999).

Tachysystole is defined as:

■ Five or more UCs in 10 minutes over a 30-minute window
■ A series of single UCs lasting 2 minutes or longer
■ UCs occurring within 1 minute of each other

Nursing actions for tachysystole with Category I (normal) FHR pattern:

■ Maternal repositioning (left or right lateral)
■ IV fluid bolus of at least 500 mL of lactated Ringer's solution
■ Decrease rate of oxytocin infusion by at least half if no response to above measures.
■ Discontinue oxytocin if the pattern persists.

Nursing actions for tachysystole with a Category II (indeterminate) or Category III (abnormal) FHR pattern would also include (Lyndon & Ali, 2008):

■ Discontinue oxytocin.
■ Maternal repositioning (left or right lateral)
■ IV fluid bolus of at least 500 mL of lactated Ringer's solution
■ Consider O_2 at 10 L/min by nonrebreather mask.
■ Notify provider of actions taken and maternal fetal response.
■ Consider terbutaline if no response to above measures.

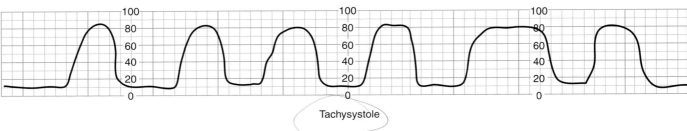

Figure 10–3 Uterine tachysystole (hyperstimulation).

CRITICAL COMPONENT

Administering Oxytocin in Labor

The goal of oxytocin use in labor is to establish uterine contraction patterns that promote cervical dilation of about 1 cm/hr once in active labor.

Generally the UC pattern consists of:

- 3 UCs in 10 minutes, lasting 40–60 seconds, intensity of 25–75 mm/Hg with IUCP with resting tone ≤ 20mm Hg with 1 minute between each UC
- Oxytocin is administered intravenously and is piggybacked to a mainline IV solution at the port most proximal to the venous site (**Fig. 10-4**).
- Oxytocin is *always* infused via a pump.
- There is variation in the concentrations of oxytocin, and it should be prepared by the pharmacy, as it is a high-alert medication.
- Typical concentrations are:

  - 10 units of oxytocin in 1000 mL of lactated Ringer's result in an infusion rate of 1 mU/min = 6 mL/hr.
  - 20 units of oxytocin in 1000 mL of lactated Ringer's result in an infusion rate of 1 mU/min = 3 mL/hr.

- Current dose recommendations are for low-dose oxytocin starting at 0.5 mU/min and increasing the dose by 1–2 mU/min every 30–60 minutes until adequate labor progress is achieved (i.e., cervical effacement or cervical dilation of 0.5–1 cm/hr) and regular UCs every 2–3 minutes lasting 45–60 seconds.
- Nursing responsibilities during oxytocin infusion involve careful titration of the drug to the maternal and fetal response.

  - The titration process includes decreasing dosage rates or discontinuing infusion when UCs are too frequent.
  - Discontinuing oxytocin when FHR is abnormal (Simpson, 2013; Simpson & O'Brien-Abel, 2013).

- Increasing doses when UCs are inadequate; however, the lowest possible dose should be used to achieve labor progress (Simpson & Atterbury, 2003).
- Once active labor is established, oxytocin should be discontinued to avoid downregulation.
- Maternal-fetal response to oxytocin is the primary consideration. If the frequency, intensity, duration, or resting tone of the contraction is increased by oxytocin, this can impede uterine blood flow and can cause fetal compromise, resulting in a Category II or Category III FHR pattern. Thus oxytocin must be administered with careful monitoring and prompt recognition and interventions for tachysystole to prevent fetal acidosis.

  - Avoid tachysystole because it frequently results in Category II (indeterminate) or Category III (abnormal) fetal heart rate pattern.
  - Continuous EFM is typically used with oxytocin administration.
  - In the absence of risk factors, intermittent auscultation is permitted with evaluation of FHR and UCs at least every 30 minutes in active labor and every 15 minutes in the second stage.
  - For Category II (indeterminate) or Category III (abnormal) FHR pattern, interventions include the following actions:

    - Discontinue oxytocin.
    - Change maternal position to lateral position.
    - Initiate IV hydration of at least 500 mL lactated Ringer's.
    - Administer O₂ by nonrebreather mask at 10 L/min.
    - Consider terbutaline if no response
    - Notify the provider and request bedside evaluations for Category III abnormal FHR.

Nursing Actions

- Ensure informed consent has been obtained by providing information about induction, discussing the agents, methods, options, and risks (Gilbert, 2011).
- Review prenatal record with woman for indication for induction of labor.

- Administer low-dose oxytocin starting at 0.5 mU/min (current dose recommendations) and increase the dose by 1–2 mU/min every 30–60 minutes (see Critical Component: Administering Oxytocin in Labor).
- In the absence of risk factors, evaluate and document FHR at least every 30 minutes in active labor and every

15 minutes in the second stage via intermittent auscultation or electronic fetal monitoring (EFM).

■ In the presence of risk factors, continuous EFM is
recommended and FHR should be evaluated and
documented every 15 minutes in active labor and every
5 minutes in the second stage.

■ Monitor strength, frequency, and duration of UCs as an
indicator of oxytocin efficacy Q 30 min.

■ Evaluate uterine resting tone by palpation or IUPC
pressure below 20 mm Hg to ensure uterine relaxation
between contractions.

■ Decrease or discontinue oxytocin in the event of uterine
tachysystole or indeterminate or abnormal fetal status.
The current recommendation when decreasing oxytocin
is to lower the dose by half.

■ Assess FHR in response to UCs (see Chapter 9).

■ For Category II (indeterminate) or Category III
(abnormal) FHR pattern, interventions include the
following actions:

■ *Change maternal position to lateral position.*

■ *IV bolus of at least 500 mL of lactated Ringer's*

■ *If no response, consider terbutaline*

■ *Administer O_2 by nonrebreather mask at 10 L/min.*

■ *Discontinue oxytocin.*

■ *Notify the provider and request a bedside evaluation if the
FHR is III.*

■ *Assess emotional response of patient and support person to
induction of labor. Provide information and reassurance as
needed to alleviate feelings of failure.*

■ *Assess patient's level of fear and provide information and
reassurance.*

■ Monitor labor progress with SVE for cervical dilation
and fetal descent. Cervical change of 1 cm/hr indicates
sufficient progress.

■ Assess the character and amount of amniotic fluid.

■ Assess the character and amount of bloody show.

■ Assess the maternal response, including level of discomfort and pain and effectiveness of pain management and
labor support Q 30 min.

■ Assess VS per policy, generally Q 2 hr.

■ Assess input and output (I&O) for fluid overload; output
should mirror intake. Signs and symptoms of fluid overload include decreased urine output, edema, increased
BP, and pulmonary edema.

■ Ensure adequate hydration, assess I&O Q 8 hr.

■ Greater than 50% of all legal settlements involved
perinatal cases, with 40%–50% of these cases related to
management of oxytocin (Jonsson, Norden-Lindeberg,
& Hanson, 2007). Nurses must minimize the risk of
patient harm by being well-educated regarding oxytocin
risks as well as being proactive with interventions
when there is evidence of tachysystole or abnormal
FHR patterns.

■ Follow the constitutions of chain of command if nursing
disagrees with the plan of care (Gilbert, 2011).

Oxytocin High Alert Medication

QSEN

Patient injury from drug therapy is the single most common type of adverse event that occurs in the inpatient
setting (Agency for Healthcare Research & Quality, 2001;
Institute for Healthcare Improvement, 2007). When medication errors result in patient injury, there are significant
costs to the patient, health care providers, and institution. Some medications that have a heightened risk of
causing significant patient harm when they are used in
error are called "high-alert medications." In 2007, the
Institute for Safe Medication Practices (ISMP) added
intravenous (IV) oxytocin to their list of high-alert medications (ISMP, 2007). Special considerations and precautions are required before and during administration of
high-alert medications (ISMP, 2007). This is significant
for perinatal care providers because oxytocin is a drug
that they use quite frequently. Errors that involve IV oxytocin administration for labor induction or augmentation
are most commonly dose related and often involve lack of
timely recognition and appropriate treatment of excessive
uterine activity (i.e., tachysystole) (Clark, Simpson, Knox,
& Garite, 2008). Other types of oxytocin errors involve
mistaken administration of IV fluids with oxytocin for IV
fluid resuscitation during Category II or III fetal heart rate
patterns and/or maternal hypotension and inappropriate
elective administration of oxytocin to women who are less
than 39 completed weeks' gestation. Oxytocin medication errors and subsequent patient harm is generally
preventable (Simpson & Knox, 2009). The perinatal team
can develop strategies to minimize risk of maternal-fetal
injuries related to oxytocin administration consistent
with safe care practices used with other high-alert
medications.

1. Requirement that women having elective labor induction
be at least 39 completed weeks' gestation
2. Standard order sets and protocols that reflect a standardized clinical approach to labor induction and augmentation based on current pharmacologic and physiologic
evidence
3. Standard concentration of oxytocin prepared by the
pharmacy
4. Standard definition of uterine tachysystole that does not
include a Category III or II (abnormal or indeterminate)
FHR pattern (a contraction frequency of more than five
in 10 minutes, a series of single contractions lasting 2
minutes or more, contractions of normal duration
occurring within 1 minute of each other)
5. Standard treatment of oxytocin-induced uterine
tachysystole guided by fetal status

Agency for Healthcare Research and Quality. (2001). Reducing and prevent-
ing adverse drug events to decrease hospital costs. (AHRQ Publication No.
01-0200). Washington, DC: Author; Institute for Healthcare Improvement.
(2007). Prevent harm from high alert medications: How to guide.
Cambridge, MA: Author; Institute for Safe Medication Practices. (2007).
High-alert medications. Huntingdon Valley, PA: Author; Simpson, K. R., &
Knox, G. E. (2009). High-Alert Medication: Implications for Perinatal Patient
Safety. Maternal Child Nursing, 34(1); Clark, S. L., Simpson, K. R., Knox, G.
E., & Garite, T. J. (2008). Oxytocin: New perspectives on an old drug.
American Journal of Obstetrics and Gynecology, 199; e-publication ahead of
print July 29.

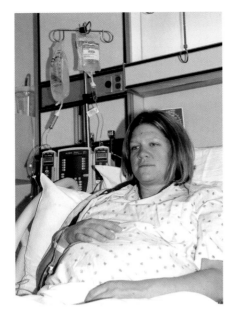

Figure 10–4   Intravenous oxytocin administration.

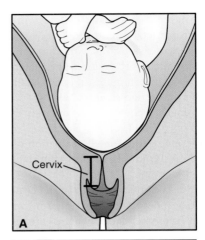

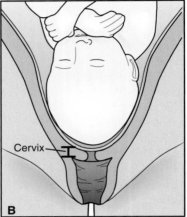

Figure 10–5   A. Unripe cervix, cervix is not effaced or dilated. B. Ripe cervix, cervix is 100% effaced and 1 cm dilated.

Cervical Ripening

The cervix, composed of connective tissue, is typically closed until labor begins. At the onset of labor it undergoes rapid changes including ripening, effacement, and dilation (**Fig. 10-5**). Cervical ripening is the process of physical softening and opening of the cervix in preparation for labor and birth. Because cervical status is the most important predictor of successful induction of labor, cervical status is assessed before induction of labor. Typically, cervical status is assessed via the Bishop score (**Table 10-2**). A score of 6 or more is considered favorable for successful induction of labor.

However, when the score is unfavorable (a Bishop score of less than 6), cervical ripening is usually considered. A mechanical or pharmacological cervical ripening agent may be used. These agents can also sometimes stimulate labor.

Mechanical Cervical Ripening

Mechanical cervical ripening methods are devices that are inserted through the vagina and into the cervix to dilate the cervix. They are among the oldest methods to initiate labor. More recently, pharmacological prostaglandins have partially replaced mechanical methods (Jozwiak, Bloemenkamp, Kelly, Mol, Irion, & Boulrain, 2012). These methods have a lower risk of tachysystole compared to pharmacological methods. Examples of mechanical cervical ripening methods are:

- Laminaria, lamicil, or dilapan
  - *These materials expand by absorbing fluid from the cervical tissues and cause the cervix to dilate and release local prostaglandin.*

- Balloon catheters
  - *The balloon is inflated after insertion into the cervix and causes pressure on the cervix and lower uterine segment and the release of prostaglandin.*

Indications

- When the woman has little or no cervical effacement
- When pharmacological methods are contraindicated, such as women with prior uterine incision

Risks Associated With Mechanical Cervical Ripening

- The infection rate is higher.
- Premature rupture of membranes (PROM)

Assessment Findings

- The cervix is unripe based on SVE and Bishop score.
- Prenatal record reflects indications for induction.

Medical Management

- The physician or midwife places the mechanical dilators, which usually stay in place for 6–12 hours before being removed by the care provider.

TABLE 10-2	BISHOP SCORE TO ASSESS CERVICAL RIPENESS			
	0	1	2	3
Dilation cm	0	1–2	3–4	5–6
Effacement %	0–30%	40%–50%	60%–70%	80%
Station	–3	–2	–1/0	+1/+2
Consistency of cervix	Firm	Medium	Soft	
Cervical position	Posterior	Medium	Anterior	
Bishop (1964).				

Nursing Actions

■ Obtain informed consent following an informative discussion as to the procedure, etc.

■ Prepare the patient and assist with the insertion procedure.

■ Instruct the patient that she might experience discomfort or cramping during insertion.

■ Provide ongoing emotional and informational support and encourage relaxation.

■ Record the type of dilator and number of dilators or the size of the balloon placed.

■ Assess onset of UCs.

■ Assess FHR.

■ Assess maternal temperature, as the woman is at higher risk for infection.

■ Assess for rupture of membranes and vaginal bleeding.

■ Assess maternal and fetal status as per institutional policy.

Pharmacological Methods of Cervical Ripening

Pharmacological methods of cervical ripening in preparation for induction of labor may use one of a variety of hormonal preparations (**Table 10-3**). These preparations, which are placed in or near the cervix, produce cervical ripening by causing softening and thinning of the cervix. Occasionally these agents can stimulate labor contractions. A review of research on the use of prostaglandins concluded there is an improvement in labor stimulation in vaginal birth rates in 24 hours, no increase in operative birth rates, and significant improvements in cervical favorability within 24–48 hours when using prostaglandins (Kelly, Kavanagh, & Thomas, 2003).

Indications

■ See indications for induction.

Risks Associated With Pharmacological Methods of Cervical Ripening

■ Tachysystole of the uterus (see Critical Component: Uterine Tachysystole)

Assessment Findings

■ Unripe cervix based on SVE and Bishop score of 6 or less

■ Prenatal record reflecting indication for induction

Medical Management

■ Determine the need for cervical ripening.

■ Insert the pharmacological agent.

■ *Administration of the agent should be done at or near the labor and birthing unit.*

Nursing Actions

■ Obtain informed consent.

■ Evaluate the prenatal record for indications and contraindications for induction (see contraindications to augmentation and induction of labor)

■ Document baseline cervical exam and Bishop score with SVE.

■ Obtain baseline FHR

■ Monitor FHR and uterine activity as indicated based on medication and institutional policies.

Stripping the Membranes

Stripping the membranes is digital separation of the chorionic membrane from the wall of the cervix and lower uterine segment during a vaginal exam done by a primary care provider to stimulate labor. The exact mechanism of action is unclear, but it is commonly believed it releases prostaglandins and also may cause maternal oxytocin release. It is most effective in first-time pregnancies with an unripe cervix. However, there is little scientific evidence of the efficacy of stripping the membranes.

■ The procedure is usually done in the care provider's office.

■ The care provider is responsible for explaining the procedure and its risks.

■ The FHR should be assessed before and after the procedure.

■ The woman might experience some spotting after the procedure.

■ The woman might experience mild cramping immediately after the procedure.

Indications

■ See indications for oxytocin induction.

PP HEMMORRHAGE

TABLE 10–3   PHARMACOLOGICAL CERVICAL RIPENING AGENTS

MEDICATION	PREPIDIL PGE₂ (DINOPROSTONE GEL)	CERVIDIL (DINOPROSTONE INSERT)	MISOPROSTOL PGE₁ (CYTOTEC)
DOSE	0.5 mg gel is placed below cervical os with speculum exam, can be repeated every 6 hours for a maximum of 3 doses	10 mg controlled released vaginal insert with string for removal after 12 hours	25 mcg inserted in the posterior vaginal fornix. A recent review reports the possibility of rare but serious adverse events, particularly uterine rupture, with misoprostol use. *Oral administration is not recommended. Further research is needed to establish the ideal route of administration and dosage, and safety. (Hofmeyr & Gülmezoglu, 2003)
NURSING ACTIONS	Inserted by MD or CNM. Woman should remain recumbent for 30 minutes after dose. Continuous FHR and UC monitoring for 30 minutes–2 hours after dose. Oxytocin should be delayed for 6–12 hours after dose.	Can be placed by perinatal nurse. Woman should remain supine or lateral position for 2 hours after insert. Continuous FHR and UC monitoring while medication is in place and for 15 minutes after removal. Oxytocin should be delayed for 30–60 minutes after removal.	Continuous FHR and UC monitoring. Oxytocin should be delayed until at least 4 hours after last dose.
CONTRAINDICATIONS		Not recommended for women with previous uterine scar	Previous cesarean section or uterine scar
ACTIONS	Uterine activity within 1 hour and peak dose 4 hours; tachysystole can occur within 1 hour in up to 5% of patients.	UCs after 5–7 hours, tachysystole can occur within 1 hour in up to 5% of patients. Remove if tachysystole or Category II or III FHR.	Wide variations in onset of UCs. Peak action 1–2 hours. Tachysystole more common with misoprostol than with prostaglandins or oxytocin.

Gilbert (2011); Simpson & O'Brien-Abel, 2013.

Risks Associated With Stripping of the Membranes

■ Infection
■ Bleeding from undiagnosed placental problem
■ Unplanned rupture of membranes (ROM)

Assessment Findings

■ Intact membranes
■ Presenting part engaged
■ Term gestation

Medical Management

■ Stripping the membranes is done by the primary care provider during a SVE by inserting a finger into the cervix and sweeping the finger around the cervix to separate the membrane from the cervix.

Amniotomy

Amniotomy is the artificial rupture of membranes (AROM) to induce or augment labor with an amnihook during a SVE (**Fig. 10-6**). Amniotic fluid release increases the conversion of prostaglandins following the amniotomy.

Amniotomy is most typically used to augment or shorten labor but may also be used to induce labor. There is insufficient evidence to support the value of this as a sole intervention for induction (Bricker & Luckas, 2000).

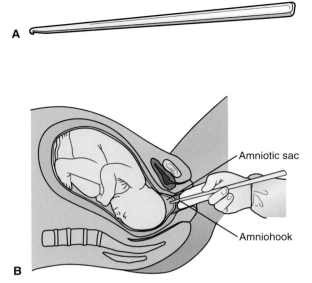

Figure 10–6 Amnihook and AROM procedure.

This procedure is done by the primary care provider and only if an emergency delivery can be performed nearby (Gilbert, 2011).

It is most effective in multiparous women who are dilated to 2 cm or more.

Amniotomy in early labor increases the risk of cesarean birth for abnormal FHR.

Indications

■ To stimulate labor

Contraindications

■ Fetal head not engaged in the maternal pelvis
■ Maternal infection such as HIV and active genital herpes

Risks Associated With Amniotomy

■ Severe variable decelerations
■ Bleeding from undiagnosed placental abnormality
■ Umbilical cord prolapse when presenting part is not engaged
■ Intra-amniotic infection increases with duration of the rupture.
■ A Cochrane Review of trials noted early intervention with amniotomy and oxytocin appears to be associated with a modest reduction in cesarean births (Wiv, Wo, Xu, Luo, Roy, & Fraiser, 2009).

Assessment Findings

■ The woman leaks amniotic fluid vaginally.

Medical Management

■ The procedure is done by the primary care provider with a SVE when head is engaged in the pelvis.

Nursing Actions

■ Assess the FHR before ROM and immediately following ROM because of the risk of umbilical cord prolapse.

■ Offer comfort and support to the woman, as the procedure may be uncomfortable.
■ Assess the color, amount, and odor of amniotic fluid.
■ Monitor UC pattern.
■ Document the time of the AROM.
■ Assess maternal temperature every 4 hours or more frequently if signs and symptoms of infection occur.
■ Administer pericare, as the woman continues to leak fluid after AROM.
■ Typically nurses do not perform an amniotomy. There may be individual institutional policies allowing nurses to perform AROM under specific criteria.

Labor Augmentation   *Oxytocin*

Wide variations in labor progress and duration occur among women in labor, and there is no consensus among experts as to the appropriate length of labor. The terms dystocia and failure to progress are sometimes used to characterize an abnormally long labor. Many providers believe there is benefit to decreasing the length of labor through augmentation with oxytocin (Simpson, 2002). The rate of augmentation of labor has increased 50% over the last decade, to a current rate of at least 18% (Martin et al., 2006). Generally, maternal-fetal status and individual clinical situations are the basis for labor management decisions. According to ACOG, contraindications to augmentation are similar to those for labor induction and may include placenta or vasa previa, umbilical cord presentation, prior classical uterine incision, active genital herpes infection, pelvic structural deformities, or invasive cervical cancer.

Labor augmentation is the stimulation of ineffective UCs after the onset of spontaneous labor to manage labor dystocia. All of the principles of oxytocin induction apply to the use of oxytocin for augmentation of labor.

Lower doses of oxytocin are required for augmentation of labor because cervical resistance is lower in women in labor who have some cervical effacement and dilation. This may not be indicated in induction protocols, as some protocols have been influenced by research on active management of labor (see Box 10-1).

Indications

■ To strengthen and regulate UCs
■ To shorten the length of labor

Contraindications

■ Any contraindications for vaginal birth
■ Previous vertical (classical) uterine scar or prior transfundal uterine scar
■ Placental abnormalities such as complete placenta previa or vasa previa
■ Abnormal fetal position
■ Umbilical cord prolapse
■ Active genital herpes
■ Pelvic abnormalities

Risks Associated With Augmentation

■ Tachysystole leading to a Category II or Category III FHR pattern is a primary complication of oxytocin in labor (see Critical Component: Tachysystole).

Assessment Findings

■ Prolonged labor
■ Inadequate UCs and inadequate labor progress

Medical Management

■ Determine the need for labor augmentation.
■ Be available to respond to complications of use of oxytocin in labor for augmentation.

Nursing Actions

■ Administer low-dose oxytocin starting at 0.5 mU/min and increasing the dose by 1–2 mU/min every 30–60 minutes as recommended.
■ Monitor FHR and UCs. FHR and UCs are typically continuously monitored, but intermittent monitoring is within the standard of care (see Chapter 9).
■ Follow the same principles of nursing care for induction of labor (see Critical Component: Tachysystole and Critical Component: Administering Oxytocin in Labor).
■ Decrease or discontinue oxytocin in the event of uterine tachysystole or Category II (indeterminate) or Category III (abnormal) fetal heart rate.

Complementary Therapies to Stimulate Labor

A variety of strategies have been proposed over many decades to initiate and/or augment labor. For example, acupuncture may stimulate the uterus. Other practices include bowel stimulation with castor oil or an enema to increase prostaglandin production. Cochrane reviews of complementary therapies indicate further research is needed to determine the effectiveness of most therapies to stimulate or induce labor (Kelly, Kavanagh, & Thomas, 2001).Therapies include:

■ Herbal preparations
   ■ *Black cohosh*
   ■ *Blue cohosh*
   ■ *Evening primrose oil*
   ■ *Raspberry leaves may be taken orally to promote prostaglandin or oxytocin production.*
■ Sexual intercourse:
   ■ *Semen contains prostaglandin to open the cervix, and orgasm may be associated with prostaglandin and oxytocin release.*

OPERATIVE VAGINAL DELIVERY

Operative vaginal delivery is a vaginal birth that is assisted by a vacuum extraction or forceps. Since 1996, the rate of cesarean birth has increased and the percentage of operative vaginal deliveries with either forceps or vacuum extraction has decreased 45% over 10 years, from 9.4% to 4.5% (Martin et al., 2011). Indications for operative vaginal delivery are to improve maternal or fetal status by shortening the second stage of labor. Facilitating birth and shortening the second stage of labor can be performed only by care providers with hospital privileges for these procedures. Although sometimes indicated, operative vaginal birth is not without risk of complications to the woman and the fetus. Specific guidelines for the use of forceps and vacuum extraction are provided, and use of only *one* method, either forceps or vacuum, for an individual patient is recommended. If attempts are unsuccessful, the physician proceeds with a cesarean birth.

Vacuum-Assisted Delivery

Vacuum-assisted delivery or vacuum extraction is a birth involving the use of a vacuum cup on the fetal head to assist with delivery of the fetal head (**Fig. 10-7**). The cup is placed on the fetal head and suction is increased gradually until a seal is formed. Gentle traction is then applied to deliver the fetal head (**Fig. 10-8**).

The rate of vacuum-assisted delivery, which had increased by 77% between 1989 (3.5%) and 1997 (6.2%), has since decreased to 4.5% for 2009 (Martin et al., 2011). Some advantages to the use of vacuum over forceps include:

■ Easier application
■ Less anesthesia required
■ Less maternal soft tissue damage
■ Fewer fetal injuries

Current guidelines for vacuum application are:

■ The fetal head needs to be engaged and the cervix completely dilated.
■ There should be a maximum of three attempts for a period of 15 minutes: the "three-pull rule."
■ Cup detachment from the fetal head (pops off of the vacuum) is a warning sign that too much pressure or ineffective force is being exerted on the fetal head.
■ The physician should proceed with a cesarean birth when vacuum attempts are not successful.

Indications

■ Suspicion of immediate or potential fetal compromise
■ Need to shorten the second stage for maternal benefit
■ Prolonged second stage
   ■ *Nulliparous woman with lack of continuing progress for 3 hours with regional anesthesia, or for 2 hours without anesthesia*

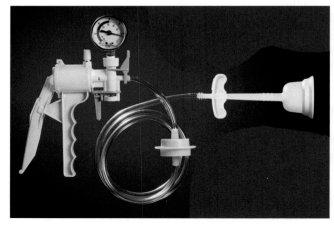

Figure 10–7   Vacuum device. Source: © CooperSurgical.

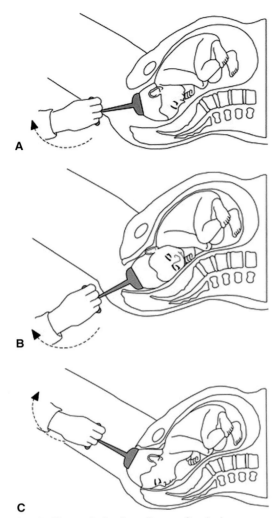

C

Used with permission from Cooper-Surgical

Figure 10-8 Vacuum delivery. Source: © CooperSurgical.

■ *Multiparous woman with lack of continuous progress for 2 hours with regional anesthesia, or for 1 hour without regional anesthesia (ACOG, 2000)*

Risks for the Woman

- Vaginal and cervical lacerations
- Extension of episiotomy
- Hemorrhage related to uterine atony, uterine rupture
- Bladder trauma
- Perineal wound infection

Risks for the Newborn

- Cephalohematoma (15%) and therefore increased risk of jaundice (**Fig. 10-9**)
- Intracranial hemorrhage and retinal hemorrhage
- Scalp lacerations or bruising (10%)

Assessment Findings

- Fetus at 36 weeks' gestation and the fetal head is engaged, at least at 0 station in the maternal pelvis (Cunningham, Leveno, Bloom, Hauth, Rouse, & Spong, 2010).

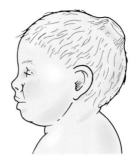

Figure 10-9 Cephalohematoma.

Medical Management

- Explain the procedure and obtain the woman's consent.
- Place the vacuum appropriately.
- After three unsuccessful attempts, proceed with a cesarean birth.
- The recommendations of the manufacturer of the vacuum device should be followed.

Nursing Actions

- Assess the woman's comfort level.
- Urinary bladder may be emptied by provider or nurse to decrease risk of trauma.
- Educate and reassure the woman and her family.
- Anticipate potential complications for the woman and the newborn.
- Pump up the vacuum pump manually to the pressure indicated on the pump, not to exceed 500–600 mm Hg.
  - *Cup detachment (pop off) is a warning sign that too much ineffective force is being exerted on fetal head.*
- Pressure should be released between contractions.
- The vacuum procedure should be timed from insertion of the cup into the vagina until the birth, and the cup should not be on the fetal head for longer than 15–20 minutes.
  - *Adherence to the guidelines for the vacuum device related to pressure and maximum time will minimize the nurse's liability in vacuum-assisted vaginal births.*

Forceps-Assisted Delivery

Forceps-assisted birth is one in which an instrument is used to assist with delivery of the fetal head, typically done to improve the health of the woman or the fetus. The rate of forceps delivery has decreased over the last 20 years from 5.55% to only 1.0% (Martin et al., 2011). Outlet forceps are used when the head is visible on the perineum and the skull has reached the pelvic floor, and rotation is less than 45 degrees (**Fig. 10-10**). Low forceps is used when the skull is at +2 station or lower in the maternal pelvis and not on the pelvic floor and rotation is greater than 45 degrees (ACOG, 2000) (**Fig. 10-11**). Only outlet and low forceps are currently recommended for use in assisting delivery.

Indications

- The fetal head engaged and the cervix is completely dilated.
- There is suspicion of immediate or potential fetal compromise.

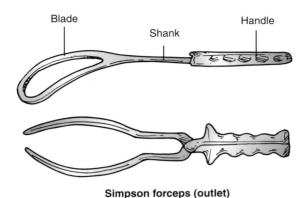

Simpson forceps (outlet)

Figure 10–10   Outlet forceps.

- To shorten the second stage for maternal benefit (e.g., maternal exhaustion and/or fetal compromise)
- Prolonged second stage
    - *Nulliparous woman with lack of continuing progress for 3 hours with regional anesthesia, or for 2 hours without anesthesia*
    - *Multiparous woman with lack of continuous progress for 2 hours with regional anesthesia, or for 1 hour without regional anesthesia*
- High level of regional anesthesia that inhibits pushing
- Maternal cardiac or pulmonary disease that contraindicates pushing efforts

Risks for the Woman

- Vaginal and cervical lacerations
- Extension of episiotomy
- Hemorrhage related to uterine atony, uterine rupture
- Perineal hematoma
- Bladder trauma
- Perineal wound infection

Risks for the Newborn

- Cephalohematoma
- Nerve injuries including craniofacial and brachial plexus injuries

- Skin lacerations or bruising
- Skull fractures
- Intracranial hemorrhage

Assessment Findings

- The cervix is completely dilated and the membranes are ruptured.
- The fetal head is engaged.
- The woman has adequate anesthesia.

Medical Management

- Use only on a fetus that is at least 36 weeks' gestation.
- Explain the procedure and obtain the woman's consent.
- Place forceps appropriately.

Nursing Actions

- Assess the woman's anesthesia level and comfort level.
- Insert a straight catheter to empty the bladder to decrease the risk of bladder trauma and increase room for the fetal head and forceps.
- Provide emotional support for the woman and her partner, since use of forceps can increase the anxiety level.
- Document the type of forceps, number of applications, and time of application.
- Anticipate potential complications for the woman and the neonate.

OPERATIVE BIRTH

Cesarean birth is a common operation performed on women, with reported rates varying across the world (**Fig. 10-12**). In developed countries, cesarean birth accounts for 21.3% of births in the United Kingdom; 23% in Northern Ireland; 23.3% in Australia; 32.9% in the United States; and more than 50% in some private hospitals in Chile, Argentina, Brazil, and Paraguay (Viswanathan et al., 2006). The cesarean section rate in the United States is 60% higher than the 1996 rate of 20.7%. Based on current data, 49.5% of women age 40 or older deliver by cesarean section (Martin et al., 2011). The benefits and harms of

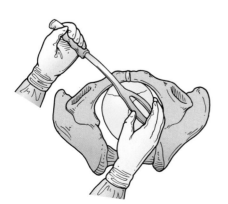
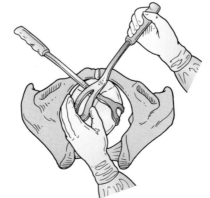
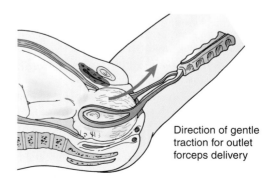

Direction of gentle traction for outlet forceps delivery

Figure 10–11   Forceps delivery.

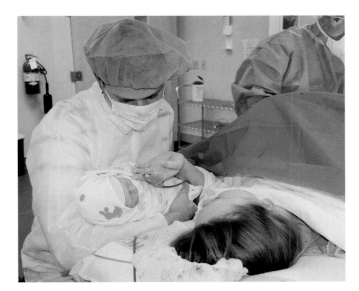

Figure 10-12 Family in cesarean birth.

elective cesarean birth, repeat cesarean birth, and vaginal birth after cesarean (VBAC) are under vigorous debate. Because cesarean birth accounts for one-third of births in the United States, Chapter 12 is devoted to care of cesarean woman and their families. Despite recommendations from ACOG on the safety of this, there has been a decrease in the rate of VBAC, which fell from 4% to 1% of all deliveries in 2008. At the same time the rate of repeat C-section nearly doubled. As a result, nearly all childbirths after a previous C-section (91%) were a repeat C-section (Podulka, Stranges, & Steiner, 2011).

Vaginal Birth After a Cesarean

Vaginal birth after a cesarean (VBAC) is used to describe labor and vaginal birth in a woman who has had a prior cesarean birth. A **trial of labor after cesarean** or **TOLAC** offer women an opportunity of achieving a VBAC. Evidence suggests that benefits of VBAC outweigh risks in women with lower uterine transverse cesarean birth who have no contraindications for a vaginal birth. Benefits of VBAC include shorter recovery time and overall lower morbidity and mortality, including less blood loss, fewer infections, and fewer thromboembolic problems (ACOG, 2010). Additionally ACOG notes for those considering larger families, VBAC may avoid potential future maternal consequences of multiple cesarean deliveries such as hysterectomy, bowel or bladder injury, transfusion, infection, and abnormal placentation such as placenta previa and placenta accreta.

According to ACOG, most women with one previous cesarean birth with a low transverse incision are candidates for vaginal birth after cesarean birth and should be counseled about VBAC and offered a trial of labor (ACOG, 2010). However, VBAC rates have fallen 67% since 1996 (Martin et al., 2006). This is reported to be related to more conservative ACOG practice guidelines, legal pressure, and the continuing debate over the harms and benefits of vaginal birth compared with cesarean birth and an increase in repeat cesarean births. Regardless of the reason for the previous cesarean birth, once a woman has had a cesarean birth there is a more than 90% chance that subsequent deliveries will be by cesarean (Martin et al., 2006). VBAC is associated with a small but important risk of uterine rupture, and that risk increases with the number of previous cesarean births.

Indications

■ One or two prior low transverse cesarean births with no other uterine scars
■ Clinically adequate pelvis
■ Physician and OR team immediately available to perform emergent cesarean birth.

Contraindications

■ Prior vertical (classical) or T-shaped uterine incision or other uterine surgery (**Fig. 10-13**)
■ Previous uterine rupture
■ Pelvic abnormalities
■ Medical or obstetric complications that preclude a vaginal birth
■ Inability to perform an emergent cesarean birth if necessary because of insufficient personnel such as surgeons, anesthesia, or facility

Risks Associated With VBAC

■ Uterine rupture and complications associated with uterine rupture (1%)
   ■ *Waiting for spontaneous labor and avoiding use of prostaglandins and oxytocin reduces the risk of uterine rupture.*
■ A failed TOLAC is associated with more complications than elective repeat cesarean delivery.

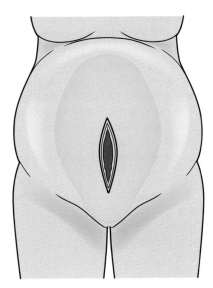

Figure 10-13 Vertical uterine incision.

■ Uterine rupture or dehiscence is the outcome associated with TOLAC that most significantly increases the chance of additional maternal and neonatal morbidity.

■ Neonatal morbidity is higher in the setting of a failed TOLAC than in a vaginal birth after cesarean delivery (VBAC).

Assessment Findings

■ Records confirm prior transverse uterine scar.

Medical Management

■ Explain the risks and benefits of VBAC.
■ Induction of labor for maternal or fetal indications remains an option in women undergoing TOLAC.
■ Use of misoprostol for cervical ripening is contraindicated.
■ The physician and surgical team must be available to perform a cesarean birth if necessary.

Nursing Actions

■ Review the prenatal record for documentation of prior uterine scar because VBAC is contraindicated in vertical uterine incisions.
■ Monitor closely and continuously uterine activity and FHR.
■ Assess the progress of labor.
■ Provide information, reassurance, and support to the woman.
■ Report any complaints of severe pain and be alert to signs of uterine rupture such as vaginal bleeding and ascending station of fetal presenting part.

POST-TERM PREGNANCY

A **post-term pregnancy** or prolonged pregnancy is one that has a gestational period of 42 completed weeks or more from the first day of the last menses (if the menstrual cycle is 28 days). The actual cause of post-term pregnancy is unclear; the etiology and pathophysiology are not completely understood (Gilbert, 2007). For 5%–10% of pregnant women, their pregnancies continue beyond 294 days (42 completed weeks) and are described as being "post-term" or "postdate" (Cunningham et al., 2010). Postmaturity refers to the abnormal condition of the newborn resulting from prolonged pregnancy. Both the woman and infant are at increased risk of adverse events when the pregnancy continues beyond term. After 41 weeks, neonatal and postneonatal death risk increase significantly (Gülmezoglu, Crowther, & Middleton, 2006).

Obstetric problems associated with post-term pregnancy include:

■ Induction of labor with an unfavorable cervix
■ Cesarean birth
■ Prolonged labor
■ Postpartum hemorrhage
■ Traumatic birth

It is likely that some of these unwanted outcomes result from intervening when the uterus and cervix are not ready for labor.

First-trimester pregnancy ultrasound is associated with a reduced incidence of post-term pregnancy, possibly by avoiding incorrect dating and misclassification of postdates. Induction of labor is widely practiced to try to prevent the problems mentioned above and to improve the health outcome for women and their infants.

■ Labor induction may itself cause problems, especially when the cervix is not ripe.
■ The ideal timing for induction of labor is not clear. In the past, there was a tendency to await spontaneous labor until 42 completed weeks.
■ Current practice is to offer induction of labor between 41 and 42 weeks.

The gestational age and the cervix being unfavorable (unripe) may affect the success of the induction of labor and result in an increase in cesarean birth rates.

■ When the cervix is favorable (usually a Bishop score of 6 or more), induction is often carried out via oxytocin and AROM.
■ If the cervix is not favorable, usually a prostaglandin gel or tablet is placed in the vagina or cervix to ripen the cervix and to initiate the UCs and labor. Many protocols are used with varying repeat intervals and transition to oxytocin and amniotomy depending on the onset of UCs and progress of cervical dilation.

Risks Associated With Post-Term Pregnancy

■ Prolonged pregnancy results in a decrease in amniotic fluid volume and may impact fetal status because amniotic fluid cushions the fetus and cord from pressure and injury and amniotic fluid volume is an indicator of placental function.
■ As the placenta begins to age, there are increased areas of infarction and deposition of calcium and fibrin within its tissue. This creates decreased placental reserve (**Fig. 10-14**).

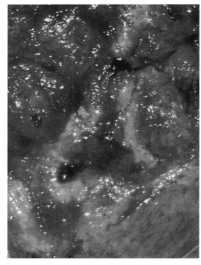

Figure 10–14   Calcified placenta are white areas in placenta.

■ Meconium-stained fluid occurs in 25%–30% of post-term pregnancies. This creates an increased risk for meconium aspiration of the neonate at birth (Cunningham et al., 2010).
■ There is an increased risk of fetal macrosomia as the fetus increases in size approximately 1 ounce per day after term.

Assessment Findings
■ Category II or III FHR related to decreased amniotic fluid and uteroplacental insufficiency with aging placenta
■ Meconium-stained fluid
■ Women report increased anxiety and frustration with prolonged pregnancy
■ Fetal macrosomia

Medical Management
■ Antenatal surveillance
■ Induction of labor offered at 41 weeks of gestation

Nursing Actions
■ Review the plan of care with the woman.
■ Confirm prolonged pregnancy on the prenatal record.
■ Anticipate management with induction of labor and possible cervical ripening agents.
■ Monitor FHR because of increased incidence of utero-placental insufficiency.
■ Assess amniotic fluid for amount and meconium staining with ROM (see Concept Map for post-term pregnancy and labor induction).

OBSTETRICAL EMERGENCIES

Obstetrical emergencies are urgent clinical situations that place either the maternal or fetal status at risk for increased morbidity and mortality. Intrapartum emergencies may be related to one or more maternal, fetal, uterine, cord, and/or placental factors. The physiological effects of intrapartum emergencies on the woman and fetus may create rapid deterioration in oxygenation and perfusion. Intrapartum emergencies may place the woman and fetus at risk of exceeding their oxygen and perfusion reserves (Curran, 2003). Interventions are directed to stabilization of maternal status, which in turn stabilizes fetal status.

Shoulder Dystocia

Shoulder dystocia refers to difficulty encountered during delivery of the shoulders after the birth of the head. The anterior shoulder or more rarely both shoulders become impacted above the pelvic rim. The first sign is a retraction of the fetal head against the maternal perineum after delivery of the head, sometimes referred to as **turtle sign**. This impaction of the fetal shoulders may lead to a prolonged delivery time of more than 60 seconds. Shoulder dystocia is an unpreventable and unpredictable obstetrical emergency that can result in serious fetal morbidity and even mortality if not recognized and successfully managed.

Neonatal morbidity includes:
■ Brachial plexus injuries
■ Clavicle fracture
■ Neurological injury
■ Asphyxia
■ Death

Reduction in the interval of time from delivery of the head to the body is crucial to fetal outcome. Most experts note that more than a 5-minute delay in head to body interval may result in fetal hypoxemia and acidosis. It is estimated that a newborn can survive for approximately 6 minutes before irreversible brain and organ damage occurs. The incidence of shoulder dystocia ranges from reports of 0.6%–1.4% (ACOG, 2002). Most cases of shoulder dystocia cannot be accurately predicted or prevented (Cunningham et al., 2010). Additionally, there is no clear evidence to support the use of prophylactic maneuvers to prevent shoulder dystocia (Atukorala, Middleton, & Crouther, 2008).

Risk Factors Associated With Shoulder Dystocia
■ Fetal macrosomia (wt >4,500 grams)
■ Maternal diabetes
■ History of shoulder dystocia
■ Prolonged second stage
■ Excessive weight gain

Risks Associated With Shoulder Dystocia
■ Delay in delivery of the shoulders results in compression of the fetal neck by the maternal pelvis, which impairs fetal circulation and results in possible increased intracranial pressure, anoxia, asphyxia, and brain damage.
■ Brachial plexus injury and clavicle fracture in the neonate can also occur.
■ Maternal complications include lacerations, infection, bladder injury, or postpartum hemorrhage.

Assessment Findings
■ The first sign is a retraction of the fetal head against the maternal perineum after delivery of the head, sometimes referred to as turtle sign.
■ Delay in delivery of shoulders after delivery of head

Medical Management
■ Downward traction may be applied to the fetal head with suprapubic pressure.
■ Extend the midline episiotomy to obtain room for maneuvers.
■ The McRoberts maneuver is a reasonable initial approach.
■ The Woods corkscrew maneuver progressively rotates the posterior shoulder 180 degrees to disimpact the anterior shoulder.
■ Deliver the posterior shoulder by sweeping the posterior arm across the fetus's chest followed by delivery of the arm.

■ Most shoulder dystocias are resolved by using the above maneuvers.
■ The Zavanelli maneuver is cephalic replacement into the pelvis and then cesarean delivery, for catastrophic cases only (ACOG, 2002).
■ Planned cesarean birth to prevent shoulder dystocia may be considered for suspected fetal macrosomia with an estimated fetal weight exceeding 5,000 grams in women without diabetes and 4,500 grams in women with diabetes (ACOG, 2002).

Nursing Actions

■ Explain the situation to the woman and the family and explain the interventions to resolve dystocia and importance of woman's assistance with maneuvers.
■ Request assistance, as additional nurses may be needed to implement maneuvers to resolve dystocia.
■ Insert a straight catheter into the woman to empty the bladder if it is distended to make more room for the fetus.
■ A variety of techniques may be used to free the impacted shoulder from beneath the symphysis pubis (Camune & Bracher, 2007); pressure can be applied above the pubic bone or laterally to the pubic bone to dislodge the anterior shoulder and push it beneath the symphysis (**Fig. 10-15A**).
■ The mother should not push except when instructed to and only when it is believed the shoulder has been released.
■ The McRoberts maneuver consists of sharply flexing the thigh onto the maternal abdomen to straighten the sacrum (**Fig. 10-15B**).
■ Use of fundal pressure is controversial and not indicated in shoulder dystocia.
■ Notify the neonatal team.
■ Prepare for neonatal resuscitation.
■ Document the series of interventions and clinical events with time intervals (Simpson & O'Brien-Abel, 2013).

Prolapse of the Umbilical Cord

Prolapse of the umbilical cord is when the cord lies below the presenting part of the fetus (**Fig. 10-16**). The cord may prolapse in front of the presenting part, into the vagina, or through the introitus. **Occult prolapse** is when the cord is palpated through the membranes but does not drop into the vagina. When cord prolapse occurs, it is typically with AROM or SROM when the presenting part is not engaged in the pelvis. The cord becomes entrapped against the presenting part and circulation is occluded, resulting in FHR bradycardia. A loop of cord may be palpated or visualized in the vagina. An emergency cesarean birth is typically done to improve neonatal outcomes with a prolapsed cord.

Risk Factors for Prolapse of the Umbilical Cord

■ Malpresentation of the fetus (such as breech)
■ Unengaged presenting part

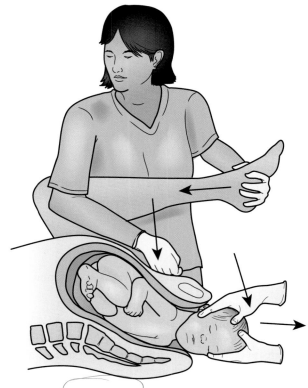

Figure 10-15 McRoberts maneuver and subrapubic pressure. When fetal shoulders become impacted under the maternal symphis pubis, the nurse should initiate McRoberts maneuver by hyperextending the birthing woman's legs onto her abdomen and simultaneously providing suprapubic pressure to assist the fetus in adducting the arms closer to the body in an attempt to release the impacted shoulders.

■ Polyhydramnios
■ Small or preterm fetus
■ Multiple gestation
■ High parity

Risks Associated With Prolapse of the Umbilical Cord

■ Total or partial occlusion of the cord, resulting in rapid deterioration in fetal perfusion and oxygenation (Curran, 2003)

Assessment Findings

■ Sudden fetal bradycardia (i.e., prolonged decelerations)
■ Prolapsed umbilical cord that may be felt with a SVE or visualized in or protruding from the vagina

Medical Management

■ Vaginal birth or operative vaginal delivery may be attempted if birth is imminent.
■ Perform emergency cesarean section.

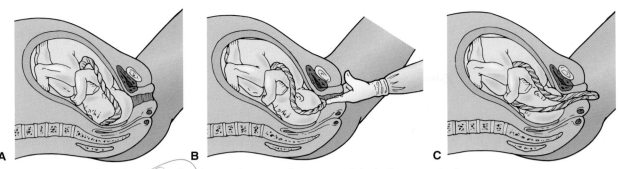

Figure 10–16 Prolapsed cord. A. Occult. The cord cannot be seen or felt during a vaginal examination. B. Complete. During a vaginal examination, the cord is felt as a pulsating mass. C. Frank. The cord precedes the fetal head or feet and can be seen protruding from the vagina.

Nursing Actions

■ Occlusion of the cord may be partially relieved by lifting the presenting part off the cord with a vaginal exam. The examiner's hand remains in the vagina, lifting the presenting part off the cord until delivery by cesarean (**Fig. 10-17**).
■ Request assistance and notify the medical provider.
■ Explain the situation to the woman and family and that interventions are necessary to expedite delivery.
■ Explain to the woman the importance of her assistance.
■ Recommend position changes such a knee-chest position or Trendelenburg to try to relieve pressure on the occluded cord (**Fig. 10-18**).
■ Administer O_2 at 10 L/min by mask.
■ Give IV fluid hydration bolus.
■ Discontinue oxytocin.
■ Administer a tocolytic agent to decrease uterine activity.
■ Move toward emergency delivery. If birth is imminent, the provider may proceed with vaginal delivery. If birth is not imminent, anticipate and prepare for emergency cesarean section.

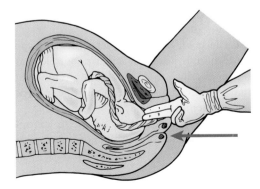

Figure 10–17 Vaginal examination with prolapsed cord, lifting presenting part off the cord.

Ruptured Vasa Previa

Vasa Previa occurs when fetal vessels unsupported by placenta or umbilical cord traverses the membranes over the cervix. The condition usually results from villimentous insertion of

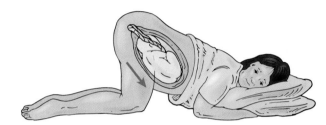

Figure 10–18 Knee-chest position with prolapsed cord.

the cord into the membranes rather than the placenta or from vessels running between lobes of the placenta with one or more accessory lobes (**Fig. 10-19**). If undiagnosed, it is associated with perinatal mortality of 60% (Oyelese, 2004). Pressure on unprotected vessels by the presenting part can lead to fetal asphyxia and death. **Ruptured vasa previa** refers to when the fetal vessels running through the membranes, over the cervix, that are unprotected rupture (Oyelese & Smulian, 2007). Rupture of membranes frequently leads to rapid fetal exsanguination (Cunningham et al., 2010).

Risk Factors for Vasa Previa

■ Low lining placenta
■ Placenta previa
■ Pregnancies in which the placenta has accessory lobes
■ Multiple gestation
■ Pregnancies resulting from IVF

Risks Associated With Vasa Previa

■ Fetal asphyxia from cord compression
■ Fetal death from exsanguination

Assessment Findings

■ Vasa previa is most commonly diagnosed when rupture of the membranes is accompanied by vaginal bleeding or fetal distress or death.

Medical Management

■ If diagnosed prenatally with ultrasound, cesarean birth prior to labor and ruptured membranes improves

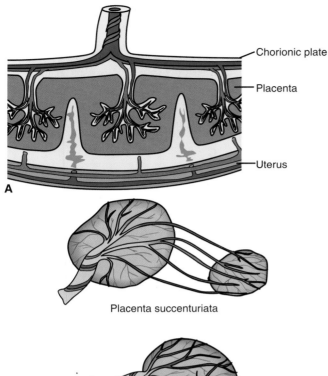

A

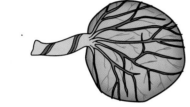

Placenta succenturiata

Marginal insertion of the cord

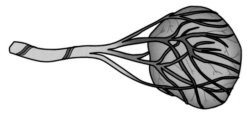

B   Velamentous insertion of the cord

Figure 10–19   A. Normal insertion of umbilical cord into chorionic plate. Normally the umbilical cord inserts near the center of the chorionic plate, which stabilizes the fetal vessels as they leave the umbilical cord. Like the roots of a tree, the fetal vessels branch over the surface of the chorionic plate and then dive into the placental parenchyma. B. Illustration depicting abnormalities of umbilical cord insertion into the placenta. With a velamentous insertion of the umbilical cord into the membranes or with a succenturiate lobe, fetal vessels, within the chorionic membranes and unprotected by the placenta, may course across the cervix and result in a vasa previa.

neonatal outcomes. Planned cesarean birth at 35 weeks improves neonatal survival to 95% (Oyelese & Smulian, 2007).

■ When acute bleeding occurs, emergent delivery is indicated. Usually cesarean birth is indicated.

■ If a woman is diagnosed by ultrasound during pregnancy, she may be admitted to the hospital for surveillance, corticosteroids to promote lung maturity, and a planned cesarean birth at 35 weeks. Nursing care related to antenatal hospitalization for high-risk pregnancy is detailed in Chapter 7.

■ If bleeding is observed upon examination by the nurse, an immediate bedside evaluation by the provider is indicated.

Rupture of the Uterus

Rupture of the uterus is a partial or complete tear in the uterine muscle.

In complete uterine rupture, all of the layers of the uterine wall are separated.

In incomplete uterine rupture (uterine dehiscence), the uterine muscle is separated but the visceral peritoneum is intact.

Signs and symptoms of uterine rupture are related to internal hemorrhage and reflected in both the maternal and fetal status, in relationship to the extent of the rupture.

■ The condition usually becomes evident because of signs of fetal compromise and maternal hypovolemia related to hemorrhage.

■ If the fetal presenting part is in the pelvis, loss of station may occur, which is detected with a vaginal exam.

Maternal and fetal survival depends on prompt identification and surgical intervention.

■ Fetal mortality with uterine rupture is reported at 50%–70%.

■ Maternal mortality is 5%.

Risks Associated With Rupture of the Uterus

■ The greatest risk factor is previous cesarean section with TOLAC 0.5–0.9% (ACOG, 2010) (Cunningham et al., 2010); others are previous vertical uterine scar, multifetal gestation, and uterine tachysystole.

■ Potential effects on woman and fetus include hypovolemic shock, infection, hypoxemia, acidosis, neurological damage, and possible death.

■ Maternal complications are primarily due to hypovolemia as a result of hemorrhage.

■ Complications to the fetus may be due to uteroplacental insufficiency, placental abruption, cord compression, asphyxia, and/or hypovolemia.

Assessment Findings

■ Maternal assessment findings may include signs and symptoms of hypovolemic shock, such as:
   ■ *Hypotension*
   ■ *Tachypnea*
   ■ *Tachycardia*
   ■ *Pallor*

■ Severe tearing sensation, burning "stabbing" pain, and contractions

■ Vaginal bleeding
■ Fetal response is related to hemorrhage and placental separation and may include late decelerations, loss of FHR variability, fetal bradycardia, or even loss of FHR.
■ Ascending station of the fetal presenting part

Medical Management

■ Perform emergency cesarean birth.
    ■ *Control maternal hemorrhage.*
    ■ *Hysterectomy may be necessary.*
■ Transfusions may be needed.

Nursing Actions

■ Request assistance and notify the medical provider.
■ Stabilize the woman with O_2 and IV fluids and blood products.
■ Prepare for emergency cesarean birth.
■ Explain the situation to the woman and her family that interventions that will expedite delivery, and the importance of their assistance.

Anaphylactic Syndrome (also known as Amniotic Fluid Embolism)

Anaphylactic Syndrome is a rare but often fatal complication that occurs during pregnancy, labor, and birth, or the first 24 hours post-birth. An embolism forms when the amniotic fluid that contains fetal cells, lanugo, and vernix enters the maternal vascular system and results in cardio respiratory collapse. This is discussed more completely in Chapter 14.

Disseminated Intravascular Coagulation

Disseminated intravascular coagulation (DIC) is a syndrome that occurs when the body is breaking down blood clots faster than it can form a clot. This quickly depletes the body of clotting factors, leads to hemorrhage, and can rapidly lead to maternal death. Women who experience DIC are transferred to the critical care unit and a perinatologist manages the care. This is discussed more completely in Chapter 14.

Critical Care in Perinatal Nursing

Critical care intrapartum nursing may be required when a woman has a preexisting condition or a maternal or fetal complication develops during pregnancy. The ability of a hospital to deliver this high level of care may vary; because high-risk and critically ill women may be encountered in any setting, all intrapartum nurses should be prepared to identify and participate in stabilizing critically ill women for transport to a tertiary care center or intensive care unit (AWHONN, 2008). Intrapartum nurses who care for critically ill women receive additional education and undergo didactic and verification of learning and clinical skills beyond the scope of this chapter. Most critically ill pregnant women are cared for in adult intensive care units or in specialized obstetric critical care units. No matter where the care is delivered, a comprehensive plan of care should address the unique physiologic needs of the pregnant woman. Therefore, it is essential that when indicated, critical care and perinatal nurses collaborate to coordinate care for this unique population. Women who have any of the disorders or diseases presented in the high-risk didactic content have the potential to become critically ill if their condition deteriorates.

OBSTETRIC COMPLICATIONS

Pregnancy-Related Complications in Labor

Most pregnancy-related complications have the potential to impact labor. For example, diabetic women in labor need continuous monitoring of glucose, in particular because hyperglycemia impacts placental perfusion. Another example is preeclampsia, where vasospasm related to the pathophysiology of preeclampsia also diminishes perfusion and impacts both maternal and fetal outcomes. Rather than repeat all the information from Chapter 7 on complications during pregnancy, we are referring you to that chapter for management and care of patients with these disorders.

Pregestational Complications Impacting Intrapartal Period

Labor complicated by cardiovascular disease is potentially dangerous to maternal and fetal outcomes. Marked hemodynamic changes in labor have a profound effect on the women in labor, placental perfusion, and fetal status. Extensive discussion of specific pregestational complications and their management in labor is beyond the scope of this text. Please refer to Chapter 7 for additional information on management of pregestational complications.

Multiple Gestation Delivery

The patient with a multiple gestation pregnancy is at higher risk for many complications during the intrapartum period, which include preterm birth, preeclampsia, and hemorrhage. With the mean gestational age of delivery being 35 weeks for twins, 32 weeks for triplets, and 29 weeks for quadruplets, preparing for the delivery of multiples is not only high risk but complex (Gilbert, 2011). Decisions on method of delivery are dependent on a number of factors, including: number of fetuses, position of presentation of fetuses, and in particular the presenting fetus (twin A) and fetal weight. If the first twin is vertex presentation, vaginal delivery may be attempted. It is common now for women to be delivered by cesarean birth with twins. High order multiple gestations are typically delivered by cesarean birth (Cunningham et al., 2010). See Chapter 7 for more on multiple gestation pregnancy and Chapter 9 for fetal monitoring with multiples.

Delivery of Intrauterine Fetal Demise

Intrauterine fetal demise is the death of the fetus in utero. Further discussion of the care of families experiencing an intrauterine fetal demise can be found related to postpartum nursing care in Chapter 17.

Causes

- Often unexplained
- Severe medical maternal complications with diabetes, renal disease, cardiovascular disease, connective tissue disease and autoimmune disease
- Placental abruption
- Labor with fetus less then 24 weeks of gestation
- Malnutrition
- Maternal trauma
- Post-term pregnancy (more then 2 weeks beyond the estimated date of delivery)
- Cord accidents
- Extreme prematurity
- Congenital or genetic abnormalities making the fetus incompatible with life

Risks Associated With Intrauterine Fetal Demise Pregnancy

- Prolonged retention of the dead fetus may lead to the development of disseminated intravascular coagulation (DIC) in the mother and puts the mother at higher risk for infection, which can result in sepsis or endometritis.

Assessment Findings

- Decreased or absent fetal movement for several hours or more

- Intrauterine Fetal Death (IUFD) is confirmed by visualization of the fetal heart with absence of heart action on ultrasound.

Medical Management

- Induction of labor within 24–48 hours of confirmed diagnosis
- Stillborn delivery

Nursing Actions

- Provide anticipatory guidance in slow, small increments
- Talk to patient and family directly.
- Give simple explanations.
- Allow the patient to grieve.
- Provide comforting touch to the patient.
- Continuity of care; prevent unnecessary moves from labor room to delivery room to recovery room.
- Allow unlimited time with infant after delivery.
- Provide the patient and family with mementos; baby clothing, photos of baby with family and patient, measuring tape, baby comb, blanket, footprints, and handprints.
- Referral Services: visits and support from social services, spiritual advisors, and hospital staff

CONCEPT MAP

Postterm Pregnancy and Labor

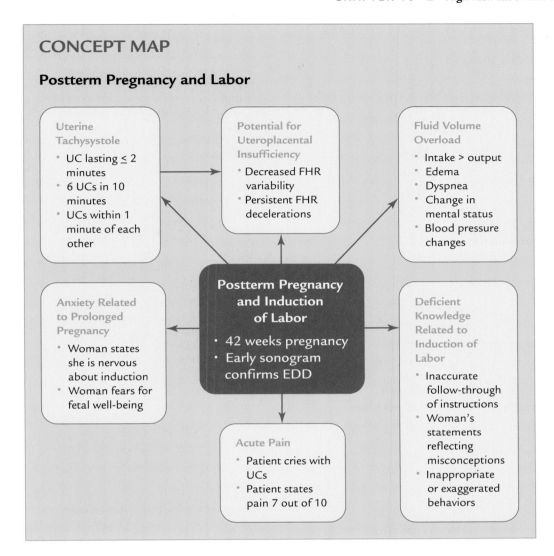

Problem No. 1: Uterine tachysystole
Goal: Decreased uterine activity
Outcome: Patient will have decreased contractions.

Nursing Actions

1. Evaluation of uterine contraction strength, frequency, and resting tone duration by palpation or IUPC
2. Evaluation of uterine resting tone by palpation or IUPC pressure below 20 mm Hg
3. Assessment of fetal heart rate in response to uterine contractions
4. Turn oxytocin down or off in the event of uterine tachysystole or indeterminate or abnormal fetal heart rate.
5. Maternal position change
6. IV bolus of at least 500 mL of lactated Ringer's
7. O_2 administration by mask at 10 L/min
8. If no response consider terbutaline.
9. Notify provider.

Problem No. 2: Knowledge deficit related to induction of labor
Goal: Patient understands indication and process of labor induction.

Outcome: Patient states she understands indication and process of induction of labor.

Nursing Actions

1. Explain all procedures.
2. Encourage verbalization of questions.
3. Practice active listening.
4. Provide emotional support.
5. Make needed referrals to social services and mental health specialists if needed.

Problem 3: Anxiety related to prolonged pregnancy
Goal: Decreased anxiety
Outcome: Patient verbalizes that she feels less anxious.

Nursing Actions

1. Explain all information and procedures in lay language and repeat information PRN.
2. Provide autonomy and choices.
3. Encourage patient and family to verbalize their feelings regarding prolonged pregnancy by asking open-ended questions.

4. Be calm and reassuring in interactions with the patient and her family.
5. Explore past coping strategies.

Problem 4: Fluid volume overload related to prolonged oxytocin
Goal: Fluid balance
Outcome: Patient maintains fluid balance.

Nursing Actions

1. Auscultate the lung sounds.
2. Assess I&O.
3. Maintain IV fluids as ordered.
4. Calculate intake of all fluids.
5. Measure output including emesis and urine.
6. Assess edema.

Problem No. 5: Acute pain related to UCs
Goal: Decreased pain
Outcome: Patient will state that pain is improved.

Nursing Actions

1. Assess level, location, and type of pain.
2. Sustaining physical presence, eye contact
3. Verbal encouragement, reassurance, and praise
4. Comfort measures such as ice chips, fluids, food, and pain medications
5. Hygiene including mouth care, pericare, and changing chux
6. Assistance with position changes
7. Reassuring touch, massage
8. Application of heat and cold
9. Hydrotherapy shower and tub if no ROM
10. Provide an environment that is conducive to relaxation, such as low lights, decreased noise.
11. Teach patient relaxation and breathing techniques.

Problem No. 6: Potential for uteroplacental insufficiency Category II or III FHR
Goal: Maintain normal FHR
Outcome: FHR pattern is Category 1, baseline is normal with moderate variability and accelerations.

Nursing Actions

1. Assess FHR baseline variability and for decelerations.
2. Change the mother's position.
3. IV bolus of at least 500 mL of lactated Ringer's
4. O_2 at 10 L/min by mask
5. Turn oxytocin down or off.
6. Notify the provider.
7. Request bedside evaluation if the FHR is Category III.

TYING IT ALL TOGETHER

As a labor and delivery nurse, this is your second shift caring for Mallory Polk. She is a 42-year-old, single, African-American attorney whom you admitted yesterday at 32 weeks' gestation with the diagnosis of preterm labor. She was treated with magnesium sulfate and Betamethasone. Tonight when you came on your shift at 7 P.M. she remained on magnesium sulfate but was contracting regularly and at 3:20 A.M. had SROM for clear fluid. At 4:00 A.M. her cervix was 5 cm/90%/+1. At that time the magnesium sulfate was discontinued and normal spontaneous vaginal birth is anticipated because of advanced preterm labor. Over the next hour Mallory is contracting every 2–3 minutes and is coping well with uterine contractions. Her sister, Allison, is at the bedside providing labor support. The FHR baseline is 140s, with average variability, occasional accelerations, and no FHR decelerations. At 5:15 A.M., Mallory feels the urge to have a bowel movement and you do an SVE. Her vaginal exam reveals that she is 10 cm/100%/+1.

Who needs to be notified of your significant assessment findings?
What would you report?

Within 15 minutes of your report, her physician arrives, confirms your assessment that Mallory is completely dilated, and wants her to start to push. You coach Mallory to begin pushing with her next contraction.

What are your priorities in nursing care for Mallory?
Discuss the rationale for the priorities.
State nursing diagnosis, expected outcome, and interventions related to this problem.
What would you anticipate as Mallory's teaching needs?

Over the next hour, Mallory's contractions slow to every 7 minutes and she is pushing with open glottis pushing and feels the urge to bear down with the peak of contractions. A sterile vaginal exam reveals that she is completely dilated and descent of the fetal head is +2 station. You request the physician to come to the bedside to evaluate fetal descent. After her physician evaluates Mallory, she requests oxytocin augmentation to increase the frequency of her contractions. You initiate oxytocin augmentation at 1 mU/min per physician orders.

Discuss the risk associated with oxytocin augmentation.
Outline nursing actions when caring for a patient with oxytocin augmentation.
What teaching would you include related to oxytocin augmentation?

Within 30 minutes of starting the oxytocin, Mallory is having UCs every 1–2 minutes lasting 45 to 55 seconds moderate to palpation with a relaxed uterus between contractions. The FHR baseline is in the 140s with variable decelerations to 90s for 40 seconds with UCs, and FHR variability is moderate.

What are your priorities in nursing care?
Discuss the rationale for the priorities and nursing actions.
What are your nursing actions based on your assessment?
State nursing diagnosis, expected outcomes.

Over the next hour, Mallory's contractions are every 3–4 minutes and she is pushing with contractions and has a strong urge to bear down with contractions. The FHR is 140s with moderate variability and variable decelerations to 100 bpm for 30 seconds with contractions and open glottis pushing. Her SVE reveals fetal descent to +3 station.

What are your immediate priorities in nursing care for Mallory?
Discuss the rationale for the priorities.

■ ■ ■   **Review Questions**   ■ ■ ■

1. Which nursing action can improve uterine blood flow, increase umbilical cord circulation, improve maternal oxygenation, and decrease uterine activity?
   A. Administering oxygen to the mother
   B. Changing the woman's position
   C. Discontinuing oxytocin
   D. Infusing intravenous fluids

2. A laboring woman reports spontaneous rupture of membranes and you assess severe decelerations in the FHR. Examination reveals a cord in the vagina. The first nursing action is to:
   A. Manually elevate the presenting part
   B. Administer a tocolytic agent
   C. Administer an IV fluid bolus
   D. Empty the patient's bladder

3. An increased risk for shoulder dystocia is associated with:
   A. Preterm labor
   B. Maternal diabetes
   C. VBAC
   D. Previous precipitous birth

4. Vacuum extractor cup placement on the fetal head should not exceed:
   A. 5 minutes
   B. 10 minutes
   C. 20 minutes
   D. 30 minutes

5. A high probability of successful induction is associated with a Bishop score of:
   A. Greater than 4
   B. Greater than 6
   C. Less than 4
   D. Less than 6

6. When fetal vessels are unsupported by placenta or the umbilical cord traverses the membranes over the cervix, below the presenting part, this is referred to as:
   A. Anterior dystocia
   B. Vasa Previa
   C. Breech
   D. Placenta Previa

7. Women 40 years or older have a cesarean rate of:
   A. 25.5%
   B. 62.5%
   C. 35.5%
   D. 49.5%

8. Preeclampsia, thrombosis, gestational and type II diabetes are associated risk factors for what?
   A. Good nutrition
   B. Maternal obesity
   C. Cardiac problems
   D. Maternal weight

9. The first sign of shoulder dystocia is referred to as:
   A. Unsuccessful vaginal delivery
   B. Breech
   C. Bishop Score
   D. Turtle sign

10. The benefits of VBACs include:
   A. Shorter recovery time, fewer infections, decreased blood loss
   B. Decreased pain, decreased fetal stress
   C. Shorter recovery time, decreased fetal stress
   D. Decreased discomfort, decreased anxiety

References

Agency for Healthcare Research and Quality. (2001). Reducing and preventing adverse drug events to decrease hospital costs (AHRQ Publication No. 01-0200). Washington, DC: Author.

American College of Obstetricians and Gynecologists (ACOG). (2010). Vaginal birth after previous cesarean delivery. Washington (DC): American College of Obstetricians and Gynecologists (ACOG); 2010 Aug. 14 (ACOG practice bulletin; no. 115).

American College of Obstetricians and Gynecologists (ACOG). (2009). Management of stillbirth. Washington (DC): American College of Obstetricians and Gynecologists (ACOG); 2009 Mar. 14 (ACOG practice bulletin; no. 102).

American College of Obstetricians and Gynecologists (ACOG). (2003). Dystocia and augmentation of labor. Washington (DC): American College of Obstetricians and Gynecologists (ACOG); 2003 Dec. 10 (ACOG practice bulletin; no. 49).

American College of Obstetricians and Gynecologists (ACOG). (1999). *Induction of labor*. Practice Bulletin No. 10, 2002. Washington, DC: Author.

American College of Obstetricians and Gynecologists (ACOG). (2000). *Operative vaginal delivery*. Practice Bulletin No. 17, June 2000. Washington, DC: Author.

American College of Obstetricians and Gynecologists (ACOG). (2002) *Shoulder dystocia*. Practice Bulletin No. 40, November, 2002.

American [...]
(2004[...]
Bullet[...]

Athukora[...]
interv[...]
*of Sys[...]
10.10[...]

AWHO[...]
Nurs[...]
Was[...]
Neor[...]

Bishop,[...]
and [...]

Bricker,[...]
of la[...]
Art.[...]

Camun[...]
Dys[...]
488-498.

1 C
2 A
3 B
4 C
5 B
6 B
7 D
8 B
9 D
10 A

Catalano, P. (2007). Management of Obesity in Pregnancy. Queenan, J. (Ed.) (2007) High Risk Pregnancy, Washington, The American College of Obstetricians and Gynecologists..

Cunningham, E. G., Leveno, K. J., Bloom, S. L., Hauth, J. C., Rouse, D. J., & Spong, C. Y. (2010). *Williams Obstetrics* (23rd ed.). New York: McGraw-Hill.

Curran, C. (2003). Intrapartum emergencies. *Journal of Obstetric, Gynecologic & Neonatal Nursing, 32,* 802–813.

Gilbert, E. (2011). Labor and Delivery at Risk. In Mattson, S., & Smith, J. (Ed.), Core Curriculum for Maternal-Newborn Nursing, Fourth Edition. Thousand Oaks, Sage.

Gilbert, E., (2010). *Manual of high risk pregnancy and delivery,* 5th Ed. St. Louis, MO: C. V. Mosby.

Gülmezoglu, A. M., Crowther, C. A., & Middleton, P. (2006). Induction of labour for improving birth outcomes for women at or beyond term. *Cochrane Database of Systematic Reviews* 2006, Issue 4. Art. No.: CD004945. DOI: 10.1002/14651858.CD004945.pub2.

Hofmeyr, G. J., & Gülmezoglu, A. M. (2003). Vaginal misoprostol for cervical ripening and induction of labour. *Cochrane Database of Systematic Reviews* 2003, Issue 1. Art. No.: CD000941. DOI: 10.1002/14651858.CD000941.

Institute for Healthcare Improvement. (2007). Prevent harm from high alert medications: How to guide. Cambridge, MA: Author.

Institute for Safe Medication Practices. (2007). High-alert medications. Huntingdon Valley, PA: Author.

Institute for Healthcare Improvement. (2010). Expedition: Improving Perinatal Safety—The Oxytocin Bundle. Retrieved from http://ihi.org/IHI/Topics/CriticalCare/IntensiveCare/ImprovementStories/WhatIsaBundleExpedition: Improving Perinatal Safety — The Oxytocin Bundle 4-16-12

Ramachenderan, J., Bradford, J., and McLean, M. (2008) Maternal obesity and pregnancy complications: A review. *Australian and New Zealand Journal of Obstetrics and Gynaecology, 48,* 228–235.

Jonsson, M., Norden-Lindeberg, S., & Hanson, U. (2007). Analysis of malpractice claims with a focus on oxytocin use in labour. *Acta Obstetricia et Gynecologica, 86,* 315–319.

Jozwiak, M., Bloemenkamp, K., Kelly, A., Mol, B., Irion, O., & Boulvain, M. (2012). Mechanical methods for induction of labour. *Cochrane Database of Systematic Reviews* 2012, Issue 3. Art. No.: CD001233. DOI: 10.1002/14651858.CD001233.pub2.

Kelly, A. J., Alfirevic, Z., Hofmeyr, G. J., Kavanagh, J., Neilson, J. P., & Thomas, J. (2009). Induction of labour in specific clinical situations: Generic protocol. (Protocol) *Cochrane Database of Systematic Reviews* 2009, Issue 2. Art. No.: CD003398. DOI: 10.1002/14651858.CD003398.pub2.

Kelly, A. J., Kavanagh, J., & Thomas, J. (2003). Vaginal prostaglandin (PGE2 and PGF2a) for induction of labour at term. *Cochrane Database of Systematic Reviews* 2003, Issue 4. Art. No.: CD003101. DOI: 10.1002/14651858.CD003101.

Kelly, A. J., Kavanagh, J., & Thomas, J. (2001). Castor oil, bath and/or enema for cervical priming and induction of labour. *Cochrane Database of Systematic Reviews* 2001, Issue 2. Art. No.: CD003099. DOI: 10.1002/14651858.CD003099.

Lyndon, A., & Ali, L. U. (Eds.). (2008). *Fetal heart rate monitoring: Principles and practice* (4th ed.). Dubuque, IA: Kendal/Hunt.

Maher, M. A. (2014). Obesity in Pregnancy In Simpson, K., & Creehan, P. *Perinatal Nursing,* 4th ed. Philadelphia, Lippincott, Williams & Wilkins.

Martin, J., Hamilton, B., Ventura, S., Osterman, M., Kirmeyer, S., Mathews, T., & Wilson, E. (2011). Birth: Final data for 2009. *National Vital Statistic Reports, 57,* 1. Hyattville, MD: National Center for Health Statistics.

Morin, K., & Reilly, L. (2007). Caring for obese pregnant women. *JOGNN: Journal of Obstetric, Gynecologic & Neonatal Nursing, 36*(5), 482–489.

Nurses' Association of American College of Obstetrics and Gynecologists (NAACOG). (1991). *Inpatient obstetrics certification review manual.* Washington, DC: Author.

O'Driscoll, K., Jackson, R. J., & Gallagher, J. (1970). Active management of labour and cephalopelvic disproportion. *Journal of Obstetrics and Gynecology of the British Commonwealth, 77,* 385–389.

O'Driscoll, K., Strange, J., & Minoque, M. (1973). Active Management of Labor. *British Medical Journal 3,* 135–137.

Oyelese, Y. (2007). Placenta Previa, Placenta Accreta and Vasa Previa. In Queenan, J. (Ed.), High Risk Pregnancy, Washington, The American College of Obstetricians and Gynecologists.

Oyelse, Y. (2004). Vasa Previa: The Impact of Prenatal Diagnosis on Outcomes. The American College of Obstetricians and Gynecologists. Lippincott Williams & Wilkins.

Podulka, J., Stranges, E., & Steiner, C. (2011). Hospitalizations Related to Childbirth, 2008. HCUP Statistical Brief #110. April 2011. Agency for Healthcare Research and Quality, Rockville, MD. Retrieved from http://hcup-us.ahrq.gov/reports/statbriefs/sb110.pdf.

Queenan, J., Hobbins, J., & Spong, C. (2005). *Protocols in high risk pregnancies.* Malden, MA: Blackwell.

Ramachenderan, J., Bradford, J., & McLean, M. (2008). Maternal obesity and pregnancy complications: a review. *Australian & New Zealand Journal of Obstetrics & Gynaecology, 48*(3), 228–235.

Simpson, K. (2013). *Cervical ripening labor induction and labor augmentation of labor* (4th ed.,). Washington, DC: Association of Women's Health, Obstetric and Neonatal Nurses.

Simpson, K., & Atterbury, J. (2003). Trends and issues in labor induction in the United States: Implications for clinical practice. *Journal of Obstetric, Gynecologic & Neonatal Nursing, 32,* 767–779.

Simpson, K. & Knox, G. (2009). High-Alert Medication: Implications for Perinatal Patient Safety. *Maternal Child Nursing, 34*(1).

Simpson & O'Brien-Abel (2013). Labor and Birth Simpson, K., & Creehan, P. *Perinatal Nursing,* 4th ed. Philadelphia, Lippincott, Williams & Wilkins.

Viswanathan, M., Visco, A., Hatmann, K., Wechter, M., Gartlehner, G., Wu, J., et al. (2006). Cesarean delivery on maternal request. Evidence Repost/Technology Assessment No. 133 (Prepared by the RTI International-University of North Carolina Evidence-Based Practice Center under Contract No. 290-02-0016.) ARHQ Publication No. 06-E009. Rockville, MD: Agency for Healthcare Research and Quality.

Wei, S., Wo, B. L., Xu, H., Luo, Z. C., Roy, C., & Fraser, W. D. (2009). Early amniotomy and early oxytocin for prevention of, or therapy for, delay in first stage spontaneous labour compared with routine care. *Cochrane Database of Systematic Reviews* 2009, Issue 2. Art. No.:CD006794. DOI: 10.1002/14651858.CD006794.pub2.

Intrapartum and Postpartum Care of Cesarean Birth Families

11

EXPECTED STUDENT OUTCOMES

On completion of this chapter, the student will be able to:

- ☐ Define key terms.
- ☐ Identify factors that place a woman at risk for cesarean birth.
- ☐ Discuss the preoperative nursing care and medical and anesthesia management for cesarean births.
- ☐ Describe the intraoperative nursing care and medical and anesthesia management for cesarean births.
- ☐ Discuss the postoperative nursing care of cesarean birth with women and their family.
- ☐ Identify potential intraoperative and postoperative complications related to cesarean birth and nursing actions to reduce risk.

Nursing Diagnoses

- At risk for low self-esteem related to perceived failure of life event
- At risk for injury related to surgical procedure and effects of anesthesia
- At risk for fluid volume deficit related to blood loss and oral fluid restriction
- At risk for acute pain related to surgical incision
- At risk for infection related to tissue trauma or prolonged rupture of membranes
- At risk for altered parent-infant attachment related to surgical intervention

Nursing Outcomes

- Parents will verbalize understanding of factors that contributed to the need for cesarean birth.
- The woman will experience an uncomplicated intraoperative period and postoperative recovery.
- The woman will have adequate urinary output and lochia within normal limits.
- The woman will verbalize a pain level below 3 on a pain scale of 0 to 10.
- The woman will be afebrile and the abdominal incision site will be free of signs of infection.
- The parents will hold the infant close to the body and demonstrate appropriate attachment behavior and care for infant needs.

INTRODUCTION

Cesarean birth, also referred to as cesarean section, C-section (C/S), or surgical birth, is an operative procedure in which the fetus is delivered through an incision in the abdominal wall and the uterus. A cesarean birth is major abdominal surgery. Approximately one-third of pregnant couples experience a cesarean birth. The percentage of cesarean births has increased from 20.7% in 1996 to 32.9% in 2009 and reflects a 60% increase over a 13-year period (Hamilton, Martin, & Ventura, 2010; Martin, Hamilton, Sutton, &Ventura, 2011). Rates have continued to increase for mothers in all age groups and among all ethnicities and races, but in particular for older

women (Hamilton et al., 2010). This increase in cesarean birth rate is partially attributed to:

- A decrease in vaginal birth after cesarean section (VBAC) rates from 30.1 per 100 live births of women with previous cesarean section in 1996 to 8.5 in 2006 (ACOG, 2010). VBACs are discussed further in Chapter 10.
- The incidence of vacuum and forceps deliveries has decreased.
- Most fetuses presenting as breech are now delivered by cesarean.
- An increase in the number of **cesarean deliveries on maternal request (CDMR). CDMR** is a cesarean section that is performed at the request of the woman before the

---

Don't have time to read this chapter? Want to reinforce your reading? Need to review for a test?
Listen to this chapter on *DavisPlus.*

start of labor and in the absence of maternal or fetal medical conditions that present a risk for labor (Grossman, Joesch, & Tanfer, 2006).

■ Rates of labor induction continue to rise, and induced labor increases the risk of cesarean birth.

■ Average maternal age is rising, and older women, in particular nulliparous, are at risk for cesarean birth. Current statistics indicate nearly half of cesarean births, 49.5%, were credited to women 40 or older. However, rates have continued to increase for mothers in all age groups and among all ethnicities and races (Hamilton et al., 2010).

■ Malpractice litigation continued to be perceived as contributing to the cesarean rate (Cunningham et al., 2010).

The needs and experiences of cesarean birth couples are distinctly different from those of couples who experience a vaginal birth. These differences include:

■ Increased length of hospitalization
■ Longer period of physical recovery
■ Increased pain
■ Increased negative emotional responses to the childbirth experience

Additionally, the experiences are also different for couples who experience a planned cesarean birth versus an unplanned cesarean birth. Women who experience an unplanned cesarean birth may experience feelings of guilt and failure for not being able to achieve a vaginal birth. Reports of these feelings have decreased as the rates of cesarean births have increased and cesarean births have become more common.

INDICATIONS FOR CESAREAN BIRTH

As shown in **Box 11-1**, repeat cesarean birth and those performed for dystocia are the leading causes in the United States. The major maternal medical indications for a cesarean birth are:

■ Previous cesarean birth
■ Placental abnormalities
■ Dystocia, difficult childbirth, or dysfunctional labor that is caused by:
  ■ *Ineffective uterine contractions that lead to prolonged first stage of labor*
  ■ *Cephalopelvic disproportion*

Cephalopelvic disproportion occurs when ineffective uterine contractions lead to prolonged first stage of labor, or it occurs when the size, shape, or position of the fetal head prevents it from passing through the maternal pelvis or when the maternal bony pelvis is not large enough or appropriately shaped to allow for fetal descent.

■ Previous uterine surgery
  ■ *Surgeries that involved an incision through the myometrium of the uterus*
■ Maternal failure to progress through labor (Berghella, 2011b; Menacker & Hamilton, 2010) termed failure to progress or dystocia.

Evidence-Based Practice: Cesarean Delivery on Maternal Request

National Institutes of Health. (2006). NIH State-of-the-Science Conference: Cesarean Delivery on Maternal Request.

Responding to the increased rates of cesarean delivery on maternal request (CDMR), NIH conducted a systematic literature review and a conference focusing on the risks and benefits of CDMR. The panel reached the following conclusions:

■ There is insufficient evidence to fully evaluate the benefits and risks of CDMR as compared to planned vaginal delivery; more research is needed.

■ Until quality evidence becomes available, any decision to perform a CDMR should be carefully individualized and consistent with ethical principles.

■ Given the risk of placenta previa, placenta accreta, and gravid hysterectomy rise with each cesarean delivery, CDMR is not recommended for women desiring several children.

■ CDMR should not be performed prior to 39 weeks of gestation or without verification of lung maturity, because of the significant danger of neonatal respiratory complications (ACOG, 2007).

■ CDMR should not be motivated by the unavailability of effective pain management.

Although some physicians have shifted their perception of CDMR risks and benefits since these conclusions were published, their practice patterns have not changed significantly, fearing risks of malpractice suits (Coleman-Cowger, Croswell, Erikson, Portnoy, Schulkin, & Spong, 2010). Women may perceive elective cesarean births as a way to control their birth experience, but may not be fully aware of negative short- and long-term implications. Educating women about informed consent requires providers to discuss the risks and benefits as well as the possible short- and long-term effects of a surgical birth.

ACOG recently published a committee opinion that may help to reduce this trend. They state that given the balance of risks and benefits in the absence of maternal or fetal indications for cesarean delivery a plan for vaginal delivery is safe and appropriate. CDMR is particularly not recommended for women desiring multiple children because of increased risk (ACOG, 2013).

National Institutes of Health. (2006). NIH State-of-the-Science Conference: Cesarean Delivery on Maternal Request. Retrieved from http://consensus.nih.gov/2006/2006CesareanSOS027main.htm

---

BOX 11–1 INDICATIONS FOR CESAREAN BIRTH

Primary Cesarean
1. Dystocia, 37%
2. Fetal intolerance of labor, 25%
3. Abnormal presentation, 20%
4. Other, 15%
5. Unsuccessful trial of forceps or vacuum, 3%

Repeat Cesarean
1. No VBAC attempt, 82%
2. Failed VBAC, 17%
3. Failed forceps or vacuum, 0.4%

Cunningham, F., Leveno, K., Bloom, S., Hauth, J., Rouse, D., & Spong, C. (2010). *Williams Obstetrics* (23rd ed.). New York: McGraw-Hill.

■ Preexisting or pregnancy-related maternal health factors such as:
  ■ *Cardiac diseases*
  ■ *Severe hypertension, preeclampsia*
  ■ *Severe diabetes mellitus*

The major fetal medical indications for a cesarean birth are:

■ Malpresentaion or malposition of fetus such as:
  ■ *Breech presentation*
  ■ *Transverse lie*
  ■ *Persistent occiput posterior position*
■ Category II or III fetal heart rate (FHR) pattern
■ Multiple gestation

The nonmedical indications for a cesarean birth include (Menacker & Hamilton, 2010):

■ Maternal demographics
■ Physician practice patterns
■ Conservative practice guidelines and legal implications
■ Maternal choice

Preventing the First Cesarean Birth

The reality is that one of three infants born in the United States is delivered by cesarean birth. The leading driver of both the rise and variation is first-birth cesarean deliveries performed during labor. Additionally with the large increase in primary cesarean deliveries, repeat cesarean delivery now has emerged as the largest single indication. The economic costs, health risks, and negligible benefits for most mothers and newborns of these higher rates highlight the need for a quality improvement multi-strategy approach, including clinical improvement strategies with careful examination of labor management practices; payment reform to eliminate negative or perverse incentives; education to recognize the value of vaginal birth; and full transparency through public reporting and continued public engagement (Main, Morton, Melsop, Hopkins, Giuliani, & Gould, 2012).

Other key points identified to assist with reduction in cesarean delivery rates include that labor induction should be performed primarily for medical indication; if done for non-medical indications, the gestational age should be at least 39 weeks or more and the cervix should be favorable, especially in the nulliparous patient. Review of the current literature demonstrates the importance of adhering to appropriate definitions for failed induction and arrest of labor progress. The diagnosis of "failed induction" should only be made after an adequate attempt. Adequate time for normal latent and active phases of the first stage, and for the second stage, should be allowed as long as the maternal and fetal conditions permit. The adequate time for each of these stages appears to be longer than traditionally estimated. Operative vaginal delivery is an acceptable birth method when indicated and can safely prevent cesarean delivery (Spong, Berghella, Wenstrom, Mercer, & Saade, 2012).

Main and colleagues concluded that national attention to the problem of unnecessary cesarean deliveries is needed as a

public health concern in the search for value and quality in U.S. health care. It is currently believed that there is no evidence to demonstrate that a 33% cesarean delivery rate is beneficial to women or their infants. Rather, this rate exposes women and infants to unnecessary risks in the perinatal period and long term and results in considerable unnecessary health-care costs.

CLASSIFICATION OF CESAREAN BIRTHS

Cesarean births are classified into two major groupings of scheduled (planned) and unscheduled (unplanned).

■ Scheduled cesarean births occur before the onset of labor. Common reasons for a scheduled cesarean birth are:
  ■ *Previous cesarean birth*
  ■ *Maternal or fetal health conditions that place the woman or fetus at risk during labor and/or vaginal birth*
  ■ *Malpresentation, such as breech presentation, diagnosed before labor*
  ■ *Cesarean delivery on maternal request (CDMR)*
■ Unscheduled cesarean births are divided into emergent, urgent, and non-urgent.
  ■ *Emergent cesarean birth* indicates an immediate need to deliver the fetus (e.g., prolapse of umbilical cord or rupture of uterus).
  ■ *Urgent cesarean birth* indicates a need for rapid delivery of the fetus such as with malpresentation diagnosed after labor has begun or placenta previa with mild bleeding and fetal heart rate with normal Category I FHR.
  ■ *Non-urgent cesarean birth* indicates a need for cesarean birth related to such complications as failure to progress (cervix does not fully dilate) and failure to descend (fetus does not descend through the pelvis) with normal Category I FHR.

RISKS RELATED TO CESAREAN BIRTH

Maternal deaths in the United States related to cesarean birth have decreased due to improved surgical techniques, anesthetic care, and the availability of blood transfusions and antibiotic therapy but still pose a risk to both the woman and her fetus. However, women who experience a cesarean birth are at higher risk for postpartum infection, hemorrhage, and thromboembolic disease and maternal death (Hacker, Moore, & Gambone, 2004). Neonates are at higher risk for respiratory morbidity (Chestnut, 2006).

One cohort study of cases found the risk of postpartum death to be 3.6 times higher after cesarean delivery than after vaginal delivery (Deneux-Tharaux, Carmona, Bouvier-Colle, & Breart, 2006). The causes of death after cesarean births in this study included venous thromboembolism (VTE), amniotic fluid embolus, puerperal infections, and complications of anesthesia. Rates of re-hospitalization are higher and costs associated with cesarean births are often double those of vaginal births.

RISKS RELATED TO REPEAT CESAREAN BIRTH

The most significant long-term complication of repeat surgical birth is placenta accreta (Hull & Resnik, 2009). The spectrum of placenta accrete includes:

- Accreta: the placenta does not penetrate the entire thickness of the uterine muscle.
- Increta: the placenta extends further into the myometrium.
- Percreta: the placenta extends fully through the uterine wall and may attach to other internal organs, such as the intestine or bladder.

In all forms of placenta accreta, the placenta does not separate from the uterine wall after delivery, potentially leading to excessive hemorrhage, disseminated intravascular coagulopathy, organ failure, and, in severe cases, death (Silver, 2010). Typically, a hysterectomy is needed to control a massive hemorrhage.

PERIOPERATIVE CARE

Perioperative perinatal nursing incorporates the skills of the specialties of obstetrics, surgery, and post-anesthesia care to provide safe and comprehensive care to promote safe and comprehensive care to women who have a cesarean birth (Simpson & O'Brien-Abel, 2013).

It is common in the United States for cesarean births to be performed in an OR in the obstetrics department and for labor and delivery nurses to care for the family throughout the perioperative experience. Preoperative care may vary somewhat based on the urgency of the cesarean birth.

Scheduled Cesarean Birth

Couples are admitted to the labor and birthing unit the day of surgery (**Fig. 11-1**). Diagnostic laboratory work, such as complete blood count (CBC), platelet count, urinalysis, blood type, and cross match may be completed a few days before admission.

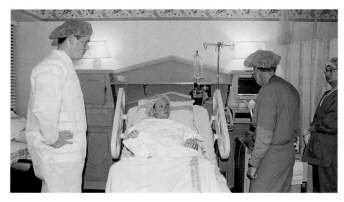

Figure 11–1   Couple awaiting scheduled cesarean section.

Medical Management

- Explain the reason for the cesarean birth and what it involves prior to hospital admission and obtain surgical consent.
- Schedule the surgery.
- Order presurgery diagnostic laboratory tests, such as CBC, blood type, and Rh.
- Send the prenatal record and orders to the birthing unit to be placed in the woman's hospital chart. (36w)
- Provide education about the woman's current medications. Identify which medications should be taken or eliminated on the day of surgery.

Skin Preparation

- Encourage women to take at least one preoperative shower using an antiseptic agent on the night prior to the scheduled procedure.

Anesthesia Management

- The anesthesiologist or certified registered nurse anesthetist (CRNA) meets with the couple during the admission process and before the woman is transferred to the operating room.
- The anesthesiologist or CRNA reviews the prenatal record.
- The anesthesiologist or CRNA completes an anesthesia history and physical, discusses anesthesia options with the couple, and answers their questions regarding anesthesia and the procedure.
- The anesthesiologist or CRNA determines, based on the woman's history, physical, and clinical signs, if a platelet count is required before administration of epidural or spinal (American Society of Anesthesiologists Task Force, 2007).

Nursing Actions

- Complete the appropriate admission assessments and required preoperative forms.
  - *Expected findings*
    - Couples and families may have an increased level of anxiety related to the surgery and method of anesthesia.
      - *Anxiety may be related to this being the woman's first surgical experience and fears of the unknown for self and fetus.*
      - *The expectant father may have concerns about injury to his partner and/or child.*

- Couples are excited about the upcoming birth of their child.
  - Couples have questions and concerns regarding the cesarean birth and method of anesthesia.
  - Vital signs are within normal limits, with a mild increase in blood pressure related to increased anxiety.
- Obtain baseline vital signs
- Obtain laboratory testing as per orders, CBC, platelets, and type and screen. A delay in lab results can result in a delay in surgery.
- Obtain a baseline fetal heart rate monitor strip before and after administration of regional anesthesia.
  - *Expected findings*
    - Category I fetal heart rate
- Review the prenatal chart for factors that place the woman at risk during or after cesarean birth and ensure that physician and anesthesiologist or CRNA are aware of risk factors such as low platelet count.
- Assess womens' knowledge and educational needs.
- Provide preoperative education.
- Identify and respect the cultural values, choices, and preferences of the woman and her family.
- Individualize care to meet needs of patient and family.
- Ensure that all required documents, such as prenatal record, current laboratory reports, and consent forms, are in the woman's chart.
- Verify that the woman has been NPO for 6–8 hours before surgery. Women without complications undergoing scheduled cesarean birth may have limited amounts of clear liquids up to 2 hours prior to induction of anesthesia (American Society of Anesthesiologists Task Force, 2007). Follow hospital policy for NPO status.
- Complete the surgery checklist, which includes removal of jewelry, eyeglasses/contact lenses, and dentures. Eyeglasses can be given to the support person to bring into the operating room so the woman can use them to see her newborn baby.
- Explain to the couple what they can expect before, during, and after the cesarean birth.
- Start an IV line and administer an IV fluid preload as per orders (see Critical Component: IV Fluid Preload before Anesthesia).
- Insert a Foley catheter as per order. Insertion may be done in the operating room after placement of the spinal or epidural and before the prep.
- Shave the abdominal and pubic regions with electric clippers.
- Administer preoperative medications per orders.
  - *This might include sodium citrate to neutralize stomach acids. Flamotidine or metoclopramide may be used to reduce the incidence of nausea or vomiting.*
- Prepare the expectant father or the support person who plans to be present for the birth for the experience by providing appropriate surgical garb to wear in the operating room.
- Instruct the expectant father or the support person as to where he or she will sit and what he or she can anticipate

regarding sights, sounds, and smells typical of an operating room.
- Provide emotional support for the couple as they wait to be transferred to the operating room.

Antibiotic and Venous Thromboembolic Prophylaxis (VTE)

- Administration of narrow-spectrum prophylactic antibiotics should occur within 60 minutes prior to the skin incision (AWHONN, 2011). Antibiotics of choice include cefazolin, or for women with penicillin and cephalosporin allergy, clindamycin with gentamicin may be given.
- Perform an assessment for risk of VTE and classify the woman according to VTE classification guidelines. Preoperative anticoagulant therapy may be necessary for women classified as moderate or high risk, or with history of recurrent thrombosis. (American Society of Anesthesiologists Task Force, 2007 and AWHONN, 2011).
- Apply sequential compression devices prior to surgery on women classified as moderate or high risk of VTE.

CRITICAL COMPONENT

IV Fluid Preload before Anesthesia

An IV fluid preload of 500–1,000 mL is given before administration of spinal or epidural anesthesia to increase fluid volume and decrease risk of hypotension related to effects of anesthetic agent *(American Society of Anesthesiologists Task Force, 2007 and AWHONN, 2011).* The use of prewarmed IV fluids in women having a cesarean birth results in an increased maternal core temperature, improved neonatal umbilical arterial pH, and improved Apgar scores (Yokoyama, Suzuki, Shimada et al., 2009).

Unscheduled Cesarean Birth

Unscheduled cesarean births are usually due to an urgent or emergent cause such as fetal intolerance of labor or placental problems. The woman and her family are usually highly anxious and have fears that either the woman and/or infant's health is in danger.

- Emergent cesarean births require immediate preparation of the woman for surgery with minimal time to spend explaining in detail what is happening. Therefore, the woman and her partner or support person need an opportunity to debrief during the immediate postpartum period.
- Urgent and non-urgent cesarean births allow the time necessary to explain fully what and why a cesarean birth is required, but the family still needs time in the postpartum unit to review the events leading up to the cesarean birth.

Medical Management

- Determine the need for a cesarean birth.
- Explain the reason for the cesarean birth.
- Explain the surgical procedure and obtain consent.

Anesthesia Management

■ The anesthesiologist or CRNA completes an anesthesia history and physical and discusses anesthesia options with the woman. This may not occur until the woman is transferred to the operating room based on the amount of time from the decision for need of cesarean birth and transfer to the operating room.

■ The anesthesiologist or CRNA explains the procedure for type of anesthesia and addresses the woman's and her partner's or support person's questions and concerns.

■ The anesthesiologist or CRNA determines the need for a platelet count.

Evidence-Based Practice: Predictive Relationship of Preoperative Anxiety With Postoperative Satisfaction

Hobson, J., Slade, P., Wrench, I., & Power, L. (2006). Preoperative anxiety and postoperative satisfaction in women undergoing elective cesarean section. *International Journal of Obstetric Anesthesia, 15*, 18–23.

The aim of this study was to determine the predictive relationship of preoperative anxiety with postoperative maternal satisfaction. The sample included 85 women scheduled for elective cesarean birth. Degree of anxiety, social support, and aspects of preoperative preparation were measured within 24 hours of the scheduled cesarean birth. Postoperative measures included the maternal satisfaction scale for cesarean section, recovery from cesarean section scale, and postoperative discharge summary form.

Results from this study indicate that the lower the preoperative anxiety, the higher the postoperative maternal satisfaction. They also indicate that postoperative satisfaction was highest when the woman was highly satisfied with the preoperative information provided by the anesthesiologist and when the woman's perceived support by her partner was high.

Implications of this study for evidence-based practice in enhancing the woman's satisfaction with her birthing experience are the importance of providing preoperative information to the woman and facilitating support to the woman from her partner.

Nursing Actions

■ Notify the anesthesia and labor and delivery team of the impending cesarean birth.

■ Initiate continuous electronic fetal heart rate monitoring.
  ■ *Expected findings*
    ■ Category II or Category III fetal heart rate pattern when the cesarean section is related to fetal intolerance of labor

■ Help ensure the woman and her support person(s) receive information appropriate to the circumstances.

■ Provide emotional support during transitional process from labor to preparation for surgery.

■ Facilitate communication with entire health care team to decrease fear, anxiety, and distress.

■ Facilitate presence of patient support person during preoperative preparation and surgical procedure because emotional support decreases anxiety.

■ Administer oxygen when indicated (i.e., signs of fetal intolerance of labor).

■ Alert neonatal personnel of the impending cesarean birth.

■ Assess the woman's vital signs.
  ■ *Expected findings*
    ■ The woman's blood pressure is elevated related to anxiety level.
    ■ There is a potential increase in temperature and pulse rate due to infection and/or dehydration related to prolonged labor and rupture of membranes.

■ Start an IV and administer IV fluid preload as per orders.

■ Ensure labs are completed as per orders; CBC, platelets, and type and screen.

■ Complete and witness surgical and anesthesia consent forms.

■ Insert a Foley catheter as per order. Insertion may be done in the operating room after placement of the spinal or epidural anesthesia and before prep.

■ Assess the couple's emotional response to the need for a cesarean birth.
  ■ *Expected findings*
    ■ Couples and family may experience high levels of anxiety based on fear of injury to the woman and/or unborn child.
    ■ Couples are not emotionally or mentally prepared for cesarean birth.
    ■ Couples and family have a knowledge deficit regarding cesarean birth and anesthesia options.
    ■ Couples and family ask questions regarding cesarean birth and anesthesia options.

■ If hair needs to be removed because it interferes with surgical site, use hair clippers on the pubic region.

■ Ensure that all required documents are in the patient's chart.

■ Complete the surgical checklist.

■ Reinforce reason for cesarean section and address questions.

■ Facilitate the transition to unscheduled surgical birth in a timely manner. Guidelines in all hospitals providing OB care should have the capability of responding to obstetrical emergencies within 30 minutes (AAP & ACOG, 2007). Hence the 30-minute "decision to incision rule."

■ Provide emotional support to the couple and family members.

■ Review with the couple what to expect during and after the cesarean birth.

■ Explain that the woman may feel pressure or pulling as her baby is being born.

■ Prepare the expectant father or support person who plans to attend the birth as to what to anticipate in the operating room and provide him or her with proper surgical garb to wear in the operating room.

INTRAOPERATIVE CARE

The cesarean birth often is the first surgical experience for most women and can increase the anxiety level for both the woman and her partner. Couples are anxious irrespective of whether this is a scheduled or unscheduled cesarean birth. To help decrease the anxiety level, ideally the nurse who admitted the woman for a scheduled cesarean section or the nurse who cared for the couple during labor continues to care for them during the surgery as the circulating nurse. The complete intraoperative team includes a surgeon, an anesthesia provider, surgical first assist, circulating nurse, and neonatal staff.

Complications

Intraoperative complications are rare owing to the advances in obstetrical anesthesia and surgical techniques. Women who are healthy during pregnancy are at low risk for complications. Intraoperative complications include:

■ Hemorrhage
  ■ *Increased morbidity and mortality rates are associated with postpartum hemorrhage, which can result in the need for emergency hysterectomy, hypovolemic shock, disseminated intravascular coagulation, and renal and hepatic failure.*
■ Bladder, ureters, and bowel trauma
■ Maternal respiratory depression related to anesthesia
■ Maternal hypotension related to anesthesia, which increases the risk for fetal distress
■ Inadvertent injection of the anesthetic agent into the maternal bloodstream
  ■ *The woman experiences ringing in her ears, metallic taste in her mouth, and hypotension that can lead to unconsciousness and cardiac arrest (Schwartz, 2006).*

Anesthesia Management
■ Determine the method of anesthesia.
  ■ *The determination of type of anesthesia is based on which one:*
    ■ Is the safest and most comfortable for the woman
    ■ Has the least effect on the fetus/neonate
    ■ Provides the optimal conditions for the surgery (Hughes, Levinson, & Rosen, 2002).
  ■ *Method of anesthesia (**Fig. 11-2**)*
    ■ Spinal anesthesia is the preferred method for scheduled cesarean sections or for laboring women who do not have an epidural in place. Spinal anesthesia, which is faster to place, provides a full sensory and motor block.
    ■ Epidural anesthesia is used for laboring women who have an epidural in place for labor pain management and then require a cesarean birth. Women with epidurals

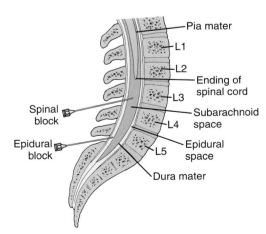

may feel tugging and pulling during the procedure because epidurals are not as dense and do not provide full sensory and motor block.
  ■ General anesthesia, which is rarely used and carries increased risks, is indicated in the following situations:
    ■ *Rapid delivery is imperative*
    ■ *Severe hemorrhage*
    ■ *Seizures*
    ■ *Failed spinal*
  ■ Gastric aspiration leading to pneumonitis is a potential complication of general anesthesia.
  ■ Additional conditions that may increase the risk of aspiration include:
    ■ *Morbid obesity*
    ■ *Diabetes*
    ■ *Difficult airway (American Society of Anesthesiologists Task Force, 2007).*
■ Contraindications for epidural or spinal anesthesia
  ■ *The woman's refusal or inability to cooperate with the procedure*
  ■ *Increased intracranial pressure*
  ■ *Infection at the site of needle insertion*
  ■ *Low platelet count*
  ■ *Uncorrected maternal hypovolemia (Chestnut, 2006)*
■ Administration of anesthesia by the anesthesiologist or CRNA
  ■ *Bupivacaine is the preferred anesthetic agent for spinal and epidural blocks.*
  ■ *Preservative-free morphine is administered intrathecally to provide postoperative analgesia (Kuczkowski, Reisner, & Lin, 2006).*
■ Position patient with a left tilt to maintain a left uterine displacement before, during, and after administration of anesthesia to decrease the risk of aortocaval compression related to compression on the aorta and inferior vena cava due to weight of the gravid uterus (Chestnut, 2006).
■ Monitor vital signs and oxygen saturation.
  ■ *Expected findings*
    ■ Vital signs and oxygen saturation within normal limits with potential mild increase in blood pressure due to anxiety
    ■ Hypotension following administration of the anesthetic agent
■ Monitor level of anesthesia and effectiveness of anesthesia.
■ Estimate blood loss (EBL). An EBL of up to 1,000 cc is expected in a cesarean birth.
■ Administer oxytocin after the delivery of the placenta.
■ Administer antibiotics when indicated.

Medical Management
■ Operative techniques:
  ■ *There are two primary operative techniques used for cesarean births.*
  ■ *Most often, a **Pfannenstiel incision** or "bikini cut" is the skin incision. This is a transverse skin incision made at the level of the pubic hairline (**Fig. 11-3A**). Typically, a lower uterine segment incision is performed on the uterus (Fig. 11-3C).*

Figure 11–2 Spinal and epidural placements.

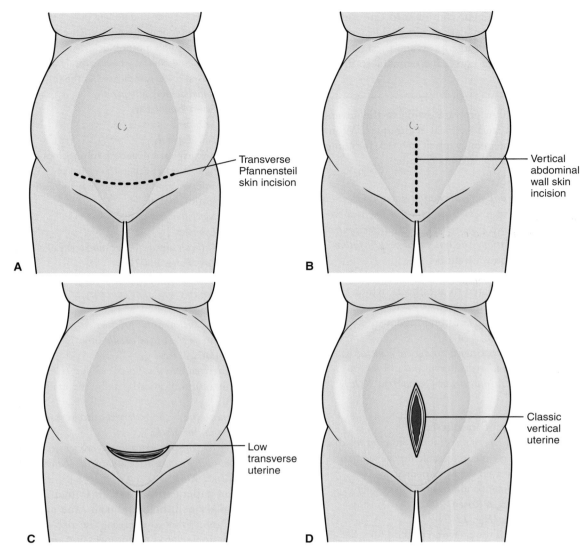

Figure 11–3   Abdominal wall and uterine incisions for cesarean births. A. Pfannenstiel incision "bikini cut", B. Vertical abdominal wall skin incision, C. Low transverse uterine incision, D. Classic vertical uterine incision.

■ *The **classical cesarean delivery** is a vertical incision in the body of the uterus (see Fig. 11-3D). This technique is rare and is used in emergent cesarean births when immediate delivery is critical.*

■ *The neonate is delivered through the uterine and abdominal incisions (**Fig. 11-4**).*

■ *The placenta is manually removed.*

■ *The uterus is lifted out of the abdominal cavity and the uterine incision is repaired.*

■ *Abdominal tissues and incision are repaired.*

Nursing Actions

■ Conduct a preprocedure informational process according to facility policy. Include assessments, comments, and lab work.

■ Position patient with a left tilt to maintain a left uterine displacement before, during, and after administration of anesthesia to decrease the risk of aorto-caval compression related to compression on the aorta and inferior vena cava due to weight of the gravid uterus (Chestnut, 2006).

■ Continue external fetal heart rate monitoring until abdominal preparation is initiated.

■ Remove the internal scalp electrode after abdominal preparation and before delivery. FSE should not be removed until MD orders removal.

  ■ Expected findings

    ■ Normal fetal heart rate unless abnormal fetal heart rate was indication for cesarean birth

■ Conduct a time-out before the administration of anesthesia for validating correct patient, site, and procedure (see QSEN Safety: Universal Protocol for Preventing Wrong Patient, Wrong Site, Wrong Person Surgery).

■ Assist the woman into the proper position for epidural or spinal anesthesia.

■ Reposition the woman after epidural or spinal anesthesia in a supine position with a left lateral tilt to decrease the pressure from the uterus on the inferior vena cava and to maintain placental perfusion.

■ Assess FHR after anesthesia placement.

- Apply the grounding device.
- Insert Foley.
- Perform abdominal skin prep.
- Secure the woman to the operating room table with a strap over her upper legs.
- Perform the duties of the circulating nurse, including instrument count, needle count, and sponge count.
- Check equipment used for the newborn to ensure it is in working order and all supplies are readily available for care of the neonate.
- Assess the couple's response to the cesarean birth.
  - *Expected findings*
    - Anxiety levels increase related to operating room environment and impeding surgery.
    - Couples may have concerns related to potential injury to the woman from anesthesia and/or surgery.
    - The woman may feel abdominal pressure as the neonate is being delivered.
- Position the expectant father or support person on a stool next to the woman's head.
- Instruct the expectant father or support person as to what he or she can and cannot touch.
- Instruct the expectant father or support person to remain seated on the stool.
- Provide emotional support to the woman and her partner or support person.
- Facilitate care for the neonate. This is done by the neonatal personnel (neonatal nurse, nurse practitioner, and/or neonatologist) who are present for the birth.
  - *At least one person skilled in neonatal resuscitation should be available whose only responsibility is to receive and care for the baby.*
  - *Expected findings*
    - The neonate's 1- and 5-minute Apgar scores are 7 or above unless there is fetal intolerance of labor before the birth.
- Record the time of delivery of the neonate and delivery of the placenta.
- Complete identification bands and place on the neonate and parents before the neonate leaves the operating room.
- Ensure that the new mother has an opportunity to see and touch her newborn and that the new father or support person has an opportunity to hold the newborn if the newborn is going to the nursery. In many birthing units the neonate, if stable, remains in the operating room, skin-to-skin contact is encouraged, and the neonate is then transferred to the L&D recovery room with the woman and her partner.
- Whenever possible, the newborn should remain in the operative suite with the mother. (AWHONN, 2011).
- Transfer unstable neonates to the nursery and encourage the new father or support person to accompany the newborn to the nursery. Neonatal personnel are responsible for transferring unstable neonates.
- Address parents' questions regarding the health of their newborn.
- Complete intraoperative documentation.

Quality and Safety Education for Nurses (QSEN): Safety

Universal Protocol for Preventing Wrong Patient, Wrong Site, Wrong Person Surgery

Utilization of the knowledge, skills, and attitudes (KSAs) of safety minimizes risk of harm to patients and providers through both system effectiveness and individual performance (QSEN, 2012). Joint Commission Standard PC 13.20 EP 9 states that "the site, procedure, and patient are accurately identified and clearly communicated using active communication techniques, during a final verification process such as time-out before the start of any surgical or invasive procedure" (Joint Commission, 2003).

The operating room circulating nurse assists in actively verifying that this is the correct patient and procedure when "time-out" is called immediately before the epidural or spinal procedure begins and immediately before the surgical incision is made to verify that it is the correct site, procedure, and patient.

POSTOPERATIVE CARE

The recovery time following a cesarean birth is longer compared to vaginal delivery due to the tissue trauma related to surgical intervention. The usual hospital stay is 3–5 days, with full recovery from surgery taking 6 weeks or longer. The maternal morbidity rate is increased twofold with cesarean delivery compared with vaginal delivery (Cunningham, Leveno, Bloom, Hanth, Ronse, & Spong, 2010). Principal sources of complications are infection, hemorrhage, and thromboembolism. There is a twofold increase in rehospitalization. Rates of complications vary based on status of cesarean, emergency versus planned. Rates of infection with emergency cesarean are reported at 12%, wound complications at 1.2%, and operative injury at 0.5% (Cunningham et al., 2010).

Complications

Women who enter pregnancy in a healthy state and have experienced a healthy pregnancy are at low risk for complications. In contrast, women who experience a prolonged labor, multiple interventions such as internal monitoring, or who have experienced prolonged rupture of membranes are at higher risk for postoperative complications. Postoperative complications include:

- Hemorrhage
- Deep vein thrombosis
- Pulmonary embolism
- Paralytic ileus
- Hematuria related to bladder trauma
- Infections of the bladder, endometrium, and incision
- Postpartum hemorrhage is most often identified in the intraoperative period or within the first few hours post-op.

CRITICAL COMPONENT

Postoperative Complications

A multidisciplinary team approach is needed to provide care to women experiencing postoperative complications (AWHONN, 2011). Nurses have a key role in recognizing deteriorating conditions in the postoperative period. The most common preventable errors related to cesarean births are: failure to recognize and act upon changes in vital signs and failure to act on postpartum hemorrhage.

■ Pulmonary embolism presents as an acute event. Signs and symptoms are dyspnea, tachypnea, chest tightness, shortness of breath, hypotension, and decreasing oxygen saturation

levels. Increased morbidity and mortality rates are associated with postpartum hemorrhage, which can result in the need for emergency hysterectomy, hypovolemic shock, disseminated intravascular coagulation, and renal and hepatic failure.
■ Surgical site infection rate is estimated to be 3%–15% and signs include serous or purulent drainage, erythema, fever, pain, and wound dehiscence.
■ Endometritis is usually diagnosed within the first few days after delivery. Fever is the most common sign. Other signs include chills, uterine tenderness, and foul smelling lochia.

Association of Women's Health, Obstetric and Neonatal Nurses (AWHONN). (2011). *Evidence-Based Clinical Practice Guideline: Perioperative care of the pregnant woman.* Washington, DC: Author.

Immediate Postoperative Care (PACU)

Immediate assessment and monitoring of maternal and newborn status is influenced by the type of anesthesia and any complications preoperatively or intraoperatively, and focuses on both maternal and fetal oxygenation, ventilation, circulation level of consciousness, and body temperature. The purpose of PACU care is to stabilize VS, bleeding, pain, itching, and nausea, and to monitor anesthesia level (see Clinical Pathway).

■ Equipment comparable to that in the main PACU should be available to care for post-op OB patients.

One RN should be assigned solely to the care of the mother until the critical elements are completed, such as report, assessments, and maternal stable vital signs (see Critical Component: Postoperative Complications).

■ Estimate blood loss in the PACU. Hospital policy may be to weigh on a scale pads and chux for more accurate measurement of EBL (1gram = 1 cc).
■ Monitor I&O
■ Active warming measures should be monitored if patient is hypothermic
■ One RN should be assigned solely to the newborn until critical elements are completed, such as report, assessment, and stable newborn vital signs.
■ Use facility-based scoring system to determine the appropriate timing for discharge from the recovery room (AWHONN, 2011).

First 24 Hours after Birth

Medical Management

■ Assess the woman for involutional changes and signs of potential complications.
■ Medical orders are usually standardized. These orders include:
■ *IV therapy*
■ *Medications such as analgesics and stool softeners*
■ *Antibiotic therapy for the woman at risk for infection related to prolonged rupture of membranes, prolonged labor, or elevated temperature during labor*
■ *Progression of diet*

■ *Removal of the Foley catheter*
■ *Activity level*
■ Immediate care of the newborn is the same for vaginal delivery and is detailed in Chapters 8 and 15.

Anesthesia Management

■ Order pain medications.
■ Order PRN medication to counteract side effects of intrathecal morphine. When intrathecal morphine is used for post-operative pain management, the anesthesia provider manages the woman's pain for the first 24 hours (see Medication: Preservative-Free Morphine).

[handwritten: Benadryl for itching]

Medication

Preservative-Free Morphine

■ Indication: Severe pain
■ Action: Alters perception of and response to painful stimuli and produces generalized CNS depression
■ Common side effects: Respiratory depression, itching, hypotension, nausea and vomiting, and urinary retention
■ Route and dose: Administered intrathecally by anesthesiologist or CRNA; 5–10 mg
(Data from Deglin & Vallerand, 2009)

CRITICAL COMPONENT

Maternal Respiratory Depression Related to Intrathecal Morphine

Severe respiratory depression (3% occurrence) is a life-threatening adverse reaction to intrathecal morphine.

■ Naloxone and resuscitative equipment need to be available whenever intrathecal morphine is administered and during the 24 hours postoperative after injection.
■ Respiratory rate and level of sedation are monitored for the first 24 hours postoperative after administration. Normal respiratory rate is 12–18 breaths per minute.
■ An initial dose of 0.4–2 mg of naloxone is administered intravenously for severe respiratory depression. Dose can be repeated every 2–3 minutes for a total of 10 mg.
■ Respiratory resuscitation is initiated immediately and continued until normal respiratory function returns.

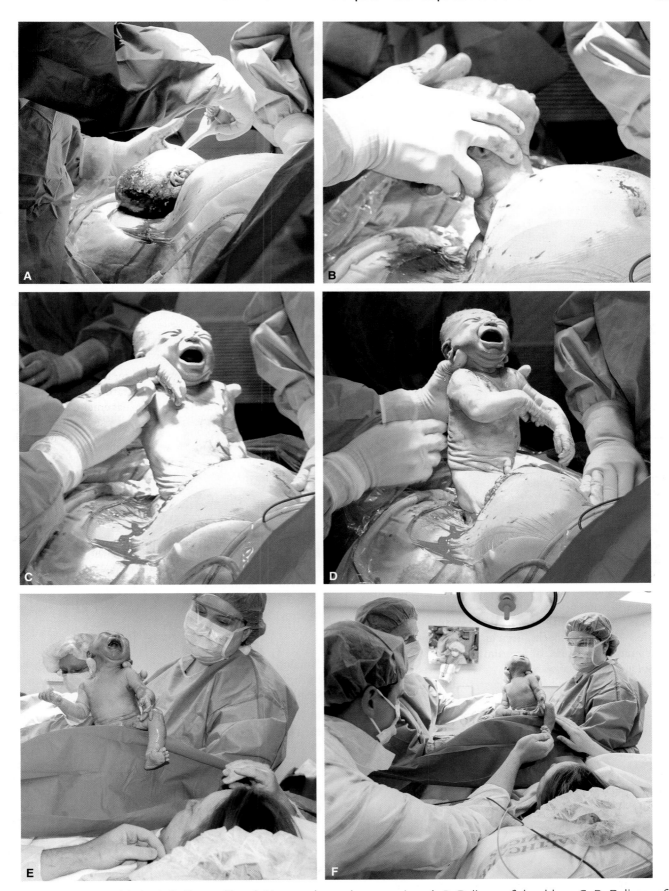

Figure 11–4 Cesarean birth. *A*. Delivery of head. Nose and mouth are suctioned. *B*. Delivery of shoulders. *C*, *D*. Delivery of body. *E*, *F*. Mom and dad meeting their daughter.

Nursing Actions

After a cesarean birth, most women recover in the labor and birthing recovery unit versus the postanesthesia unit of the main OR. Nursing actions are similar to care of women with vaginal birth and/or emphasis on the following (see Clinical Pathway):

■ Review prenatal, labor, and intrapartal records for risk factors. Monitor vital signs as per protocol.
  ■ *Monitor respiratory rate and level of sedation every hour for the first 24 hours after administration of intrathecal morphine (see Critical Component: Maternal Respiratory Depression Related to Intrathecal Morphine).*
■ Assess woman for pain.
■ Use pharmacological and non-pharmacological interventions for pain relief.
■ Reassess pain at appropriate levels.
■ Monitor the level of sensation.
■ Monitor for side effects of intrathecal morphine and provide appropriate interventions. The primary side effects and interventions are:
  ■ *Pruritus (80%): Administer medication as per order, such as naloxone or diphenhydramine.*
  ■ *Nausea/vomiting (53%): Administer medication as per order, such as naloxone or metoclopramide.*
  ■ *Urinary retention (43%) that occurs after removal of catheter: Administer naloxone or catheterize as per order.*
  ■ *Respiratory depression (3%): Administer oxygen as needed and/or naloxone as per order (Hughes, Levinson, & Rosen, 2002).*
■ Monitor for complications of anesthesia. These are:
  ■ *Postpartum hemorrhage related to uterine atony*
  ■ *Seizures*
  ■ *Neurological deficits (e.g., prolonged decreased sensation in legs)*
  ■ *Postdural puncture headaches*
■ Assess the fundus and lochia as per protocol.
■ Auscultate lungs, encourage coughing and deep breathing, and assist patient in using incentive spirometry.
■ Assess the abdominal dressing for signs of bleeding.
■ Assess for paralytic ileus. Sign and symptoms include abdominal distention, diffuse and persistent abdominal pain, and nausea or vomiting.
■ Monitor for signs of hemorrhage, such as increased bleeding, increased pulse, and decreased blood pressure.
■ Monitor intake and urinary output (per Foley catheter).
■ Advance diet as tolerated.
■ Regulate IV fluids as per order.
  ■ *Oxytocin is usually added to IV fluids to reduce the risk of postpartum hemorrhage related to uterine atony.*
■ Assist the woman into a comfortable position for infant feeding. Breastfeeding mothers may be more comfortable in a side lying position or using the football hold, which prevents pressure on her abdomen.
■ Assist with infant care.
■ Provide emotional support by actively listening to the couple recalling their birth experience and by addressing their questions and concerns.

Expected Assessment Findings

■ Vital signs are within normal limits.
■ Lochia is moderate to scant.
■ The fundus is firm and midline and generally 1–2 cm above the umbilicus.
■ The abdominal dressing is dry.
■ The catheter is draining clear/yellow urine.
  ■ *Blood in the urine occurs when there has been trauma to the bladder.*
■ The IV site is free of signs of infiltration or inflammation.
■ The pain level is below 3 on a pain scale of 0–10.
■ The woman gradually regains full motor and sensory function as the effects of anesthetic agent decrease.
  ■ *The woman sits at the bedside for short periods of time.*
■ The woman may experience itching, nausea, or decreased respirations related to side effects of morphine.
  ■ *Itching and nausea are the most common side effect of morphine.* BENADRYL
    ■ Itching varies from a facial rash to a full body rash. Antihistamines are given to promote comfort.
■ The woman feeds her newborn with assistance.
■ The partner and family assists in care of the newborn.
■ The couple may be tired and need time to rest.
■ Women with unplanned cesarean births may experience guilt feelings or a sense of failure or disappointment.
■ Couples with unplanned cesarean births may ask questions about the cesarean birth and the events leading up to it.
■ The couple will want time alone with their newborn child.
■ The couple will call family and friends, informing them of the birth.

24 Hours Postoperative to Discharge

Medical Management

■ Assess the woman for involutional changes and signs of potential postoperative complications.
■ Remove abdominal dressing. The dressing is usually removed on the first postoperative day.
■ Provide discharge instructions.

Nursing Actions

Nursing actions are similar to the care of women with vaginal birth with addition to and/or emphasis on the following (see Clinical Pathway):

■ Monitor vital signs as per protocol, generally every 8 hours.
■ Assess breath sounds.
■ Instruct the woman to deep breathe and cough every 2 hours.
■ Instruct the woman on the use of an incentive spirometer if ordered.
■ Assess postoperative pain and medicate as indicated.
■ Use non-pharmacological pain management strategies.
■ Assess the fundus and lochia as per protocol. Use gentle pressure when assessing the fundus due to the woman's abdomen being tender.
■ Monitor for signs of hemorrhage and infection.
■ Assess the abdominal dressing or surgical wound for drainage and signs of infection.

■ Administer antibiotics as per order. Women who experience a prolonged labor, prolonged rupture of membranes, or increased temperature may be placed on antibiotic therapy.

■ Remove the Foley catheter as per order when the woman is able to ambulate to bathroom. This generally occurs 8–12 hours postsurgery. Ensure woman voids after urinary catheter removal at least 200-300 cc.

■ Assist the woman with ambulation and encourage her to ambulate to reduce risk of abdominal pain related to gas buildup.

■ Encourage fluid intake to assist in hydration.

■ Discontinue IV fluids per order when the woman is able to take fluids by mouth and the fundus and lochia are within normal limits.

■ Assess bowel sounds and advance to a regular diet as per order based on the presence of bowel sounds and absence of nausea and vomiting.

■ Provide information on nutrition to promote tissue healing.

■ Assist the woman into a comfortable position for infant feeding. Breastfeeding mothers may be more comfortable in a side lying position or football hold, which prevents pressure on the abdomen.

■ Assist the woman with infant care.

■ Provide opportunities for the family to ask questions about their cesarean birth experience.

■ Facilitate mother-infant attachment by bringing the infant to the woman and ensuring the woman's comfort.

■ Instruct the family that they need to assist the woman with infant care and housework as she needs 6 weeks to recover from surgery.

■ Provide teaching on infant care, postoperative care, and postpartum care.

■ Remove staples before discharge per protocol.

Expected Assessment Findings

■ Vital signs are within normal limits.
  ■ *Temperature elevations may be a sign of infection.*

■ Lung sounds are clear bilaterally.

■ The woman deep breathes and coughs every 2 hours while awake.

■ The pain level is 3 or below on a pain scale of 0–10 with the use of nonpharmacological and pharmacological interventions.

■ The fundus is firm and midline at one finger breadth below the umbilicus.

■ The lochia is moderate to scant.

■ The abdominal incision is clean, intact, approximated, and free of redness, edema, ecchymosis, and drainage.

■ The woman spontaneously voids at least 200 mL within 4–6 hours of removal of the Foley catheter.

■ The woman ambulates to the bathroom and in hallways.

■ Bowel sounds are present and the woman reports passing gas.

■ The woman is able to tolerate oral fluids and food.

■ Negative Homan's sign.

■ The mother is able to feed her newborn with assistance.

■ The couple cares for the needs of their newborn.

■ The woman may remain in the taking-in phase longer related to her focus being on pain control and integration of the birthing experience.

■ Couples talk about their cesarean birth experience with staff, family, and friends.

Clinical Pathway for Scheduled Cesarean Birth

Focus of Care	Preoperative	Intraoperative	Immediate Postoperative First 2 hours	First 24 Postoperative Hours	Postoperative 24 Hours to Discharge
Assessments	Review prenatal record for risk factors. Complete admission assessments as per protocol. Assess the couple's emotional responses. Complete the surgical checklist.	Vital signs are monitored by the anesthesiologist or CRNA. Apgar score on neonate by neonatal personnel. Assess the neonate per protocol.	Assess per protocol-level of consciousness (orientation to time, place, person, or to preoperative level). Monitor VS, color, and O2 sat every 15 minutes for the first 2 hours. Assess fundus-height, tone, location, lochia, urinary output, and bladder distention together with VS. Monitor dressing condition, intake and output, and sensory motor function.	Monitor VS, usually every hour x 4, then every 4 hours until stable, and then every 8 hours until discharge. Monitor respirations and sedation level as per post intrathecal morphine administration protocol — usually every hour for the first 24 hours. Assess the level and location of pain. Assess abdominal dressing for bleeding and/or drainage.	Assess as per protocol, usually every 4 hours. Assess incisional site for drainage and signs of infection. Assess for signs of urinary disturbances.

Continued

Clinical Pathway for Scheduled Cesarean Birth—cont'd

Focus of Care	Preoperative	Intraoperative	Immediate Postoperative First 2 hours	First 24 Postoperative Hours	Postoperative 24 Hours to Discharge
			Newborn assessment, as per protocol usually every 30 minutes for the first 2 hours.	Monitor intake and output. Monitor ability to void. Monitor for signs of potential postpartum hemorrhage. Review laboratory test reports such as H&H, CBC. Monitor for signs of potential infections. Complete post-anesthesia assessments. Assess for adverse reaction related to intrathecal morphine, such as decreased respirations, itching, and vomiting, and intervene as per protocol.	
Activity Level	Ambulatory until Foley inserted	Bed rest	Bed rest	Bed rest until complete return of motor and sensory sensation/function. Following return of motor and sensory sensation, the woman is assisted in short walks and sitting in chair or on bedside. Assistance is required for peri-care and ADLs.	Up ad libitum. Encourage the woman to ambulate to reduce risk of gas pains. May require assistance with pericare and ADLs.
Education	Provide information on surgical procedure, anesthesia, and what to expect during cesarean birth and postoperatively.	Provide information to the woman and her support person on woman's and fetus's/neonate's condition.	Provide information to the woman and her support person on woman's and fetus's/neonate's condition.	Begin teaching on care of the neonate and of the woman's needs during the postpartum period.	Continue teaching and preparing the couple for discharge. Provide postoperative discharge teaching.
Elimination	Insert the Foley catheter and connect to continuous drainage.	Insert the Foley catheter if not done previously. Connect the Foley catheter to continuous drainage.	Monitor I & O	Connect the Foley catheter to continuous drainage for the first 8–12 hours. Remove the Foley catheter as per order. Assist the woman to the bathroom and measure voiding.	Assist the woman to the bathroom and measure voiding.
Emotional Needs	The couple may be anxious and excited.	The couple may be anxious and excited.	The couple may be anxious and excited. Address the couple's concerns and questions.	Couples may be excited and tired. Address the couple's concerns regarding cesarean	Provide opportunities for couples to share their thoughts and feelings regarding

Clinical Pathway for Scheduled Cesarean Birth—cont'd

Focus of Care	Preoperative	Intraoperative	Immediate Postoperative First 2 hours	First 24 Postoperative Hours	Postoperative 24 Hours to Discharge
	Provide emotional support and address questions and concerns. Keep the couple informed on surgical time.	Address the couple's concerns and questions. Provide an opportunity for the family to see and touch the neonate if the neonate is transferred to the nursery. Encourage the new father or support person to accompany the neonate to the nursery.	Provide an opportunity for the family to be with their neonate.	birth and the woman's and neonate's condition. Provide opportunities for the couple to share their experience and emotional responses to the birth.	the birthing experience and care of their neonate.
Medications	Administer preoperative medications as per protocol.	The CRNA or anesthesiologist administers antibiotics as indicated. The CRNA or anesthesiologist administers oxytocin.	Administer medications per anesthesia including medications for treatment of intrathecal morphine side effects such as pruritus and nausea/vomiting	Administer interventions including medications for treatment of intrathecal morphine side effects such as pruritus and nausea/vomiting. Administer medications as per orders (i.e., stool softener, vitamins).	Administer medications as per orders (i.e., stool softeners, vitamins).
Nutrition	NPO Insert IV. Administer IV fluid preload.	NPO IV fluids	NPO IV fluids	NPO and advancing to regular diet. IV fluids until bowel sounds are present and the woman is tolerating fluids by mouth.	Diet as tolerated. Provide information on the role of nutrition in postpartum recovery and breastfeeding.
Pain Management	CRNA or anesthesiologist meets with the couple to discuss anesthesia options.	The CRNA or anesthesiologist inserts the epidural catheter. The CRNA or anesthesiologist administers anesthetic agents via epidural catheter. The CRNA, anesthesiologist, or nurse removes the epidural catheter.	The anesthesiologist or CRNA responsible for prescribing medication for pain management in PACU	Intrathecal morphine administered via epidural catheter by CRNA or anesthesiologist after the birth of the neonate The anesthesiologist or CRNA responsible for prescribing medication for pain management and treatment of intrathecal morphine side effects for the first 24 hours postop.	Per MD orders

AWHONN, 2011

TYING IT ALL TOGETHER

You are assigned to care for a couple who is scheduled to have a repeat cesarean birth. Lisa is a gravida 2 para 1, 25-year-old woman. Her husband, Joe, is 27 years old and plans to accompany Lisa in the operating room. Their first cesarean birth was due to CPD. Lisa and Joe have a healthy 3-year-old daughter, Sara, who is excited about having a baby brother.

Describe the nursing action for the preoperative period.

You transfer the couple to the operating room on the labor and birthing unit. You will be the circulating nurse. Spinal anesthesia is used for the cesarean birth.

Describe the major nursing action during the intraoperative period.
Describe the anesthesia management during this period of time.

Lisa experiences an uncomplicated cesarean birth and delivers a 3,800-gram baby boy with Apgar scores of 9 and 9. Lisa and her son are transferred to the OB recovery room where you continue to care for the family. Lisa plans to breastfeed her son.

Describe the major nursing actions during the immediate postoperative recovery period.

The following day you are assigned to Lisa and her family in the postpartum unit. The shift report indicates that Lisa's lungs are clear; BS positive, fundus firm at 1 above U. Lisa ambulated to the bathroom and voided 450 mL. She is tolerating fluids. Her H&H are 30 and 10.2. She is having difficulty with breastfeeding. She complained of pain of 6 on a 10-point pain scale.

List the expected assessment findings for this period of time.
Discuss the nursing actions based on the shift report.
Discuss the major nursing action for couples and their newborn in preparation for discharge.

■ ■ ■ Review Questions ■ ■ ■

1. Indication for a cesarean delivery on maternal request is:
   A. Nonreassuring fetal heart rate
   B. Placenta previa
   C. Woman's desire to have a cesarean birth versus vaginal birth
   D. Obstetrician preference for cesarean delivery

2. The experiences of cesarean birth parents differ from those of vaginal birth parents in which of the following?
   A. Emotional responses to the childbirth experience
   B. Ability to breastfeed
   C. Nutritional needs
   D. Maternal hormonal changes

3. In the operating room, the circulating nurse calls a "time-out" before the surgery begins. The purpose of the time-out is to:
   A. Confirm that the surgeon is ready to begin
   B. Verify that it is the correct site, procedure, and patient
   C. Verify that the anesthesia is adequate
   D. Confirm that the neonatal team is in attendance

4. The most serious complication of the use of intrathecal morphine in the first 24 hours postoperative is:
   A. Urinary retention
   B. Nausea and itching
   C. Decreased sensation in legs
   D. Respiratory depression

5. You are assigned to take care of a woman, Lisa, who is 24 hours postoperative after an emergent cesarean birth related to fetal intolerance of labor. Lisa tells you that she is upset about having a cesarean birth. Your best initial nursing action is to:
   A. Inform her she has a healthy newborn
   B. Inform her that most women experience disappointment in having a cesarean birth
   C. Ask her to tell you more about her feelings
   D. Explain why she had a cesarean birth

6. You are caring for a woman having surgical birth who is low risk for developing a postpartum venous thromboembolism. The recommended treatment would include:
   A. Bilateral sequential compression devices and early ambulation
   B. Low molecular weight heparin 12–24 hours after birth
   C. Warfarin 24 hours after birth
   D. Daily low-dose aspirin

7. Evidence describes the best time for prophylactic antibiotic administration for women having a surgical birth to be:
   A. After the first postoperative assessment
   B. After cord clamping
   C. Within 60 minutes after birth of the infant
   D. Within 60 minutes prior to incision

8. The best intervention to help maintain maternal normothermia in the operating room is to:
   A. Preheat the radiant warmer and have an insensible fluid loss barrier available
   B. Provide warm blankets, warmed IV fluids, and maintain the temperature in the operating room between 20–30° C (68–73° F)
   C. Increase the operating room temperature to 26.7° C (80° F)
   D. Have the woman wear a heavy cloth gown and slippers to the operating room

9. When assessing a woman's pain after a surgical birth, the nurse should:
   A. Recognize pain management is the responsibility of the nurse, the anesthesia provider, and the primary physician
   B. Ensure that the prescribed pain medications are effective
   C. Implement non-pharmacologic interventions for promoting maternal comfort before administering pain medications
   D. Determine whether the pain is visceral or somatic

10. A common indication for an urgent surgical birth includes:
   A. Fetal intolerance of labor
   B. Posterior vertex position
   C. Failed assisted vaginal birth without fetal stress
   D. Maternal request for the procedure

References

American College of Obstetricians and Gynecologists. (2010). *Vaginal birth after previous cesarean delivery* (Committee Opinion No. 115). Washington, DC: Author.

American College of Obstetricians and Gynecologists. (2007). *Cesarean Delivery on Maternal Request* (Committee Opinion No. 394). Washington, DC: Author.

American College of Obstetricians and Gynecologists (2013) *Cesarean Delivery on Maternal Request.* (Committee Opinion No. 559. *Obstetrics & Gynecology 121*, 904–907.

American Society of Anesthesiologists Task Force. (2007). *Anesthesiology, 106,* 843–863.

Association of Women's Health, Obstetric and Neonatal Nurses (AWHONN). (2011). *Evidence-Based Clinical Practice Guideline: Perioperative care of the pregnant woman.* Washington, DC: Author.

Berghella, V. (2011b). Cesarean delivery: Preoperative issues. In D. S. Basow (Ed.), *UpToDate.* Waltham, MA: UpToDate.

Chestnut, D. (2006). Cesarean delivery on maternal demand: Implications for anesthesia providers. *International Journal of Obstetric Anesthesia, 15,* 269–272.

Coleman-Cowger, J., Erickson, K., Portnoy, B., Schulkin, J., & Spong, C. Y. (2010). Current practice of cesarean delivery on maternal request following the 2006 state-of-the-science conference. *Journal of Reproductive Medicine, 55(1-2),* 1–5.

Cunningham, F., Leveno, K., Bloom, S., Hauth, J., Rouse, D., & Spong, C. (2010). *Williams Obstetrics* (23rd ed.). New York: McGraw-Hill.

Declercq, E., MacDorman, M., & Menacker, F. (2011). Recent trends and patterns in cesarean and vaginal birth after cesarean (VBAC) deliveries in the United States. *Clinics in Perinatology, 38(2),* 179–192.

Deglin, J., & Vallerand, A. (2009). *Davis's drug guide for nurses* (11th ed). Philadelphia: F. A. Davis.

Deneux-Tharaux, C., Carmona, E., Bouvier-Colle, M. H., & Breart, G. (2006). Postpartum maternal mortality and cesarean delivery. *Obstetrics & Gynecology, 108,* 541–547.

Grossman, G., Joesch, J., & Tanfer, K. (2006). Trends in maternal request cesarean delivery from 2001 to 2004. *The American College of Obstetricians and Gynecologists, 108,* 1506–1516.

Hacker, N., Moore, J., & Gambone, J. (2004). *Essentials of obstetrics and gynecology* (4th ed). Philadelphia: W.B. Saunders.

Hamilton, B., Martin, J., & Ventura, S. (2011). Births: Preliminary data for 2010. *National Vital Statistics Reports, 60,* no. 2. [online].

Hyattsville, MD: National Center for Health Statistics. Retrieved from www.cdc.gov/nchs/products/pubs/pubd/hestats/prelimbirths05/prelimbirths05.htm

Hobson, J., Slade, P., Wrench, I., & Power, L. (2006). Preoperative anxiety and postoperative satisfaction in women undergoing elective cesarean section. *International Journal of Obstetric Anesthesia, 15,* 18–23.

Hughes, S., Levinson, G., & Rosen, M. (2002). *Shnider and Levinson's anesthesia for obstetrics* (4th ed). Philadelphia: Lippincott, Williams & Wilkins.

Hull, A. D., & Resnik, R. (2009). Placenta previa, placenta accrete, abruption placentae, and vasa previa. In R. K. Creasy, R. Resnik, & J. D. Iams (Eds.), *Maternal-fetal medicine: Principles and practice* (6th ed., pp. 725–737). Philadelphia: Saunders, Elsevier.

Joint Commission. (2003). Universal protocol for preventing wrong site, wrong procedure, wrong person surgery. Retrieved from www.jointcommission.org/patientsafety/universalprotocol/

Kuczkowski, M., Reisner (Ed.), L., & Lin, D. (2006). Anesthesia for cesarean section. In D. Chestnut (Ed.), *Obstetric anesthesia: Principles and practice* (3rd ed.). Philadelphia: C. V. Mosby.

Main, E. K., Morton, C. H., Melsop, K., Hopkins, D., Giuliani, G., & Gould, J. B. (2012). Creating a public agenda for maternity safety and quality in Cesarean delivery. *Obstetrics & Gynecology, 120,* 1194–1198.

Martin, J., Hamilton, B., Sutton, P., Ventura, S., Menacker, F., & Kirmeyer, S. (2011). Preliminary Data for 2010. *National Vital Statistics Reports, 60,* no. 2. Retrieved from www.cdc.gov/nchs/data/nvsr/nvsr55/nvsr545_11.pdf

National Institutes of Health. (2006). NIH State-of-the-Science Conference: Cesarean Delivery on Maternal Request. Retrieved from www.consensus.nih.gov/2006/2006CesareanSOS027main.htm

Quality and Safety Education for Nurses (2011). Innovations for Integrating Quality and Safety in Education and Practice: The QSEN Project. Retrieved from www.qsen.org/about_qsen.php

Silver, R. M. (2010). Delivery after previous cesarean: Long term maternal outcomes. *Seminars in Perinatology, 34,* 258–266.

Simpson & O'Brien-Abel (2013). Labor and Birth in Simpson K & Creehan. *Perinatal Nursing* (4th ed). Philadelphia: Lippincott.

Schwartz, A. (2006). Learning the essentials of epidural anesthesia. *Nursing 2006, 36,* 44–49.

Spong, C. Y., Berghella, V., Wenstrom, K. D., Mercer, B. M., & Saade, G. R. (2012). Preventing the f sarean delivery. *Obstetrics & Gynecology 1*

Yokoyama of pre-warmed nia following l of Clincal

Postpartal Period

Postpartum Physiological Assessments and Nursing Care

EXPECTED STUDENT OUTCOMES

On completion of this chapter, the student will be able to:
- ☐ Define key terms.
- ☐ Describe the physiological changes that occur during the postpartum period.
- ☐ Identify the critical elements of assessment and nursing care during the postpartum period.
- ☐ Describe the critical elements of discharge teaching.

Nursing Diagnosis

- Pain related to tissue trauma secondary to vaginal delivery
- Pain related to uterine involution secondary to vaginal delivery
- Pain related to congestion, increased vascularity, and milk accumulation secondary to breast engorgement
- At risk for infection related to tissue trauma
- At risk for infection (mastitis) related to altered skin integrity and milk stasis
- At risk for fluid volume deficit related to uterine atony
- At risk for impaired urinary elimination related to decreased sensation; tissue trauma
- At risk for constipation related to hormonal effects on smooth muscles
- At risk for knowledge deficit regarding health promotion post-birth related to lack of information

Nursing Outcomes

- The woman will report adequate pain control.
- The woman will remain free from symptoms of infection.
- The woman's fundus will remain firm with scant to moderate lochia.
- The woman will spontaneously void within 6–8 hours post-birth.
- The woman will eat a diet high in fiber and roughage and will drink a minimum of 10 glasses of fluid per day.
- The woman will verbalize an understanding of major components of health promotion.
- The woman will identify signs of complications that must be reported to the health care provider.

INTRODUCTION

The **postpartum** period is the 6-week period after childbirth. It is a time of rapid physiological changes within the woman's body as it returns to a pre-pregnant state. Women who enter pregnancy in a healthy state and experience a low-risk pregnancy and labor and birth are at low risk for complications during the postpartum period (see Critical Component: Physiological Aspects of Postpartum Nursing Care *and* Critical Component: Overview of the Postpartum Assessment).

The CDC and the Department of Health and Human Services Office of Disease Prevention and Health Promotion have set national health goals that are published in Healthy People 2020, several of which relate to the postpartum period (**Table 12-1**).

Don't have time to read this chapter? Want to reinforce your reading? Need to review for a test? Listen to this chapter on DavisPlus.

TABLE 12–1   HEALTHY PEOPLE 2020 OBJECTIVES RELATED TO THE POSTPARTUM PERIOD

OBJECTIVE	BASELINE	TARGET
Reduce the rate of maternal mortality	12.7 maternal deaths per 100,00 live births	11.4 maternal deaths per 100,000
Reduce maternal illness and complications due to pregnancy (complications during hospital labor and delivery)	31.1% of pregnant females experienced complications during hospitalized labor and delivery.	28%
Increase the proportion of infants that are breastfed:		
Ever	74%	81.9%
At 6 months	43.5%	60.6%
At 1 year	22.7%	34.1%
Reduce postpartum smoking relapse among women who quit smoking during pregnancy	No baseline data provided	No target provided
Increase the number of women giving birth who attend a postpartum care visit with a health care worker	No baseline data provided	No target provided
Increase the proportion of pregnancies that are intended	51.0%	56%
Reduce the proportion of females experiencing pregnancy despite use of reversible contraceptive method	12.4%	9.9%
Reduce the proportion of pregnancies conceived within 18 months of a previous birth	35.3%	31.7%
Reduce pregnancy rates among adolescent females	40.2%	36.2%

U.S. Department of Health and Human Services Office of Disease Prevention and Health Promotion, 2012.

CRITICAL COMPONENT

Physiological Aspects of Postpartum Nursing Care

The focus of the physiological aspect of postpartum nursing care is:

- Assessing for early signs of potential complications
- Providing comfort and restoring physiologic functions affected by childbirth
- Health promotion
- Family education

THE REPRODUCTIVE SYSTEM

The reproductive system, which includes the uterus, cervix, vagina, and perineum, undergoes dramatic changes during the 6 weeks after the birthing experience. Women are at risk for hemorrhage and infection. Nursing assessments and interventions are aimed at reducing these risks.

Uterus

After delivery of the placenta, the uterus begins the process of **involution,** by which the uterus returns to a pre-pregnant size, shape, and location; and the placental site heals. This occurs through uterine contractions, atrophy of the uterine muscle, and a decrease in the size of uterine cells. Primiparous women usually do not experience discomfort related to uterine contractions during the postpartum period. Multiparous women or women who are breastfeeding may experience "afterpains" during the first few postpartum days. **Afterpains** are moderate to severe cramp-like pains that are related to the uterus working harder to remain contracted and/or to the increase of oxytocin that is released in response to infant suckling. The uterus needs to be in a contracted state during the postpartum period to decrease the risk of postpartum hemorrhage. The contracted uterine muscle compresses the open vessels at the placental site and decreases the amount of blood loss.

Nursing Actions

- Assess the uterus for location, position, and tone of the fundus.
  - *After the third stage of labor, assess the uterus:*
    - Every 15 minutes for the first hour
    - Every 30 minutes for the second hour
    - Every 4 hours for the next 22 hours
    - Every shift after the first 24 hours or as stated in hospital/unit protocols
    - More frequently if the assessment findings are not within normal limits
      - *Rationale: Frequent assessment of uterine tone and placement allows for the identification of potential complications such as uterine atony (decreased uterine muscle tone) that may lead to postpartum hemorrhage (James, 2008). The risk for postpartum hemorrhage is the greatest within the*

first hour following delivery (James, 2008). Primary (early) postpartum hemorrhage occurs during the first 24 hours after birth, and secondary (late) postpartum hemorrhage is most prevalent during the first 6–14 days following birth (James, 2008). See Chapter 14 for more information about the care of the woman with postpartum hemorrhage.

- ■ *Before assessment:*
  - ■ Inform the woman that you will be palpating her uterus.
  - ■ Explain the procedure.
  - ■ Instruct the woman to void.
    - ▪ *Rationale: An overdistended bladder can result in uterine displacement and atony (James, 2008). Encouraging the woman to void prior to uterine assessment will allow for an accurate assessment of uterine placement and tone.*
  - ■ Provide privacy.
  - ■ Lower the head and foot of the bed so that the woman is in a supine position and flat.
  - ■ Support the lower uterine segment by placing one hand just above the symphysis pubis (**Fig. 12-1**).
    - ▪ *Rationale: During pregnancy there is stretching of the ligaments that hold the uterus in place. Fundal pressure could result in uterine inversion (James, 2008). Supporting the lower uterine segment may prevent uterine inversion during fundal assessment or massage.*
- ■ Locate the fundus with the other hand using gentle downward pressure.
- ■ Determine the tone of the fundus: Firm (contracted) or soft (boggy).
  - ■ *A boggy uterus indicates that the uterus is not contracting and places the woman at risk for excessive blood loss (see Critical Component: Boggy Uterus). If the uterus is boggy, the nurse should:*
    - ■ Massage the fundus with the palm of the hand.
      - ▪ *Rationale: Fundal massage stimulates contraction of the uterus (James, 2008; Katz, 2012).*
    - ■ Give oxytocin as per the physician's or midwife's orders.
      - ▪ *Rationale: Oxytocin promotes contraction of the uterus by stimulating the smooth muscle of the uterus (Vallerand & Sanoski, 2013).*
    - ■ Notify the physician or midwife if the uterus does not respond to massage.
      - ▪ *Rationale: Lack of response to fundal massage and oxytocin administration may indicate complications such as retained placental tissue, or birth trauma. Continued uterine atony can lead to postpartum hemorrhage and requires assessment and potentially further treatment by the woman's health care provider.*
- ■ Measure the distance between the fundus and umbilicus with your fingers.
  - ■ *Each finger breadth equals 1 cm.*
- ■ Determine the position of the uterus.
  - ▪ Rationale: A uterus that is shifted to the side may indicate a distended bladder. A distended bladder interferes with uterine contractibility, which places the woman at risk for uterine atony and increases her risk of hemorrhage.
  - ▪ If the uterus is deviated, soft, or elevated above the umbilicus, the immediate action is to explain to the

patient the need for her to void and to assist her to the bathroom. Reassess the uterine position after the woman has voided and returned to her bed. If the patient is unable to void, urinary catheterization may be necessary.

- ■ *Expected assessment findings (**Fig. 12-2**)*
  - ■ After birth, the uterine fundus is palpated midway between the umbilicus and symphysis pubis and is firm and midline.
  - ■ Within 12 hours after birth of the placenta, the fundus is located at the level of the umbilicus or 1 cm above the umbilicus and is firm and midline.
  - ■ 24 hours after birth of placenta, the fundus is located at 1 cm below the umbilicus and is firm and midline.
  - ■ The uterus descends 1 cm per day; by day 14 the fundus has descended into the pelvis and is not palpable.
- ■ *Document the location, position, and tone of the fundus and interventions.*

CRITICAL COMPONENT

Boggy Uterus

- ■ A boggy uterus is a sign that the uterus is not in a contracted state.
- ■ Risk of excessive blood loss and/or hemorrhage is increased.
- ■ The immediate action is to massage the fundus with the palm of your hand in a circular motion until firm and reevaluate within 30 minutes.
- ■ If the uterus does not respond to massage, follow the standing order for oxytocin and notify the physician or midwife.

Medication

Oxytocin (Pitocin, Syntocinon)

- ■ Indication: Postpartum control of bleeding
- ■ Action: Stimulates uterine smooth muscle to produce uterine contraction
- ■ Adverse reactions with IV use: Coma, seizures, hypotension, water intoxication
- ■ Route and doses: 10 units in a liter of IV solution or 10 units IM
- ■ Nursing actions/implications: Monitor vital signs frequently, assess for signs of water intoxication (drowsiness, headache, anuria), administer with an infusion pump, teach patient that medications will cause uterine cramping.

(Data from Vallerand & Sanoski, 2013)

The Endometrium

The **endometrium,** the mucous membrane that lines the uterus, undergoes exfoliation and regeneration after the birth of the placenta through the process of necrosis of the superficial layer of the decidua and regeneration of the decidua basalis into endometrial tissue. **Lochia,** a bloody discharge from the uterus

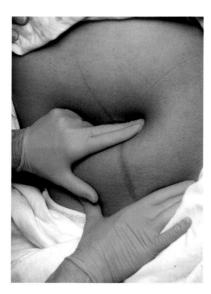

Figure 12–1 Nurse supporting lower uterine segment while assessing the postpartum uterus.

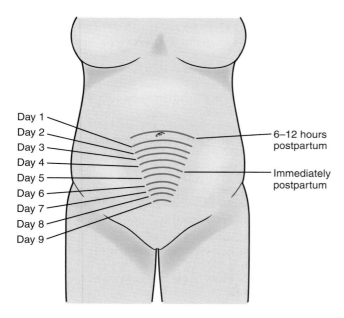

Day 1
Day 2
Day 3
Day 4
Day 5
Day 6
Day 7
Day 8
Day 9

6–12 hours postpartum

Immediately postpartum

Figure 12–2 Location of fundus at 6–12 hours postpartum, 2, 4, 6, and 8 days postpartum.

that contains sloughed off necrotic tissue, undergoes changes that reflect the healing stages of the uterine placental site (Table 12-2). Uterine contractions constrict the vessels around the placental site and help decrease the amount of blood loss. A primary complication is **metritis,** which is an infection of the endometrial tissue (see Chapter 14).

Nursing Actions

- Assess lochia each time the uterus is assessed.
  - *Rationale: Frequent assessment of lochia in the early postpartum period allows the nurse to monitor blood loss and identify if bleeding is excessive.*

- *Lower the peripad for inspection and determine the amount of lochia.*
  - The amount of flow is determined by the amount of lochia on a perineal pad after 1 hour (AWHONN, 2006).
  - *Lochia is assessed as scant, light, moderate, or heavy* **(Fig. 12-3).**
    - Scant is less than 1 inch on the pad.
    - Light is less than 4 inches on the pad.
    - Moderate is less than 6 inches on the pad.
    - Heavy is when the pad is saturated within 1 hour (Whitmer, 2011).
- Assess for clots.
  - *Rationale: It is common for lochia to contain clots, which occur when the lochia has been pooling in the lower uterine segment.*
  - *Small clots should be noted in the patient chart.*
  - *Large clots should be weighed and findings reported to the physician or midwife.*
    - 10 grams equals 10 milliliters of blood loss.
    - Rationale: Large clots can interfere with uterine contractions.
  - *Clots should be examined for the presence of tissue.*
    - Retained placental tissue can interfere with uterine involution and lead to excessive bleeding (Katz, 2012) (see Critical Component: Excessive Bleeding).
  - *Expected assessment findings* **(Table 12-2)**

CRITICAL COMPONENT

Excessive Bleeding

- Heavy lochia is a sign of excessive bleeding and/or postpartum hemorrhage.
- Assess the tone of uterus.
- If the uterus is boggy, massage.
- If the uterus is boggy and displaced to the side, instruct the patient to void and reevaluate.
- If firm, change the pad and reevaluate in 15 minutes.
- In case of continued excessive bleeding, notify the physician or midwife.
- Continued heavy bleeding with good fundal tone may indicate the presence of a genitourinary tract laceration or hematoma of the vulva or vagina (Katz, 2012).

- Patient education
  - *Teach the woman how to assess the uterus and explain the normal process of involution.*
  - *Teach the woman how to massage her uterus if boggy and instruct her to notify the nurse while in the hospital and health care provider after discharge.*
    - Rationale: Secondary hemorrhage often occurs after the patient has been discharged. To prevent serious complications, women should understand the normal progression of lochia and uterine involution, and report abnormal amounts of bleeding.

■ *Provide information regarding "afterpains."*
- Uterine cramps are caused by the contraction and relaxation of the uterus as it decreases in size.
- Afterpains occur within the first few days and last 36 hours.
- They occur more commonly with multiparous women and increase with each additional pregnancy/birth.
- The condition may increase when breastfeeding during the first few postpartum days.
- Comfort measures (see Critical Component: Assessment and Management of Pain in the Postpartum Period):
  - *Empty bladder*
    - Rationale: A distended bladder can increase afterpains.
  - *Warm blanket to abdomen*
  - *Analgesia (ibuprofen is commonly used for postpartum discomfort)*
    - Rationale: Analgesics alter the perception and response to pain (Vallerand & Sanoski, 2013).
  - *Relaxation techniques*
    - Rationale: According to the gate control theory of pain, interventions such as applying warm compresses and promoting relaxation may interfere with the transmission and sensation of pain.
■ *Provide information on the stages of lochia.*
■ *Explain that the flow of lochia can increase when getting up in the morning or after sitting for prolonged periods of time due to vaginal pooling of lochia, or from excessive physical activity.*
■ *Instruct the woman to notify the nurse, physician, or midwife if she experiences:*
- A sudden increase in the amount of lochia
- Bright red bleeding after the rubra stage
- Foul odor
  - *Rationale: Foul smelling lochia could indicate the development of an infection. An increase in lochia or the return of bright red bleeding may be signs of secondary hemorrhage (James, 2008).*
■ *Provide information for reducing the risk of infection.*
- Instruct the patient to change the peripad frequently from the front to back, and to wash hands before and after changing pads.
  - *Rationale: Lochia is a medium for bacterial growth. Frequent pad changes and hand washing are actions aimed at preventing infection.*
■ Document the stage and amount of lochia and interventions.

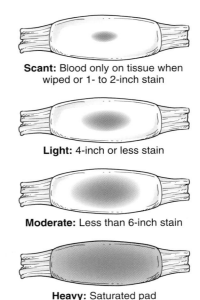

Scant: Blood only on tissue when wiped or 1- to 2-inch stain

Light: 4-inch or less stain

Moderate: Less than 6-inch stain

Heavy: Saturated pad

Figure 12–3 Comparison of heavy, moderate, light, and scant lochia on pads.

TABLE 12–2	STAGES AND CHARACTERISTICS OF LOCHIA		
STAGE	**TIME FRAME**	**EXPECTED FINDINGS**	**DEVIATIONS FROM NORMAL**
LOCHIA RUBRA	Day 1–3	Bloody with small clots Moderate to scant amount Increased flow on standing or breastfeeding Fleshy odor	Large clots Heavy amount; saturates pad within 15 minutes (sign of possible hemorrhage) Foul odor (sign of infection) Placental fragments
LOCHIA SEROSA	Day 4–10	Pink or brown color Scant amount Increased flow during physical activity Fleshy odor	Continuation of rubra stage after day 4 Heavy amount; saturates pad within 15 minutes (sign of possible hemorrhage) Foul odor (sign of infection)
LOCHIA ALBA	Day 10	Yellow to white in color Scant amount Fleshy odor	Bright red bleeding (sign of possible late postpartum hemorrhage) Foul odor (sign of infection)

Medication

Ibuprofen (Motrin)

- Indication: Mild to moderate pain
- Action: Decreased pain and inflammation by inhibiting prostaglandin synthesis
- Common side effects: Headaches, constipation, dyspepsia, nausea, vomiting, edema
- Route and dose: PO; 600–800 mg every 6 hours PRN
- Nursing actions/implications: May be administered with food or milk to decrease GI upset. Give with a full glass of water. Patients with asthma, nasal polyps, or who are allergic to aspirin are at risk for hypersensitivity to ibuprofen. Assess pain before and 1 hour after administration.

(Data from Vallerand & Sanoski, 2013)

Vagina and Perineum

- The vagina and perineum experience changes related to the birthing process ranging from mild stretching and minor lacerations to major tears and episiotomies.
- The woman may experience mild to severe pain depending on the degree and type of vaginal and/or perineal trauma.
- The primary complication is infection at the lacerations or episiotomy sites.
- The vagina and perineum undergo healing and restoration during the postpartum period.

Nursing Actions

- The perineum is assessed when the fundus and lochia are checked in the post-delivery period (James, 2008). After that, the perineum is assessed every shift using the acronym REEDA (redness, edema, ecchymosis, discharge, approximation of edges of episiotomy or laceration).
  - *Rationale: Frequent assessment of the perineum using the REEDA scale will allow identification of potential complications such as infection, hematoma, and excess bleeding (James, 2008). See Chapter 14 for more information about lacerations and hematoma.*
  - *Explain the procedure.*
  - *Provide privacy.*
  - *Assist the woman to her side.*
  - *Lower the peripad and separate the buttocks to expose the perineum for assessment.*
    - Rationale: Positioning the woman in the side lying position and removing the peripad will allow for visualization of the perineal area. It also allows for the assessment of the amount of lochia present on the entire peripad. While the woman is in the side lying position, assess the rectal area for hemorrhoids.
- Expected assessment findings:
  - *Mild edema*
  - *Minor ecchymosis*
  - *Approximation of the edges of the episiotomy or laceration*
  - *Mild to moderate pain*
- Assess for discomfort (see Critical Component: Assessment and Management of Pain in the Postpartum Period).

- Provide comfort measures:
  - *Apply ice to the perineum, or encourage the use of cold sitz baths for the first 24 hours.*
    - Rationale: Ice causes local vasoconstriction, which decreases edema and provides an anesthetic effect (Katz, 2012).
  - *Encourage the woman to lie on her side.*
    - Rationale: The side lying position decreases pressure on the perineum.
  - *Instruct the woman to tighten her gluteal muscles as she sits down and to relax muscles after she is seated.*
    - Rationale: This helps cushion the perineum and increases comfort when assuming a sitting position.
  - *Instruct the woman to wear peripads snugly to prevent rubbing.*
  - *Instruct the woman to take warm sitz baths starting 24 hours after delivery twice a day for 20 minutes.*
    - Rationale: Warm sitz baths promote circulation, healing, and comfort (James, 2008). According to the gate control theory of pain, a sitz bath using warm water can alter a patient's perception of pain (Wilkinson and Treas, 2011).
  - *Administer analgesia per the physician's or midwife's order.*
    - Rationale: Analgesics such as ibuprofen are effective in treating perineal pain (Katz, 2012).
  - *Administer a topical anesthetic per the physician's or midwife's order.*
    - Rationale: Topical anesthetics may relieve localized discomfort.
- Reduce the risk for infection.
  - *Instruct the woman to use a peri-bottle with warm water and rinse the perineum after elimination.*
  - *Instruct the woman to change the peripad frequently.*
  - *Instruct the woman to properly dispose of soiled pads and to wash her hands.*
    - Rationale: Lochia is a medium for bacterial growth. Frequent pad changes and hand washing will reduce the risk for infection.
- Document findings and interventions.

Breasts

During pregnancy, the breasts undergo changes in preparation for lactation (see Critical Component: Breast Engorgement). Breast fullness is normal and is manifested by swelling of the breast tissue; however, the breast tissue remains soft and nontender (James, 2008). Around the third postpartum day, all women, breastfeeding and non-breastfeeding, experience some degree of primary breast engorgement. **Primary engorgement,** which is an increase in the vascular and lymphatic system of the breasts, precedes the initiation of milk production. The woman's breasts become larger, firm, warm, and tender, and the woman may feel a throbbing pain in the breasts. Primary engorgement subsides within 24–48 hours. Women who breastfeed experience **subsequent breast engorgement** related to distention of milk glands that is relieved by having the baby suckle or by expressing milk. The primary complication is **mastitis,** which is an infection of the breast (see Chapter 14).

CRITICAL COMPONENT

Assessment and Management of Pain in the Postpartum Period

- Pain in the postpartum period may result from uterine contractions, perineal trauma, lacerations, episiotomy, nipple pain caused by improper infant latch, breast engorgement, hemorrhoids, and procedures (James, 2008).
- Pain is considered the fifth vital sign and should be assessed routinely when vital signs are done, when the patient complains of pain, before and after a painful procedure, and before and after implementation of a pain management intervention (Wilkinson & Treas, 2011).
- Assess pain using an appropriate pain scale per agency protocol. Many scales measure pain intensity, duration, quality, location, factors that make pain better or worse, and acceptable level of pain.
- Pharmacologic interventions

  - Non-steroidal anti-inflammatory medications such as ibuprofen can be used for mild to moderate pain.
  - Opioid analgesics can be used for moderate to severe pain. These medications are often used in combination with a non-opioid medication for added analgesic affect.

- Non-pharmacological interventions. Examples of non-pharmacologic interventions are as follows:

  - Ice packs
  - Warm compresses
  - Sitz baths
  - Repositioning
  - Topical treatments such as witch hazel pads and anesthetic sprays can be applied to decrease localized discomfort.

Colostrum, a clear, yellowish fluid, precedes milk production. It is higher in protein and lower in carbohydrates than breast milk. It contains immunoglobulins G and A that provide protection for the newborn during the early weeks of life.

Lactation is further addressed in Chapter 16.

Nursing Actions for the Breastfeeding Woman

- Assess the breasts for engorgement.
  - *Inspect the breasts for signs of engorgement: tenderness, firmness, warmth, and/or enlargement.*
  - *Expected assessment findings:*
    - In the first 24 hours postpartum, the breasts are soft and non-tender.
    - On postpartum day 2, the breasts are slightly firm and non-tender.
    - On postpartum day 3, the breasts are firm, tender, and warm to touch.
- Assess the nipples for signs of irritation and nipple tissue breakdown.
  - *Rationale: Signs of irritation and tissue breakdown are cracked, blistered, or reddened areas. Skin breakdown of the nipples is often associated with an improper infant latch. (See Chapter 16 for interventions to prevent/treat nipple irritation and breakdown.)*
- Assess for plugged milk ducts (see Critical Component: Plugged Milk Ducts).

Nursing Actions for the Non-Breastfeeding Woman

- Assess the breasts for primary engorgement.
  - *Inspect the breasts for signs of engorgement: Tenderness, firmness, warmth, and/or enlargement.*
    - Rationale: In women who choose not to breastfeed, milk leakage, breast pain, and engorgement may be experienced between 1–4 days post-delivery (James, 2008).
  - *Expected assessment findings*
    - During the first 24 hours postpartum, the breasts are soft and non-tender.
    - On postpartum day 2, the breasts are slightly firm and non-tender.
    - On postpartum day 3, the breasts are firm and tender.

CRITICAL COMPONENT

Breast Engorgement

- Breast engorgement is caused by an increase in the vascular and the lymphatic systems within the breast and milk accumulation.
- Engorgement typically occurs 2–3 days after birth.
- Physiological engorgement:

  - Breasts are swollen.

- Pathological engorgement:

  - Breasts are hard, swollen, red, and tender/painful.
  - Breasts feel warm to the touch.
  - Woman may feel a throbbing sensation in the breasts.
  - Woman may have an elevated temperature.
  - Infant may have difficulty latching on due to the severe engorgement (James, 2008).

- Treatment for breastfeeding women

  - Frequent feedings to empty the breasts and to prevent milk stasis

  - Warm compresses to the breast and breast massage to facilitate the flow of milk prior to feeding sessions
  - Express milk by breast pump or manually if the infant is unable to nurse, i.e., preterm infant.
  - Ice packs after feedings to reduce inflammation and discomfort
  - Analgesics for pain management
  - Wear a supportive bra

- Prevention and treatment for non-breastfeeding women

  - Wear a supportive bra.
  - Avoid stimulating the breast.
  - Ice packs to breast
  - Analgesics for pain management
  - Subsides within 24 hours.

CRITICAL COMPONENT

Plugged Milk Ducts

- Plugged milk ducts are associated with inadequate emptying of the breast, wearing overly tight bras, and/or failure to change the infant into different feeding positions (Balkam, 2010; James, 2008).
- Symptoms: palpation of tender breast lumps the size of peas (James, 2008)
- Treatments:
    - *Frequent feedings*
    - *Changing feeding positions (Mass, 2004; Whitmer, 2011)*
    - *Application of warm compresses to breast or taking a warm shower prior to feeding session*
    - *Massaging the breasts prior to feeding session*
- Continued milk stasis or unresolved plugged milk ducts can lead to mastitis and potential breast abscess (Mass, 2004; Whitmer, 2011).
- Patient education
    - *Apply heat to the breasts to increase circulation and comfort.*
    - *Encourage the woman to wear a supportive bra.*
    - *Instruct the woman to examine her nipples before feedings for signs of irritation.*
    - *Instruct the woman to feed her infant frequently on demand or express milk if she is experiencing breast engorgement.*
    - *Provide information on mastitis.*
        - Mastitis typically occurs at 3–4 weeks post-birth.
        - The infection may be due to bacterial entry through cracks in the nipples, and is associated with milk stasis, stress, and fatigue (James, 2008; Mass, 2004).
        - Symptoms: Fever, chills, malaise, flu-like symptoms, unilateral breast pain, and redness and tenderness in the infected area
        - The woman needs to report symptoms to her health care provider.
        - Treatment: Antibiotic therapy, analgesia, rest, and hydration
        - The woman should continue to breastfeed or pump her breasts as per the physician's or midwife's recommendation.
        - The woman should apply moist heat to the affected breast before breastfeeding.
- Document findings and interventions.

- Patient education
    - *Instruct the woman to wear a supportive bra or sports bra 24 hours a day until her breasts become soft. Teach the woman to avoid expressing milk or stimulating the breasts.*
        - Rationale: Atrophy in milk secreting cells of the breasts can be caused by back pressure in the milk ducts that occurs when the breasts are not emptied (James, 2008).
    - *Instruct the woman who is experiencing engorgement to:*
        - Apply ice to the breasts.
        - Not express milk because this stimulates milk production.
        - Avoid heat to the breast because this can stimulate milk production.
        - Take an analgesic for pain.
- Document findings and interventions.

CRITICAL COMPONENT

Overview of the Postpartum Assessment

The following should be assessed per the health care provider's order or unit protocol.
- Vital signs, pain, breath sounds
- Laboratory findings, such as, CBC, rubella status, and Rh status
- Breasts
- Uterus
- Bladder
- Bowel
- Lochia
- Episiotomy, lacerations, perineum, hemorrhoids
- Lower extremities
- Emotions, bonding with infant, fatigue

THE CARDIOVASCULAR SYSTEM

Women have an average blood loss of 200–500 mL related to the vaginal birthing experience.

This has a minimal effect on a woman's system due to pregnancy-induced hypervolemia. There is an increase in cardiac output during the first few postpartum hours related to blood that was shunted through the uteroplacental unit returning to the maternal system. Cardiac output returns to pre-pregnant levels within 48 hours. White blood cell (WBC) levels may increase to 25,000/mm within a few hours of birth as the result of stress related to labor and birth, and return to normal levels within 7 days.

Women are at risk for thrombosis related to the increase of circulating clotting factors during pregnancy. Clotting factors slowly decrease after the birth of the placenta and return to normal ranges within the first 2 postpartum weeks. A potentially life threatening complication of thrombus formation is pulmonary emboli (James, 2008).

There is an increased risk of **orthostatic hypotension,** a sudden drop in the blood pressure when the woman stands up, which is due to decreased vascular resistance in the pelvis. Most women will experience an episode of feeling cold and shaking during the first few hours following birth. This phenomenon is referred to as **postpartum chills** and is related to vascular instability.

Nursing Actions

- Assess pulse and blood pressure:
    - *Every 15 minutes for the first hour*
    - *Every 30 minutes for the second hour*
    - *Every 4 hours for the next 22 hours*
    - *Every shift after the first 24 hours or as stated in hospital/ unit protocols*
        - Rationale: Hemodynamic changes occur during labor and delivery and in the postpartum period. There are rapid changes in blood volume and cardiac output. Assessment of pulse and blood pressure is important in identification of potential complications such as

excessive blood loss, orthostatic hypotension, infection, and gestational hypertension/preeclampsia. An elevated pulse may indicate excessive blood loss, fever, or infection (James, 2008).

■ *Expected assessment findings:*
■ Pulse and blood pressure within normal ranges. After delivery there may be a transient 5% elevation in the woman's systolic and diastolic blood pressure (Katz, 2012).
■ Bradycardia may occur 6–10 days post-delivery (Whitmer, 2011).
■ Assess for orthostatic hypotension (see Critical Component: Orthostatic Hypotension).
■ *Expected assessment findings:*
■ May experience orthostatic hypotension during the first few postpartum days when moving from a sitting or lying position to a standing position. During first 24 hours postpartum, women need assistance when ambulating.

CRITICAL COMPONENT

Orthostatic Hypotension

■ Women are at risk for orthostatic hypotension during the first postpartum week.
■ Explain cause and incidence of orthostatic hypotension.
■ Instruct the woman to rise slowly to a standing position.
■ Assist the woman when ambulating during the first few hours post-birth.
■ Assist the woman to a sitting position if she becomes dizzy or faint.
■ Use an ammonia ampule if the woman faints.
■ Assess for excessive blood loss.

■ *Check lab values such as a complete blood count (CBC) if ordered.*
■ Rationale: Components of the CBC, such as the hematocrit and hemoglobin, are assessed in cases where excessive blood loss has occurred. The hematocrit measures the concentration of red blood cells in the blood (Kee, 2009). Hemoglobin decreases by 1.0 to 1.5 g/dL and hematocrit decreases 3%–4% per 500 mL of blood loss (AWHONN, 2006).
■ *Expected assessment findings:*
■ Blood loss within normal ranges
■ Hemoglobin and hematocrit within normal ranges
■ Pulse rate normal, blood pressure within normal limits. An increase in pulse rate may be an indicator of excessive blood loss.
■ Assess lower extremities for venous thrombosis.
■ *Rationale: Increased coagulability associated with pregnancy continues into the post-delivery period. Additionally, venous stasis may occur when there is limited mobility in the immediate postpartum period. These factors lead to an increased risk of venous thrombosis (James, 2008; Katz, 2012).*

■ *Some postpartum units may include assessment for the Homan's sign each shift. However, evidence suggests that the Homan's sign is not an accurate or useful assessment for deep vein thrombosis (James, 2008).*
■ *Assess the legs for calf tenderness, edema, and sensation of warmth each shift. Compare pulses in both extremities.*
■ Rationale: Symptoms of deep vein thrombosis include muscle pain, tenderness, palpation of a hard cordlike vessel, swelling of veins, edema, and decreased blood circulation to the affected area (James, 2008).
■ *Expected assessment findings:*
■ No tenderness or sensation of warmth
■ Assess for postpartum chills.
■ *Assess temperature.*
■ Women who are experiencing chills with temperature within normal ranges should be offered a warm blanket and reassurance that it is normal.
■ Women who are experiencing chills with elevated temperature need to be evaluated further for possible infection, and the physician or midwife needs to be notified.
■ Patient education
■ *Instruct the woman on ways to reduce risk of orthostatic hypotension. Women should be accompanied by the nurse during ambulation in the early postpartum period.*
■ Rationale: Orthostatic hypotension places the patient at risk for fainting and falls.
■ *Instruct the woman to take her temperature if she experiences chills and report temperature elevations to her physician or midwife.*
■ Rationale: An elevated temperature over 100.4°F on two occasions that are 6 hours apart is a symptom of infection (James, 2008).
■ *Encourage frequent ambulation.*
■ Rationale: Early and frequent ambulation prevents deep vein thrombosis by preventing stasis of blood in the lower extremities.
■ *Instruct the woman not to cross her legs.*
■ *Apply TED hose as per orders for women with a history of blood clots (James, 2008).*
■ Document findings and interventions.

THE RESPIRATORY SYSTEM

There is a return of chest wall compliance after the birth of the infant due to reduction of pressure on the diaphragm. The respiratory system returns to a pre-pregnant state by the end of the postpartum period.

Nursing Actions

■ Assess the respiratory rate:
■ *Every 15 minutes for the first hour*
■ *Every 30 minutes for the second hour*
■ *Every 4 hours for the next 22 hours*
■ *Every shift after the first 24 hours or as stated in hospital/unit protocols*

■ Assess breath sounds
  ■ *Rationale: Women who received oxytocin; large amounts of intravenous fluids; tocolytics such as magnesium sulfate or terbutaline; had multiple birth; an infection; preeclampsia; or who were on bed rest are at risk for pulmonary edema (James, 2008).*
■ Expected assessment findings:
  ■ *Within normal limits. The respiratory rate in the postpartum period is typically in the range of 16–24 breaths per minute (Whitmer, 2011).*
  ■ *Breath sounds clear*
■ Document findings and intervention.

THE IMMUNE SYSTEM

■ Temperature
  ■ *It is common for the postpartum woman to experience mild temperature elevations during the first 24 hours post-birth related to muscular exertion, exhaustion, dehydration, or hormonal changes.*
  ■ *A temperature greater than 100.4°F (38°C) after the first 24 hours on two occasions may be indicative of postpartum infection and requires further evaluation.*
■ Immunizations
  ■ *Women who are rubella non-immune should be immunized for rubella before discharge (see Critical Component: Rubella Immunization). Women may be required to sign a consent form prior to administration of the vaccine.*
  ■ *Women may also receive vaccinations such as Tdap (tetanus, diphtheria, and pertussis), hepatitis B, varicella, and influenza if needed (ACOG, 2012; CDC, 2011; Katz, 2012).*

CRITICAL COMPONENT

Rubella Immunization

■ Women who contract rubella during the first trimester have a 90% chance of transmitting the virus to their fetuses.
■ Fetuses exposed to rubella during the first trimester are at risk for birth defects that include deafness, blindness, heart defects, and mental retardation.
■ Postpartum women who are rubella-nonimmune should be immunized for rubella before discharge. The measles, mumps, and rubella vaccine is often given.
■ Women who are immunized should avoid pregnancy for 4 weeks, although the risk of the fetus developing birth defects from the vaccine is extremely low.

(Centers for Disease Control, 2011)

■ Rh isoimmunization
  ■ *Rh isoimmunization occurs when an Rh-negative woman develops antibodies to Rh-positive blood related to exposure to Rh-positive blood either by blood transfusion or during pregnancy with an Rh-positive fetus.*

  ■ *Women who are sensitized produce IgG anti-D (antibody), which crosses the placenta and attacks the fetal red blood cells, causing hemolysis.*
  ■ *Rh isoimmunization is preventable (see Critical Component: Prevention of Rh Isoimmunization).*

CRITICAL COMPONENT

Prevention of Rh Isoimmunization

■ Rho immune globulin is given to Rh-negative women at 28 weeks' gestation.
■ Rh-negative women who gave birth to an Rh-positive neonate are screened for anti-Rh antibodies (Coombs' test).
■ A second injection of Rho immune globulin is given to the woman if she is Coombs' negative.

Medication

Rho(D) Immune Globulin (RhoGAM)

■ Indication: Administered to Rh-negative women who have given birth to an Rh-positive neonate
■ Action: Prevents production of anti-Rh (D) antibodies
■ Adverse reactions: Pain at the injection site, anemia
■ Route and dose: 300 mcg (Rhopylac, 1500 IU) IM within 72 hours post-birth

(Vallerand & Sanoski, 2013)

Nursing Actions

■ Assess temperature:
  ■ *Every 15 minutes for the first hour*
  ■ *Every 30 minutes for the second hour*
  ■ *Every 4 hours for the next 22 hours*
  ■ *Every shift after the first 24 hours or as stated in hospital/unit protocols*
    ■ Rationale: Assessing the postpartum patient's temperature allows health care providers to monitor for complications such as infection.
■ Temperature elevations less than 100.4°F (38°C) during the first 24 hours post-birth:
  ■ *Hydrate the woman.*
  ■ *Promote relaxation and rest.*
  ■ *Reassess in 1 hour after interventions.*
    ■ Rationale: Slight temperature elevations during the first 24 hours postpartum are likely associated with dehydration (Whitmer, 2011).
■ Temperature elevation 100.4°F (38°C) or higher after 24 hours post-birth:
  ■ *Hydrate the woman.*
  ■ *Notify the physician or midwife for further evaluation.*
    ■ Rationale: A temperature of 100.4°F on two different occasions after the first 24 hours post-delivery is a sign of infection (James, 2008).
■ Administer rubella vaccine as indicated.
■ Administer other needed vaccines as ordered.
■ Administer Rho(D) immune globulin (RhoGAM) as indicated.
■ Document findings and interventions.

THE URINARY SYSTEM

Bladder distention, incomplete emptying of the bladder, and inability to void are common during the first few days post-birth. These are related to a decreased sensation of the urge to void and/or edema around the urethra. Diuresis, caused by decreased estrogen and oxytocin levels, occurs within 12 hours post-birth and aids in the elimination of excess tissue fluids. Primary complications are bladder distention and cystitis (see Critical Component: Cystitis).

CRITICAL COMPONENT

Cystitis

- Bladder inflammation/infection
- Symptoms: Frequency, urgency, pain/burning on urination, and malaise
- Treatment: Antibiotic therapy, increased hydration, rest

Nursing Actions

- Assist the woman to the bathroom and encourage her to void within 6 hours post-birth.
  - *Rationale: Early voiding decreases the risk of cystitis. In addition, it prevents bladder distention, which could lead to uterine atony and postpartum hemorrhage (James, 2008).*
- Assess for urinary disturbances.
  - *Measure voidings during the first 24 hours post-birth.*
    - Rationale: Various birth related factors, such as the stretching of the urethra, displacement of the bladder, birth trauma associated neural dysfunction, and anesthesia, may interfere with the return of urinary function. Rapid filling of the bladder associated with the administration of IV fluids during labor and delivery, and postpartum diuresis can lead to overdistention of the bladder (James, 2008). Measuring voidings allows the nurse to identify inadequate output and problems with urinary elimination.
    - If voiding is less than 150 mL, the nurse needs to palpate for bladder distention. Signs of bladder distention include uterine atony, displacement of the uterus above the umbilicus to the right, increased lochia, and fullness in the suprapubic area (James, 2008).
    - Voiding less than 150 mL of urine is indicative of urinary retention with overflow (Whitmer, 2011).
      - *Incomplete emptying of the bladder can lead to uterine atony and postpartum hemorrhage. Urinary retention may also lead to cystitis.*
    - The woman should be able to void within 4–8 hours of delivery (Whitmer, 2011).
      - *If unable to void within 12 hours post-birth, the woman may need to be catheterized.*
        - A Foley catheter is recommended when inability to void is related to edema.
          - *Rationale: After 24 hours, edema associated with trauma of the bladder and urethra related to birth should decrease (James, 2008).*

- A straight or "in and out" catheterization may be done if there is little or no edema present and repeated catheterizations are not needed.
  - An alternative method when a woman is unable to void is the use of peppermint oil.
    - *Saturate a cotton ball with peppermint oil.*
    - *Place the saturated cotton ball in the "hat" (urine collection container) with a small amount of water.*
    - *Place the "hat" on the toilet.*
    - *Instruct the woman to sit on the toilet.*
    - *The vapors of the peppermint oil have a relaxing effect on the urinary sphincter.*
  - *Assess for frequency, urgency, and burning on urination.*
    - Notify the physician or midwife if the patient reports frequency, urgency and/or burning on urination.
      - *Rationale: These are signs of possible cystitis.*
  - *Expected assessment findings:*
    - The woman spontaneously voids within 6–8 hours post-birth.
    - Each voiding is a minimum of 150 mL.
    - The woman does not experience frequency, urgency, and burning on urination.
- Instruct the woman to increase fluid intake to a minimum of 8 glasses per day.
- Document findings and interventions.

THE ENDOCRINE SYSTEM

Abrupt changes occur in the endocrine system after the delivery of the placenta. Estrogen, progesterone, and prolactin levels decrease. Estrogen levels begin to rise after the first week of postpartum.

- Nonlactating women: Prolactin levels continue to decline throughout the first 3 postpartum weeks. Menses begins 7–9 weeks post-birth. The first menses is usually anovulatory. Ovulation usually occurs by the fourth cycle.
- Lactating women: Prolactin levels increase in response to the infant's suckling. Lactation suppresses menses. Return of menses depends on the length and amount of breastfeeding. Ovulation is suppressed longer for lactating women than for nonlactating women.

CRITICAL COMPONENT

Contraception

- Women, nonlactating and lactating, are advised to use a form of contraception when they resume sexual intercourse as ovulation can precede their first menses.
- Breastfeeding is not an effective means of contraception.

Diaphoresis

Diaphoresis occurs during the first few postpartum weeks in response to the decreased estrogen levels. This profuse sweating, which often occurs at night, assists the body in excreting the increased fluid accumulated during pregnancy.

Nursing Actions

- ■ Assess for diaphoresis.
  - ■ If present, assess for infection by taking the woman's temperature.
  - ■ Expected assessment findings:
    - ■ *Diaphoresis with temperature within normal ranges*
- ■ Patient education
  - ■ *Instruct the woman regarding the cause of diaphoresis.*
  - ■ *Discuss comfort measures such as wearing cotton nightwear.*
  - ■ *Instruct the woman to check the temperature and notify the physician or midwife if elevated.*
    - ■ Rationale: Feelings of warmth, sweating, and chills are signs of fever, which is a cardinal sign of infection. Women with these symptoms need to differentiate between fever and diaphoresis, which is a normal physiologic process.
  - ■ *Provide information regarding return of menses and ovulation.*
  - ■ *Encourage the couple to use contraception when they resume sexual intercourse (see Critical Component: Contraception).*
    - ■ Rationale: Some couples may decide to resume sexual intercourse prior to the postpartum follow-up appointment. It is recommended that women wait 24 months after birth until the next pregnancy is attempted. Couples should be counseled to use contraception to prevent unintended pregnancy from occurring in the postpartum period (Kennedy & Trussel, 2011).
- ■ Document findings and interventions.

THE MUSCULAR AND NERVOUS SYSTEMS

After birth, the abdominal muscles have a reduction in tone and the abdomen appears soft and flabby. Some women experience a separation of the rectus muscle, which is noted as **diastasis recti abdominis** (**Fig. 12-4**). This separation becomes less apparent as the body returns to a pre-pregnant state.

- ■ Women may experience muscular soreness related to the labor and birth experience.
- ■ Lower body nerve sensation may be diminished for women who have received an epidural during labor.
  - ■ *Delay ambulation until full sensation returns.*

Nursing Actions

- ■ Assess for diastasis recti abdominis.
  - ■ *The nurse can feel the separation of the rectus muscle when assessing the fundus.*
  - ■ *Reassure the woman that this is normal and will diminish over time.*
- ■ Assess for muscle tenderness.
  - ■ *Rationale: Muscle soreness may result from positioning during labor and delivery, and generalized muscle use during second stage labor/pushing.*
  - ■ *Expected assessment findings:*
    - ■ None to mild muscle soreness
  - ■ *Comfort measures for muscle soreness:*
    - ■ Ice pack to area for 15 minutes
    - ■ Heat to area
    - ■ Warm shower
    - ■ Analgesia
      - ■ *Rationale: Applying heat increases circulation, which facilitates healing. Cold packs result in vasoconstriction and decreased swelling. These interventions may alter the woman's perception of pain according to the gate control theory of pain modulation (Wilkinson and Treas, 2011). Analgesics alter a patient's perception of pain.*
- ■ Assess for decreased nerve sensation.
  - ■ *Rationale: Epidural or spinal anesthesia causes lack of sensation that may last several hours into the early postpartum period. Regional anesthesia may interfere with urinary elimination and mobility until the effects wear off.*
  - ■ *Expected assessment findings:*
    - ■ Full sensation of lower extremities for women who did not receive an epidural during labor
    - ■ Diminished lower body sensation for women who received an epidural during labor with full sensation returning within a few hours post-birth
  - ■ *Delay ambulation or assist the woman when ambulating until full sensation has returned.*
    - ■ Rationale: Women who have received spinal or epidural anesthesia are at risk for falls until full sensation has returned.
- ■ Assess for headache.
  - ■ *If the woman complains of headache, assess the location and quality of the headache (James, 2008).*
  - ■ *Notify the woman's health care provider if the headache is associated with signs and symptoms of preeclampsia, or if a post-epidural/spinal headache is suspected.*
    - ■ Rationale: Women who have had spinal or epidural anesthesia may develop headaches related to dural

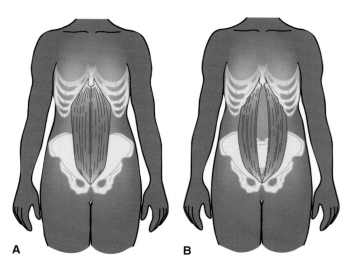

Figure 12–4 Diastasis recti abdominis. *A.* Normal location of rectus muscles of the abdomen. *B.* Diastasis recti. There is separation of the rectus muscles.

puncture, and subsequent leakage of cerebrospinal fluid (CSF) leading to decreased levels of CSF. Headaches related to epidural or spinal anesthesia tend to be worse when the patient is in an upright position and improved when the patient is lying down (Klein & Loder, 2010). Headache may also be associated with preeclampsia (Klein & Loder, 2010; James, 2008).

■ Assess for fatigue
  ■ *Rationale: Fatigue is a common complaint among women during the postpartum period. Discomfort, and lack of sleep related to infant care activities contribute to feelings of fatigue (James, 2008; Katz, 2012).*
■ Promote rest and sleep
  ■ *Provide teaching about the importance of sleep and rest.*
  ■ *Encourage the woman to sleep/nap while the baby is sleeping, and to prioritize activities, with a focus on self- and infant care.*
  ■ *Cluster nursing care such as assessments, interventions, and medication administration.*
    ■ Rationale: This minimizes disruptions to the woman's sleep/naps.
  ■ *Medicate the woman for pain as per orders and/or offer non-pharmacologic interventions if appropriate.*
    ■ Rationale: Pain interferes with sleep (Wilkinson & Treas, 2011).
■ Document findings and interventions.

Evidence-Based Practice: Maternal Fatigue

Kurth, E., Kennedy, H., Spichiger, E., Hosli, I., & Zemp Stutz, E. (2011). Crying babies, tired mothers: What do we know? A systematic review. *Midwifery, 27,* 187–94.

The purpose of this study was to synthesize evidence about the relationship between infant crying and maternal tiredness and fatigue during the first 3 months after birth. This study was a systematic review of both quantitative and qualitative studies published between 1980 and 2007. Initially 100 studies were retrieved, and 10 of the studies met specific criteria for the systematic review.

Results

■ The amount of infant crying during the first 3 months after birth is related to maternal tiredness and fatigue.
■ Infant crying disrupts the mother's circadian rhythm and decreases time for maternal rest.
■ Exhaustion decreases the mother's ability to concentrate, which leads to concerns about harming the baby. Fatigue may also trigger depressive symptoms and interfere with infant-parent interaction.

Recommendations

■ Teach parents soothing techniques, and how to cope with infant crying.
■ Give parents a realistic view of parenting an infant.
■ Help parents identify strategies to decrease maternal fatigue.

THE GASTROINTESTINAL SYSTEM

There is a decrease in gastrointestinal muscle tone and motility post-birth with a return to normal bowel function by the end of the second postpartum week.

■ Constipation
  ■ *Women are at risk for constipation due to:*
    ■ Decreased GI motility due to the effects of progesterone
    ■ Decreased physical activity
    ■ Dehydration and fluid loss from labor
    ■ Fear of having a bowel movement after perineal lacerations or episiotomy
    ■ Perineal pain and trauma
■ Hemorrhoids
  ■ *It is common for women to develop hemorrhoids during pregnancy and/or the birthing process.*
  ■ *Hemorrhoids will slowly resolve but can be painful.*
■ Appetite
  ■ *Women are hungry after the birthing experience and can be given a regular diet, unless they are on a prescribed diet such as for diabetes.*
  ■ *Women are exceptionally hungry during the first few postpartum days and may require snacks.*
■ Weight loss
  ■ *Most women will experience a significant weight loss during the first 2–3 weeks postpartum.*
  ■ *The average American woman at the end of 6 months postpartum is approximately 3–4 pounds above her pre-pregnancy weight (Olson et al., 2003).*

Nursing Actions

■ Assess bowel sounds at each shift.
  ■ *Notify the physician or midwife if bowel sounds are faint or absent.*
    ■ Rationale: Decreased motility can lead to diminished peristalsis and intestinal obstruction.
■ Assess for constipation.
  ■ *Ask the woman if and when she had a bowel movement.*
    ■ Rationale: Constipation is common in the postpartum period. Bowel function usually returns in 2-3 days after delivery (James, 2008). Decreased frequency of bowel movements and the passage of hard, dry stools indicate constipation (Wilkinson and Treas, 2011).
  ■ *Instruct the woman to increase fluid intake and increase fiber and roughage in diet to decrease risk of constipation.*
    ■ Rationale: A diet that includes fiber-rich foods (fruits, vegetables, whole grains, and legumes) promotes intestinal peristalsis. Adequate fluid intake is necessary when women are encouraged to increase dietary fiber to prevent constipation. Intake of 2,000-3,000 mL of fluids a day will soften bowel movements and provide adequate mucus to lubricate the colon (Whitmer, 2011; Wilkinson and Treas, 2011).
  ■ *Ask the woman what she did for constipation during pregnancy or in the past and implement these strategies.*

■ *Encourage ambulation.*
　■ Rationale: Ambulation promotes intestinal peristalsis and reduces the risk for constipation (Wilkinson and Treas, 2011).
■ *Administer a stool softener as per health care provider's orders.*
　■ Rationale: Stool softeners prevent constipation by increasing water in the stool, promoting stool softening and elimination (Vallerand & Sanoski, 2013).

Medication

Docusate (Colace)

- Indication: Prevention of constipation
- Action: Promotes incorporation of water into the stool
- Common side effects: Mild abdominal cramps, diarrhea
- Route and dose: PO; 100 mg twice a day
- Nursing actions/implications: Administer with a full glass of water or juice; do not administer within 2 hours of other laxatives, such as mineral oil.

(Data from Vallerand & Sanoski, 2013)

■ Assess for hemorrhoids.
　■ *Rationale: Hemorrhoids may increase in size during labor and cause discomfort in the postpartum period (James, 2008).*
　■ *Instruct the woman to lie on her side, then separate the buttocks to expose the anus.*
　■ *If hemorrhoids are present:*
　　■ Encourage the woman to avoid sitting for long periods of time by lying on her side.
　　■ Instruct the woman to take sitz baths.
　　　■ *Rationale: Sitz baths are helpful in promoting circulation and reducing pain.*
■ Assess appetite.
　■ *Assess the amount of food eaten during meals.*
　■ *Ask the woman if she is hungry.*
　　■ Rationale: In most cases, after a vaginal delivery women can resume eating a regular diet (James, 2008).
　■ *Ask the woman if she is nauseous or has vomited.*
　　■ Rationale: Nausea and vomiting may occur during labor. Additionally, nausea is a common side effect of opioid analgesics commonly used for pain management during labor and delivery (Wilkinson & Treas, 2011).
■ Patient education
　■ *Instruct the woman to increase fluid intake, and increase fiber and roughage in diet to decrease risk of constipation.*
　■ *Provide nutritional education. This is especially important for lactating women and women who had a cesarean bith.*
　■ *Encourage the woman to ambulate to increase GI motility and decrease risk of gas pains.*
　■ *Instruct the woman to increase fluid intake to a minimum of 8–10 glasses per day.*
■ Document findings and interventions.

CULTURAL AWARENESS: Food Preferences Across Cultures

- Foods and how they are prepared can be significant to women of different cultures.
- Ask women of different cultures if there are foods that they prefer to eat based on their cultural beliefs; if not available in the hospital, encourage patients to have family members bring them to the woman.
- Ask women of Japanese or Chinese cultures if they prefer hot water versus ice water at the bedside.
- In-service training should be provided to staff about cultures that are common to that unit.

DISCHARGE TEACHING

Discharge teaching for the woman and her partner focuses on:

■ Signs of complications that need to be reported to the physician or midwife:
　■ *Excessive lochia (saturating more than one pad in an hour); indicates possible secondary postpartum hemorrhage (Whitmer, 2011).*
　■ *The return of bright red, heavy bleeding after lochia has diminished or has become serosa or alba, or the passage of clots; indicates possible secondary postpartum hemorrhage.*
　■ *Foul smelling lochia; indicates possible infection.*
　■ *Increased temperature (100.4°F [38°C] or higher); indicates possible infection.*
　■ *Pelvic or abdominal tenderness/pain; indicates possible infection.*
　■ *Frequency, urgency, or burning on urination; indicates possible cystitis.*
　■ *Breasts tender, warm, and reddened; indicates possible mastitis (AWHONN, 2006).*
　■ *Blurry vision, severe headaches may be associated with preeclampsia.*
　■ *Leg pain may indicate venous thrombosis. Chest pain and difficulty breathing may be associated with pulmonary embolism.*
　■ *Thoughts of harming infant or self, and persistent feelings of depression and sadness, are associated with postpartum depression.*
■ Expected physical changes
　■ *Uterine involution, afterpains, progression of lochia*
　■ *Breast changes, engorgement*
　■ *Diaphoresis and diuresis*
　■ *Weight loss*
　　■ Women can expect to lose approximately 12 pounds immediately after delivery, and an additional 5-8 pounds due to fluid losses associated with uterine involution and diuresis (Mattson and Smith, 2011).
■ Self-care
　■ *Hygiene*
　■ *Perineal care*
　■ *Breast care for lactating and non-lactating women*
　■ *Pharmacologic and non-pharmacologic pain control measures*

- Health promotion
  - *Nutrition and fluids*
    - Instruct the woman about nutritional needs for lactating and nonlactating women.
      - *Lactating women should increase their caloric intake by 500 calories per day and have a fluid intake of approximately 2 liters per day.*
      - *Teach the woman how to use "MyPlate" (www. ChooseMyPlate.gov) and how this can assist the woman in meeting her nutritional needs (**Fig.12-5**).*
  - *Smoking cessation and relapse prevention*
    - A goal of Healthy People 2020 is to reduce postpartum relapse of smoking among women who quit during pregnancy (Healthy People 2020).
    - Ask women about tobacco use.
    - Teach women about the dangers of smoking (cancer, lung problems such as chronic obstructive pulmonary disease, osteoporosis).
    - Teach women to never allow smoking around their infant/children as secondhand smoke is associated with problems such as ear infections and respiratory problems.
    - Encourage women who quit smoking for pregnancy to remain abstinent.
      - *The majority of women who quit smoking during pregnancy relapse after delivery.*
    - Advise all women who currently smoke to quit. Provide information about resources to assist with cessation, such as counseling services/classes, cessation help lines, and medications.

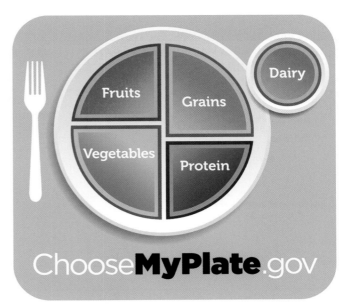

Figure 12–5 MyPlate illustrates the five food groups using a familiar mealtime visual, a place setting. Source: United States Department of Agriculture, www.ChooseMyPlate.gov.

AWHONN POSITION STATEMENT

Smoking and Women's Health
"Women and girls should not initiate smoking cigarettes, and current smokers should pursue smoking cessation. There is no known level of smoking that is considered a safe consumption level. Health care professionals should educate all women about the risks of cigarette smoking and secondhand smoke, screen women for tobacco use, and support smoking cessation efforts. Focusing attention on these efforts before, during, and after pregnancy is also critically important because of the harmful effects of smoking and exposure to secondhand smoke on the fetus and newborn."

Association of Women's Health, Obstetric and Neonatal Nurses (AWHONN). (2010b). Smoking and women's health. *Journal of Obstetric, Gynecologic, & Neonatal Nurses, 39,* 611-613.

- *Activity and exercise*
  - Explain the importance of activity to decrease risk of constipation and to promote circulation and a sense of well-being.
  - Instruct the woman about appropriate exercises in the postpartum, such as walking.
- *Rest and comfort*
  - Teach the woman the importance of rest in promoting healing and lactation.
  - Problem-solve with the woman ways to increase rest time (e.g., nap when the baby is napping, prioritizing activities).
  - Encourage the woman to take pain medication as ordered by the physician or midwife.

- *Routine health check-ups*
  - Stress the importance of following through with follow-up visits to her physician or midwife.
- Contraception
  - *Assess the couple's desire for future pregnancies.*
  - *Assess satisfaction with previous method of contraception.*
  - *Encourage the patient to discuss contraceptive options with the health care provider.*
  - *Provide information on various methods of contraception (**Table 12-3**).*

AWHONN POSITION STATEMENT

Insurance Coverage for Contraceptives
"AWHONN supports legislation and policies that mandate insurance coverage for the range of U.S. Food and Drug Administration-approved contraceptive drugs and devices, as well as related services. AWHONN considers access to affordable and acceptable health care, which includes safe and reliable contraceptives, a basic human right."

Association of Women's Health, Obstetric and Neonatal Nurses (AWHONN). (2010a). Insurance coverage for contraception. *Journal of Obstetric, Gynecologic, & Neonatal Nurses, 38,* 743-744.

- Sexual activity
  - *Instruct the couple to discuss with the physician or midwife when they can resume sexual intercourse.*
    - General guidelines are to resume sexual intercourse when the lochia has stopped, perineum has healed, and the woman is physically and emotionally ready.

TABLE 12–3   METHODS OF CONTRACEPTION

METHOD	FAILURE RATE	AVAILABILITY	ADVANTAGES	DISADVANTAGES
NATURAL METHOD				
Abstinence	0%	Handouts and information from care provider	Readily available	Must have knowledge and be willing to frequently monitor body functions: temperature, vaginal mucus production and consistency
Natural family planning	24%		Personal	
Withdrawal	22 %	Internet access of information	No cost	
Lactational amenorrhea method (LAM)			No cost	Requires *exclusive* breastfeeding/infant suckling
				Using a barrier method with LAM increases effectiveness
BARRIER METHODS				
Condoms (male and female)	18%–21%	OTC purchase	Readily available	Allergic reactions
				Barrier methods have higher rate of protection when combined with spermicides.
Vaginal sponges	12% if no prior births	OTC available	One-time use	
	24% if previous births	Most have spermicide added	May be placed before intercourse	
			May leave in for up to 30 hours	
			Protects repeated acts of IC	
Cervical caps	9.5% no prior birth	Prescription	Fits snugly over cervix	Must be left in place for at least 6 hours post-intercourse (IC)
	20.5% women with prior birth	Must be fitted by provider	Can remain in place >24 hours for repeated IC	Irritation and allergic reaction
		If birth or large weight change, needs to be refitted		May be difficult to insert and remove
Diaphragms	12%	Prescription, must be fitted after birth, large change in weight	Fits over cervix	Need additional doses of spermicide for repeated IC
			Can remain in place >24 hours for repeated IC	May be difficult to insert and remove
				Irritation
				Allergic reaction
Spermicidal gels, cream suppository, or foam	28%	OTC	Readily available	Irritation
			Use at time of IC	Allergic reaction
HORMONAL METHODS				
Combination estrogen/ progesterone oral contraception	9%	Prescription only	Suppresses ovulation	May have multiple side effects (nausea, headache, spotting weight gain, breast tenderness, chloasma).
		91-day option available; 12-week pill cycle with menses only 4 times per year	Take one pill a day.	

TABLE 12–3   METHODS OF CONTRACEPTION—cont'd

METHOD	FAILURE RATE	AVAILABILITY	ADVANTAGES	DISADVANTAGES
Emergency contraceptives (Not to be used as regular form of birth control)	20%	Postcoital ingestion of hormones Must take within 72 hours of incident OTC for women aged >17 years old. Prescription only for women less than 17 years old.	Reduces risk of pregnancy for one-time unprotected IC	Increased risks for blood clots, heart disease, and strokes Due to high dose of hormones, may have headache, nausea, vomiting, or abdominal pain
Progestin only	6%	Prescription only	Take one pill at same time every day. Can be used during lactation	Irregular bleeding Weight gain
Depo-Provera	3%	Injectable every 3 months	One injection 4 times a year, can be used during breastfeeding once lactation is established.	Irregular bleeding Weight gain, decreased bone density
Contraceptive patch	9%	Prescription only	Place patch for 3 weeks, then remove for one week	Risk same as for oral contraceptives Possibly less effective for larger women Possible skin irritation
Vaginal ring	9%	Prescription only	Flexible hormone-filled ring inserted and left in the vagina for 3 weeks, then removed for 1 week	Side effects similar to oral contraceptives Vaginal irritation and discharge If ring falls out, need to use alternative protection for at least 1 week
LONG ACTING REVERSIBLE CONTRACEPTIVES Intrauterine contraceptives (IUCs) Copper material or hormone releasing	0.8%	Prescription Office procedure to insert	Long-term contraceptive method; good for 1–10 years Copper-releasing IUCs can be used as emergency contraceptive; must be inserted within 5 days of intercourse.	Risk of uterine perforation Risk of pelvic inflammatory disease (PID) Increase of cramping and bleeding in the first few cycles
Hormone implants	>0.5%	One rod implanted in the arm Office procedure	Once in place, there is minimal discomfort Last for several years Can be used with lactation	Side effects similar to oral contraceptives Skin irritation at site Must be removed

Continued

TABLE 12–3   METHODS OF CONTRACEPTION—cont'd

METHOD	FAILURE RATE	AVAILABILITY	ADVANTAGES	DISADVANTAGES
STERILIZATION				
Vasectomy	0.15%–1%	Surgical procedure done under local anesthesia in the office or clinic	Discomfort for 2–3 days Difficult to reverse High rate of effectiveness	Discomfort for 2–3 days Difficult to reverse Need to use alternative contraceptive method until two post-surgery sperm tests indicate procedure is effective.
Tubal ligation	0.5%	Surgical procedure done under general anesthesia	High rate of effectiveness	Bleeding or pain at incision site Difficult to reverse
Sterilization implant	0.5%–1%	Office procedure	Metallic implants placed in the fallopian tubes, which causes scar tissue that eventually block the tubes.	Another contraceptive method needs to be used until blockage is confirmed, usually 3 months.

■ *Explain that an artificial vaginal lubricant might be needed to increase comfort during intercourse due to changes in hormone levels that result in vaginal dryness.*
■ *Explain the importance of using contraception when the couple resumes sexual activity.*

■ Prescribed medications
  ■ *Explain all discharge medications, including dose, frequency, action, and side effects.*

Evidence-Based Practice: Discharge Teaching Methods

Wagner, D. L., Bear, M., & Davidson, N. (2011). Measuring patient satisfaction with postpartum teaching methods used by nurses within the interaction model of client health behaviors. *Research and Theory for Nursing Practice, 25,* 176–190.

The purpose of this study was to determine the relationship between new mothers' interaction with the nurse using different teaching methods. The design of this study was quasi-experimental with two study groups to examine patient satisfaction with different teaching methods used to deliver postpartum discharge teaching. Thirty-five women were assigned to each group. The first group received traditional discharge teaching. This consisted of verbal teaching using a discharge teaching form designed by the hospital as a guide. The teaching included information on self-care, infant care, safety, vaccine schedules, and follow up. The patients also received a New Mom's Handbook. The second group received the traditional discharge teaching and demonstration, and return demonstration on selected self-care and infant care skills. The patients were allowed a 30-minute time period during which they performed returned demonstration on selected skills. A client satisfaction instrument was used to measure the participants' satisfaction with the postpartum teaching method received.

Results

■ Satisfaction with both methods of postpartum teaching was high.
■ There was no difference in client satisfaction scores between groups.
■ Recommendations
■ Traditional methods of teaching postpartum discharge information (verbal instruction, providing written materials) as well as demonstration/return demonstration methods of teaching should be used to prepare patients for discharge.

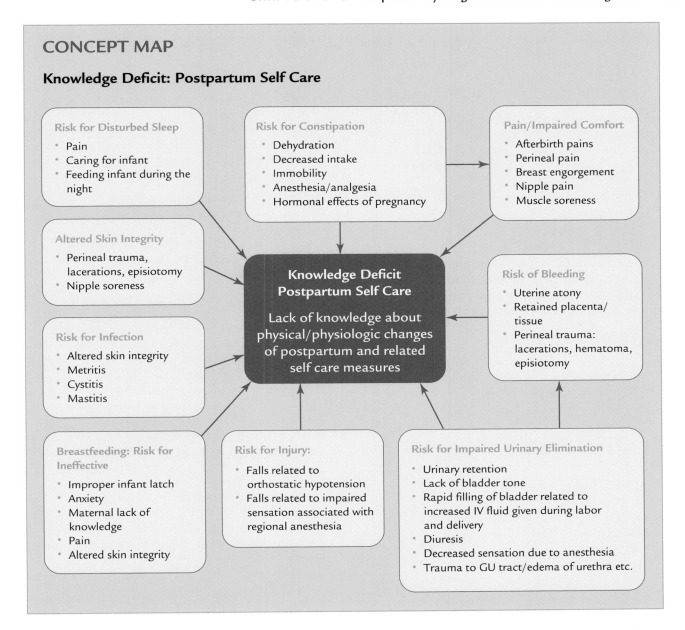

CONCEPT MAP

Knowledge Deficit: Postpartum Self Care

Risk for Disturbed Sleep
- Pain
- Caring for infant
- Feeding infant during the night

Altered Skin Integrity
- Perineal trauma, lacerations, episiotomy
- Nipple soreness

Risk for Infection
- Altered skin integrity
- Metritis
- Cystitis
- Mastitis

Breastfeeding: Risk for Ineffective
- Improper infant latch
- Anxiety
- Maternal lack of knowledge
- Pain
- Altered skin integrity

Risk for Constipation
- Dehydration
- Decreased intake
- Immobility
- Anesthesia/analgesia
- Hormonal effects of pregnancy

Risk for Injury:
- Falls related to orthostatic hypotension
- Falls related to impaired sensation associated with regional anesthesia

Pain/Impaired Comfort
- Afterbirth pains
- Perineal pain
- Breast engorgement
- Nipple pain
- Muscle soreness

Risk of Bleeding
- Uterine atony
- Retained placenta/tissue
- Perineal trauma: lacerations, hematoma, episiotomy

Risk for Impaired Urinary Elimination
- Urinary retention
- Lack of bladder tone
- Rapid filling of bladder related to increased IV fluid given during labor and delivery
- Diuresis
- Decreased sensation due to anesthesia
- Trauma to GU tract/edema of urethra etc.

Knowledge Deficit Postpartum Self Care

Lack of knowledge about physical/physiologic changes of postpartum and related self care measures

---

Problem No. 1: Risk for bleeding

Goal: The amount of vaginal bleeding will be within normal limits.

Outcome: The woman's lochia amount will be moderate to small; the woman's fundus is firm and midline. The woman's vital signs will be within normal limits. Urine output will be within normal limits. The woman will verbalize when she will notify the provider if her bleeding is excessive.

Nursing Actions

1. Teach the woman the purpose of fundal checks.
2. Teach the woman to palpate her fundus and massage it if soft.
3. Teach the woman about the normal progression of lochia; what to expect in regards to amount, color, and flow.
4. Instruct the woman to notify the nurse or provider if she soaks more than one pad an hour or passes clots.
5. Instruct the woman about the purpose of Pitocin administration; provide information about afterpains.
6. Teach the woman the importance of emptying her bladder every 3–4 hours.

Problem No. 2: Risk for impaired urinary elimination

Goal: Spontaneous voids of a sufficient quantity (at least 150 mL per void)

Outcome: The woman will spontaneously void at least 150 ml per void. The woman will state the importance of voiding frequently and adequately. The woman will identify that she will notify the nurse or provider of burning, frequency, or urgency with voiding.

Nursing Actions

1. Explain to the woman that voidings will be measured during the first 24 hours after delivery.
2. Encourage the woman to voidings within 6 hours after delivery.
3. Explain to the woman that if she is unable to void, she will need to have a catheter placed to empty her bladder.
4. Instruct the woman to notify the nurse or health care provider if she experiences frequency, burning, or urgency during urination.
5. Encourage the woman to drink 8–10 glasses of fluids a day.
6. Teach the woman that diuresis is a normal process and often begins within 12 hours of delivery.

Problem No. 3: Pain/Impaired Comfort
Goal: Pain or discomfort is adequately controlled.
Outcome: The woman will identify pharmacological and non-pharmacological methods to treat pain and discomfort. The woman's pain/discomfort is adequately controlled.

Nursing Actions

1. Teach the woman to report pain by providing information about the intensity, location, and quality of her discomfort.
2. Teach the woman about medications ordered and administered for pain (action, dose and frequency, potential side effects).
3. Teach the woman about non-pharmacological methods of pain control:
   a. Ice packs
   b. Sitz baths/warm compresses
   c. Peri-bottle
   d. Repositioning
   e. Deep breathing and relaxation
   f. Warm shower

Problem No. 4: Risk for infection
Goal: Reduce risk of infection.
Outcome: The woman will remain free from signs of infection. The woman will identify ways to prevent infection and when to call the nurse or health care provider for signs of infection.

Nursing Actions

1. Explain the importance of monitoring vital signs.
2. Instruct the woman to call the provider if she has signs of infection such as temperature over 100.4°F, chills, pain in her abdomen, perineum, or breasts; burning, frequency or urgency with urination; foul smelling lochia.
3. Teach the woman the importance of hand washing before and after peri-care, and pad changes.
4. If indicated, teach the woman about immunizations that will be given prior to discharge.

Problem No. 5: Risk for injury
Goal: Reduced risk for injury
Outcome: The woman will call for assistance with ambulation until sensation returns to her lower extremities (post-epidural)

and her blood pressure and pulse are within normal limits. The woman will remain free from injury associated with falls.

Nursing Actions

1. Explain orthostatic hypotension and the importance of requesting assistance in the initial postpartum period.
2. Instruct the woman to rise slowly to a standing position.
3. Advise the woman to ambulate with assistance.
4. Instruct the woman to return to bed/sitting position if she becomes dizzy.

Problem No. 6: Altered skin integrity
Goal: Regain skin integrity through healing
Outcome: The woman will identify perineal care and comfort measures. The woman will identify signs of perineal infection and will notify her health care provider if she experiences signs of infection.

Nursing Actions

1. Teach the woman that her perineal area will be assessed for redness, bruising, swelling, and drainage. Explain the procedure and position the woman on her side for better visualization of the area.
2. Teach the woman about comfort measures for perineal lacerations/episiotomy such as ice packs during the first 24 hours and warm sitz baths after the first 24 hours.
3. Instruct the woman on how to use topical treatments that may be ordered by the health care provider.
4. Teach the woman to rinse the perineum with the peri-bottle using warm water after each elimination.
5. Encourage the woman to change peri-pads frequently, and to wash her hands before and after pad changes to reduce risk of infection.
6. Teach the woman to lie on her side to decrease pressure on her perineum.
7. Instruct the woman to take ordered analgesics as directed to decrease perineal pain.
8. Teach the woman to report signs of perineal infection such as drainage, swelling, pain, and fever to the health care provider.

Problem No. 7: Risk for constipation
Goal: The woman will have regular, soft bowel movements.
Outcome: The woman will state ways to promote regular, soft bowel movements. The woman will not develop constipation.

Nursing Actions

1. Teach the woman the importance a diet high in fruits, vegetables, and whole grains.
2. Teach the woman the importance of drinking 2,000–3,000 ml of fluids daily.
3. Teach the woman the importance of ambulating several times daily.
4. Instruct the woman to have a bowel movement when she feels the urge.

5. If ordered, teach the woman about stool softeners, laxatives, etc. Discuss the action, dose and frequency, and potential side effects.

Problem No. 8: Risk for disturbed sleep
Goal: Adequate sleep and rest
Outcome: The woman will be report adequate sleep patterns, and report feeling rested. The woman will identify strategies for getting enough rest and sleep.

Nursing Actions

1. Teach the woman the importance of sleep and rest in healing and recovery from childbirth.
2. Encourage the woman to identify strategies for getting enough sleep, such as sleeping when the baby sleeps and naps, prioritizing activities to focus on self- and infant care, and occasionally delegating infant care and feeding to other family members if possible so that she can rest.
3. Teach the woman ways to treat pain and discomfort to facilitate rest and sleep.

Problem No. 9: Breastfeeding: Risk for Ineffective
Goal: Effective breastfeeding
Outcome: The woman will identify how to tell if the baby is breastfeeding effectively. The woman will demonstrate proper positioning and technique for breastfeeding her infant. The baby will latch to the mother's nipple properly and demonstrate signs of adequate feedings. The woman will identify community resources to contact for support and assistance with breastfeeding.

Nursing Actions

1. Teach the woman to recognize cues that the baby is hungry.
2. Teach the woman to prepare for a feeding by getting into a comfortable position.
3. Teach the woman infant positioning for breastfeeding (cradle hold, cross cradle hold, football hold, etc.).
4. Teach the woman how to properly get the infant latched to the nipple, and signs of correct latch on.
5. Teach the woman about the frequency and duration of feedings.
6. Teach the woman how to remove the baby from the breast and how to burp the baby.
7. Teach the woman how to recognize that the baby is receiving adequate feedings.
8. Provide the woman with information about lactation consultant services, and community resources available to support breastfeeding after discharge.

Clinical Pathway for Uncomplicated Vaginal Delivery

Focus of Care	Postpartum: Admission	Postpartum: First 4 hours	Postpartum: Greater than 4 hours → discharge	Expected Outcomes/ Discharge Criteria
Diagnostic Tests	RPR, HBSag, rubella, blood type and Rh status documented or drawn if no prenatal record available GBS status documented with appropriate interventions Urine toxicology screening as per policy	Fetal Rh study as indicated (woman Rh-negative and neonate Rh-positive)	Hemogram as ordered Notify CNM/MD of abnormal results or if the woman is symptomatic.	Rubella status known and MMR vaccine given if indicated Rh status known—Rh₀ immune globulin given if indicated Hemogram within normal ranges Needed vaccinations are given as ordered (flu shots, Tdap, varicella etc.).
Activity and Safety	Moves legs Lifts bottom off bed Needs assistance with initial ambulation Infant security and safety reviewed	Women who received an epidural for labor and/or birth will need assistance with ambulation until return of sensory and motor sensation.	Able to stand and walk with minimal assistance	Ambulates without assistance

Continued

Clinical Pathway for Uncomplicated Vaginal Delivery—cont'd

Focus of Care	Postpartum: Admission	Postpartum: First 4 hours	Postpartum: Greater than 4 hours → discharge	Expected Outcomes/ Discharge Criteria
Treatments and Patient Care	Assess vital signs Assess level of consciousness Assess fundus, lochia, and perineum Ice to perineum Assess lower extremities for edema, pain, pulses Assess Foley catheter if in place Assess IV site and fluids if in place Assess breast for potential breastfeeding problems	Vital signs as per orders Postpartum physical assessment as per orders/unit protocol Peri care with each voiding Ice to perineum Input and output while Foley catheter or IV in place Measure first 2 voidings; notify CNM/MD if urine output <30 mL/hr	Vital signs as per orders Postpartum physical assessment as per orders Peri care with each voiding Ice to perineum for first 24 hours Assess breast for signs of engorgement and nipple irritation	Vital signs stable and within normal limits Fundus firm, midline, and descending by 1 cm per day Lochia moderate to scant Perineum healing without signs of infection Breasts exhibit physiological changes of lactation. Breastfeeding without difficulty Bowel and bladder function within normal limits
Medications	Maintain IV patency if indicated. Oxytocin as indicated to reduce risk of or treat postpartum hemorrhage Analgesics and/or comfort measure as indicated for pain management	IV discontinued if fundus firm and lochia within normal limits Oxytocin discontinued if fundus firm and lochia within normal limits Analgesics and/or comfort measures as indicated for pain management	Analgesics and/or comfort measure as indicated for pain management Rubella vaccine administered, if indicated, at least 30 minutes before discharge $Rh_o(D)$ immune globulin administered as indicated Stool softener as ordered	Mild to moderate pain relieved with comfort measures and/or PO analgesia Rubella vaccine administered when indicated $Rh_o(D)$ immune globulin administered as indicated Discharge medication teaching provided
Nutrition	Regular diet as tolerated PO fluids	Regular diet as tolerated PO fluids	Regular diet as tolerated PO fluids	Maintains adequate diet and fluid intake
Discharge Planning/ Evaluation of Social Support	Evaluate need for referrals such as social worker, lactation specialist, and dietitian. Explain physical changes. Teach self-care and health promotion.	Continue to evaluate need for referrals. Initiate referrals as indicated. Explain physical changes. Teach self-care and health promotion.	Review discharge preparation with the woman and her family. Explain physical and emotional changes. Teach self-care and health promotion.	The woman and her family have appropriate support on discharge. The woman can provide appropriate self-care. The woman and her family verbalize the importance of follow-up care for both the woman and infant.

Clinical Pathway for Uncomplicated Vaginal Delivery—cont'd

Focus of Care	Postpartum: Admission	Postpartum: First 4 hours	Postpartum: Greater than 4 hours → discharge	Expected Outcomes/ Discharge Criteria
Patient/Family Education	Initiate discharge teaching by assessing immediate learning needs. Assist with breastfeeding.	Continue discharge teaching based on the woman's/family's learning needs.	Complete discharge teaching.	The woman and her family verbalize understanding of infant needs and the woman's needs. The woman and her family demonstrate basic well baby care skills. The woman and her family verbalize understanding of signs and symptoms that warrant contact with the health care provider.

Nursing Care Plan

Problem (Check appropriate line)	Actual or Potential	Action (Initial care provided)	Expected Outcome/ Discharge Criteria (Initial outcomes obtained)
Potential or actual postpartum hemorrhage related to: _____ Uterine atony _____ Retained placenta _____ Laceration _____ Hematoma _____ Full bladder _____ Other _____	Initiated by: RN: _____ Date/Time _____ ☐ Actual ☐ Potential Change in status Date/Time _____ RN: _____ ☐ Actual ☐ Potential Resolved: Date/Time _____ RN: _____	_____ Monitor and assess vital signs including blood pressure and woman's mental status, lochia flow, and uterine tone per policy. _____ Encourage voiding every 2–3 hours. _____ Massage fundus as needed and instruct the woman on self-assessment. _____ Notify CNM/MD for heavy bleeding/ saturation of one pad in <1 hour. _____ Give medications such as oxytocin, Methergine, or Hemabate per CNM/MD order. _____ Assist with activity PRN. _____ Notify the provider if the woman has continued excessive bleeding and/or dizziness.	_____ Lochia scant to moderate rubra _____ Fundus firm and at midline _____ No signs or symptoms of postpartum hemorrhage

Continued

Nursing Care Plan—cont'd

Problem (Check appropriate line)	Actual or Potential	Action (Initial care provided)	Expected Outcome/ Discharge Criteria (Initial outcomes obtained)
Potential or actual alteration in comfort related to: _____ Uterine cramping _____ Incision _____ Perineal/rectal pain _____ Breast discomfort _____ Other _____ Potential or actual alteration in effective breastfeeding related to: Poor latch Previous breast surgery Twins or higher order multiples Infant with cleft lip/palate Nearly term infant _____ Infant in NICU _____ Patient's health status _____ Other _____ Potential or actual impaired parent–infant bonding related to: _____ Adolescent parents _____ Substance abuse _____ Domestic violence _____ Social risk factors _____ Infant's health status _____ Mother's health status _____ Other _____	Initiated by: RN: _____ Date/Time _____ ☐ Actual ☐ Potential Change in status Date/Time _____ RN: _____ ☐ Actual ☐ Potential Resolved: Date/Time _____ RN: _____	_____ Pain assessment _____ Provide or assist with nonpharmacological comfort measures for relief. _____ Provide analgesics as ordered.	_____ Pain will be adequately controlled by analgesics and nonpharmacological comfort measures.

Nursing Care Plan—cont'd

Problem (Check appropriate line)	Actual or Potential	Action (Initial care provided)	Expected Outcome/ Discharge Criteria (Initial outcomes obtained)
Potential or actual postpartum infection related to: _____ Perineum _____ Uterus _____ Breast _____ GBS _____ Other _____	Initiated by: _____ Date/Time _____ ☐ Actual ☐ Potential Change in status Date/Time _____ RN: _____ ☐ Actual ☐ Potential Resolved: Date/Time _____ RN: _____	_____ Vital signs monitored per policy _____ CNM/MD notified immediately if any signs or symptoms of infection are present _____ Woman instructed in self-care including peri care, incisional care, and breast care _____ Woman instructed in signs and symptoms of infection	_____ Woman will exhibit no signs or symptoms of infection (i.e., temperature <100.4°F (38°C), no abnormal discharge, incision clean and dry if present, breasts without redness) _____ Woman will verbalize understanding of signs and symptoms of infection and aware of when to notify CNM/MD.
Potential or actual alteration in elimination related to: _____ Loss of bladder and/or bowel sensation/function following childbirth _____ Other _____	Initiated by: _____ Date/Time _____ ☐ Actual ☐ Potential Change in status Date/Time _____ RN: _____ ☐ Actual ☐ Potential Resolved: Date/Time _____ RN: _____	_____ Assess and monitor for bladder distention as needed. _____ Assess and document initial voidings after delivery to ensure >30 mL/hr without retention in first 6–12 hours. _____ If unable to void catheterize per CNM/MD order. _____ Provide instructions on Kegel exercises. _____ Encourage early ambulation, adequate fluid intake, diet with roughage to prevent constipation. _____ Provide stool softener as ordered.	_____ Woman is voiding without difficulty. _____ Fundus is firm and midline. _____ Woman is able to verbalize methods of avoiding constipation and to notify CNM/MD if no stool in 4 days.

TYING IT ALL TOGETHER

As the nurse, you admit Margarite Sanchez to the postpartum unit at 1050 and receive the transfer report from Labor and Delivery stating the following:

■ Patient is a 28-year-old G3 P2 Hispanic woman who gave birth at 0839, vaginal delivery with a second-degree laceration.
■ She received two doses of Nubain in labor at 0215 and 0440 for pain relief in active labor.
■ Both mother and baby are stable.
■ The mother's bleeding in labor and delivery was moderate.
■ V.S. 120/68-72-20-98.2
■ Ms. Sanchez did not void in labor and delivery.
■ Ms. Sanchez nursed her baby for 15 minutes on each breast after the birth.

José, her husband, has accompanied her to the unit.

Detail the aspects of your initial assessment.

As part of the physical assessment you discover her fundus is 2 cm above the umbilicus and deviated to the left, her lochia is moderate, saturating one third of the pad during transfer, and her perineum is swollen.

What are your immediate priorities in nursing care for Margarite Sanchez? Discuss the rationale for the priorities.
Initial teaching would include the following:

At 5 hours postpartum Margarite rates her perineal pain at 6 on a scale of 0–10.

State the nursing diagnosis, expected outcome, and interventions related to this problem.

The next day you are assigned to care for the Sanchez family. Your report from the previous shift indicated that:

■ Her vital signs were within normal limits.
■ She had voided once during the night.
■ Her fundus was 1 cm below the umbilicus.
■ Lochia was scant to moderate.
■ She breastfed her infant twice.

Margarite informs you that she experienced night sweats.

Discuss your nursing actions including rationales.

You are anticipating that she will be discharged in the afternoon.

Discuss your plan for discharge teaching indicating the priority needs with rationales.

■ ■ ■ Review Questions ■ ■ ■

1. Your patient, who gave birth to a 7-pound baby boy 24 hours ago, is complaining of uterine cramping (afterpains). This is her second baby and she is breastfeeding. Your assessment reveals a firm fundus at midline at 1 cm below the umbilicus. Select all of your initial nursing actions.
   A. Instruct the patient to bottle-feed for 36 hours or until the cramping has stopped.
   B. Place a warm blanket on her abdomen.
   C. Explain that these are normal for second-time mothers to experience.
   D. Offer the patient acetaminophen with codeine so she can continue to breastfeed.

2. Your patient gave birth to a 6-pound baby girl 6 hours ago. It was a spontaneous delivery. You note on your assessment of her perineum that there is some edema and slight bruising. She stated that her pain was at 1 on the pain scale. Your nursing action would be to:
   A. Continue applying ice to the perineum.
   B. Assist her with a sitz bath.
   C. Encourage her to keep her bladder empty.
   D. Administer ibuprofen 800 mg.

3. To decrease the risk of orthostatic hypotension during the first few hours after the birth, the nurse should:
   A. Assist the patient to the bathroom by using a wheelchair.
   B. Break open an ammonia ampule and have the patient take a deep breath before getting up.
   C. Have the patient sit on the side of the bed for a few minutes before standing.
   D. Check the patient blood pressure before assisting her to the bathroom.

4. Select the statements that are true regarding primary engorgement.
   A. Only women who are lactating will experience primary engorgement.
   B. It is caused by an increase in the vascular and lymphatic system of the breast.
   C. The breasts become large, firm, and warm to touch.
   D. It subsides within 24–36 hours.

5. During your discharge teaching, you are evaluating if your patient needs information on contraception. Select the responses that indicate she needs additional information.
   A. "I will be breastfeeding for the next 6 months. We will start using a condom after I have my first period."
   B. "My husband is getting a vasectomy. We will be using condoms until his second semen analysis is negative for sperm."
   C. "I plan to have an IUD. We will be using condoms until I get an IUD."
   D. "I used a diaphragm prior to this pregnancy and plan to use my old one."

6. The nurse is preparing a woman in the early postpartum period for a fundal check. Select all appropriate nursing actions:
   A. Provide for privacy.
   B. Position the woman in high Fowler's position.
   C. Have the patient empty her bladder.
   D. Position the patient in the supine position.

7. A nurse is providing discharge teaching to a postpartum patient who is bottle feeding. The patient asks the nurse when she should expect to have her period return. The nurse's best response is:
   A. "You can expect to have your period in 3–4 weeks."
   B. "Many women who choose not to breastfeed will have a period in 7–9 weeks after childbirth."
   C. "Your period will return at about 6 months post-delivery."
   D. "Bottle feeding suppresses ovulation, so as long as you bottle feed, you will not have a period."

8. A patient who delivered 20 hours ago reports a transient increase in her lochia when she ambulated to the bathroom to void this morning after sleeping for a few hours. The nurse performs an assessment and documents scant rubra, lochia with no clots, fundus firm 1 cm below the umbilicus. Which of the following nursing actions are appropriate at this time?
   A. Report this finding to the patient's health care provider immediately.
   B. Begin weighing and counting pads.
   C. Reassure the patient that this is normal.
   D. Obtain a physician's order to administer oxytocin.

9. The nurse assists a patient who delivered vaginally 6 hours ago to the bathroom to void for the first time since delivery. The patient voids 65 mL of urine. The nurse's initial action is to:
   A. Document this as a normal finding.
   B. Encourage the patient to try to void again within the next 4–6 hours.
   C. Insert an indwelling Foley catheter.
   D. Palpate for bladder distention.

10. A patient who delivered vaginally and has a third-degree laceration is being prepared for discharge. Which of the following instructions should the nurse include in her discharge teaching? Select all that apply.
   A. Drink at least 2 liters of fluid a day.
   B. Ambulate several times a day.
   C. Eat plenty of whole grain foods, and fruits and vegetables.
   D. Use suppositories to help promote regular, soft bowel movements.

References

American College of Obstetrics and Gynecology (ACOG). (2012). *Committee opinion: Update on immunization and pregnancy: Tetanus, diphtheria, and pertussis vaccination.* Retrieved from www.acog.org/Resources_And_Publications/Committee_Opinion/Committee_on_obstetric practice/UpdateonImmunization

Association of Women's Health, Obstetric and Neonatal Nurses (AWHONN). (2006). *The compendium of postpartum care.* Washington, DC: Author.

Association of Women's Health, Obstetric and Neonatal Nurses (AWHONN). (2010a). Insurance coverage for contraception. *Journal of Obstetric, Gynecologic, & Neonatal Nurses, 38,* 743–744.

Association of Women's Health, Obstetric and Neonatal Nurses (AWHONN). (2010b). Smoking and women's health. *Journal of Obstetric, Gynecologic, & Neonatal Nurses, 39,* 611–613.

Balkam, J. (2010). Painful breast lumps in nursing mothers. *American Journal of Nursing, 110,* 65–67.

Centers for Disease Control. (2011). General recommendations of the advisory committee on immunization practices. *MMWR, 60,* 1–60. Retrieved from www.cdc.gov/mmwr/preview/mmwrhtml/rr6002a1.htm?s_cid=rr6002a1_e

James, D. (2008). Postpartum care. In K. Simpson & P. Creehan (Eds.), *AWHONN: Perinatal nursing* (3rd ed). Philadelphia: Lippincott, Williams & Wilkins.

Katz, V. (2012). Postpartum care. In S. Gabbe et al. (Eds.), *Obstetrics: Normal and Problem Pregnancies* (6th ed) Philadelphia: Saunders, Elsevier.

Kee, J. (2009). Laboratory and diagnostic tests with nursing implications (6th ed.). Upper Saddle River, NJ: Pearson.

Kennedy, K., & Trussell, J. (2011). Postpartum contraception and lactation. In R. Hatcher et al., (Eds.), *Contraceptive technology* (20th ed.). Montvale, NJ: PDR Network.

Klein, A., & Loder, E. (2010). Postpartum headache. *International Journal of Obstetric Anesthesia, 19,* 422–430.

Kurth, E., Kennedy, H., Spichiger, E., Hosli, I., & Zemp Stutz, E. (2011). Crying babies, tired mothers: What do we know? A systematic review. *Midwifery, 27,* 187–94.

Mass, S. (2004). Breast pain: Engorgement, nipple pain, and mastitis. *Clinical Obstetrics and Gynecology, 47,* 676–682.

Olson, C., Strawderman, M., Hinton, P., & Pearson, T. (2003). Gestational weight gain and postpartum behaviors associated with change from early pregnancy to 1 year postpartum. *International Journal of Obesity, 27,* 7–127.

U.S. Department of Health and Human Services Office of Disease Prevention and Health Promotion. (2012). Healthy people 2020 topics and objectives. Retrieved from www.Healthypeople.gov/2020/topicsobjectives2020/objectives

Vallerand, A., and Sanoski, C. (2013). *Davis's drug guide for nurses* (13th ed.). Philadelphia: F.A. Davis.

Wagner, D., Bear, M., & Davidson, N. (2011). Measuring patient satisfaction with postpartum teaching methods used by nurses within the interaction model of client health behaviors. *Research and Theory for Nursing Practice, 25,* 176–190.

Whitmer, T. (2011). Physical and psychological changes. In S. Mattson & J. Smith (Eds.), *Core curriculum for maternal-newborn nursing* (4th ed). St. Louis, MO: Elsevier.

Wilkinson, J., & Treas, L. S. (2011). *Fundamentals in nursing* (2nd ed). Philadelphia: F.A. Davis.

Transition to Parenthood

13

EXPECTED STUDENT OUTCOMES

On completion of this chapter, the student will be able to:

- [ ] Define key terms.
- [ ] Describe the process of "becoming a mother."
- [ ] Identify factors that influence women and men in their role transitions to mother or father.
- [ ] Discuss bonding and attachment.
- [ ] Identify factors that affect the family dynamics.
- [ ] Describe nursing actions that support couples during their transition to parenthood.

Nursing Diagnoses

- Knowledge deficit related to role of parent due to being a first-time parent
- At risk for situational self-esteem disturbance due to new parenting role
- At risk for altered family processes related to incorporation of a new family member
- At risk for altered parent-infant attachment related to anxiety of being a new parent

Nursing Outcomes

- Parents will verbalize an understanding of parental role expectations and responsibilities.
- Parents will verbalize stressors of new role.
- Parents will demonstrate positive comments and actions when interacting with family members.
- Parents will hold the newborn close to the body, attend to the newborn's needs, and interact with the newborn.

INTRODUCTION

The postpartum period is a time of both physiological and psychological adjustments. As the woman is adjusting to the numerous physiological changes within her body, she and her partner are adjusting to their new roles as parents and the effect these new roles have on the couple's relationship and the family unit (**Fig. 13-1**). This chapter focuses on the psychological, emotional, and developmental changes that take place during the transition to parenthood.

TRANSITION TO PARENTHOOD

The **transition to parenthood** is a dynamic developmental process that begins with the knowledge of pregnancy and continues throughout the postpartum period as the couple takes on their new or expanded roles of mother and father. Whether this is the first child or tenth child, this transition is a major life event that is both exciting and stressful, and produces developmental challenges for the individual, the couple's relationship, and family members. Each individual deals with the growth, realization, and preparation of becoming a parent in different ways, and cultural beliefs have an effect on how the individual takes on the role of parent (**Table 13-1**).

The transition to parenthood is fostered or hampered by many factors, some of which include:

- Previous life experiences: Previous experiences with caring for infants and children can foster a smoother transition to parenthood.
- Length and strength of the relationship between partners: A strong relationship between the couple can foster a smoother transition to parenthood.
- Financial considerations: Financial concerns can hamper the transition to parenting.
- Educational levels: Decreased ability to read and comprehend information regarding child care may hamper the couple's ability to gain knowledge in the care of the infant.
- Support systems: A lack of positive support in the care of the woman and infant may hamper the transition to parenting.

Don't have time to read this chapter? Want to reinforce your reading? Need to review for a test? Listen to this chapter on DavisPlus.

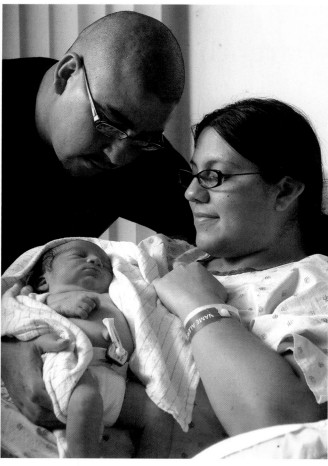

Figure 13–1 Mother and father getting acquainted with their new son.

■ Desire to be a parent: A lack of desire to be a parent can hamper the transition to parenting.
■ Age of parents: Adolescent parents may have a more difficult transition to parenting.

The transition to parenthood involves taking on the role of mother or father, viewing the child as an individual with his or her own personality, and incorporating the new child into the family system.

Parental Roles

Individuals have many roles throughout their lifetimes. As a child, the individual has the roles of son or daughter, sister or brother, grandchild, and student. Additional roles are acquired as the individual ages. Roles change over time as the individual matures and new roles are added. The role of mother or father evolves and changes over time as the child grows and additional children are added to the family. Each new role has expectations and responsibilities that the individual must learn in order to be successful in the role.

Couples are given the title of mother and father with the birth of their child, but must learn the expectations and responsibilities of these roles.

■ Examples of parental role expectations are that others will acknowledge the person as being a parent or that the child will obey the parents.
■ Examples of responsibilities are that the parents will love and protect their child.

Knowledge of these expectations and responsibilities is acquired through intentional learning (formal instructions) and incidental learning (observing others in the role). Most individuals have little intentional/instructional learning regarding the role of mother or father. The majority of learning of the expectations and responsibilities for these roles occurs through incidental learning. Examples of incidental learning of the parental role are:

■ Observing other individuals who are mothers and fathers
■ Recalling how they were parented
■ Watching movies or television programs that have mothers and/or fathers as characters

The process of learning and developing parental roles should start during the pregnancy. Partners who learn together during the pregnancy have better outcomes when they take on the role of parents. Providing couples with written information regarding different styles of parenting roles allows the expectant couple to learn about parenting behaviors. The expectant couple can then discuss parenting issues and mutually agree on expectations and responsibilities for their new roles.

Evidence-Based Practice: Maternal Adaptation During the Early Postpartum Period

In the 1960s, Reba Rubin conducted qualitative research studies focusing on maternal adaptation during the early postpartum weeks. Her research is the foundation of our understanding of the psychosocial experience of women during the postpartum period. Two concepts identified through her research are "maternal phases" and "maternal touch." Rubin (1984) refined and modified the process as more evidence was linked to maternal adjustments and behaviors and identified areas of development that women progress through to "becoming a mother."

Ramona Mercer, a student and colleague of Rubin, added to and expanded this body of nursing knowledge through numerous research studies that focused on the maternal role. Based on these studies, Mercer (1995) developed the theory of "maternal role attainment" that describes and explains the process women progress through as they become a mother. Based on her previous research and the research of others, Mercer (2004) supports replacing the term "maternal role attainment" with "becoming a mother." The term "becoming a mother" reflects that the process is not stagnant but continually evolving as the woman and her child are changing and growing.

The theories generated by Rubin's and Mercer's research agendas are the cornerstone of evidence-based knowledge used in establishing nursing guidelines for the care of postpartum women and families.

TABLE 13–1 CULTURAL BELIEFS AND THE POSTPARTUM FAMILY

CULTURE	BELIEFS AND PRACTICES
ARAB HERITAGE	Children are dearly loved and indulged. Care of the newborn includes wrapping the infant's abdomen at birth to prevent cold or wind from entering the body.
	The call to pray is recited in the newborn's ear.
	Male circumcision is a religious requirement of Muslims.
	Breastfeeding is delayed 2–3 days based on the belief that the woman requires rest, and that nursing immediately after birth causes "colic" pain for the mother.
CHINESE HERITAGE	Pregnancy and childbirth are viewed as women's business.
	Postpartum care includes 1 month of recovery, and women eat specific foods and avoid exposure to cold air to decrease the yin (cold) energy.
	Female relatives care for the newborn so that the woman can rest.
	Women, during the postpartum period, avoid drinking and touching cold water to decrease the yin (cold) energy.
FILIPINO HERITAGE	The mother often is the major decision maker regarding health, children, and finances.
	Older relatives such as grandparents share in the responsibility for the care and discipline of younger family members.
	The woman and her infant remain at home for the first 4 weeks except to go to the doctor.
HINDU HERITAGE	Older female relatives are considered to have expert knowledge in the use of home remedies during pregnancy and the postpartum period.
	The birth of a son is a blessing because he will carry the family name and take care of aging parents.
	The birth of a daughter may be cause of concern because of the traditions associated with a dowry.
	Exposure to cold air is considered dangerous.
	The mother and infant undergo purification rites on the 11th day after the birth.
	The baby is officially named on the 11th day.
	There are prescribed foods to eat and to avoid when the woman is breastfeeding.
JAPANESE HERITAGE	The primary relationship within the family is the mother-child relationship.
	It is customary for a mother to sleep with the youngest child until that child is 10 years old.
	Babies are not allowed to cry. Women constantly hold their babies.
	Women often return to their mother's home during the last 2 months of pregnancy and stay there for the first 2 months after birth.
	Female relatives assist with the care of the newborn so that the woman can rest.
	Maternal rest is viewed as important for successful breastfeeding.
	Women do not bathe, shower, or wash their hair for the first month after birth.
MEXICAN HERITAGE	Women care for the children and the home.
	Cutting the baby's hair or nails during the first 3 months is believed to cause blindness or deafness.
	Women are discouraged from taking baths or washing their hair for 6 weeks post-birth.
NAVAJO INDIAN HERITAGE	Grandmothers and mothers are at the center of Navajo society.
	Children may be named at birth, but the name is not revealed until their first laugh, when they are considered to officially have a soul.
	Infants are often kept in cradleboards until they can walk.
	It is taboo to purchase clothes for the baby before he or she is born.
	The placenta is buried soon after the birth as a symbol of the child being tied to the land.
	The newborn is given a mixture of juniper bark to cleanse his or her insides and dispel mucus.

Adapted from Purnell & Paulanka (2008).

Expected Findings

- Parents identify changing roles and are willing to make lifestyle changes to accommodate the changes.
- Parents identify with the parental roles.
- Parents discuss what the roles mean to them.
- Couples incorporate a third person, the newborn, into their relationship.
- Couples support each other in mutual caregiving tasks.

Nursing Actions

Nursing actions are directed at supporting the couple as they take on their role of mother or father. Nursing actions include:

- Provide an environment that is conducive to rest, such as uninterrupted periods of time so that parents can sleep.
    - *Adequate rest can increase the couple's ability to take in new information and develop new skills.*
- Provide culturally sensitive care.
    - *Mother and father role expectations and responsibilities vary based on cultural backgrounds.*
- Encourage, through active listening, the parents to talk about their expectations of each other in their respective role of mother or father.
    - *Having realistic and mutually agreed upon expectations decreases the level of stress within the relationship.*
- Provide parental education on care of the newborn by using a variety of educational strategies such as handouts, videos, and demonstrations of procedures (burping, swaddling, entertaining, and stimulating the infant).
    - *Information needs to be appropriate and relevant for the couple.*
- Provide positive feedback for parent's infant care behaviors.
    - *New parents are insecure regarding infant care and need to know they are correctly interacting with and caring for their infant.*
- Provide information on community parenting classes and support groups.
    - *This will provide parents opportunities for both intentional and incidental learning.*

Becoming A Mother

Becoming a mother is a relatively new term used to describe and explain the process that women undergo in their transition to motherhood and establishment of their maternal identity (Mercer, 2004).

Mercer describes four stages through which women progress in "becoming a mother." These are:

- Commitment, attachment, and preparation for an infant during pregnancy
- Acquaintance with and increasing attachment to the infant, learning how to care for the infant, and physical restoration during the early weeks after birth
- Moving toward a new normal during the first 4 months
- Achievement of a maternal identity around 4 months (Mercer, 2006, p. 649)

Evidence-Based Practice: Transition to Motherhood

Nelson, A. (2003). Transition to motherhood, *JOGNN, 32*, 465–477.

In a meta-synthesis of nine qualitative studies that focused on the transition to motherhood, Nelson (2003) identified actions of women that facilitate the transition to motherhood:

Mercer describes four stages through which women progress in "becoming a mother":

- The woman's commitment to mothering: The higher the woman's commitment to being a mother, the smoother the transition.
- Prenatal discussion of realistic expectations for the transition to motherhood: The more realistic the woman's expectations of motherhood, the smoother the transition.
- The woman being actively involved in caring for her infant: Early and continuous involvement in infant care facilitates the transition.
- Support during the first 6 postpartum months: The greater the perceived support, the smoother the transition.
- The use of role models: The availability of positive motherhood role models facilitates a smoother transition.

Nursing care during the postpartum period that facilitates the transition to motherhood is based on knowledge of these identified maternal actions.

The process of becoming a mother begins during pregnancy but can occur before pregnancy. Some women begin preparing for this role as children when they fantasize about being mothers and role-play being mothers with dolls. Others, before pregnancy, actively improve their health in preparation for the pregnancy (Mercer, 2006).

The process of "becoming a mother" is influenced by:

- How the woman was parented
- Her life experiences
- Her unique characteristics
- The pregnancy experience
- The birth experience
- Support from partner, family, and friends
- The woman's willingness to assume the role of mother
- The infant's characteristics such as appearance and temperament (Mercer, 1995, 2006).

Nursing Actions

- Review prenatal and labor records for risk factors such as complications during pregnancy and labor and birth.
    - *Pregnancy and birth experiences can either enhance or impede the process of "becoming a mother."*
- Assess the stages of "becoming a mother."
    - *Assessment data assists in developing individualized nursing actions.*
- Expected assessment findings:
    - *Positive feelings toward being pregnant*
    - *Positive health behaviors*
    - *Nurturing behaviors toward the infant*
    - *Protective feelings toward the infant*
    - *Increasing confidence in knowing and caring for the infant*
    - *Establishment of new family routines (Mercer, 2006)*

- Provide rooming-in or couplet care to facilitate bonding and attachment.
- Provide private time for the parents to interact with their newborn.
- Provide comfort measures for the woman to promote rest and healing.
- Listen to the woman's concerns in order for her to process the incorporation of the newborn into her life.
- Provide information on the care of newborns.
- Praise the woman for the care she provides to her newborn.

MATERNAL PHASES

Maternal phases, as defined by Rubin (1963, 1967), is a three-phase process that occurs during the first few weeks of the postpartum period (**Table 13-2**). A delay in transitioning through the phases may indicate that the woman is experiencing difficulty in becoming a mother. Factors that can affect the woman's transition through the maternal phases are:

- Medications (e.g., magnesium sulfate or analgesics) that depress the central nervous system (CNS), leading to a sense of tiredness and a slow response to stimuli.
- Complications during pregnancy, labor and birth, and/or postpartum (e.g., preterm labor, chronic illness, difficult birth, or cesarean birth) can cause the woman's focus to shift to her health and well-being, and/or to resolving feelings of disappointment.
- Cesarean births can cause increased discomfort that interferes with the woman's ability to care for her infant.
- Pain causes a shift of maternal attention from focusing on caring for baby to seeking pain relief for self.

TABLE 13–2 MATERNAL PHASES

TAKING-IN PHASE	TAKING-HOLD PHASE	LETTING-GO PHASE
The **taking-in phase**, a period of dependent behaviors, occurs during the first 24–48 hours after birth and includes the following maternal behaviors: • The woman is focused on her personal comfort and physical changes. • The woman relives and speaks of the birth experience. • The woman adjusts to psychological changes. • The woman is dependent on others for her and her infant's immediate needs. • The woman has a decreased ability to make decisions. • The woman concentrates on personal physical healing (Rubin, 1963, 1967).	The **taking-hold phase**, the movement between dependent and independent behaviors, follows the taking-in phase and can last up to weeks and includes the following maternal behaviors: • The focus moves from self to the infant. • The woman begins to be independent. • The woman has an increased ability to make decisions. • The woman is interested in the newborn's cues and needs. • The woman gives up the pregnancy role and initiates taking on the maternal role. • The woman is eager to learn; it is an excellent time to initiate postpartum teaching. • The woman begins to like the role of "mother." • The woman may have feelings of inadequacy and being overwhelmed. • The woman needs verbal reassurance that she is meeting her newborn's needs. • The woman may show signs and symptoms of baby blues and fatigue. • The woman begins to let more of the outside world in (Rubin, 1963, 1967).	In the **letting-go phase**, the movement from independence to the new role of mother is fluid and interchangeable with the taking-hold phase. Maternal characteristics during this phase are: • Grieving and letting go of old relationship behaviors in favor of new ones • Incorporating the newborn into her life whereby the baby becomes a separate entity from her • Accepting the newborn as he or she really is • Giving up the fantasy of what it would/could have been • Independence returning; may go back to work or school • May have feelings of grief, guilt, or anxiety • Reconnection/growth in relationship with partner (Rubin, 1963, 1967)

- Preterm infants or infants who experience complications can cause additional stresses on the woman and delay her transition through the phases.
- Mood disorders, such as depression, cause the woman's focus to be more on self and less on the infant.
- Lack of support from the partner and/or support system may lead to maternal exhaustion.
- Adolescent mothers are more focused inwardly and on peer relationships than on care of the newborn.
- The lack of financial resources forces the woman to focus on obtaining basic needs rather than on her infant.
- Cultural beliefs can have an effect on the behaviors the woman takes on and the amount of time the woman spends in each phase. In some cultures, such as traditional Asian cultures, it is an expectation that the woman rest and not be actively involved in the care of her infant or in decision making during the first few months following the birth of her infant.

Nursing Actions

- Review prenatal and labor records for factors that might delay progression through the maternal phases.
- Assess for maternal phases.
  - *Assessment data assists in developing individualized nursing actions.*
- Expected assessment findings:
  - *Taking-in behaviors during the first 24– 48 hours*
  - *Taking-hold behaviors from 24–48 hours through the first few weeks after birth*
- Nursing care during the taking-in phase is directed by the nurse because the woman is more dependent during this phase and has difficulty making decisions.
- Nursing care during the taking-hold phase is directed more by the woman as she is becoming more independent and has an increased ability to make decisions.
- Provide comfort measures such as backrubs, uninterrupted periods of rest, and analgesics.
- Adapt teaching to reflect the maternal phase.
  - *During the taking-in phase, teaching is directed to immediate learning needs and provided in short sessions as the woman's focus is on self versus learning about the care of the newborn.*
  - *During the taking-hold phase, praise the woman for her learning as she is eager to learn but can become frustrated with not being able to master a new task quickly.*

FATHERHOOD

Men's preparation for the role of father is vastly different from women's preparation for motherhood. In general, men do not fantasize about being a father, nor do they role-play being a father during childhood. During pregnancy, men mentally evaluate how they were fathered and how they want to father, but the reality of becoming a father may not occur until the child is born (May, 1982). Men are less likely than women to read about infant care and parenting during and after the pregnancy; yet during the postpartum period they report that they do not feel they have the knowledge, skills, and support for this new role (Jordan, 1990).

The meaning of "father" varies based on the man's interpretation of the role and its expectations and responsibilities. This is influenced by:

- How he was fathered
- How his culture defines the role
  - *In some cultures, men are not expected to be involved in the birthing process and/or care of the newborn.*
- By friends and family, and by his partner.

The man's partner/wife has a major influence in the degree of the man's involvement in infant and child care. For the man to be an involved father, his partner/wife needs to share this desire and to be supportive.

Becoming a father evolves over time as the man has increasing contact with his infant, increasing knowledge of infant and infant care, and increasing experiences in infant care. Factors that influence the man's transition to fatherhood are:

- Developmental and emotional age
- Cultural expectations
- Relationship with his partner/wife
- Knowledge and understanding of fatherhood
- Previous experiences as a father
- The manner in which he was fathered
- Financial concerns
- Support from partner/wife, friends, and family

Nursing Actions

- Provide information on infant care and infant behavior.
- Demonstrate infant care such as diapering, feeding, and holding.
  - *Providing information and demonstrating infant care skills enhances the father's comfort in caring for his infant.*
- Praise the father for his interactions with his infant.
  - *Praising can encourage continued interactions with his infant.*
- Provide opportunities for the father to talk about the meaning of fathering.
  - *Talking about the meaning of fathering assists in identifying his beliefs regarding the role of father.*
- Facilitate a discussion with the father and his partner to identify mutual expectations of the fathering role.
  - *Mutually agreed upon expectations can decrease the level of stress within the relationship.*

ADOLESCENT PARENTS

Adolescence is the transition between childhood and adulthood. This transition is a very challenging time as the individual experiences many physiological, psychological, and social changes. Adolescent parenting is a stressful life experience in that the adolescent is taking on the role responsibilities of being a mother or father while at the same time working through the developmental tasks of being a teenager.

■ Adolescent parents have had few life experiences that prepare them for the role conflicts and strain that is experienced by first-time parents.
■ Adolescent motherhood is viewed by the adolescent woman as either a positive turning point or a hardship (Clemmens, 2003).
■ A majority of adolescent mothers live with their family of origin until their infant is 1 year old.
■ The adolescent mother's relationship with her own mother affects the adolescent mother's feelings of competency in parenting. A supportive mother-daughter relationship has a positive effect on the adolescent's competency level of parenting (DeVito, 2007).
■ An adolescent father's involvement with his infant is positively affected by support for father involvement from his parents and from the infant's mother (Fagan et al., 2007).
■ Adolescent fathers who are involved during the prenatal period have a higher involvement with their child following birth (Fagan et al., 2007).

Nursing Actions

Nursing actions are directed at supporting the adolescent parents in developing child care behaviors and learning to cope with the stress of parenting. Additionally, nursing actions are directed at increasing the adolescent father's involvement in the support, care, and nurturing of his child. These nursing actions include:

■ Assess level of knowledge.
  ■ *Information needs to be appropriate and relevant for the individual and/or couple for learning to occur.*
■ Present information at an age appropriate level.
  ■ *Learning styles and teaching strategies are different for young teens and older teens. Information needs to be provided in a manner that will engage the teen in the learning process.*
■ Include the adolescent father in infant care teaching sessions.
  ■ *Adolescent fathers need information and encouragement in developing care behaviors.*
■ Involve the maternal grandparent in teaching sessions focused on infant care.
  ■ *Grandparents need a review of infant care since the majority of teen mothers live with their parents during the first year.*
■ Discuss with the adolescent parents their expectations of each other regarding child care and support.
  ■ *Realistic and mutually agreed upon expectations decrease the level of stress within the relationship.*
■ Involve adolescent fathers in prenatal care based on adolescent mother's comfort level.
  ■ *Adolescent fathers who are involved during the prenatal period have greater involvement with infants following the birth.*

Evidence-Based Practice: Teen Fathers

Paschal, A., Lewis-Moss, R., and Hsiao, T. (2011). Perceived fatherhood roles and parenting behaviors among African American teen fathers. *Journal of Adolescent Research, 26,* 61–83.

In the qualitative study, 30 African American fathers ages 14–19 were interviewed to examine how they defined and performed the role of father. Three themes emerged from the data:

■ Provider role
  ■ 53% of the teen fathers indicated that the primary attribute of being a good father was being a good provider.
  ■ Most of these fathers provide some form of tangible goods such as diapers, baby clothes, and baby food.
  ■ Economic support to the mother and child was sporadic.
■ Nurturer role
  ■ 27% of the teen fathers indicated that the primary attributes that made a good father were emotional involvement, physical presence, and/or nurturing.
  ■ Older teens were more likely to display involved, nurturing, and caregiving behaviors.
■ Autonomous fathers
  ■ 20% of the teen fathers expressed opposition to the idea of fatherhood.
  ■ These teen fathers did not feel they had an obligation to be involved in the lives of their children or provide financial support.

BONDING AND ATTACHMENT

Bonding and attachment are two phenomena that parents encounter during their transition to parenting and parental role attainment. **Bonding** is defined as the emotional feelings that begin during pregnancy or shortly after birth between the parent and the newborn (Klaus & Kennell, 1982). Bonding is unidirectional from parent to newborn. **Attachment** is an emotional connection that forms between the infant and his or her parents (Bowlby, 1969). It is bidirectional from parent to infant and infant to parent. Attachment has a lifelong impact on the developing individual. The quality of this attachment influences the person's physical and emotional development and is the foundation for the formation of future relationships. With each interaction, the parent and infant become more acquainted with each other, recognizing and becoming sensitive to each other's behaviors. This leads to reciprocal behaviors and emotional bonds between parent and newborn over time (**Table 13-3**).

Bonding and Attachment Behaviors

Bonding and attachment are affected by time, proximity of parent and infant, whether the pregnancy is planned/wanted, and the ability of the parents to process through the necessary development tasks of parenting. Other factors that influence bonding and attachment behaviors are:

■ The knowledge base of the couple
■ Past experience with children

TABLE 13–3   BONDING AND ATTACHMENT BEHAVIORS

BONDING BEHAVIORS UNIDIRECTIONAL: PARENT → INFANT	ATTACHMENT BEHAVIORS BIDIRECTIONAL: PARENT ↔ INFANT
En face	Parents respond to the infant's cry.
Calls baby by name	
Cuddles baby close to chest	The infant responds to the parents' comforting measures.
Talks/sings to baby	Parents stimulate and entertain the infant while awake.
Kisses the baby	
Breastfeeds the baby or holds the baby close when bottle-feeding	Parents become "cue sensitive" to the infant's behavior.

- Maturity and educational levels of the couple
- Type of extended support system
- Maternal/paternal expectations from this pregnancy
- Maternal/paternal expectations of the infant
- Cultural expectations

Risk Factors for Delayed Bonding and/or Attachment

- Maternal illness during pregnancy and/or the postpartum period that interferes with the woman's ability to interact with her infant
- Neonatal illness such as prematurity that necessitates separation of the infant from the parents
- Prolonged or complicated labor and birth that leads to exhaustion for both the woman and her partner
- Fatigue during the postpartum period related to lack of rest and sleep
- Physical discomfort experienced by women post-birth
- Age and developmental age of the woman, such as adolescent or developmentally challenged
- Outside stressors not related to pregnancy or childbirth (e.g., concerns with finances, poor social support system, or need to return to work soon after the birth)

Nursing Actions

- Review the prenatal and labor record for risk factors that place woman/couple at risk for delayed bonding/attachment.
- Assess for risk factors that could delay bonding and attachment.
  - *Early identification of couples at risk can lead to early interventions to enhance bonding/attachment.*
- Assess cultural beliefs.
  - *Type of interactions between parents and infants can vary based on cultural beliefs.*
- Assess for bonding and attachment by observation of parent-infant interaction.
  - *Assessment data provides information for individualizing nursing actions.*

- Expected assessment findings:
  - *Parents hold the infant close.*
  - *Parents refer to the infant by name or proper sex.*
  - *Parents respond to the infant's needs.*
  - *Parents speak positively about the infant.*
  - *Parents appear interested in learning about the infant.*
  - *Parents ask appropriate questions about infant care.*
  - *Parents appear comfortable holding and caring for the infant.*
- Maladaptive assessment findings:
  - *Parents call the infant "it."*
  - *Parents avoid eye contact with the infant (this can be viewed as adaptive based on culture).*
  - *Parents do not respond to the infant's cries.*
  - *Parents are emotionally unavailable to the infant.*
  - *Parents allow others to care for the infant, showing no interest (this can be viewed as adaptive based on culture).*
  - *Parents demonstrate poor feeding techniques such as propping bottles, not burping the infant, or seeming to be uncomfortable and/or irritated when nursing.*
- Teach parents about bonding and attachment and the importance of these to the child's development of future relationships.
  - *Understanding why it is important enhances likelihood of increased bonding and attachment behaviors by parents.*
- Instruct parents regarding the importance of parents responding to the infant's cues such as crying, cooing, and movement.
  - *Attachment is bidirectional.*
- Promote bonding and attachment by:
  - *Initiating early and prolonged contact between the parent and infant.*
  - *Initiating rooming-in or couplet care.*
  - *Providing positive comments to parents regarding their interactions with the infant.*
  - *Encouraging mothers to breastfeed.*
  - *Encouraging the woman and her partner to talk about their birth experience and feelings regarding becoming parents.*
- Promote attachment between mothers and infants separated due to either maternal illness or neonatal complications by:
  - *Recommending that family members take pictures of the newborn and bring them to the mother to keep in her room.*
  - *Assisting parents to the NICU or nursery so that they can see and touch their infant.*
  - *Providing opportunities for parents to care for the infant in the NICU or nursery.*
  - *Instructing the woman on breast milk pumping and encouraging her to bring breast milk to the NICU for use with her infant.*
  - *Informing parents that they can call the NICU or nursery any time of the day or night and talk with the nurse caring for their infant.*

PARENT-INFANT CONTACT

Early contact between the parents and their infant fosters the development of attachment of parents and infant and integration of the newborn into the maternal and paternal relationship.

Continued contact and interaction provide the avenue for the parents and infant to learn more about each other. As they interact and perform for each other, they find themselves becoming more aware of the cues that make them respond to each other. This interaction cycle of behavior is called **reciprocity.** It is a **biorhythmic** or inherent rhythm that exists between the parents and newborn that becomes stronger with each interaction and the passing of time. This sequence of events strengthens the bonding and attachment processes that are the foundation for all other relationships the infant will establish throughout his or her life.

Maternal Touch

Maternal touch is a process that new mothers transition through beginning with the first physical contact with their newborns (Rubin, 1963). Most mothers do not instantly feel close to their newborns. Feeling comfortable holding her newborn close to her body occurs over time with a progression through three stages. These stages, as described by Rubin, are:

■ Initial stage: The woman touches her newborn tentatively with her fingertips.
■ Second stage: The woman, as she becomes more comfortable with herself as a mother, uses her hand to stroke her newborn's head or body.
■ Final stage: The mother holds her newborn in her arms and brings her newborn close to her body.

Rubin's maternal touch is a component of the acquaintance process through which mothers and newborns transition. Mothers go through multiple stages of awareness during early contacts with their newborns. The first time the new mother touches and meets her newborn, she is excited about her infant's features and verbally responds to sounds and expressions the baby makes. Later, after the new mother enters the final stage of maternal touch, she will hold her newborn **en face,** a position in which the mother and newborn are face-to-face with eye contact (**Fig. 13-2**). The en face position provides a positive connection that facilitates the bonding process. Some cultures believe that you should not gaze into the newborn's eyes.

CRITICAL COMPONENT

Paternal-Infant Contact

The new father, when holding his child for the first time, may feel awkward and uncomfortable and have a fear of injuring the baby. These feelings will decrease over time with continued contact with the newborn.

Paternal-Infant Contact

In the 1980s, studies provided data that promoted and supported fathers' involvement in the birth of their infants. When expectant fathers participated in the labor and birth of their children in roles that were comfortable for them, they had a greater sense of belonging, which led to their being more

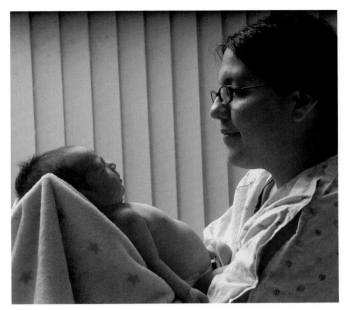

Figure 13-2   Mother and son in en face position.

engaged in the father role (Chapman, 1991). Reinforcement of this type of involvement has had positive benefits to the family unit and has strengthened early and positive parental involvement in the bonding and attachment process. Early physical contact with the newborn provides an opportunity for the new father to become comfortable touching and holding, which fosters a more active role in caring for his infant (see Critical Component: Paternal-Infant Contact).

New fathers experience an intense preoccupation about and interest in their newborn. Greenberg and Morris (1974) identified these behaviors as **engrossment** (**Fig. 13-3**). These behaviors can vary based on the cultural beliefs of the couple.

Evidence-Based Practice: The Newborn's Impact on the Father

Greenberg, M., & Morris, N. (1974). Engrossment: The newborn's impact upon the father. *American Journal of Orthopsychiatry, 44,* 520–531.

In their research of new fathers, Greenberg and Morris identified the concept of engrossment that new fathers experience during the postpartum period in relationship to their newborns. They defined engrossment as an absorption, preoccupation, and interest with their newborns. New fathers can be observed gazing at their newborns for prolonged periods of time as if they are in a hypnotic trance. Greenberg and Morris described seven characteristics of engrossment:

■ A visual awareness of the newborn: Seeing their newborn as being attractive
■ A tactile awareness of the newborn: Having a desire to touch the newborn
■ An awareness of their newborn's distinct features: Positive comments about their newborn's features
■ A perception that their newborn is perfect
■ A strong attraction to their newborn
■ A feeling of strong elation
■ An increase of self-esteem

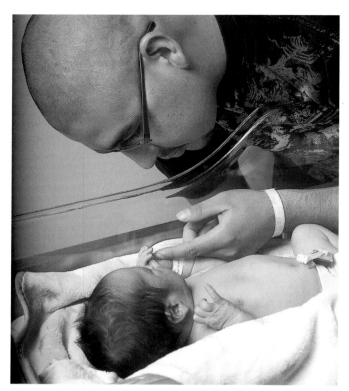

Figure 13–3 Father exhibiting sign of engrossment by gazing at his newborn son.

Nursing Actions for Parent-Infant Contact

- Assess for stages of maternal touch.
    - *Assessment data assists in developing individualized nursing care.*
    - *Expected findings*
        - Tentatively touching her infant's extremities with her fingertips
        - Progressing to fuller touch and examination of the infant
        - Verbalizing positive comments about the infant
        - Snuggling and providing comfort to the infant
        - En face positioning to interact with the infant (varies based on cultural beliefs)
- Assess paternal-newborn interactions.
    - *Expected findings (varies based on cultural beliefs)*
        - Spends prolonged periods of time gazing at the newborn
        - Assists with infant care
        - Holds the newborn close to the body
        - Expresses delight in his infant's features
        - Verbally and physically expresses love and joy for both his newborn and his partner
    - *Maladaptive findings (may be viewed as adaptive based on cultural beliefs)*
        - Displays little or no interest in the infant
        - Makes negative comments about or to the infant
        - Ignores the infant's needs and cues
        - Displays sadness or anger to the partner or infant

- Does not spend time with the infant or is emotionally absent
- Experiences mood swings
- Has conflict between family members over the infant
- Provide early, continuous, and uninterrupted periods of time for parents to see, hold, and interact with their newborn.
    - *Bonding and attachment occur over time and continued contact.*
- Facilitate rooming-in, which provides the opportunity for the newborn and father to stay in the mother's room throughout the hospital stay.
- Promote parental interaction with the newborn by delaying unnecessary procedures.
- Provide adequate rest periods (2–4 hours every 12 hours) for the parents. This ensures they have the stamina and rest to take care of and provide emotional support to each other.
- Provide comfort measures to assist the parents in feeling rested and relaxed.
- Explain to new parents that they may not feel comfortable holding the newborn close and that these feelings will decrease with increasing contact with their newborn.
- Role model en face positioning.
- Role model appropriate behaviors by calling the infant by name and identifying normal infant behaviors.
- Use therapeutic listening and provide positive feedback to parents when they are verbalizing their feelings about their newborn.
- Educate parents about the newborn's unique behaviors and temperament.
- Educate and give information to both parents using multiple models of learning.
    - *Teaching strategies need to fit the learning style of the parents.*
- Provide culturally sensitive care to the family unit.
    - *The way parents interact with their infant can vary based on cultural beliefs.*

CULTURAL AWARENESS: Cultural Beliefs Influence Parents

Cultural beliefs influence the ways parents relate to and care for their newborns, and the role of fathers during the postpartum period and care of infants. An awareness of variations across cultural practices is an important component in providing appropriate care. Cultural beliefs can influence:

- The degree of father involvement in infant care
- The role extended family members have in the care of the infant and new mother
- The method of infant feeding
- Foods that are eaten and foods that are avoided during the postpartum period
- When a woman can bathe and wash her hair
- When the baby is named and who names the baby

COMMUNICATION BETWEEN PARENT AND CHILD

Communication is a bidirectional process that involves a sender and a receiver. People communicate through the use of verbal and written words, and through the use of their eyes, ears, faces, and body gestures. Newborns have the ability to see, hear, and smell; to respond to their environment; and to display displeasure. They engage in behaviors designed to evoke a response from individuals in their environments. They rely on vocal noises such as crying and cooing, as well as facial expressions and body movements, to participate actively in relationship-building with other human beings. The challenge to parents and care providers is to learn the cues newborns and infants use to communicate their needs and pleasures.

Nurses are in the unique position to provide information about the newborn's ability to communicate. Nurses can help parents identify infant behaviors and offer appropriate interventions to promote positive interactions (see Critical Component: Positive Interactions between Parents and Newborns). Examples of newborn and infant communication styles and cues are:

■ Crying
■ Cooing
■ Facial expressions
■ Eye movements
■ Smelling
■ Cuddling
■ Arm and leg movements
■ **Entrainment:** A phenomenon in which the newborn and infant moves his or her arms and legs in rhythm with speech patterns of an adult.

Responding to and encouraging newborn and infant communication assists the infant in developing communication and language skills. The parents' ability to recognize their infant's positive response cues fosters the parents' confidence in their parenting skills. Teaching parents how to identify their newborn's unique cues and behaviors promotes a positive relationship that empowers the dyad to continue to grow and learn as the newborn matures and adds new skills and insights into the relationship.

Parents who are aware of and start to understand infant behaviors by becoming cue-sensitive will be able to identify:

■ The best time to communicate with their newborn
■ Ways to comfort
■ Methods to assist infant to self-comfort
■ When the infant is overstimulated and how to provide quiet times during these periods of fussiness (White, Simon, & Bryan, 2002)

Newborns have very acute senses when interacting with their parents. Newborns who are placed on their mothers' abdomens will crawl to the breast. Newborns also interact with their parents by responding to voices and touch. They look en face and root when stimulated. These initial interactions and ongoing interactions lead to **synchrony** events, which are reciprocal actions between parents and infants that show mutual expressions of contentment. These interactions are very pleasurable for parents and infants. Examples of synchrony events are:

■ The mother holds the infant in an en face position. The response to this action is that they gaze into each other's eyes and talk, coo, or smile at each other.
■ The father places his finger in the infant's hand. The infant grabs the father's finger and they gaze at each other.

CRITICAL COMPONENT

Positive Interactions Between Parents and Newborns

Newborns have the ability to communicate, to interact, and to be stimulated by early interactions. Depending on the state of awareness, newborns have the ability to respond positively by becoming more alert, or negatively by crying. Nurses who understand newborn behaviors, infant state of awareness, and communication cues can identify and promote positive interactions between parents/caregivers and their newborns through role modeling and parent education (**Table 13-4**).

Nursing Actions

■ Review prenatal, labor and birth, and postpartum records for factors that might delay or hinder parent-infant communication and provide early interventions.
■ Assess parent-infant interactions.
   ■ *Expected findings*
      ■ Parents gently touch their newborn and hold the newborn close to the body.
      ■ Parents talk to or sing to their newborn.
      ■ Parents, when culturally acceptable, hold their newborn en face.
      ■ Parents respond to their newborn's cues for interaction and care.
      ■ The newborn responds to his or her parents' touch and voice.
   ■ *Role model communication with infant.*
      ■ Parents learn through incidental and intentional learning
   ■ *Praise parents for their interactions with their infant.*
   ■ *Provide teaching on infant communication:*
      ■ The infant's ability and need to communicate
      ■ Eye contact, when culturally appropriate
      ■ Synchronized interactions
      ■ Recognizing and interpreting the infant's cues
      ■ Entrainment
      ■ Infant alertness states

FAMILY DYNAMICS

Family dynamics are unique ways in which family members interact and participate within the family. Adaptation to these dynamics determines the cohesiveness, or lack of such, in the family unit.

TABLE 13–4   INFANT STATES

STATES	BEHAVIORS	ACTIONS
DEEP SLEEP	Minimal body twitches and eye movement. Cycles between deep and light sleep	Do not try to wake up or feed infant.
LIGHT SLEEP	More active body movement; may smile	More easily aroused and stimulated
DROWSY	Awakens easily; can be rocked back to sleep or made more awake	May enjoy being held and cuddled Responds to gentle stimuli May self-comfort by sucking
QUIET ALERT	Eyes open; quiet and attentive	Best time for interacting
ACTIVE ALERT	More sensitive to stimuli, active body movement; may be tired or hungry or need changing	Decrease stimuli. Provide a quiet environment. Provide comfort measures. The infant may attempt to self-comfort.
CRYING	Grimaces, cries, or whimpers	The infant may self-comfort. Meet infant needs.

There are several types of relationships and family compositions. The family structure can be as small as the mother and newborn, or as large as two or more generations plus extended family members. Each has its own unique dynamics and structure that present challenges and offers rewarding experiences to nurses who come into contact with these various family compositions. Examples of family compositions include:

■ Married or non-married male-female couples
■ Same-sex couples
■ Adoptive couples
■ Adolescent women with partner, mother, and/or grand-mother as support system
■ Adolescent women without support system
■ Single adult women with no partner
■ Blended families

The time immediately after childbirth is filled with many emotional changes for the partners and family members. Family members are redefining who they are as individuals and their roles within the family. Adjustments within the couple's relationship and family unit occur as the couple and family members incorporate and make room for the newest family member. Couples make adjustments within their relationship and learn how to support each other in their roles as parents. They reprioritize their other responsibilities and roles to fit their new roles and responsibilities. Siblings take on the role of older brother or sister and adjust to the decreased amount of time the parents have available to interact with and care for them.

The family unit is affected and influenced by changes both within the family and outside the family. Outside influences, such as friends and relatives, may have positive or negative effects on the family. The couple needs to determine which resources are helpful and which are stressful, and whom they can seek for positive assistance. Nursing care is directed at assisting families in identifying their needs and adjustment during this period of transition.

Coparenting

Coparenting is "a conceptual term that refers to the ways that parents and/or parental figures relate to each other in the role of parents" (Feinberg, 2003, p. 96).

Coparenting:

■ Occurs when the parents have shared responsibilities in child rearing
■ Consists of support for each other and coordination they exhibit in child rearing
■ Does not imply that parenting roles are or should be equal in responsibilities or authority (Feinberg, 2003).

Coparenting develops during the transition to parenthood and is influenced by:

■ The parent's beliefs, values, desires, and expectations.
■ The individual's cultural background and the dominant culture of the society (Feinberg, 2009).
■ The infant's temperament (Davis et al., 2009).

Multiparas

The maternal role changes and becomes more complex with each additional child. Multiparas may have more knowledge and practice regarding the care of newborns, but they usually experience more exhaustion and have less help than with their first child. In a classic 1979 article, Ramona Mercer described the unique concerns of multiparas:

■ Concerns for her other children
   ■ *Will her other children feel abandoned?*

Evidence-Based Practice: Effect of Infant Temperament on Coparenting

Davis, E., Schoppe-Sullivan, S., Mangelsdorf, S., and Brown, G. (2009). The role of infant temperament in stability and change in the coparenting across the first year of life. *Parenting: Science and Practice, 9,* 143–159.

In this longitudinal study of 56 two-parent families, the researchers collected data at infants' age of 3.5 months and 13 months. Data included (1) observational assessments of coparenting and (2) mothers' and fathers' perceptions of their infant's temperament difficulties.

Results:

- Infant difficulty reported by fathers at 3.5 months was associated with a decrease in supportive coparenting behavior.
- Supportive coparenting behaviors observed in fathers at 3.5 months was associated with a decrease in reported infant difficulties.

Recommendations:

- Early interventions to enhance coparenting are essential for families with temperamentally difficult infants.

- Concerns about being able to love the new child
  - *Does she have the capacity to love this new child as she does her other children?*
- Concerns for her ability to care for more than one child
  - *Does she have the time and energy to care for an additional child?*
- Concerns about her ability to get rest and sleep
  - *Will she be able to find time for sleep and rest?*
- Concerns about having help at home to care for her and her expanding family
  - *Will family members and friends be willing to help her with a second child?*

It is important that nurses who care for multiparous women provide the women with opportunities to express their concerns, fears, and doubts in caring for and loving another child. Nurses can facilitate this transition by providing reassurance and suggesting strategies in caring for an additional child. Strategies for caring include:

- Spend quality time with older child when newborn is sleeping.
- Carry infant in a sling to free hands for doing things with older child.
- Have prepared meals ready to use during the day.
- Encourage the partner to take on more responsibility for cleaning, cooking, and caring for older child.

Sibling Rivalry

The addition of a new family member can be a stressful life event for siblings within the family unit. They will need to make adjustments in their young lives in response to the incorporation of the newborn within the family (see Critical Component: Sibling Adjustment). Depending on the age of the siblings and birth order, they have varying degrees of feeling displaced. Younger children experience a sense of loss over

no longer being the "baby" of the family. Older children may have a sense of increased responsibility due to their parents' expectation that they assist in the care of younger children.

Preparing for the new family addition should begin during pregnancy as the parents talk about the expected new baby (see Chapter 5). Providing opportunities for the children to feel the fetus move and hear the fetal heartbeat are concrete ways to assist the children in understanding the upcoming event. Discussion on what it will mean to have a new baby in the family can also help in their adjustments.

Siblings should be introduced to their new brother or sister as soon as possible and spend time with mother and baby during the postpartum hospitalization. They should be allowed to hold and touch the new baby with supervision (**Fig. 13-4**).

CRITICAL COMPONENT

Sibling Adjustment

The addition of a new member to the family can be stressful for siblings. Actions that can facilitate their adjustment are:

- Spending time during the prenatal period talking about the upcoming arrival of a new baby
- Providing opportunities for siblings to feel the baby move and hear the heartbeat during the pregnancy
- Providing opportunities for siblings to spend time with their new brother or sister during the hospital stay
- Encouraging siblings to lie in bed with their mother during hospital visits
- Giving siblings a present that is from their new brother or sister
- Explaining to parents the importance of quality time with other children, such as sitting and reading books with them, playing games, and listening to them
- Taking siblings on a special outing while the newborn stays at home with a babysitter
- Explaining why babies cry and how they communicate

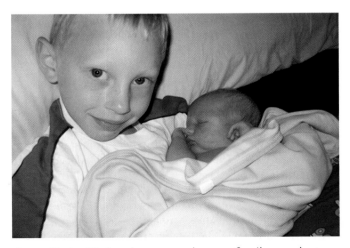

Figure 13–4 Big brother meets the new family member.

Nursing Actions for Family Dynamics

Introducing a new member into the family can be stressful for each member of the family. The majority of nursing actions are aimed at reducing stress within the family and family members. Nursing actions include:

■ Review the records for relationship issues, pregnancy history, and delivery summary.
  ■ *Complications encountered during pregnancy and/or labor and birth can have a negative effect on family dynamics.*
■ Assess for prior experiences with a newborn.
■ Assess for maladaptive behaviors and make referrals to social services or the community health nurse as indicated.
■ Respect cultural beliefs and incorporate them in the nursing care.
  ■ *How an individual interacts within the family unit is influenced by his cultural beliefs.*
■ Provide information of the potential adjustments parents, couples, and siblings will encounter as they incorporate the newborn into the family.
■ Assist parents in identifying ways to assist their other children in their adjustments to the new family member.
■ Provide positive verbal reinforcement for their family interactions.
■ Provide opportunities for family members to talk about the adjustments within the family.
  ■ *Increased communication can decrease misunderstanding.*
■ Provide opportunities for couples to talk about the adjustments within their couple relationship and ways to enhance their relationship.

PARENTS WITH SENSORY OR PHYSICAL IMPAIRMENTS

Parents with sensory impairments such as visual loss or diminished hearing, or those with physical impairments such as decreased mobility, present challenges to nurses and other health care professionals. These challenges can turn into opportunities to creatively adapt nursing care to meet the needs of these parents. It is important that health care professionals be aware of the rights of disabled individuals, provide information in ways they can understand, and provide care that is sensitive to their needs (see Critical Component: Working with Parents with a Sensory or Physical Impairment *and* Critical Component: Assisting Parents with an Impairment).

There are ranges in the degree of visual impairment, auditory impairment, and physical impairment. Visual impairment/blindness ranges from visual loss, where the person can read large print, to complete blindness, where the person has no usable vision. Auditory impairment ranges from mild to profound hearing loss. Those with mild hearing loss have enough hearing to carry on a conversation under ideal conditions. People with profound hearing losses usually rely on sign language as their form of communication and will not be able to converse orally with hearing people. Physical impairment can range from a person being dependent on a cane to people who do not have motor control of their arms and/or legs.

Nursing Actions

Visually Impaired Parents

■ When reporting, use the person's name. Do not refer to her as the "blind woman in room 211."
■ When entering a room, address the person by name and introduce yourself and anyone else who is in the room.
■ When leaving a room, announce your departure and indicate if others are staying or leaving.
■ Speak directly to the person in a clear manner. Do not exaggerate word pronunciation or speak in a loud voice.
■ Keep doors, cabinets, and closets closed to prevent injury.
■ Use sighted-guide when assisting with ambulation (the visually impaired person holds the elbow of the sighted person when walking). Avoid shoving, pushing, or grabbing unless in an emergency.
■ Do not pull on the person's cane to direct her.
■ Do not play with a seeing-eye dog while it is in harness. Ask permission to touch the dog.
■ Orient the person to the area of the room or new location after you have guided her to this new area.
■ At a given point (the door or bed), orient the room by describing its contents in logical sequence of progressive order (e.g., "To the right as you lie in the bed is the nightstand with the phone and call button; beside that is the bed curtain and then a chair. Next to the chair is the door to the bathroom").
■ Describe the location of food on a plate according to the clock face (e.g., "Potatoes are at 2:00, meat is at 5:00"). Ask the woman if she needs assistance.
■ Offer to read printed material or ask for the preferred manner for receiving information that is in printed form.
■ Provide space for Braillers and other special equipment used by the woman.
■ Provide teaching in a manner the parents can understand. Example of teaching instructions:
  ■ *Instruct the parents in diapering by having them diaper their child while you explain the steps.*
■ Provide discharge teaching and instructions in Braille or on audiotape.

Hearing Impaired Parents

■ Face the parents when speaking to them.
■ Be articulate but do not exaggerate pronunciation.
■ Speak in a normal voice volume.
■ Be within 6–8 feet of the parents when speaking to them. Make sure that light from windows is behind the parents.
■ Avoid putting your hand over your mouth or turning your back to the parents when you are speaking.

■ When communicating information with the use of illustrations, provide time for parents to study the illustrations.

■ If there is more than one speaker, take turns speaking with clear indications as to who is speaking.

■ Minimize background noises (e.g., turn off volume of TV, close the door to the room).

■ If there is misunderstanding, do not repeat words louder; instead use synonyms or other words that mean the same thing.

■ Provide discharge teaching and information in written form that parents can easily understand.

■ Use graphics and visuals when available.

■ Ensure a registered interpreter for the deaf person is present when discussing medical information and teaching. When using an interpreter:
  ■ *Allow sufficient time for the interpreter to complete a thought.*
  ■ *Speak directly to the patient and not to the interpreter.*
  ■ *Avoid saying, "Tell him/her...."*
  ■ *Check the parent for understanding or if he or she is getting too much information.*
  ■ *Allow time for questions and concerns.*

■ A head nod by the parent may have different meanings, such as "yes" or "continue"; it may not mean that the parent understands.

■ Flick lights on and off to get the attention of the parent. Do not shout, wave, or touch for the purpose of getting attention.

■ Be aware that hearing aids amplify sound 6–10 times, so shouting and loud noises can be uncomfortable.

■ Provide closed-captioned TV, TDD/TTY (telephone device for deaf), writing pad, and implements.

■ Discuss with the parents how they have adapted their home for the newborn.
  ■ *Some parents will use a device that causes a light to flash in response to the infant's cry, thus alerting parents to check on their infant.*
  ■ *Some parents might use closed-circuit TV to monitor the infant while in another room.*

Parents With Physical Impairments

■ Provide standard ADA-required facilities, such as raised toilets, wheelchair accessible rooms and hallways, and easy-to-use call buttons.

■ Keep the environment free of clutter.

■ Assess the type of assistance needed by asking him or her.

■ Discuss the type of assistance parents will need in caring for their newborn at home.

■ Assist parents in infant care.

■ Assist parents in developing strategies to adapt infant care to their limitations.

■ Make referrals to social services when indicated for additional assistance.

CRITICAL COMPONENT

Assisting Parents with an Impairment

Nurses can best assist parents who have sensory or physical impairments by exploring, identifying, and implementing techniques, tools, and alternative ways to:

■ Facilitate bonding and attachment
■ Teach parents about infant care
■ Promote a safe environment for the newborn
■ Enhance the family dynamics.

POSTPARTUM BLUES

Postpartum blues, also known as baby blues, occur during the first few postpartum weeks, last for a few days, and affect a majority of women. During this period of time, the woman feels sad and cries easily, but she is able to take care of herself and her infant. (Postpartum psychological complications are discussed in Chapter 14.)

Possible causes of postpartum blues are:

■ Changes in hormonal levels
■ Fatigue
■ Stress from taking on the new role of mother

Signs and symptoms of postpartum blues are:

■ Anger
■ Anxiety
■ Mood swings
■ Sadness
■ Weeping
■ Difficulty sleeping
■ Difficulty eating

Nursing Actions

■ Provide information to the couple regarding postpartum blues.
  ■ *Explain that this occurs in the majority of postpartum women.*
  ■ *Explain the importance of rest in reducing stress.*
  ■ *Explain to the woman's partner the importance of emotional and physical support during this period of time.*
  ■ *Explain that the woman or family should seek assistance from the health care provider if the symptoms persist beyond 4 weeks or if it is of concern for her or her family, as she may be experiencing postpartum depression.*

Clinical Pathway for Transition to Parenthood

Focus of Care	Postpartum Admission	Postpartum 4–24 Hours	Postpartum 24–48 Hours	Discharge Criteria
Emotional status	Taking-in phase	Progressing toward the taking-hold phase	Taking-hold phase. The woman shows more independence in managing her own and the infant's care.	The woman is able to provide self-care. The woman demonstrates increased confidence in infant care.
Nursing action	Provide care and comfort to the woman. Provide positive reinforcement of appropriate behaviors. Discuss the infant's unique capabilities. Provide early and consistent contact with the infant to facilitate bonding.	Encourage the woman and her family to participate in self- and infant care. Encourage extended infant contact. Observe for bonding and attachment behaviors. Begin discharge education.	Observe for bonding and attachment behaviors, noting any signs of maladaptive behaviors. Provide written/visual information on infant behaviors and characteristics. Teach methods for comforting the infant.	Positive bonding and attachment behaviors noted. Parents express understanding of infant behaviors and cues. Parents express positive understanding of how to care for the infant Provide resources for parents to call as needed.
Family dynamics	Parents demonstrate beginning bonding behaviors. Parents begin introducing the infant to the extended family.	Parents demonstrate positive bonding and attachment behaviors. Extended family demonstrate positive/supportive behaviors toward the newborn.	Parents continue to demonstrate bonding and attachment behaviors. Extended family demonstrates positive behaviors towards newborn and parents.	Parents demonstrate positive adaptive behaviors.

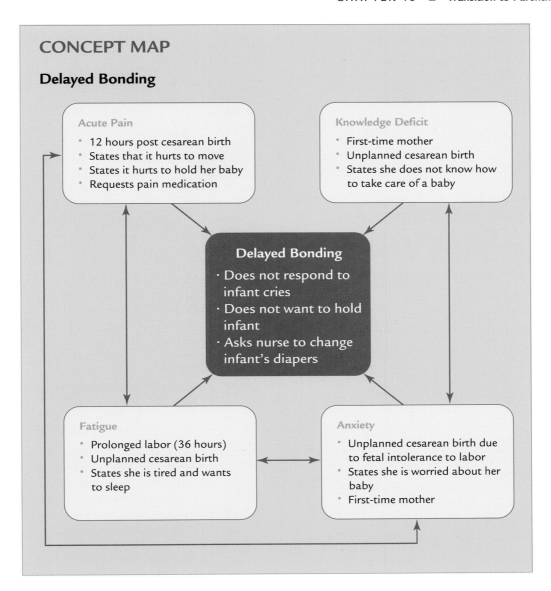

CONCEPT MAP

Delayed Bonding

Acute Pain
- 12 hours post cesarean birth
- States that it hurts to move
- States it hurts to hold her baby
- Requests pain medication

Knowledge Deficit
- First-time mother
- Unplanned cesarean birth
- States she does not know how to take care of a baby

Delayed Bonding
- Does not respond to infant cries
- Does not want to hold infant
- Asks nurse to change infant's diapers

Fatigue
- Prolonged labor (36 hours)
- Unplanned cesarean birth
- States she is tired and wants to sleep

Anxiety
- Unplanned cesarean birth due to fetal intolerance to labor
- States she is worried about her baby
- First-time mother

Problem No. 1: Acute Pain

Goal: Minimal pain

Outcome: Woman reports that her pain is controlled at a level at or below 2 on a 10-point scale.

Nursing Actions

1. Assess level, location, and type of pain.
2. Assist woman into a comfortable position.
3. Administer pain medications based on assessment data as per orders.

4. Provide an environment that is conducive to relaxation, i.e., low lights, decreased noise, and uninterrupted rest periods.
5. Teach woman relaxation techniques.
6. Demonstrate position when holding infant that promotes maternal comfort, i.e., woman lying on her side with infant next to her, avoiding external pressure on woman's abdomen.

Problem No. 2: Knowledge Deficit

Goal: Improved knowledge of infant care

Outcome: By time of discharge, mother will state she feels comfortable caring for her infant.

Nursing Actions

1. Assess women's level of knowledge regarding infant care and cesarean births to identify learning needs and level of understanding.
2. Provide information at woman's level of understanding.
3. Create an environment that is conducive of learning, i.e., turn off TV, close door to room, help mother into a comfortable position.
4. Medicate for pain, if needed, prior to teaching sessions to promote comfort.
5. Provide information on infant care, bonding and attachment, and post-cesarean birth recovery during several short teaching sessions.
6. Assist woman with infant care, i.e., bring infant to her so she can change diaper.
7. Praise mother for infant care behaviors.

Problem No. 3: Fatigue
Goal: Increased level of energy
Outcome: Woman states that she feels rested.

Nursing Actions

1. Assess level of fatigue.
2. Create an environment that is conducive to rest and sleep by:
   a. Clustering nursing activities to increase the amount of uninterrupted time
   b. Providing pain management techniques, i.e., pain medications, back rubs
   c. Closing door to room and dimming lights
   d. Assisting woman into comfortable position
3. Explain importance of rest in the healing process.
4. Provide information on high-energy foods.

Problem No. 4: Anxiety
Goal: Decreased level of anxiety
Outcome: Woman states that she feels comfortable holding and caring for infant.

Nursing Actions

1. Assess the woman's beliefs, attitudes, concerns, and questions regarding infant care and mothering.
2. Discuss with the woman her labor and birth experience and clarify reasons for cesarean birth and any misconceptions.
3. Discuss with the woman the health of her infant and address the woman's concerns.
4. Encourage the woman to hold infant by:
   a. Explaining the importance of mother-infant contact
   b. Helping her into a comfortable position
   c. Bringing infant to her.
5. Praise the woman for her infant care behaviors.

TYING IT ALL TOGETHER

As the nurse in the postpartum unit, you are caring for the Sanchez family. Margarite gave birth to a healthy boy 5 hours ago. Both she and her son are stable. She breastfed her son for 15 minutes after the birth.

You notice that she is lightly touching the top of her newborn's head with her fingertips. She comments that she does not feel comfortable holding her baby close to her body for breastfeeding.

Discuss your nursing actions that are based on your knowledge of maternal touch.

List the maternal phase and expected maternal behaviors for this period of time.

List five expected bonding behaviors for this period of time.

The next day you are again assigned to care for the Sanchez family. Mom and baby are stable. José, Margarite's husband, is present during the shift. Margarite and José voice concern about integrating their newborn into the family.

Discuss your nursing actions that reflect an understanding of the couple's transition to parenthood.

Discuss specific strategies to decrease sibling rivalry.

Margarite tells you that she thinks she experienced postpartum depression with her first baby. She tells you that she cried a lot during the first week at home, but was able to care for herself and her newborn.

Discuss the appropriate nursing actions in response to her concerns.

■ ■ ■ Review Questions ■ ■ ■

1. Your postpartum patient is 10 hours post-birth. She experienced an uncomplicated labor and birth and her newborn is full term with Apgar scores of 9 at 1 minute and 9 at 5 minutes. During your assessment, you note that she was hungry and very interested in telling you about her birth experience. You had to remind her to change her baby's diaper and to feed her baby. Based on this assessment you determine that she is:
   A. Having difficulty bonding with her baby
   B. Not concerned about her baby's needs
   C. In the taking-in phase
   D. In the taking-hold phase

2. Your postpartum patient is a 25-year-old, white, single woman who gave birth to a healthy infant. She is 36 hours post-birth. You note that she holds her infant at a distance and refers to her infant as "it." Based on this assessment, your initial nursing actions include:
   A. Obtain referral for a social worker.
   B. Ask the woman to tell you about her pregnancy and childbirth experience.
   C. Teach her the importance of holding her baby close to her body.
   D. Take her baby to the nursery so she can have some uninterrupted sleep.

3. Which 2-day postpartum woman has an abnormal finding that requires intervention?
   A. A 23-year-old Arabic woman who plans to breastfeed but wants to bottle feed her newborn until her milk comes in
   B. A 28-year-old Chinese woman who refuses to take a shower
   C. A 20-year-old Japanese woman who has her mother care for her baby
   D. A 19-year-old Caucasian woman who requests that her baby stay in the nursery so she can sleep

4. You are providing discharge teaching to your patient. In addition to her newborn son, she has a 2-year-old daughter. Which of the following will you include in your teaching? Select all that apply.
   A. Stressing the importance of quality time with her 2-year-old daughter
   B. Instructing the woman to include the 2-year-old in the care of her baby brother
   C. Explaining that all children experience some degree of sibling rivalry
   D. Instructing the woman to explain to her daughter the reasons babies cry

5. Factors that can hamper a couple's transition to parenthood include which of the following? Select all that apply.
   A. First experience with newborns
   B. Change of employment
   C. Adolescent father

6. Factors that influence a man's transition to fatherhood include which of the following? Select all that apply.
   A. Educational level
   B. Cultural expectations
   C. Socioeconomic status
   D. Support from partner

7. Your postpartum assignment includes a 15-year-old first-time mother who gave birth to a healthy baby girl 6 hours ago. The 16-year-old father of the baby was present for the birth and is present while you are caring for the new mother. Which of the following nursing actions are appropriate for this couple? Select all that apply.
   A. Include the new father in infant care teaching sessions.
   B. Ask the new father to tell you about his labor and birth experience.
   C. Include the new father in teaching session on contraception.
   D. Include the new father in teaching session on postpartum blues.

8. You are assigned a hearing impaired first-time mother. When you enter the room, your patient is looking away from you. Which of the following is the most appropriate way to get the woman's attention?
   A. Flick the overhead lights on and off.
   B. Make a loud noise as you enter the room.
   C. Tap the woman on her shoulder.
   D. Walk to her bed and wave your hand.

9. You observe a new father gently touching his newborn son and spending time gazing at his son. These behaviors are characteristics of _____.
   A. Entrainment
   B. Attachment
   C. Engrossment
   D. Bonding

10. Which statements are true regarding coparenting? Select all that apply.
   A. Implies that the parenting roles are equal in the amount of child care responsibilities
   B. Consists of parental figures supporting each other in the rearing of their child
   C. Can be affected by the infant's temperament.
   D. Can be affected by the man's cultural beliefs.

References

Bowlby, J. (1969). *Attachment and loss. Vol. 1. Attachment.* New York: Basic Books.

Chapman, L. (1991). Searching: Expectant fathers' experiences during labor and birth. *Journal of Perinatal Neonatal Nursing, 4,* 21–29.

Clemmens, D. (2003). Adolescent motherhood: A meta-synthesis of qualitative studies. *The American Journal of Maternal Child Nursing, 28,* 93–99.

Davis, E., Schoppe-Sullivan, S., Mangelsdorf, S. and Brown, G. (2009). The role of infant temperament in stability and change in coparenting across the first year of life. *Parenting: Science and Practice, 9,* 143–159.

DeVito, J. (2007). Self-perceptions of parenting among adolescent mothers. *The Journal of Perinatal Education, 16,* 16–23.

Fagan, J., Bernd, E., and Whiteman, V. (2007). Adolescent fathers' parenting stress, social support, and involvement with infants. *Journal of Research on Adolescence, 17,* 1–22.

Feinberg, M. (2003). The internal structure and ecological context of coparenting: A framework for research and intervention. *Parenting: Science and Practice, 3,* 95–131.

Greenberg, M., & Morris, N. (1974). Engrossment: The newborn's impact upon the father. *American Journal of Orthopsychiatry, 44,* 520–531.

Klaus, M., & Kennell, J. (1982). *Parent–infant bonding.* St. Louis, MO: C. V. Mosby.

May, K. (1982). Three phases of father involvement in pregnancy. *Nursing Research, 31,* 337–342.

Mercer, R. (1986). *First-time motherhood.* New York: Springer Publishing.

Mercer, R. (1995). *Becoming a mother: Research from Rubin to the present.* New York: Springer Publishers.

Mercer, R. (1997). Having another child: "She's a multip....she knows the ropes." *Journal of Maternal Child Nursing, 4,* 301–304.

Mercer, R. (2004). Becoming a mother versus maternal role attainment. *Journal of Nursing Scholarship, 36,* 226–232.

Mercer, R. (2006). Nursing support of the process of becoming a mother. *Journal of Obstetric, Gynecologic and Neonatal Nursing, 35,* 649–651.

Paschal, A., Lewis-Moss, R., and Hsiao, T. (2011). Perceived fatherhood roles and parenting behaviors among African American teen fathers. *Journal of Adolescent Research, 26,* 61–83.

Purnell, L., and Paulanka, B. (2008). *Transcultural Health Care.* Philadelphia: F.A. Davis Company.

Rubin, R. (1963a). Maternal touch. *Nursing Outlook, 11,* 828–831.

Rubin, R. (1963b). Puerperal change. *Nursing Outlook, 9,* 753–755.

Rubin, R. (1967). Attainment of the maternal role. Part 1. Processes. *Nursing Research, 16,* 237–346.

Rubin, R. (1984). *Maternal identity and the maternal experience.* New York: Springer Publishing.

White, C., Simon, M., & Bryan, A. (2002). Using evidence to educate birthing center nursing staff about infant states, cues, and behaviors. *Maternal Child Nursing, 27,* 294–298.

High-Risk Postpartum Nursing Care

14

EXPECTED STUDENT OUTCOMES

On completion of this chapter, the student will be able to:
- ☐ Define key terms.
- ☐ Describe the primary causes of postpartum hemorrhage and the related nursing actions and medical care.
- ☐ Describe the primary postpartum infections and the related nursing actions and medical care.
- ☐ Describe the primary postpartum psychological complications and the related nursing actions and medical care.

Nursing Diagnoses

- At risk for hemorrhage related to uterine atony, lacerations, retained placental tissue, or hematoma
- At risk for infection related to tissue trauma or prolonged rupture of membranes
- At risk for mood disorders related to stress, hormonal changes, lack of rest, or lack of social support

Nursing Outcomes

- The woman's fundus will remain firm and lochia within normal ranges.
- The woman will remain free from symptoms of infection.
- The woman will indicate that she feels supported by her family and is getting adequate rest.

INTRODUCTION

Most women do not experience a complication during the postpartum period, but when they do, it can be life threatening and disruptive to the family unit. A majority of complications occur after discharge and may require readmission to the hospital. Most hospitals do not allow the infant to be readmitted with the mother. Thus, readmission to the hospital for treatment of complications can interfere with the attachment process and increase stress within the family unit.

A focus of postpartum nursing care is to reduce women's risks for complications related to childbirth and to identify complications early for prompt interventions (see Critical Component: Risk Reduction for Postpartum Complications). Women need to be evaluated by their health care provider when a complication is suspected.

Hemorrhage, coagulation disorders, and infections are the primary physiological complications. Postpartum depression and postpartum psychosis are the primary psychological complications.

CRITICAL COMPONENT

Risk Reduction for Postpartum Complications

Reducing a woman's risk for postpartum complications is a major component of postpartum nursing care. Nursing actions to reduce risk are:

- Reviewing the prenatal and intrapartal records for risk factors such as anemia, long labor, and operative vaginal delivery and addressing these risk factors in planning care.
- Assessing for signs of a postpartum complication and intervening appropriately.
  - *Early identification and treatment decreases the impact of the complication.*
- Assisting the woman with ambulation.
  - *Ambulation assists in uterine drainage.*
- Preventing overdistended bladder.
  - *Overdistended bladder can place the woman at risk for uterine atony and/or cystitis.*
- Using good hand washing techniques by health care workers, patients, and visitors.
- Promoting health with appropriate diet, fluids, activity, and rest.

Don't have time to read this chapter? Want to reinforce your reading? Need to review for a test?
Listen to this chapter on *DavisPlus*.

Hemorrhage

Hemostasis following the separation of the placenta is affected by the following physiologic changes:

■ Blood volume increases during pregnancy.
■■ *Healthy women can lose 500 mL without adverse effects due to the normal pregnancy blood volume increase of 1,000–2,000 mL or 30% to 60%.*
■ Contractions of the uterine myometrium
■■ *The blood vessels that supply the placental site pass through the myometrium, which is an interlacing network of smooth muscle fibers.*
■■ *Contractions of the myometrium compress the blood vessels at the placental site, thus decreasing the amount of blood loss.*
■ Hypercoagulability during childbirth
■■ *Factor VIII complex increases during labor and birth.*
■■ *Factor V increases following placental separation.*
■■ *Platelet activity increases at delivery.*
■■ *Fibrin formation increases at delivery.*

Postpartum hemorrhage (PPH) is a blood loss greater than 500 mL for vaginal deliveries and 1,000 mL for cesarean deliveries with a 10% drop in hemoglobin and/or hematocrit (Harvey & Dildy, 2013). The primary causes of PPH are uterine atony, retained placental fragments, and lower genital track lacerations (see Critical Component: Indications of Primary PPH and Maternal Vital Signs). It is estimated that 10% of postpartum women will experience a PPH. A major complication of PPH is hemorrhagic shock related to hypovolemia.

Postpartum hemorrhage (PPH) is classified into primary (early) and secondary (late) hemorrhage. Primary PPH occurs within the first 24 hours after childbirth and is due to uterine atony, lacerations, or hematomas. Secondary PPH occurs after 24 hours post-birth and is due to hematomas, subinvolution, or retained placental tissue.

LATE PPH INF *CAUSE*

Risk Factors

■ Neonatal macrosomia: Birth weight greater than 4,000 grams
■ Polyhydramnios
■ High parity
■ Prior PPH
■ Operative vaginal delivery: Use of forceps or vacuum extractor
■ Augmented or induced labor
■ Ineffective uterine contractions during labor: Prolonged first and second stage of labor
■ Precipitous labor and/or birth
■ Chorioamnionitis
■ Maternal obesity
■ Congenital or acquired coagulation defects

CRITICAL COMPONENT

Maternal Vital Signs

"Careful assessment and interpretation of maternal vital signs are critical in patient care during active bleeding. Obstetric patients, however, may not show signs and symptoms usually observed in non-pregnant patients with hemorrhage until approximately one-third of the woman's entire blood volume is lost" (Harvey & Dildy, 2013, pp. 249 and 251).

CRITICAL COMPONENT

Indications of Primary PPH

■ A 10% decrease in the hemoglobin and/or hematocrit post-birth
■ Saturation of the peripad within 15 minutes
■ A fundus that remains boggy after fundal massage
■ Tachycardia (late sign)
■ Decrease in blood pressure (late sign)

Uterine Atony

Uterine atony, a decreased tone of the uterine muscle, is the major cause of primary PPH. Uterine contractions constrict the open vessels at the placental site and assist in decreasing the amount of blood loss. When the uterus is relaxed, the vessels are less constricted and the woman experiences an increase of blood loss.

Assessment Findings

■ Soft (boggy) fundus versus firm fundus
■ Saturation of the peripad within 15 minutes
■ Bleeding is slow and steady or sudden and massive
■ Blood clots may be present
■ Pale color and clammy skin
■ Anxiety and confusion
■ Tachycardia
■ Hypotension

Medical Management

■ Bimanual compression of the uterus (**Fig. 14-1**)
■ Medications: Oxytocin, methylergonovine, and carboprost to stimulate uterine contractions
■■ *Dinoprostone and misoprostol may be ordered but are not FDA approved for treatment of uterine atony.*
■ IV therapy to reduce risk of hypovolemia
■■ *Isotonic, non-dextrose crystalloid solutions (normal saline or lactated Ringer's solution)*
■■ *A ratio of 3 to 1: 3 liters of IV solution for each liter of estimated blood loss*
■■ *Blood replacement to reduce risk for hemorrhagic shock*
■ Platelet transfusion and fibrinogen replacement in management of massive obstetric hemorrhagic shock

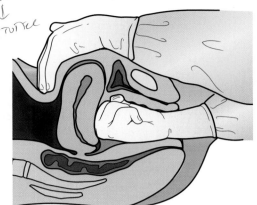

mother-nurse *if hemorrhage PP*
↓ *fluids (polyvolemia)*
oxytocin
↓
cytotec

Figure 14–1 Bimanual compression of the uterus.

■ Non-surgical interventions such as uterine packing with gauze or uterine tamponade

　■ *Uterine tamponade: A 24F Foley catheter with a 30 mL balloon is inserted into the uterus via the vagina. The catheter balloon is filled with 60 to 80 mL of saline, causing pressure on vessels at placental site.*

■ Surgical interventions such as hysterectomy may be indicated when all other treatments have failed to contract the uterus.

Nursing Actions (see Critical Component: Management of Uterine Atony)

■ Review prenatal and intrapartal records for risk factor for PPH and monitor more frequently women who are at risk for uterine atony. *(p 358)*

■ Assess for a displaced uterus. An overdistention of the bladder can displace the uterus and cause it to relax. When uterus is displaced:

　■ *Assist the woman to the bathroom to void, then reassess the location and firmness of the fundus and the amount and characteristics of the lochia.*

　■ *Catheterize the woman if she is unable to void or is experiencing small, frequent voidings.*

■ Assess the fundus for degree of firmness. If boggy:

　■ *Massage uterus and reassess (Fig. 14-2).* #1 ACTUAL

　■ *Put baby to breast to initiate release of oxytocin.*

■ Assess lochia for amount and for clots.

　■ *Express clots: Clots can interfere with uterine contraction.*

　■ *Weigh bloodied pads and linens to obtain an accurate amount of blood loss: 1 mL of blood = 1 gram.*

■ Review laboratory tests such as hemoglobin and hematocrit (H & H).

■ Notify physician or midwife of assessment findings and abnormal test results.

■ Establish IV site with large-bore intracatheter.

■ Administer oxytocin, methylergonovine, and/or carboprost to stimulate uterine contractions as per orders.

■ Start and monitor blood transfusions as per orders and protocol.

■ Provide emotional support and teaching to both the woman and her support system, as PPH increases the anxiety and stress levels of the woman and her family.

CRITICAL COMPONENT

Management of Uterine Atony

■ Fundal massage is the first action to initiate when the uterus is midline and boggy (**Fig. 14-2**).

■ The physician or midwife is notified when the fundus does not respond to fundal massage.

■ Oxytocin therapy is initiated as per orders.

　■ An IV is started with 1,000 mL of Ringer's lactate solution with 20–40 units of oxytocin added as per orders; and

　■ 14 G or 16 G intracatheters are used for IV and blood access.

　■ The IV infusion rate is started at 10 mL/min (200 mU/min) and regulated by the firmness of the fundus (You & Zahn, 2006).

■ If bleeding continues, methylergonovine or carboprost is administered as per order.

Medication

Methylergonovine (Methergine)

■ Indication: PPH due to uterine atony or subinvolution

■ Action: Stimulates contraction of the uterine smooth muscle

■ Common side effects: Nausea, vomiting, and cramps.

■ Route and dose: IM or IV; 200 mcg every 2–4 hours (only one IV dose)

■ Precaution: Check blood pressure before injection; if elevated, do not give until the physician or midwife has been notified. Use with caution with women who have PPH. This medication can increase the blood pressure.

(Data from Vallerand & Sanoski, 2013)

Medication

Carboprost Tromethamine (Hemabate)

■ Indication: PPH that has not responded to oxytocin or methylergonovine therapy

■ Action: Uterine contractions

■ Common side effects: Diarrhea, nausea, vomiting, and fever

■ Route and dosage: IM; 250 mcg, which can be repeated every 15 to 90 minutes. Total dose should not exceed 2 mg.

(Data from Vallerand & Sanoski, 2013)

Lacerations

Lacerations, which are the second most common cause of primary PPH, can occur during childbirth. Common sites are the cervix, vagina, labia, and perineum.

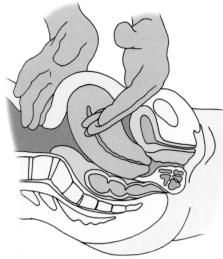

Figure 14–2 Fundal massage.

Risk Factors

- Fetal macrosomia
- Operative vaginal delivery: Use of forceps or vacuum extraction
- Precipitous labor and/or birth → UN ATTENDED

Assessment Findings

- A firm uterus that is midline with heavier than normal bleeding
- Bleeding is usually a steady stream without clots.
- Tachycardia
- Hypotension (Higgins, 2004)

Medical Management

- Visual inspection of cervix, vagina, perineum, and labia
- Surgical repair of laceration

IV PAIN MED BEFORE EXAM

Nursing Actions

- Review labor and birth records for possible risk factors and monitor more frequently women who are at higher risk for lacerations.
- Monitor vital signs.
- Monitor blood loss.
  - *Weigh bloodied pads and linens to obtain accurate amount of blood loss: 1 mL of blood = 1 gram.*
- Notify the physician or midwife of increased bleeding with a firm fundus.
- Administer medications for pain management as per order.
- Prepare the woman for a pelvic examination.
- Provide emotional support to the woman and her family.

Hematomas

Hematomas occur when blood collects within the connective tissues of the vagina or perineal areas related to a vessel that ruptures and continues to bleed (**Fig. 14-3**). It is difficult to

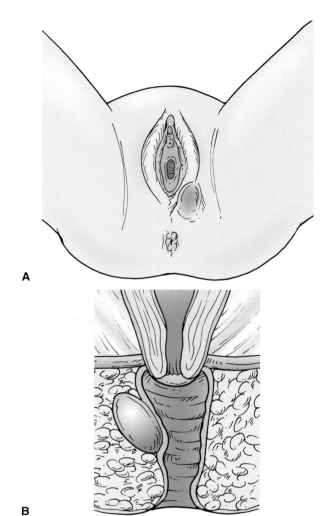

A

B

Figure 14–3 *A.* Vulvar hematoma. *B.* Vaginal wall hematoma.

determine the degree of blood loss since the blood is retained within the tissue; thus, PPH may not be diagnosed until the woman is in hypovolemic shock.

Risk Factors

- Episiotomy is the major risk factor (You & Zahn, 2006)
- Use of forceps
- Prolonged second stage (HEAD PRESSURE) — △ POSITIONS

Assessment Findings

- Women express severe pain in the vagina/perineal area, and the intensity of pain cannot be controlled by standard postpartum pain management.
- Presence of tachycardia and hypotension.
- Hematomas that are located in the vagina cannot be visualized by the nurse. When located in the vaginal area, women will express severe pain, a heaviness or fullness in the vagina, and/or rectal pressure.
- Hematomas in the perineal area present with swelling, discoloration, and tenderness.

■ Hematomas with an accumulation of 200 to 500 mL can become large enough to displace the uterus and cause uterine atony, which can increase the degree of blood loss. *HRT BP ↓, UNILATERAL SWELL*

Medical Management

■ Small hematomas are evaluated and monitored without surgical intervention.
■ Large hematomas are surgically excised and the blood evacuated. The open vessel is identified and ligated.
  ■ *Women experience immediate relief from pain once the blood has been evacuated.* *I + D INCISION + DRAINAGE*

Nursing Actions

■ Review the chart for risk factors and monitor more frequently women who are at risk for a hematoma.
■ Apply ice to the perineum for the first 24 hours to decrease the risk of hematoma. *NOT TREATMENT*
■ Assess the degree of pain by use of a pain scale.
■ Severe vaginal/perineal pain is a primary symptom of hematomas.
■ Ask women who indicate either verbally or nonverbally an increase of pain if they are experiencing any heaviness or fullness in their vaginal or rectal areas.
■ Monitor for decrease in blood pressure and an increase in pulse rate.
■ Administer prescribed analgesia for pain management.
■ Review laboratory reports such as H & H: A decrease in H & H may be an indication of blood loss.
■ Notify the physician or midwife of nursing assessment findings for further evaluation.
■ Provide emotional support and teaching to both the woman and her family, as increasing pain can increase the anxiety and stress levels of the woman and her family.

Subinvolution of the Uterus

Subinvolution of the uterus is a term used when the uterus does not decrease in size and does not descend into the pelvis. This usually occurs later in the postpartum period. Before the diagnosis of subinvolution, the uterus and lochia had been undergoing normal involution.

Risk Factors

■ Fibroids → *METHERGINE*
■ Metritis
■ Retained placental tissue

Assessment Findings

■ The uterus is soft and larger than normal for the days postpartum.
■ Lochia returns to the rubra stage and can be heavy.
■ Back pain is present.

Medical Management

■ Ultrasound evaluation to identify intrauterine tissue or subinvolution of the placental site (ACOG, 2006).

■ Medical intervention depends on the cause of the subinvolution.
  ■ *A dilation and curettage (D&C) is performed for retained placental tissue.*
  ■ *Methergine PO is prescribed for fibroids.*
  ■ *Antibiotic therapy is initiated for metritis.*

Nursing Actions

■ Review prenatal and labor records for risk factors.
■ Monitor women who are at risk for subinvolution of the uterus more frequently.
■ Patient education is the primary action, as PPH from subinvolution usually occurs after discharge.
  ■ *Provide education on involution and signs to report, such as increased bleeding, clots, or a change in the lochia to bright red bleeding.*
  ■ *Provide education on ways to reduce risk for infection, such as changing peripads frequently, hand washing, nutrition, adequate fluid intake, and adequate rest.*
  ■ *Explain to women who have fibroids that they are at risk for subinvolution. Provide instruction on the proper use of discharge medication, since these women are usually discharged with an order for Methergine PO.*

Retained Placental Tissue

Retained placental tissue is the primary cause of secondary postpartum hemorrhage. It occurs when small portions of the placenta, referred to as cotyledons, remain attached to the uterus during the third stage of labor. The retained placental tissue can interfere with involution of the uterus and can lead to metritis. *COMMON CAUSE PPH*

Risk Factor

■ Manual removal of the placenta

Assessment Findings

■ Profuse bleeding that suddenly occurs after the first postpartum week
■ Subinvolution of the uterus
■ Elevated temperature and uterine tenderness if metritis is present *ENDO*
■ Pale skin color
■ Tachycardia
■ Hypotension

Medical Management

■ D&C is performed to remove retained placental tissue.
■ IV antibiotic therapy may be prescribed because of the increased risk for metritis.

Nursing Actions

■ Patient education is a primary intervention, as PPH from retained placental fragment usually occurs after discharge.
  ■ *Instruct women to report to their health care provider any sudden increase in lochia, bright red bleeding, elevated temperature, or uterine tenderness.*

Nursing Actions Following a PPH

- Assess the fundus and lochia every hour for first 4 hours and PRN after hemorrhage.
- Assess orthostatic vital signs.
- Instruct the woman on how to assess the fundus and how to do fundal massage, and the signs of PPH that should be reported to the health care provider.
- Increase oral and IV fluid intake to decrease risk of hypovolemia.
- Explain the importance of preventing an overdistended bladder to reduce the risk for further PPH.
- Assist with ambulation since there is an increase of orthostatic hypotension related to blood loss.
- Explain the importance of rest to decrease the risk of fatigue related to blood loss.
- Provide uninterrupted rest periods while in the hospital.
- Provide an opportunity for the woman and her support system to talk about their feelings and experiences with PPH, as this experience can cause feelings of fear, anxiety, and stress.
- Provide information on foods high in iron and the importance of eating a high-iron diet to decrease the risk of anemia.
- Review the H&H laboratory report. Notify the physician or CNM of abnormal results.

COAGULATION DISORDERS

A variety of complications can occur during the postpartum period related to alterations in the clotting mechanisms. Three of these complications are disseminated intravascular coagulation, amniotic fluid embolism, and thrombosis.

Disseminated Intravascular Coagulation

Disseminated intravascular coagulation (DIC) is a syndrome in which the coagulation pathways are hyperstimulated (Venes, 2009). When this occurs, the woman's body breaks down blood clots faster than it can form them, thus quickly depleting the body of clotting factors and leading to hemorrhage and death.

- DIC is a complication of an underlying pathological process, i.e., amniotic fluid embolism.
- Women who experience DIC are transferred to critical care units, and a perinatologist, when available, manages the care.

Risk Factors

SEPSIS

- Abruptio placenta   *PROLONGED PTL*
  - This is the primary cause of DIC.
- HELLP syndrome
- Amniotic fluid embolism (Cunningham et al., 2010)
  HTN PIH INDUCED

Assessment Findings

- Prolonged, uncontrolled uterine bleeding
- Bleeding from the IV site, incision site, gums, and bladder

NURSE TRICK

- Purpuric areas at pressure sites, such as blood pressure cuff site
- Abnormal clotting study results, such as platelets and activated partial thromboplastin time (PPT)
- Increased anxiety
- Signs and symptoms of shock related to blood loss:
  - *Pale and clammy skin*
  - *Tachycardia*
  - *Tachypnea*
  - *Hypotension*

Medical Management

The focus of medical management is on optimizing hemodynamic function and improving overall tissue oxygenation while identifying and eliminating the underlying pathology (Cunningham et al., 2010; Sisson & Mann, 2013).

- Laboratory tests (e.g., fibrinogen levels, prothrombin time [PT], partial thromboplastin time [PTT], and platelet count) to assess for abnormal clotting. *BEST INDICATOR*
- Identification of the primary cause of bleeding and intervention based on this knowledge
- IV therapy
- Blood replacement
- Platelet transfusion
- Fresh frozen plasma
- Oxygen therapy

Nursing Actions

- Reduce risk of DIC.
  - *Review prenatal and labor records for risk factors.*
  - *Monitor women more frequently who are at risk for DIC.*
  - *Assess for PPH and intervene appropriately. Early intervention can decrease the risk of DIC.*
  - *Monitor vital signs and immediately report to the MD or CNM abnormal findings, such as an increase in heart rate, a decrease in blood pressure, and a change in quality of respirations.*
- Obtain IV site with large-bore intracatheter as per orders.
  - *Administer IV fluids as per orders.*
- Administer oxygen as per orders.
- Obtain laboratory specimens as per orders.
- Review laboratory results and notify the physician of results.
- Start a blood transfusion as per orders.
- Provide emotional support and information to the woman and her family to decrease level of anxiety.
- Facilitate transfer to intensive care unit.

Amniotic Fluid Embolism

Amniotic fluid embolism (AFE), also referred to as anaphylactoid syndrome of pregnancy, is a rare but often fatal complication that occurs during pregnancy, labor and birth, and the first 24 hours post-birth. Amniotic fluid that contains fetal cells, lanugo, and vernix enters the maternal vascular system and initiates a cascading process that leads to cardiorespiratory collapse and disseminated intravascular coagulation (DIC).

The process that causes the fluid to enter into the maternal vascular system is not clearly understood.

- Areas of potential entry points of amniotic fluid are:
  - *Cervix following rupture of amniotic membranes.*
  - *Site of placental separation.*
  - *Site of uterine trauma—lacerations that occur during the labor and delivery process (Jones & Clark, 2013).*
- AFE is a two-stage process (**Table 14-1**).
- Women with AFE usually die within 1 hour of onset of symptoms.
- It is estimated that there is one case per 8,000 to 30,000 pregnancies (Moore, 2012).

Risk Factors

Numerous risk factors, such as induction of labor, abruptio placenta, and placenta previa, have been postulated, but there are no reliable risk factors that predict AFE (Jones & Clark, 2013).

Assessment Findings

- Dyspnea
- Seizures
- Hypotension
- Cyanosis
- Cardiopulmonary arrest
- Uterine atony that causes massive hemorrhage and leads to disseminated intravascular coagulation (DIC)
- Cardiac and respiratory arrest

Medical Management

- There are no scientific data to support any intervention that improves maternal prognosis with AFE (Cunningham et al., 2010).
- The focus is on maintaining cardiac and respiratory function, stopping the hemorrhage, and correcting blood loss.
- Complete blood count (CBC), platelet count, arterial blood gases, fibrinogen, and PT are a few of the laboratory tests that might be ordered.
- Blood type and screen for possible transfusion.

- Chest x-ray exam
- Blood replacement, packed red blood cells, and platelets.
- Transfer the woman to the critical care unit.
- A heart-lung bypass machine, when available, may be used to help stabilize the woman.

Nursing Actions

- Monitor for signs of AFE. (NEW CARDIO, BREATHING TROUBLE)
- Notify the physician, immediately, of assessment data, so that early interventions can be initiated.
- Administer oxygen.
- Establish 2 IV sites with large-bore intracatheters: one for IV fluid replacement and one for blood replacement.
- Obtain laboratory specimens as per orders.
- Administer blood replacement as per order.
- Provide emotional support to the woman and her support system.
- Call code and initiate CPR when indicated.
- Facilitate transfer to intensive care unit (Kramer, Rouleau, Baskett, & Joseph, 2006; Schoening, 2006).

Thrombosis

PMH = HYPER COAGULATORY STATE → TRANES TO HEPARIN 6w

Thrombosis is a blood clot within the vascular system. During pregnancy and the first 6 weeks post-birth, women are at risk for forming blood clots. This is related to the normal physiological changes that occur during pregnancy. During pregnancy, there is an increase in clotting factors I, II, VII, IX, X, and XII, as well as an increase in fibrinogen. These components of clotting remain elevated during the postpartum period.

- Thrombosis during pregnancy and/or the postpartum period usually occurs in a vein of the legs and is referred to as a deep vein thrombosis (DVT).
- A major concern is that the clot will detach, becoming an embolism, and travel to a vital organ; an example is a pulmonary embolism.
- Nursing actions focus on decreasing the risk for formation of thrombosis and risk of embolism.

Risk Factors

- Normal physiological changes in coagulation related to pregnancy
- Cesarean birth, which has a risk five times greater than vaginal birth
- Metritis, which can spread to the vascular system, causing thrombophlebitis, and can lead to thrombosis
- Decreased mobility, which increases the risk for venous stasis
- Obesity, which places extra pressure on pelvic vessels, causing venous stasis

Assessment Findings

- Tenderness and heat over the affected area
- Leg pain with walking
- Swelling in the affected leg

TABLE 14–1	AMNIOTIC FLUID EMBOLISM: A TWO-STAGE PROCESS
Stage 1	
Amniotic fluid and fetal cells enter the maternal circulation → release of endogenous mediators → pulmonary vasospasm and pulmonary hypotension → elevated right ventricular pressure and hypoxia → myocardial and pulmonary capillary damage → left heart failure and acute respiratory distress	
Stage 2	
Hemorrhage and DIC	
Schoening, 2006	

Medical Management

- Doppler ultrasonography to confirm the diagnosis
- Coagulation therapy of IV heparin and warfarin
- Antibiotic therapy if thrombosis is related to infection
- Bed rest with the affected leg elevated
- Compression stockings

Nursing Actions

- Review prenatal and labor records for risk factors.
- Monitor women who are at greater risk for thrombosis more frequently.
- Apply compression stockings as per orders; compression stockings reduce venous stasis and risk of DVT.
- Assist with ambulation. Early ambulation increases circulation and decreases the risk of venous stasis.
- Report assessment finding of possible signs of thrombosis to the physician or CNM for further evaluation.
- Administer medications as per orders.
- Provide discharge teaching regarding use of heparin and/or warfarin.

INFECTIONS

It is estimated that 1% to 8% of postpartum women will experience a postpartum infection (Wong, 2012). It is also estimated that 0.6 maternal deaths per 100,000 live births are attributed to postpartum infections (Wong, 2012). The most common sites for infections during the postpartum period are the uterus, bladder, breast, and incisional site. Most infections that occur during the postpartum period can be easily treated when identified at an early stage. Infections that are not identified and treated at an early stage can lead to serious complications such as abscess formation, cellulitis, thrombophlebitis, and septic shock (see Critical Component: Postpartum Infections: Risk Reduction).

CRITICAL COMPONENT

Postpartum Infections: Risk Reduction

- Good hand washing techniques by staff and patients
- Fluid intake of a minimum 3,000 mL per day, to rehydrate the woman from fluid loss during labor and birth
- Diet high in protein and vitamin C to assist in tissue healing
- Early ambulation to promote circulation and uterine drainage

---

Metritis

Metritis is the most common postpartum infection. It is an infection of the endometrium, myometrium, and/or parametrial tissue that usually starts at the placental site and spreads to encompass the entire endometrium. Approximately 2% of women who experience a vaginal birth and 15% of women who experience a cesarean birth develop metritis.

Risk Factors

- Cesarean birth: Primary risk factor
- Prolonged rupture of membranes
- Prolonged labor
- Internal fetal and uterine monitoring
- Meconium-stained fluid
- Multiple cervical exams during labor
- Obesity

Assessment Findings

- Elevated temperature greater than 38°C (100.4°F) with or without chills
- Lower abdominal pain or discomfort
- Uterine tenderness
- Tachycardia
- Subinvolution
- Malaise
- Lower abdominal pain or discomfort
- Lochia heavy and foul smelling when anaerobic organisms are present
  - *Foul smelling lochia is a later sign that occurs when the entire endometrium is involved.*
- Lochia is scant and odorless when beta-hemolytic *Streptococcus* is present.

Medical Management

- CBC to assess for leukocytosis (white blood cell [WBC] count >20,000/mm³).
- Endometrial cultures
- Blood cultures
- Urinalysis to rule out urinary tract infection, which can present with similar symptoms
- Antibiotic therapy
  - *Mild cases: Oral antibiotic therapy*
  - *Moderate to severe cases: IV antibiotic therapy, which is discontinued after the woman is afebrile for 24 hours.*
  - *Improvement should be noted within 72 hours of initiation of antibiotic therapy.*

Nursing Actions

- Reduce risk of metritis:
  - *Educate the woman regarding proper hand washing techniques to reduce spread of bacteria.*
  - *Instruct the woman in proper pericare and to wipe front to back. Instruct woman to change her peripads every 3 to 4 hours or sooner because lochia is a medium for bacterial growth.*
  - *Encourage early ambulation by explaining how ambulation reduces the risk of infection by promoting uterine drainage.*
  - *Encourage intake of fluids to rehydrate by explaining to the woman that maintaining adequate hydration can reduce her risk for infections. Woman should have a minimum fluid intake of 3,000 mL/day (James, 2008).*
  - *Educate the woman on a diet high in protein and vitamin C, which aids in tissue healing.*

■ Monitor for signs and symptoms of metritis.
  ■ *Report assessment data of possible metritis and abnormal laboratory reports to physician and/or midwife for further evaluation.*
■ Administer antibiotics as per orders.
■ Provide pain management measures.
■ Provide emotional support to the woman and her family.
■ Discharge teaching
  ■ *Provide teaching on discharge medications.*
  ■ *Provide information on signs and symptoms to report to health care provider.*

Cystitis

Cystitis, an infection of the bladder, is a common occurrence in the postpartum period. Cystitis is easily treated, but if left untreated or if there is a delay in treatment, the woman is at risk for pyelonephritis.

Risk Factors

■ Epidural anesthesia, which decreases the woman's ability to feel the urge to void, leading to an increased risk for an overdistended bladder
■ Overdistended bladder or incomplete emptying of the bladder, which can cause an increase of bacterial growth in the bladder
■ A Foley catheter inserted during the labor process
■ Neonatal macrosomia, which can cause edema around the urethra
■ Operative vaginal deliveries, forceps, or vacuum extractor, which can cause edema around the urethra
■ Intrapartal vaginal exams and the birth process, which can contaminate the urethra with bacteria

Assessment Findings

■ Low-grade fever (< 38.5°C/101.3°F)
■ Burning on urination
■ Suprapubic pain
■ Urgency to void
■ Small, frequent voidings—less than 150 mL per voiding

Medical Management

■ Urinalysis, CBC, and urine culture and sensitivity
■ Antibiotics (usually PO) started before culture results

Nursing Actions

■ Risk reduction for cystitis
  ■ *Assist the woman to the bathroom to void within a few hours after birth. This will flush bacteria out of the urethra.*
  ■ *Catheterize the woman if she is unable to void within 12 hours post-birth as per orders.*
  ■ *Remind the woman to void every 3–4 hours; woman may not feel urge to void during the first 24–48 hours following birth.*
  ■ *Measure voidings for the first 24 hours, assessing for complete emptying of the bladder. Each voiding should be equal to or greater than 150 mL.*
  ■ *Change peripads at least every 3–4 hours. Soiled peripads can encourage growth of bacteria that can enter the urethra.*

  ■ *Remind postpartum women to drink a minimum of 3,000 mL/day (AWHONN, 2006).*
  ■ *Encourage foods that increase acidity in urine, such as cranberry juice, apricots, and plums.*
■ Monitor for signs and symptoms of cystitis.
  ■ *Report findings of possible urinary tract infection (UTI) to the physician or CNM for further evaluation.*
■ Obtain laboratory specimens as per orders.
■ Administer antibiotics as per orders.
■ Discharge teaching
  ■ *Provide information on proper use of discharge medications.*
  ■ *Provide information on signs and symptoms of cystitis to report to the health care provider.*

Mastitis

Mastitis is an inflammation/infection of the breast that is common among lactating women. It usually occurs in just one of the breasts and within the first 2 postpartum weeks after milk flow has been established. Infection resolves within 24–48 hours of antibiotic therapy. Abscess formation can occur in 10% of women who develop mastitis.

Risk Factors

■ History of mastitis with a previous infant
■ Cracked and/or sore nipples
■ Use of antifungal nipple cream, which is often applied when the newborn has thrush.

Assessment Findings

■ A hard, tender palpable mass
■ Redness in the area around the mass
■ Acute pain in affected breast
■ Temperature elevation
■ Tachycardia
■ Malaise
■ Purulent drainage

Medical Management

■ Culture of expressed milk from affected breast
■ Oral antibiotics therapy for 10–14 days

Nursing Actions

■ Risk reduction
  ■ *Explain to the woman the importance of washing her hands before feeding to decrease spread of bacteria.*
  ■ *Proper hand washing technique by hospital personnel*
  ■ *Teach the woman methods to decrease nipple irritation and tissue breakdown, such as correct infant latch on and removal from the breast, and air-drying nipples after feedings (refer to Chapter 16 for additional information).*
  ■ *Teach the woman the importance of a healthy diet and adequate fluids to decrease risk for any infection.*
■ Palpate and inspect the breasts for signs of mastitis.
  ■ *Report assessment data of possible mastitis to physician or CNM.*
■ Administer antibiotics as per orders.
■ Administer analgesia as per orders.

- Apply warm compresses to the affected area for comfort and promotion of circulation.
- Instruct the woman to continue to breastfeed or to massage and express milk from the affected breast to promote continuation of milk flow.
- Explain to the woman that it is very common for lactating women to experience mastitis and that it is easily treated when identified early.

Wound Infections

Wound infections can occur at the episiotomy site, cesarean incision site, and laceration site.

Risk Factors

- Obesity
- Diabetes
- Malnutrition
- Long labor
- Premature rupture of membranes
- Preexisting infection
- Immunodeficiency disorders
- Corticosteroid therapy
- Poor suturing technique

Assessment Findings

- Erythema
- Redness
- Heat
- Swelling
- Tenderness
- Purulent drainage
- Low-grade fever
- Increased pain at incision or laceration site

Medical Management

- Obtain a culture specimen from the wound or laceration.
- For mild to moderate wound infections that do not have purulent drainage:
  - *Administer oral antibiotic therapy.*
  - *Apply warm compresses to area.*
- Wound infections with purulent drainage:
  - *Open and drain the wound.*
  - *IV antibiotic therapy.*

Nursing Actions

- Assess perineum or surgical incision for REEDA. Inform physician or midwife of abnormal assessment data.
- Assess vital signs.
- Obtain laboratory specimens such as cultures as per orders.
- Review laboratory reports and notify the physician or midwife of abnormal results.
- Administer antibiotics as per orders.
- Pain management
  - *Administer analgesia for fever and discomfort as per order.*
  - *Apply hot packs for abdominal wounds or sitz bath for perineal wounds to promote comfort and circulation.*
- Use proper hand washing technique before and after contact with the wound.

- Provide education on proper diet, fluids, and rest that can decrease the risk for infection and assist in the healing process.
- Provide information on proper use of discharge medications.

POSTPARTUM PSYCHOLOGICAL COMPLICATIONS

A women's psychological state is affected during the postpartum period by hormonal changes, lack of sleep, and stress of integrating a new person within the woman's life and within the family unit. A majority of women will experience postpartum blues, which are short term and require no medical intervention (see Chapter 13). Approximately 15% of women will experience major mood disorders that have a profound effect on their ability to care for themselves and/or their infants. Mood disorders during the first year after childbirth have a negative effect on the mother-infant relationship (AWHONN, 2006). Two major mood disorders are postpartum depression and postpartum psychosis. These disorders require management by mental health care professionals. The primary role of the perinatal nurse is assessing for early signs of potential mood disorders and reporting these findings to the woman's health care provider for further evaluation and treatment.

Evidence-Based Practice: Mother/Infant Skin-to-Skin Contact

Bigelow, A., Power, M., MacLellan-Peters, J., Alex, M., and McDonald, C. (2012). Effects of mother/infant skin-to-skin contact on postpartum depressive symptoms and maternal physiological stress. *JOGNN, 41,* 369–382.

The purpose of this longitudinal quasi-experimental study was to examine the effects of mother/infant skin-to-skin contact (SSC) on the mothers' postpartum depressive symptoms during the first 3 postpartum months and their physiological stress during the first postpartum month.

The study included 30 mothers in the SSC group and 60 mothers in the control group. Mothers in the SSC group provided 5 hours per day of SSC with their infants in the first week postpartum and then more than 2 hours per day until infants were age 1 month. Mothers in the control group provided little or no SSC.

Mothers completed self-reported depression scales at 1 week, 1 month, 2 months, and 3 months of infant age. Salivary samples were collected and assayed for cortisol.

Results: Mothers in the SSC group had lower scores on the depression scales at 1 week and 1 month. There was no significant difference at 2 and 3 months. During the first 4 weeks the SSC mothers had a greater reduction in their salivary cortisol than mothers in the control group.

Conclusion: Mother/infant SSC benefits mothers by reducing their depressive symptoms and physiological stress during the first postpartum month.

Postpartum Depression

Postpartum depression (PPD) is a mood disorder characterized by severe depression that occurs within the first 6–12 months postpartum. PPD is classified as a major depressive disorder when the woman has a depressed mood or a loss of interest or pleasure in daily activities for at least 2 weeks plus four of the following symptoms:

- *Significant weight loss or gain: a change of more than 5% of body weight in a month*
- *Insomnia or hypersomnia*
- *Changes in psychomotor activity: agitation or retardation*
- *Decreased energy or fatigue*
- *Feelings of worthlessness or guilt*
- *Decreased ability to concentrate; inability to make decisions*
- *Recurrent thoughts of death or suicide attempt (American Psychiatric Association, 1994)*

- It is estimated that this occurs in 14.5% of postpartum women (AWHONN, 2008).
- PPD has an effect on the woman, her partner, and other children within the family unit.
- A major difference between postpartum blues and PPD is that PPD is disabling; the woman is unable to safely care for herself and/or her baby (**Table 14-2**).
- Women who receive proper treatment will recover from PPD, but they grieve over the lost time with their infants (AWHONN, 2006).

Risk Factors

- History of depression before pregnancy
- Depression or anxiety during pregnancy
- Inadequate social support
- Poor quality relationship with partner
- Life and child care stresses
- Complications of pregnancy and/or childbirth

Assessment Findings

- Sleep and appetite disturbance
- Fatigue greater than expected for caring for a newborn
- Despondency
- Uncontrolled crying
- Anxiety, fear, and/or panic
- Inability to concentrate
- Feelings of guilt, inadequacy, and/or worthlessness
- Inability to care for self and/or baby
- Decreased affectionate contact with the infant

TABLE 14–2	MAJOR DIFFERENCES BETWEEN POSTPARTUM BLUES AND POSTPARTUM DEPRESSION	
POSTPARTUM BLUES	**POSTPARTUM DEPRESSION**
Symptoms disappear without medical intervention.	Requires psychiatric interventions.
Occurs within the first 2 weeks postpartum.	Occurs within the first 12 months postpartum.
Able to safely care for self and baby.	Unable to safely care for self and/or baby.

- Decreased responsiveness to the infant
- Thoughts of harming baby
- Thoughts of suicide

Medical/Psychiatric Management

- Mild PPD
  - *Interpersonal psychotherapy (Yonkers et al., 2011)*
- Moderate PPD
  - *Interpersonal psychotherapy*
  - *Antidepressants (Yonkers et al., 2011)*
- Severe PPD or suicidal ideation
  - *Intense psychiatric care*
  - *Crisis interventions*
  - *Interpersonal psychotherapy*
  - *Antidepressants*
  - *Electroconvulsive therapy (Yonkers et al., 2011)*

Nursing Actions

- Review prenatal record for risk factors.
- Monitor mother-infant interactions more closely for women at risk for PPD.
- Teach the woman and her partner signs of PPD that should be reported to her health care provider.
- Be supportive and encouraging in interactions.
- Provide the woman with information regarding postpartum support groups and other community resources to assist her with parenting issues and to provide support.
  - *Postpartum support by health care professionals can mitigate the onset of postpartum mood disorders (Yonkers, 2011).*

Postpartum Psychosis

Postpartum psychosis (PPP) is a variant of bipolar disorder and is the most serious form of postpartum mood disorders. This is a rare postpartum mood disorder that occurs in 1–2 women per 1,000 births (AWHONN, 2006). Onset of symptoms can be as early as the third postpartum day. Women with PPP require immediate hospitalization and evaluation, as they are at risk for injuring themselves or their infants.

Risk Factors

- Women with known bipolar disorder
- Personal or family history of bipolar disorder (Sit, Rotherschild, & Wisner, 2006)

Assessment Findings

- Paranoia, grandiose or bizarre delusions usually associated with the baby
- Mood swings
- Extreme agitation
- Depressed or elated moods
- Distraught feelings about ability to enjoy infant
- Confused thinking
- Strange beliefs, such as that she or her infant must die
- Disorganized behavior (Engqvist et al., 2009; Sit et al., 2006)

Medical/Psychiatric Management

- Hospitalization to the psychiatric unit
- Psychiatric evaluation
- Antidepressant and antipsychotic drug treatment
- Psychotherapy
- Electroconvulsive therapy

Nursing Actions

- Review the prenatal record for risk factors.
- Educate women who are at risk and their support system of early signs of PPP, such as mood swings, hallucinations, and strange beliefs, and instruct them to contact the health care provider if symptoms are present.
  - *Early detection and treatment can prevent a major episode (Born, 2004).*

Paternal Postnatal Depression

The majority of new fathers experience feelings of happiness and excitement, but some will experience depression. Paternal postnatal depression (PPND) is estimated to occur in 1%–8% of new fathers during the first 6 months following childbirth (see Critical Component: Paternal Postnatal Depression [PPND]).

- During the first few months of postpartum, the man's testosterone levels decrease and estrogen levels increase.
  - *Lower levels of testosterone are linked with depression in men.*
- Signs and symptoms are not as apparent as they are with maternal PPD.
  - *The man may withdraw from social interactions.*
  - *The man may be cynical in his interactions and experience irritable moods.*

PROFESSIONAL POSITION STATEMENT: AWHONN POSITION STATEMENT ON THE ROLE OF THE NURSE IN POSTPARTUM MOOD AND ANXIETY DISORDERS

Position

Health care facilities that serve pregnant women, new mothers, and newborns should have routine screening protocols and educational mechanisms for staff training and client education related to postpartum mood and anxiety disorders.

Background

Postpartum depression (PPD) is a catchall phrase for many emotional symptoms associated with pregnancy and childbirth. The literature has described several postpartum anxiety disorders: postpartum obsessive compulsive disorder; postpartum panic disorder; and post-traumatic stress disorder due to childbirth. Postpartum mood disorders include: postpartum psychosis; bipolar II disorder, the postpartum depression impostor; and postpartum depression.

Postpartum mood and anxiety disorders affect the whole family. The mother-infant relationship is often adversely affected. A mother's postpartum mood and anxiety disorder can negatively influence her infant's cognitive, social, and emotional development; in some cases this impact may extend into early and middle childhood. Depressive symptoms are also associated with early cessation of breastfeeding. Additionally, the relationship between the father/partner and mother may be strained.

Postpartum depression, specifically, is a non-psychotic depressive episode that begins in the postpartum period, includes at least 2 weeks of depressed mood or loss of interest in almost all activities, and at least four of the following symptoms: changes in appetite or weight, sleep, and psychomotor activity; decreased energy; feelings of worthlessness or guilt; difficulty thinking, concentrating, or making decisions; or recurrent thoughts of death or suicidal ideation, plans, or attempts. Incidence rates for major and minor postpartum depression combined are estimated at up to 14.5%.

Role of Nurses

Registered nurses and members of the multidisciplinary health care team working with pregnant women and new mothers can optimize the level of service they provide postpartum women by:

- Obtaining knowledge about the distinctions among postpartum mood and anxiety disorders to differentiate postpartum depression from other mental health illnesses occurring after birth;
- Familiarizing themselves with the risk factors associated with postpartum mood and anxiety and disorders, including prenatal depression, child care stress, life stress, lack of social support, prenatal anxiety, maternity blues, marital dissatisfaction, history of previous depression, difficult infant temperament, low self-esteem, low socioeconomic status, unplanned/unwanted pregnancy, single marital status, preterm birth and multiple births;
- Recognizing the symptoms for the spectrum of postpartum mood and anxiety disorders ranging from "baby blues" to life-threatening postpartum psychoses;
- Gaining a thorough knowledge of the screening methodologies that help identify women at risk for developing postpartum mood and anxiety disorders;
- Being knowledgeable about the range of treatment options available for the variety of postpartum mood and anxiety disorders;
- Providing women and their families/support systems with resource materials that include appropriate referral information for the treatment of postpartum mood and anxiety disorders; referral information for the treatment of postpartum mood and anxiety disorders;
- Educating women about the myth that equates motherhood with total happiness and fulfillment;
- Encouraging women to engage in a dialogue with a health care provider about any negative feelings they may be experiencing during pregnancy or after the birth of a child.

Nurses serve a vital role in maximizing the health and health care experiences of pregnant women and new mothers. New mothers often perceive the following nursing themes to be caring and helpful in their diagnosis and recovery:

- Having sufficient knowledge about postpartum mood and anxiety disorders that result in a quick, correct diagnosis
- Using astute observations and intuition that lead to an awareness that something might be wrong with a mother
- Providing hope that the mothers' postpartum mood or anxiety disorder will end

PROFESSIONAL POSITION STATEMENT: AWHONN POSITION STATEMENT ON THE ROLE OF THE NURSE IN POSTPARTUM MOOD AND ANXIETY DISORDERS—cont'd

- Sharing valuable time
- Making the appropriate referrals so that the mother is started on the right path to recovery
- Making an extra effort to provide continuity of care for the mother
- Understanding what the mother is experiencing

Screening and Treatment

Screening mechanisms for potential risks for postpartum mood and anxiety disorders should begin during a woman's prenatal care. In fact, screening should not be limited to the postpartum or prenatal periods but should be available for women across the life span with incorporation possible in annual well women care visits. Health care providers can prepare women and their families with information on risk factors by educating them on the symptoms, providing valuable educational materials, and arranging for follow-up mechanisms, including phone calls and/or home visits to track their progress after giving birth.

A significant factor in the duration of postpartum mood and anxiety disorders is the length of delay to adequate treatment. Many new mothers are reluctant to admit that they are not experiencing motherhood's idealized standard of perfection, complicating the ability to express all of their feelings—including negative emotions—about their role as mothers.

While postpartum depression usually appears in the first 3 months postpartum, it can occur any time during the first 12 months after delivery; therefore, screening mechanisms should be available in all health care facilities where new mothers typically may be, including obstetric, neonatal, and pediatric settings. Even if a new mother screens negatively for PPD in the early postpartum months, she may develop PPD sometime later the first year after the birth of her baby. Extreme postpartum mood disorders such as postpartum psychosis can be life threatening for mothers and newborns; therefore, the importance of appropriate screening and early intervention strategies cannot be overstated. If a woman is contemplating her death or contemplating harming her infant, immediate formal mental health interventions are necessary.

Association of Women's Health, Obstetric and Neonatal Nursing (AWHONN). (2008). Position statement: The role of the nurse in postpartum mood and anxiety disorders, Washington, DC: Author.

- *The man may demonstrate avoidance behaviors such as spending more time away from the family.*
- *The man's affect may appear to be anxious or mad versus sad.*
- PPND has a negative effect on the couple's relationship and on the father-child relationship.
- PPND can have a long-term negative effect on the mental well-being of the child (Melrose, 2010).

Risk Factors

- Maternal PPD: this is the primary risk factor.
- Depressive symptoms during pregnancy
- Unplanned and/or unexpected pregnancy
- Baby with health or feeding problems
- Lack of social support
- Excessive stress about becoming a father
- Pre-existing mental health disorder
- Stressful life event, e.g., death of his parent (Bradley & Slade, 2011).

Assessment Findings

- Irritable
- Overwhelmed
- Frustrated
- Indecisive
- Avoidance of social situations
- Cynical
- Alcohol: increased consumption
- Drug use
- Domestic violence

Medical Management

- Interpersonal psychotherapy
- Antidepressant medications

Nursing Actions

- Provide information on PPND to the man and his partner.
- Stress the importance of seeking professional help if he is experiencing symptoms of PPND.
  - *Explain that PPND can have negative long-term effects on his child.*

CRITICAL COMPONENT

Paternal Postnatal Depression (PPND)

PPND often goes undiagnosed and untreated due to:

- The man or health care provider failing to recognize signs and symptoms of PPND.
  - Lack of guidelines for assessing and treating PPND.
- The man downplaying the degree to which the symptoms affect his life and relationships.
- The man being reluctant to discuss his depression symptoms with friends, family, or health care professionals.
- The man resisting mental health treatment; worried about stigma of depression.
- Few programs existing that address PPND.

CONCEPT MAP

Postpartum Hemorrhage

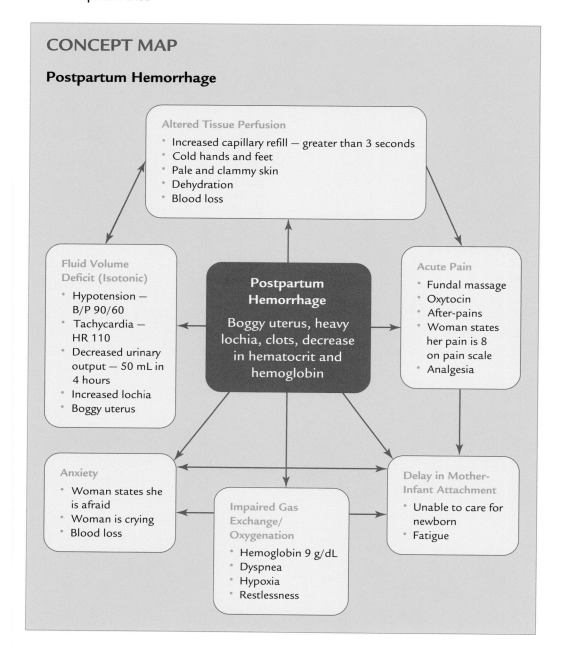

Altered Tissue Perfusion
- Increased capillary refill — greater than 3 seconds
- Cold hands and feet
- Pale and clammy skin
- Dehydration
- Blood loss

Fluid Volume Deficit (Isotonic)
- Hypotension — B/P 90/60
- Tachycardia — HR 110
- Decreased urinary output — 50 mL in 4 hours
- Increased lochia
- Boggy uterus

Postpartum Hemorrhage
Boggy uterus, heavy lochia, clots, decrease in hematocrit and hemoglobin

Acute Pain
- Fundal massage
- Oxytocin
- After-pains
- Woman states her pain is 8 on pain scale
- Analgesia

Anxiety
- Woman states she is afraid
- Woman is crying
- Blood loss

Impaired Gas Exchange/ Oxygenation
- Hemoglobin 9 g/dL
- Dyspnea
- Hypoxia
- Restlessness

Delay in Mother-Infant Attachment
- Unable to care for newborn
- Fatigue

Problem No. 1: Fluid volume deficit (isotonic)
Goal: Increase fluid volume
Outcome: The woman's blood pressure and heart rate will be within normal ranges, and intake and output will be within 200 mL of each other by the end of the shift.

Nursing Actions

1. Assess fundus for firmness: Massage if boggy.
2. Assess lochia for amount, color, and clots.
3. Instruct and remind the woman to drink a minimum of one glass of fluid per hour.
4. Initiate IV therapy as per orders.
5. Initiate oxytocin therapy as per orders.
6. Assess intake and output.
7. Assist the woman to the bathroom every 3–4 hours.
8. Monitor blood pressure and pulse every 2 hours.
9. Assess skin turgor and mucous membranes every 4 hours.

Problem No. 2: Altered tissue perfusion
Goal: Normal tissue perfusion
Outcome: Blood pressure and pulse within normal limits; capillary fill less than 3 seconds

Nursing Actions

1. Every 2 hours, monitor vital signs, capillary refill, and motor and sensory status.
2. Compare post-hemorrhage Hb/Hct with results on admission to labor.
3. Administer oxygen as per orders and monitor oxygen saturation levels.

Problem No. 3: Anxiety
Goal: Decreased anxiety
Outcome: The woman verbalizes that she feels less anxious.

Nursing Actions

1. Be calm and reassuring in interactions with the woman and her family.
2. Explain all procedures.
3. Teach the woman relaxation breathing techniques.
4. Encourage the woman and family to verbalize their feelings regarding recent hemorrhage by asking open-ended questions.

Problem No. 4: Delay in mother-infant attachment
Goal: Positive mother-infant attachment
Outcome: The woman will hold the infant close, respond to the infant's needs, and state she enjoys her baby.

Nursing Actions

1. When the woman is stable, have the infant remain in the woman's room.
2. Assist the woman with infant care as needed.
3. Encourage holding of infant by assisting the woman into a comfortable position and placing the infant in the woman's arms.
4. Praise the woman for positive mother-infant interactions.
5. Provide information on infant care.

Problem No. 5: Acute pain
Goal: Decreased pain
Outcome: The woman will state that pain is less than 3 on pain scale.

Nursing Actions

1. Assess level, location, and type of pain.
2. Prevent overdistention of the bladder by reminding the woman to void every 3–4 hours.
3. Administer pain medications based on assessment data as per orders.
4. Provide an environment that is conducive to relaxation, such as low lights, decreased noise, and uninterrupted rest periods.
5. Teach the woman relaxation techniques.

Problem No. 6: Impaired gas exchange/oxygenation
Goal: Maintain oxygenation
Outcome: Oxygen saturation is 98% and respiratory rate and pattern are within normal limits.

Nursing Actions

1. Monitor respirations, breath sounds, and oxygen saturation.
2. Provide oxygen by mask as per orders.
3. Instruct and assist the woman with deep breathing and coughing to decrease the risk of pneumonia.
4. Initiate iron replacement therapy as per orders.
5. Provide nutritional information on food high in iron such as green leafy vegetables.

TYING IT ALL TOGETHER

You are a nurse working in the postpartum unit. You are assigned Mallory Polk, a 42-year-old African American woman. (Refer to Tying It All Together in Chapters 7 and 10 for antepartum and intrapartum data.)

Summary of Labor and Delivery Record

Mallory was admitted 2 days ago at 32 weeks' gestation and managed in the birthing unit for preterm labor with magnesium sulfate and antibiotics. She received betamethasone. The magnesium sulfate was discontinued 3 hours before delivery. Her labor was augmented during the transitional phase. She spontaneously delivered a 1559-gram (3 lb., 7 oz.) boy with Apgar scores of 5 and 7 at 1 and 5 minutes. Her baby is experiencing mild signs of respiratory distress and is in the NICU.

Postpartum Report

Mallory is 4 hours post-birth and has an IV of D_5W lactated Ringer's solution with 10 units of oxytocin running in her left arm. She voided in the recovery unit 2 hours post-birth.

Assessment Findings

Vitals signs: Temperature 37°C; pulse 98 bpm; respirations 14 breaths/min; blood pressure 110/70 mm Hg
Fundus is at the umbilicus and boggy.
Lochia is heavy.
Based on your assessment findings and Mallory's history, what are your immediate nursing actions?
Discuss the rationale for your nursing actions.

You reevaluate Mallory 10 minutes after your initial nursing actions. Her fundus is firm, midline, and 1 finger breadth below the umbilicus with scant lochia. You continue to monitor Mallory and 15 minutes later her fundus is boggy with heavy lochia. The fundus becomes firm after massage. Her pulse is 100 bpm and blood pressure is 100/60 mm Hg. You notify her CNM and report your findings.

Detail the aspects of your assessment findings that you will report to the CNM.

The CNM orders 20 units of oxytocin in 1,000 mL of lactated Ringer's solution. The ordered infusion rate is 10 mL/min, to be regulated by firmness of the uterus.

Discuss your nursing actions and rationale for actions.
Discuss the assessment data needed to determine effectiveness of medical and nursing actions.

You note that in her prenatal chart she has a diagnosis of fibroids.

Discuss the implications of the diagnosis as it relates to your nursing care and discharge teaching plan.

■ ■ ■ ■ **Review Questions** ■ ■ ■ ■

1. Your patient is a 25-year-old gravida 1 woman who is 2 hours postpartum. You note on assessment that her fundus is firm and midline. She is experiencing a steady stream of blood. The bed linen under her is soaked in blood. Based on these findings and observations, you suspect that she is exhibiting early signs/symptoms of a postpartum hemorrhage related to:
   A. Uterine atony
   B. Laceration of the cervical or vaginal area
   C. Retained placental tissue
   D. Fibroids

2. Mrs. Fischer is 4 days post-birth. She calls the clinic and tells the triage nurse that she has a temperature and does not feel well. What additional assessment findings does the triage nurse need to obtain to assist in her nursing assessment? Select all that apply.
  A. When did she notice an increase in temperature and what is her temperature?
  B. Is she experiencing pain, and if so, where is it located?
  C. What is the amount of her fluid intake within the past 24 hours?
  D. What is the color and amount of her bleeding?

3. Foul-smelling lochia occurs:
  A. When beta-hemolytic *Streptococcus* is the primary organism associated with metritis
  B. Within the first 24 hours post-birth related to metritis
  C. When the entire endometrium is infected
  D. During the normal involution process

4. Women who experience mastitis should be instructed to:
  A. Stop breastfeeding until 48 hours after the start of antibiotic treatment.
  B. Continue to breastfeed or massage and express milk from the affected breast.
  C. Wash nipples with antibiotic soap before each feeding session.
  D. Apply cream to nipples after each feeding until mastitis has resolved.

5. Signs and symptoms of postpartum depression include which of the following? Select all that apply.
  A. Sleep and appetite disturbance
  B. Uncontrolled crying
  C. Delusions
  D. Feelings of guilt and/or worthlessness

6. During a six-week postpartum clinic visit, your patient tells you she is concerned about her husband. She tells you that he either stays late at work or goes out after work with his friends. When he is home, he is usually drinking beer while watching sports on TV. Which of the following is the most appropriate response?
  A. "These are common behaviors of men as they process the meaning of fatherhood. You just need to give him time to work through this life change."
  B. "These behaviors can indicate that your husband does not want to take on the responsibilities of being a father. You need to talk to him about his feelings regarding fatherhood."
  C. "These behaviors indicate that your husband is concerned about the added cost of having a newborn. You and your husband need to sit down and set up a budget."
  D. "These behaviors might indicate that your husband is depressed. You need to encourage him to see a mental health professional."

7. Which of the following should be included in postpartum discharge teaching regarding risk reduction for cystitis? Select all that apply.
  A. Drink a minimum of 3,000 mL of fluid per day.
  B. Change peripads at least every 3–4 hours.
  C. Eat foods low in acidity.
  D. Avoid caffeinated fluids.

8. Which of the following factors place a woman at risk for thrombosis? Select all that apply.
  A. Obesity
  B. Physiological changes of pregnancy
  C. Metritis
  D. Cesarean birth

9. You are assigned a woman who is 2 hours post birth. She had an emergency cesarean section for an abruptio placenta. Based on this history, the woman is at risk for _____. Fill in the blank.
  A. Disseminated intravascular coagulation
  B. Retained placenta fragments
  C. Thrombosis
  D. Subinvolution of the uterus

10. You are assigned a woman who is 5 hours post-birth. She gave birth to an 8-pound girl and experienced a 4th degree tear of the perineum. During your postpartum assessment, she informed you that she has rectal pressure and severe pain where she tore. Her level of pain is 10 on a pain scale of 0–10. You note her perineum is intact with minimal bruising. Her blood pressure is 100/60 and pulse is 98. Based on this assessment data, select the best initial nursing action.
  A. Medicate her for pain.
  B. Notify her physician of your assessment data.
  C. Place an ice pack on the perineum.
  D. Assist her in ambulating to the bathroom.

References

ACOG Practice Bulletin. (2006). Postpartum hemorrhage. *Obstetrics & gynecology, 108*, 1039–1046.

American Psychiatric Association. (1994). Diagnostic and statistical manual of mental disorders (4th ed.). Washington, DC: American Psychiatric Association.

Association of Women's Health, Obstetric and Neonatal Nursing (AWHONN). (2008). The role of the nurse in postpartum mood and anxiety disorders. Washington, DC: Author.

Association of Women's Health, Obstetric and Neonatal Nursing (AWHONN). (2006). *The compendium of postpartum care.* Philadelphia: Medical Broadcasting Company.

Born, L., Zinga, D., and Steiner, M. (2004). Challenges in identifying and diagnosing postpartum disorders. *Primary psychiatry, 11*, 29–36.

Engqvist, I., Ferszt, G., Ahlin, A., and Nilsson, K. (2009). Psychiatric nurses' descriptions of women with postpartum psychosis and nurses' response—an exploratory study in Sweden. *Issues in mental health nursing, 30*, 23–30.

Harvey, C., and Dildy, G. (2013) Obstetric hemorrhage. In Troiano, N., Harvey, C., and Chez, B. High risk and critical care obstetrics (3rd ed., pp. 246–273). Philadelphia, PA: Wolters Kluwer/Lippincott, Williams & Wilkins.

James, D. (2008). Postpartum care. In Simpson, K. and Creehan, P. Perinatal nursing (3rd ed., pp. 473–520). Philadelphia, PA: Wolters Kluwer/Lippincott, Williams & Wilkins.

Jones, R., and Clark, S. (2013). Amniotic fluid embolus. In Troiano, N., Harvey, C., and Chez, B. High risk and critical care obstetrics (3rd ed., pp. 316–325). Philadelphia, PA: Wolters Kluwer/Lippincott, Williams & Wilkins.

Melrose, S. (2010). Parental postpartum depression: How can nurses help? *Contemporary nurse, 34,* 199–210.

Moore, L. (2007). Amniotic fluid embolism. *eMedicine.* [Online] Retrieved from http:/emedicine.medscape.com/article/2553068-overview

Schoening, A. (2006). Amniotic fluid embolism: Historical perspective and new possibilities. *MCN, The American Journal of Maternal Child Nursing, 31,* 78–83.

Sisson, M., and Mann, M. (2013). Disseminated intravascular coagulation in pregnancy. In Troiano, N., Harvey, C., and Chez, B. High risk and critical care obstetrics (3rd ed., pp. 274–284). Philadelphia, PA: Wolters Kluwer/Lippincott, Williams & Wilkins.

Sit, K., Rotherschild, A., & Wisner, K. (2006). A review of postpartum psychosis. *Journal of Women's Health, 15,* 352–368.

Vallerand, A., and Sandoski, C. (2013). *Davis's drug guide for nurses* (13th ed.). Philadelphia: F.A. Davis.

Venes, D. (2009). *Taber's cyclopedic medical dictionary* (21st ed.). Philadelphia: F.A. Davis.

Yonkers, K., Vigod, S., and Ross, L. (2011). Diagnosis, pathophysiology, and management of mood disorders in pregnancy and postpartum women. *Obstetrics & gynecology, 117,* 961–977.

Wong, A. (2012). Pregnancy, postpartum infections. *eMedicine.* [Online] Retrieved from: http://emedicine.medscape.com/article/796892-overview

You, W., & Zahn, C. (2006). Postpartum hemorrhage: abnormally adherent placenta, uterine inversion, and puerperal hematomas. *Clinical Obstetrics and Gynecology, 49,* 184–197.

Neonatal Period

Physiological and Behavioral Responses of the Neonate

EXPECTED STUDENT OUTCOMES

On completion of this chapter, the student will be able to:

- ☐ Define key terms.
- ☐ Identify the changes that occur during the transition from intrauterine to extrauterine life and the related nursing actions.
- ☐ List the critical elements of neonatal assessment.
- ☐ List the critical elements of neonatal gestational age assessments.
- ☐ Discuss methods used in neonatal pain management.
- ☐ Describe the nursing care for neonates during the first week of life.
- ☐ Describe the common laboratory and diagnostic tests for neonates.
- ☐ Discuss the nursing actions that support parents in the care of their newborn.
- ☐ Describe the most common therapeutic and surgical procedures used for neonates and the related nursing care.

Nursing Diagnoses

- ☐ At risk for altered body temperature related to decreased amounts of subcutaneous fat and/or large body surface
- ☐ At risk for infections related to tissue trauma and/or poor hand washing techniques by health care providers and parents
- ☐ At risk for impaired gas exchange related to transitioning from fetal to neonatal circulation, cold stress, and/or excessive mucus production
- ☐ At risk for fluid volume deficit related to limited oral intake
- ☐ At risk for knowledge deficit related to first-time parenting and/or limited learning resources

Nursing Outcomes

- ☐ The neonate's temperature will be within normal limits, and the skin will be pink and feel warm to touch.
- ☐ The neonate will not exhibit signs or symptoms of an infection.
- ☐ The neonate's respiratory rate and heart rate will be within normal ranges; the skin will be pink and the airway will remain clear.
- ☐ The neonate will void six times daily.
- ☐ Parents will respond to their newborn's needs.

Don't have time to read this chapter? Want to reinforce your reading? Need to review for a test?
Listen to this chapter on DavisPlus.

INTRODUCTION

The **neonatal period** is from birth through the first 28 days of life. During these few weeks, the neonate transitions from intrauterine to extrauterine life and adapts to a new environment. Most neonates who are term and whose mothers experienced a healthy pregnancy and low-risk labor and birth accomplish this transition with relative ease (**Fig. 15-1**).

The focus of nursing care during this time is to protect and support the neonate as he undergoes numerous physiological changes and adapts to extrauterine life. This is accomplished by:

■ Maintaining body heat
■ Maintaining respiratory function
■ Decreasing risk for infection
■ Assisting parents in providing appropriate nutrition and hydration
■ Assisting parents in learning to care for their newborn

TRANSITION TO EXTRAUTERINE LIFE

The transition to extrauterine life begins at birth when the umbilical cord is clamped and the neonate takes his first breath. This initiates various changes within the neonate's physiological systems. Each system needs to adapt to the changes that occur during this transition. The most critical and dynamic changes occur in the respiratory and cardiovascular systems. Thermoregulatory, metabolic, hepatic, gastrointestinal, renal, and immune systems also undergo significant changes.

The Respiratory System

The establishment of extrauterine respirations is the most critical and immediate physiological change that occurs in the transition from fetus to neonate. This change is initiated by compression of the thorax, lung expansion, increase in alveolar oxygen concentration, and vasodilatation of the pulmonary vessels.

■ Mechanical and chemical stimuli are the primary factors that initiate extrauterine respirations (**Figs. 15-2** and **15-3**).
■ Sensory stimuli such as exposure to temperature changes, sounds, lights, and touch also influence respirations by stimulating the respiratory center of the medulla.
■ In utero, the lungs are filled with amniotic fluid. Approximately 30 mL of amniotic fluid is forced out of the lungs during the delivery process.

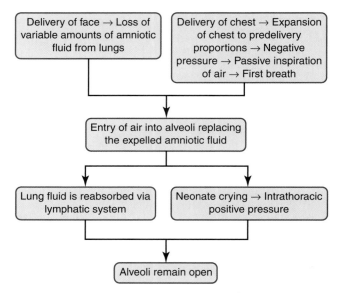

Figure 15-2   Transition to extrauterine pulmonary function: Mechanical stimuli.

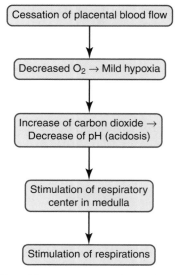

Figure 15-3   Transition to extrauterine pulmonary function: Chemical stimuli.

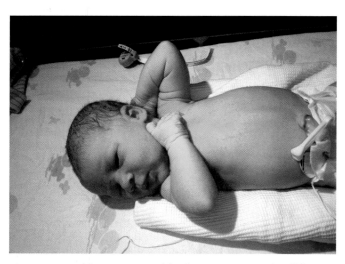

Figure 15-1   Neonate transitioning to extrauterine life.

- The presence of surfactant, a phospholipid, within the alveoli assists in the establishment of functional residual capacity. This residual capacity assists in keeping the alveolar sacs partially open at the end of exhalation, which decreases the amount of pressure and energy required on inspiration (see Chapter 17).
- The initiation of respiration has an effect on the pulmonary circulation and gas exchange:
  - *First breath → ↑ alveolar oxygen tension (PaO_2) and ↓ arterial pH → dilation of pulmonary arteries → ↓ pulmonary vascular resistance → ↑ blood flow through pulmonary vessels → ↑ oxygen and carbon dioxide exchange within the lungs*
- Two factors that negatively affect the transition to extrauterine respirations are:
  - *Decreased surfactant levels related to immature lungs*
  - *Persistent hypoxemia and acidosis that leads to constriction of the pulmonary arteries*
- Approximately 10% of neonates require some degree of assistance with respirations at the time of delivery, and 1% require extensive resuscitation (see Critical Component: Signs of Respiratory Distress).

CRITICAL COMPONENT

Signs of Respiratory Distress

- Cyanosis
- Abnormal respiratory pattern such as apnea and tachypnea
- Retractions of the chest wall
- Grunting
- Flaring of nostrils
- Hypotonia

The Circulatory System

The transition from fetal circulation to neonatal circulation begins rapidly within seconds of the clamping of the umbilical cord and the initiation of the first breath. The transition to neonatal circulation is strongly influenced by the changes within the respiratory system. Fetal circulation is discussed in Chapter 3.

- The decrease in pulmonary vascular resistance causes an increase in pulmonary blood flow, and the increase in systemic vascular resistance influences the cardiovascular changes (**Fig. 15-4**).

The three major fetal circulatory structures that undergo changes are the ductus venosus, foramen ovale, and the ductus arteriosus.

- The **ductus venosus,** which connects the umbilical vein to the inferior vena cava, closes by day 3 of life and becomes a ligament. Blood flow through the umbilical vein stops once the cord is clamped.
- The **foramen ovale,** which is an opening between the right atrium and the left atrium, closes when the left

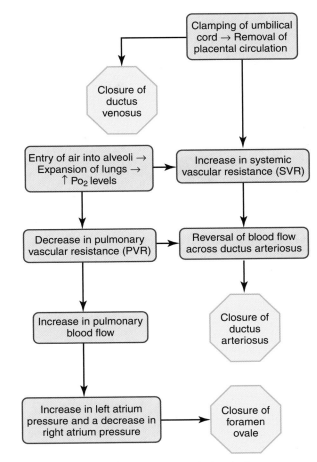

Figure 15-4 Transition to neonatal circulation.

atrial pressure is higher than the right atrial pressure. This closure occurs when:

- *Increased PaO_2 → decreased pulmonary pressure → increased pulmonary blood flow → increased pressure in left atrium → closure of foramen ovale*
- *Significant neonatal hypoxia can cause a reopening of the foramen ovale*
- The **ductus arteriosus,** which connects the pulmonary artery with the descending aorta, usually closes within 15 hours post-birth.
  - *This closure occurs when the pulmonary vascular resistance becomes less than system vascular resistance → left to right shunt → closure of ductus arteriosus.*
  - *It will remain open if lungs fail to expand or PaO_2 levels drop.*

The Thermoregulatory System

The fetus is surrounded in amniotic fluid that maintains a fairly constant environmental temperature based on the maternal body temperature. Once the neonate enters the extrauterine world, he must adapt to changes in the environmental temperatures. The neonate's responses to extrauterine temperature changes during the first few weeks are delayed and place the neonate at risk for cold stress.

The neonate responds to cold by:

- An increase in metabolic rate,
- An increase of muscle activity,
- Peripheral vascular constriction, and
- Metabolism of brown fat.
- **Neutral thermal environment (NTE)** is an environment that maintains body temperature with minimal metabolic changes and/or oxygen consumption.
  - *A neutral thermal environment (NTE) decreases possible complications related to the delayed response to environmental temperature changes.*
- **Brown adipose tissue (BAT),** also referred to as brown fat or nonshivering thermogenesis, is a highly dense and vascular adipose tissue. Neonates possess large amounts of BAT, while children and adults have smaller amounts (Blackburn, 2012).
  - *BAT is located in the neck, thorax, axillary area, intrascapular areas, and around the adrenal glands and kidneys.*
  - *BAT promotes:*
    - An increase in metabolism
    - Heat production
    - Heat transfer to the peripheral system (Blackburn, 2012)
  - *Heat is produced by intense lipid metabolic metabolism of BAT.*
  - *BAT reserves are rapidly depleted during periods of cold stress.*
  - *Preterm neonates have limited BAT.*
- Neonates are at higher risk for thermoregulatory problems related to:
  - *Higher body surface-area-to-body-mass ratio*
  - *Higher metabolic rate*
  - *Limited and immature thermoregulatory abilities*
- Factors that negatively affect thermoregulation are:
  - *Decreased subcutaneous fat*
  - *Decreased BAT in preterm neonates*
  - *Large body surface*

- *Loss of body heat from convection, radiation, conduction, and/or evaporation (Fig. 15–5):*
  - **Evaporation:** Loss of heat that occurs when water on the neonate's skin is converted to vapors, such as during bathing or directly after birth
  - **Conduction:** Transfer of heat to cooler surface by direct skin contact, such as cold hands of caregivers or cold equipment
  - **Convection:** Loss of heat from the neonate's warm body surface to cooler air currents, such as air conditioners or oxygen masks
  - **Radiation:** Transfer of heat from the neonate to cooler objects that are not in direct contact with the neonate, such as cold walls of the isolette or cold equipment near the neonate

Cold Stress

Cold stress is a term that describes excessive heat loss that leads to hypothermia and results in the utilization of compensatory mechanisms to maintain the neonate's body temperature (**Fig. 15-6**).

- Cold stress occurs when there is:
  - *A decrease in environmental temperatures → a decrease in the neonate's body temperature → an increase in respiratory rate, heart rate → an increase in oxygen consumption, a depletion of glucose, and a decrease in surfactant → respiratory distress*
- Cold stress can delay the transition from fetal to neonatal circulation.

Risk Factors

- Prematurity
- Small for gestational age
- Hypoglycemia
- Prolonged resuscitation efforts
- Sepsis
- Neurological, endocrine, or cardiorespiratory problems

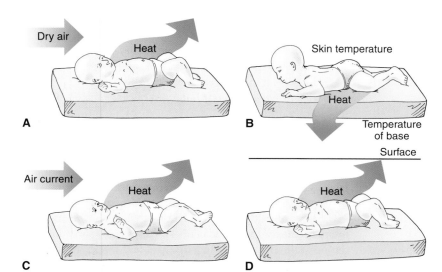

Figure 15–5 The four mechanisms of heat loss in the newborn. *A.* Evaporation. *B.* Conduction. *C.* Convection. *D.* Radiation.

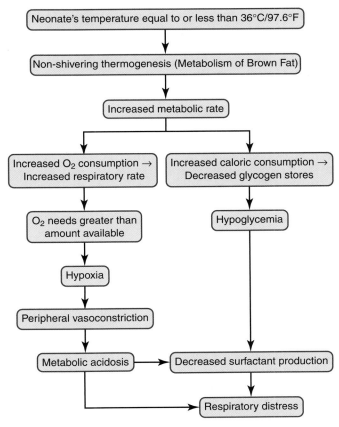

Figure 15-6 Cold stress.

Signs and Symptoms

- Axillary temperature at or below 36.5°C (97.7°F)
- Cool skin
- Lethargy
- Pallor
- Tachypnea
- Grunting
- Hypoglycemia
- Hypotonia
- Jitteriness
- Weak suck

Nursing Actions

- Preventative actions
  - *Dry the neonate thoroughly immediately after birth to decrease heat loss due to evaporation.*
  - *Remove wet blankets from the neonate's direct environment to decrease heat loss due to radiation, evaporation, and conduction.*
  - *Place a stocking cap on the neonate's head to decrease heat loss due to radiation and convection (**Fig. 15-7**).*
  - *Skin-to-skin contact with the mother with a warm blanket over the mother and neonate decreases heat loss due to radiation and conduction.*
  - *Use pre-warmed blankets and clothing to decrease heat loss due to conduction.*

- *Swaddle in warm blankets to decrease heat loss due to convection and radiation.*
- *Pre-warm radiant warmers and heat shields to decrease heat loss due to conduction.*
- *Delay initial bath until the neonate's temperature is stable to decrease heat loss due to evaporation.*
- *Place the neonate away from air vents to decrease heat loss due to convection.*
- *Place the neonate away from outside walls and windows to decrease heat loss due to convection radiation.*
- *Maintain a NTE to decrease heat loss due to convection and radiation.*
- Actions when the neonate displays signs/symptoms of cold stress
  - *Place a stocking cap on the neonate's head.*
  - *Skin-to-skin contact with the mother with a warm blanket over both the mother and neonate when there is a mild decrease in temperature; reassess temperature as per institutional protocol.*
  - *Swaddle in warm blankets; reassess temperature as per institutional protocol, which is generally every 30 minutes until stable.*
  - *Place the naked neonate under a preheated radiant warmer.*
    - Attach the servo-controlled probe on the neonate's abdomen or other body surface that is closest to the radiant source.
      - *It is recommended not to place probe over BAT areas, but there are too few research studies to view this as evidenced-based practice (Blackburn, 2012).*
    - Set the control to 36.5°C.
    - Monitor the neonate's temperature, respiratory rate, and heart rate every 5 minutes when rewarming.
    - Assess and adjust the neonate's fluid requirement; fluids may need to be increased to compensate for insatiable water loss.
  - *Monitor temperature as per institutional protocol.*
  - *Obtain a heel stick to assess for hypoglycemia (glucose <40 mg/dL).*
    - Treat hypoglycemia.

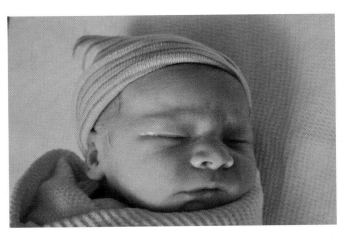

Figure 15-7 Stocking cap is placed on the neonate's head to reduce heat loss due to radiation and convection.

The Metabolic System

Large quantities of glycogen are stored by the fetus during pregnancy in preparation for meeting energy requirements when transitioning from intrauterine to extrauterine life. Immediately after birth, the neonate becomes independent of the mother's metabolism and must balance the amount of insulin production with glucose availability.

- Glucose values normally decrease about 1 hour post-birth, and then values rise and stabilize by 2 to 3 hours post-birth (Blackburn, 2012).
- Optimal range for plasma glucose is 70–100 mg/dL.
- Hypoglycemia (blood glucose level under 40 mg/dL in the neonate) is common during this transitional time, especially in neonates of diabetic mothers (see Critical Component: Hypoglycemia).
  - *During intrauterine life, neonates of diabetic mothers produce high levels of insulin in response to the high levels of circulating maternal glucose. During the first few hours of extrauterine life, the neonate's insulin level remains higher than normal, leading to hypoglycemia.*

CRITICAL COMPONENT

Hypoglycemia

Hypoglycemia is defined as a blood glucose level <40 mg/dL in the neonate.

Risks for Hypoglycemia

- Neonates of diabetic mothers
- Neonates weighing >4,000 grams or large for gestational age
- Post-term neonates
- Preterm neonates
- Small for gestational age neonates
- Hypothermia
- Neonatal infection
- Respiratory distress
- Neonatal resuscitation
- Birth trauma

Signs and Symptoms

- Jitteriness
- Hypotonia
- Irritability
- Apnea
- Lethargy
- Temperature instability

Nursing Actions

- Monitor for signs and symptoms of hypoglycemia.
- Assess blood glucose level with use of glucose monitor.
- Assist the woman with breastfeeding.
- Feed the neonate either formula or dextrose water when the glucose level is <40 mg/dL as per institutional protocol, generally 5 mL/kg.
- Maintain NTE to decrease risk of cold stress.

The Hepatic System

Functions of the liver include:

- Carbohydrate metabolism
  - *The liver regulates the blood glucose levels by:*
    - Converting excessive glucose to glycogen (insulin and cortisol facilitate this process)
    - Converting glycogen to glucose when glucose levels are low.
- Amino acid metabolism
- Lipid metabolism
- Synthesis of plasma proteins
- Blood coagulation
  - *Coagulation factors II, VII, IX, and X are synthesized in the liver.*
  - *Vitamin K influences the activation of these factors. During intrauterine life, the fetus receives vitamin K from his mother. After birth, the neonate experiences a decrease in vitamin K and is at risk for delayed clotting and for hemorrhage.*
  - *Vitamin K is synthesized in the intestinal flora, which is absent in the newborn. The intestinal flora develops after the introduction of microorganisms, which usually occurs with the first feedings.*
  - *A vitamin K injection is given as a prophylaxis to decrease the risk of bleeding related to vitamin K deficiency.*
  - *The decline of maternally acquired vitamin K levels is greater in breastfed neonates, neonates with a history of perinatal asphyxia, and neonates of mothers who are on warfarin (Blackburn, 2012).*
- Conjugation of bilirubin
  - *There is an increase in the neonate's RBC turnover (shorter RBC life span) and an increased RBC count at birth. These factors contribute to a proportionally greater amount of bilirubin production.*
  - *There are two forms of bilirubin: indirect and direct.*
  - ***Indirect bilirubin** (unconjugated bilirubin), a fat-soluble substance, is produced from the breakdown of red blood cells (RBCs). It is converted to **direct bilirubin** (conjugated bilirubin), a water-soluble substance, by liver enzymes. Direct bilirubin is in a form that can be excreted in the urine and stool.*
  - ***Hyperbilirubinemia** is a condition in which there is a high level of unconjugated bilirubin in the neonate's blood related to the immature liver function, high RBC count that is common in neonates, and an increased hemolysis caused by the shorter life span of fetal RBCs (see Chapter 17 for information on hyperbilirubinemia/jaundice).*
- Phagocytosis by Kupffer cells (macrophages)
- Storage of fat-soluble vitamins A, D, E, and K and iron
  - *The formation of new RBCs is suppressed during the first few weeks post-birth. During this time the liver stores iron from destroyed RBCs. This iron is used when RBC formation is resumed (Blackburn, 2012).*

■ Detoxification
  ■ *The smooth endoplasmic reticulum (SER) of the liver produces enzymes that detoxify harmful substances such as medications (Blackburn, 2012).*
  ■ *The neonate has a reduced number of SER → decreased ability to detoxify medication → ↑ risk of toxic effects from medications.*

Medication

Phytonadione (Vitamin K, AquaMEPHYTON)

■ Indication: Prevention of hemorrhagic disease in neonate
■ Action: Vitamin K is required for the hepatic synthesis of blood coagulation factors II, VII, IX, and X.
■ Common side effects: Erythema, pain, and swelling at injection site
■ Route and dose: IM; 0.5–1 mg within 1 hour of birth

(Data Vallerand & Sanoski, 2013)

The Gastrointestinal System

The neonate's gastrointestinal system is functionally immature but rapidly adapts to demands for growth and development through ingestion, digestion, and absorption of nutrients, as well as eliminations of waste.

■ Gastric capacity for the first few days is approximately 5–10 mL and increases to 60 mL by day 7.
■ Stomach emptying time is 2–4 hours.
  ■ *Neonates should feed every 2–4 hours.*
■ Neonates may appear uninterested in feeding during the first few days.
  ■ *Decreased interest during this time may be related to a quiet sleep state.*
■ The characteristics of stools and stool pattern vary depending on the type, frequency, and amount of feeding and the age of the neonate (**Table 15-1**). The types of stools are:
  ■ *Meconium stool begins to form during the 4th gestational month and is the first stool eliminated by the neonate. It is sticky, thick, black, and odorless. It is first passed within 24–48 hours.*
  ■ *Transitional stool begins around the 3rd day and can continue for 3 or 4 days. The stool transitions from black to greenish black, to greenish brown, to greenish yellow. This phase of stool characteristics occurs in both breastfed and formula-fed neonates.*
  ■ *Breastfed stool is yellow and semiformed. Later it becomes a golden yellow with a pasty consistency and has a sour odor.*
  ■ *Formula-fed stool is drier and more formed than breastfeed stools. It is a paler yellow or brownish yellow and has an unpleasant odor.*
  ■ *Diarrheal stool is loose and green.*
■ Breastfed neonates tend to have more stools per day than do formula-fed neonates. It is not uncommon for the neonate to pass 4–8 stools per day.

TABLE 15–1 MINIMUM NUMBER OF WET DIAPERS AND STOOLS DURING FIRST MONTH

NEONATE'S AGE	NUMBER OF WET DIAPERS	NUMBER OF STOOLS	TYPE OF STOOL
Day 1	1	1	Meconium – sticky, thick and black
Day 2	2	3	Meconium – sticky, thick and black
Day 3	5-6	3	Transitional – looser greenish black-greenish brown
Day 4	6	3	Yellow, soft, watery
Day 5 → 1 month	6	3	Breastfed stool or formula-fed stool

DHHS, 2009.

■ Constipation usually does not occur in breastfed neonates.
■ Constipation can occur in bottle-fed infants when formula is not properly diluted.

The Renal System

Two major functions of the kidneys are control of fluid and electrolyte balance and excretion of metabolic waste. During fetal life, these functions are assumed by the placenta. Once the cord is clamped, the neonate's kidneys must take on these functions.

■ Initially the neonate's kidneys are immature and place the neonate at risk for:
  ■ *Over-hydration*
  ■ *Dehydration*
  ■ *Electrolyte disorders such as hyponatremia and hypernatremia (Blackburn, 2012)*
■ There is higher risk for complications for preterm neonates.
■ The glomerular filtration rate (GFR) is initially low in the neonate but doubles by 2 weeks of age (Blackburn, 2012).
  ■ *Decreased GFR →↓ability to excrete water →↑risk of over-hydration and water intoxication*
■ Dehydration can occur due to the neonate's kidneys' limited ability to concentrate urine.
■ The limited abilities of the kidneys can affect the excretion of drugs from the neonate's systems and increase the risk of side effects and toxicity (Blackburn, 2012).
■ Full-term neonates excrete 15–60 mL/kg of urine per day for the first few days of life. Urinary output increases

to 250–400 mL by end of the first month of life (Blackburn, 2012).

■ *A delay or decrease in urinary output can occur in neonates whose mothers received magnesium sulfate during labor. Magnesium sulfate blocks neuromuscular transmissions and can cause urinary retention (Blackburn, 2012).*

■ Neonates usually lose 5%–10% of birth weight during the first week of life due to diuresis.

The Immune System

The immune system protects the body from invasion by foreign materials such as bacteria and viruses (Scanlon & Sanders, 2011). Before rupture of membranes, the fetus lives in the sterile environment of the maternal uterus and relies on the maternal immune system to protect him from pathogenic organisms. During the transition from extrauterine life, the neonate begins the process of developing normal microbial flora and must respond to colonization by potential pathogenic bacteria (Blackburn, 2012).

■ Major components of the immune system:
  ■ *Active humoral immunity is the process in which B cells detect antigens and produce antibodies against them. Active humoral immunity is further classified as:*
    ■ Acquired immunity that develops from vaccination
    ■ Natural immunity that develops from exposure to antigens, after which the individual produces antibodies
  ■ *Passive immunity, which is not permanent, is acquired either naturally or artificially.*
    ■ An example of natural passive immunity is the placental transmission of antibiotics from the mother to the fetus. This provides protection for the neonate during the first few months of life from the pathogens to which the mother has been exposed.
    ■ An example of artificial passive immunity is gamma globulin, which provides immediate protection for a short time.
  ■ *Lymphocytes are white blood cells that are primarily composed of T cells and B cells.*
    ■ The number of T cells within the neonate's system is comparable to that in adults, but their functional abilities are decreased, which delays the response to microorganisms (Blackburn, 2012).
    ■ The functional abilities of B cells are also hyporesponsive (Blackburn, 2012).
  ■ *Immunoglobulins are classified as IgG, IgA, IgM, IgD, and IgE (**Table 15-2**).*
    ■ Maternal IgGs are the primary antibodies that cross the placenta and enter the fetal system and provide passive immunity for the neonate (Blackburn, 2012).
    ■ The maternal transfer of IgG antibodies protects the neonate from bacterial and viral infections for which the mother has developed antibodies, such as rubella, tetanus, and diphtheria (Blackburn, 2012).
■ Neonates are at risk for infection related to:
  ■ *Immature defense mechanism*
  ■ *Lack of experience with and exposure to organisms, which leads to a delayed response to antigens*

TABLE 15–2	CLASSES OF IMMUNOGLOBULINS	
NAME	LOCATION	FUNCTION
IgG	Blood Extracellular fluid	Crosses the placenta to provide passive immunity for newborns Provides long-term immunity after recovery or a vaccine
IgA	External secretions (tears, salvia, etc.)	Present in breast milk to provide passive immunity for breast-fed infants Found in secretions of all mucus membranes
IgM	Blood	Produced first by the maturing immune system of infants Produced first during an infection (IgG production follows) Part of the ABO blood group
IgD	B lymphocytes	Receptors on B lymphocytes
IgE	Mast cells or basophils	Important in allergic reaction (mast cells release histamine)

Scanlon & Sanders (2011).

  ■ *Breakdown of skin and mucous membranes that provides a portal of entry for bacteria (Blackburn, 2012)*
■ During the transitional period, the neonate's immune system begins to:
  ■ *Develop normal microbial flora of the skin, respiratory tract, and gastrointestinal tract*
  ■ *Respond to bacterial colonization of potential pathogens (Blackburn, 2012)*
■ Neonates are first exposed to organisms from the maternal genital tract during the birthing process.
  ■ *The maternal genital tract may contain group B Streptococcus and E. coli, which can result in neonatal sepsis (see Chapter 17).*

Neonatal Assessment

A neonatal assessment should be done within 2 hours after birth. This initial assessment provides the baseline data for the neonate and assists in determining the course of nursing and medical care.

CRITICAL COMPONENT

Methods of Reducing Heat Loss

The thermoregulatory systems of neonates respond more slowly to external temperature changes than those of adults. Prevention of heat loss is critical when doing assessments. Methods to reduce heat loss during assessments are:

- Ensure that the room is warm and free of air drafts.
- Place the infant under a warming unit to help maintain a NTE **or** assess the neonate in the mother's arms. Skin-to-skin contact between the mother and neonate can decrease the amount of heat loss.
- When doing assessments in an open crib or in a parent's arms, keep the neonate wrapped and expose only the body area that is being assessed.

Preparation for Assessment

- Gather the equipment needed for the assessment: Latex gloves, measuring tape, infant stethoscope, thermometer, scale for weighing, and documentation records.
- Ensure that assessment is done in a NTE (i.e., close doors to prevent drafts and regulate room temperature). (See Critical Component: Methods of Reducing Heat Loss.)
- Inform the parents of the assessment and invite them to watch. This is especially helpful for new fathers when the initial assessment is done in the labor/delivery/recovery room.

General Survey

- Review the prenatal record and birth record for factors that could place the neonate at risk for complications. Examples of risk factors are:
  - *Maternal malnutrition prior to and/or during pregnancy*
  - *Maternal age younger than 16 and older than 35 years*
  - *Chronic maternal illnesses such as diabetes and hypertension*
  - *Hypertensive disorders of pregnancy*
  - *Labor and birth before 38 weeks of gestation*
  - *Long labor: Greater than 24 hours*
  - *Operative delivery: Use of forceps or vacuum extractor*
  - *Medications during labor that have an effect on the central nervous system (CNS; e.g., magnesium sulfate and analgesia/anesthesia)*
  - *Prolonged rupture of membranes (longer than 24 hours)*
  - *Meconium-stained amniotic fluid*
  - *Placental abnormalities*
  - *Apgar score 7 or below at 5 minutes*
- Complete a general survey of the neonate before the head-to-toe assessment.
  - *Observe the respiratory pattern and assess respirations and breath sounds.*
    - It will become more difficult to assess respiratory rate once the neonate responds (cries) to being handled during the assessment.
  - *Observe posture.*
  - *Assess the skin for color, birth trauma, and birthmarks.*
  - *Observe the level of alertness/activity.*
  - *Assess muscle tone and posture.*
- The complete assessment begins after this initial overall observation.

Neonatal Assessment by Area/System

See **Tables 15-3**, **15-4**, and **15-5**.

Gestational Age Assessment

Gestational age assessment of the newborn is based on the mother's menstrual history, prenatal ultrasonography, and/or neonatal maturational examination. The calculation

(Text continues on page 394)

TABLE 15–3 NEONATAL ASSESSMENT BY AREA/SYSTEM			
AREA OR SYSTEM	**TECHNIQUE AND ASSESSMENT**	**EXPECTED FINDINGS FOR TERM NEONATE**	**DEVIATIONS FROM NORMAL**
POSTURE	Unwrap the newborn and observe posture when the neonate is quiet.	Extremities are flexed.	Extension of extremities often related to prematurity; effects of medications given to mother during labor such as magnesium sulfate and analgesics/anesthesia; birth injuries; hypothermia; or hypoglycemia

Continued

TABLE 15–3   NEONATAL ASSESSMENT BY AREA/SYSTEM—cont'd

AREA OR SYSTEM	TECHNIQUE AND ASSESSMENT	EXPECTED FINDINGS FOR TERM NEONATE	DEVIATIONS FROM NORMAL
HEAD CIRCUMFERENCE	Measure by placing tape around the head just above the ears and eyebrows. Measurement is usually recorded in centimeters.	33–35.5 cm (13–14 inches)	Microcephaly: Head circumference is below the 10th percentile of normal for newborns gestational age. This is often related to congenital malformation, maternal drug or alcohol ingestion, or maternal infection during pregnancy. Macrocephaly: Head circumference is >90th percentile. This can be related to hydrocephalus.
CHEST CIRCUMFERENCE	Measure by placing tape around the chest over the nipple line.	30.5–33 cm (12–13 inches) or 2–3 cm less than head circumference	
LENGTH	Measure the length of body by securing tape on a flat surface. Place the top of neonate's head at the top of the tape. Extend the body and one leg. Measurement is taken from the top of the head to the bottom of the heel.	45–53 cm (19–21 inches)	Molding may interfere with accurate assessment of length. Neonates whose length is <45 cm should be further assessed for causes such as intrauterine growth restriction or prematurity.
WEIGHT	Clean scale before use. Place clean paper on the scale. Set the scale at zero. Place the naked neonate on the scale. Record the neonate's weight. Do not leave the neonate unattended while weighing.	2,500–4,000 g (5 lbs. 8 oz.–8 lbs. 13 oz.) Weight loss of 5%–10% of birth weight during the first week is normal. This is due to water loss through urine, stools, and lungs and an increase in metabolic rate. It is also related to limited fluid intake. The neonate will regain birth weight within 10 days	Weight above the 90th percentile are common in neonates of diabetic mothers. Weight below the 10th percentile is due to prematurity, intrauterine growth restriction, malnutrition during the pregnancy.
TEMPERATURE	Place a clean temperature probe in the axillary area. Axillary temperatures are preferred because of the risks of tissue trauma, perforation, and cross-contamination associated with the rectal temperature method (Blackburn, 2012).	36.5°–37.2°C (97.7°–99°F) Axillary	Hypothermia or hyperthermia is related to infection, environmental extremes, and/or neurological disorders.

TABLE 15–3 NEONATAL ASSESSMENT BY AREA/SYSTEM—cont'd

AREA OR SYSTEM	TECHNIQUE AND ASSESSMENT	EXPECTED FINDINGS FOR TERM NEONATE	DEVIATIONS FROM NORMAL
RESPIRATIONS	Assess respiratory rate by observing the rise and fall of the chest and abdomen for one full minute.	30–60 breaths per minute Slightly irregular Diaphragmatic and abdominal breathing Rate increases when crying and decreases when sleeping.	Periods of apnea >15 seconds Tachypnea that may be related to sepsis, hypothermia, hypoglycemia, or respiratory distress syndrome Respirations <30; may be related to maternal analgesia and/or anesthesia during labor.
PULSE	Assess apical pulse rate by auscultating for one full minute. Assess rate and rhythm. Use of a stethoscope designed for neonates is recommended.	120–160 bpm Rate increases (to 180 bpm) with crying and decreases (to 100 bpm) when asleep. Murmurs may be heard; most are not pathological and disappear by 6 months.	Tachycardia (> 160 bpm) indicates possible sepsis, respiratory distress, congenital heart abnormality. Bradycardia (<100 bpm) indicates possible sepsis, increased intracranial pressure, or hypoxemia.
BLOOD PRESSURE	Blood pressure is not a routine part of neonatal assessment. Requires the use of specially designed equipment for neonates. The blood pressure is obtained from either the arm or the leg of the neonate.	50–75/30–45 mm Hg	
INTEGUMENTARY/SKIN	Inspect the skin for color, intactness, bruising, birth marks, dryness, rashes, warmth, texture, and turgor. Inspect nails. Stork bite	Skin is pink with acrocyanosis (cyanosis of hands and feet). Milia are present on the bridge of the nose and chin (see Table 15-4). Lanugo is present on the back, shoulders, and forehead, which decreases with advancing gestation (see Table 15-4). Peeling or cracking is often noted on infants >40 weeks' gestation. Mongolian spots (see Table 15-4) Hemangiomas such as salmon-colored patch (stork bites), nevus flammeus (port-wine stain), and strawberry hemangiomas are developmental vascular abnormalities. Stork bites are found at the nape of the neck, on the eyelid, between the eyes, or on the upper lip. They deepen in color	Jaundice within the first 24 hours is pathological (see Chapter 17). Pallor occurs with anemia, hypothermia, shock, or sepsis. Greenish/yellowish vernix indicates passage of meconium during pregnancy and/or labor. Persistent ecchymosis or petechiae occurs with thrombocytopenia, sepsis, or congenital infection. Abundant lanugo is often seen in preterm neonates. Thin and translucent skin, and increased amounts of vernix caseosa are common in preterm neonates. Nails are longer in neonates >40 weeks' gestation. Pilonidal dimple: A small pit or sinus in the sacral area at top of crease between the

Continued

TABLE 15–3   NEONATAL ASSESSMENT BY AREA/SYSTEM—cont'd

AREA OR SYSTEM	TECHNIQUE AND ASSESSMENT	EXPECTED FINDINGS FOR TERM NEONATE	DEVIATIONS FROM NORMAL
		when the neonate cries. They disappear within the first year of life. Nevus flammeus are purple- to red-colored flat areas that can be located on various portions of the body. These do not disappear. Strawberry hemangiomas are raised bright red lesions that develop during the neonatal period. They spontaneously resolve during early childhood. Erythema toxicum, newborn rash (see Table 15-4).	buttocks; the sinus can become infected later in life.
HEAD	Note the shape of the head. Inspect and palpate fontanels and suture lines. Inspect and palpate the head for caput succedaneum and/or cephalo-hematoma (see Table 15-4). 	Molding present (see Table 15-4). Fontanels are open, soft, intact, and slightly depressed. They may bulge with crying. The anterior fontanel is dia-mond shaped, approximately 2.5–4 cm (closes by 18 months of age). The posterior fontanel is a triangle shape that is approxi-mately 0.5–1 cm (closes between 2 and 4 months). May be difficult to palpate due to excessive molding. There are overriding sutures when there is increased molding.	Fontanels that are firm and bulging and not related to crying are a possible indica-tion of increased intracra-nial pressure. Depressed fontanels are a possible indication of dehydration. Bruising and laceration at the site of the fetal scalp elec-trode or vacuum extractor Presence of caput succeda-neum and/or cephalohe-matoma (see Table 15-4).
NECK	Lift the chin to assess the neck area. 	The neck is short with skin folds. Positive tonic neck reflex (see Table 15-5).	Webbing is a possible indica-tion of genetic disorders. Absent tonic neck reflex is an indication of nerve injury.

TABLE 15–3 NEONATAL ASSESSMENT BY AREA/SYSTEM—cont'd

AREA OR SYSTEM	TECHNIQUE AND ASSESSMENT	EXPECTED FINDINGS FOR TERM NEONATE	DEVIATIONS FROM NORMAL
EYES	Assess the position of the eyes. Open the eyelids and assess color of sclera and pupil size. Assess for blink reflex, red light reflex, and pupil reaction to light.	Eyes are equal and symmetrical in size and placement. The neonate is able to follow objects within 12 inches of the visual field. Edema may be present due to pressure during labor and birth and/or reaction to eye prophylaxes. The iris is blue-gray or brown. The sclera is white or bluish-white. Subconjunctival hemorrhages related to birth trauma. Pupils are equally reactive to light. Positive red light reflex and blink reflex. No tear production (tear production begins at 2 months). Strabismus and nystagmus related to immature muscular control	Absent red light reflex indicates cataracts. Unequal pupil reactions indicate neurological trauma. Blue sclera is a possible indication of osteogenesis imperfecta.
EARS	Inspect the ears for position, shape, and drainage. Hearing test is done before discharge.	Top of the pinna is aligned with external canthus of the eye. Pinna without deformities, well formed and flexible. The neonate responds to noises with positive startle signs. Hearing becomes more acute as Eustachian tubes clear. Neonates respond more readily to high-pitched vocal sounds.	Low-set ears are associated with genetic disorders such as Down's syndrome. Absent startle reflex is associated with possible hearing loss.
NOSE	Observe the shape of the nose. Inspect the opening of the nares. Assess patency of the nares by inserting a small soft catheter. (This may not be done on all infants. Check hospital policy and procedure manual.)	The nose may be flattened or bruised related to the birth process. Nares should be patent. Small amount of mucus. Neonates primarily breathe through their noses.	Large amounts of mucus drainage can lead to respiratory distress. A flat nasal bridge is seen with Down's syndrome. Nasal flaring is a sign of respiratory distress.

Continued

TABLE 15–3   NEONATAL ASSESSMENT BY AREA/SYSTEM—cont'd

AREA OR SYSTEM	TECHNIQUE AND ASSESSMENT	EXPECTED FINDINGS FOR TERM NEONATE	DEVIATIONS FROM NORMAL
MOUTH	Inspect lips, gums, tongue, palate, and mucous membranes. Open the mouth by placing gentle pressure on the lower lip. Test for rooting, sucking, swallowing, and gag reflexes (see Table 15-5).	Lips, gums, tongue, palate, and mucous membranes are intact, pink, and moist. Reflexes are positive. Epstein's pearls are present (see Table 15-4). Thrush	Natal teeth, which can be benign or related to congenital abnormality (see Table 15-4). Thrush, a fungal infection, can be contracted during vaginal birth. It appears as white patches on the mucous membranes of the mouth. Cleft lip and/or palate, which is a congenital abnormality in which the lip and/or palate does not completely fuse (see Chapter 17).
CHEST/LUNGS	Inspect shape, symmetry, and chest excursion. Inspect the breast for size and drainage. Auscultate breath sounds. 	The chest is barrel-shaped and symmetrical. Breast engorgement is present in both male and female neonates related to the influence of maternal hormones. This resolves within a few weeks. Clear or milky fluid from nipples related to maternal hormones. Lung sounds are clear and equal. Scattered crackles may be detected during the first few hours after birth. This is due to retained amniotic fluid which will be absorbed through the lymphatics.	Funnel chest is a congenital abnormality. Pigeon chest can obstruct respirations. Chest retractions are a sign of respiratory distress. Persistent crackles, wheezes, stridor, grunting, paradoxical breathing, decreased breath sounds, and/or prolonged periods of apnea (>15–20 seconds) are signs of respiratory distress. Decreased or absent breath sounds are often related to meconium aspiration or pneumothorax.
CARDIAC	Auscultate heart sounds; listen for at least one full minute. Palpate peripheral pulses. 	Point of maximal impulse (PMI) at the 3rd or 4th intercostal space. S_1 and S_2 are present. Normal rhythm with variation related to respiratory changes. Murmurs in 30% of neonates which disappear within 2 days of birth. Peripheral pulses are present and equal. The femoral pulse may be difficult to palpate.	Dextrocardia: Heart on the right side of the chest. Displaced PMI occurs with cardiomegaly. Persistent murmurs indicate persistent fetal circulation or congenital heart defects.

TABLE 15–3   NEONATAL ASSESSMENT BY AREA/SYSTEM—cont'd

AREA OR SYSTEM	TECHNIQUE AND ASSESSMENT	EXPECTED FINDINGS FOR TERM NEONATE	DEVIATIONS FROM NORMAL
ABDOMEN	Inspect size and shape of the abdomen. Palpate the abdomen, assessing for tone, hernias, and diastasis recti. Auscultate for bowel sounds. Inspect the umbilical cord. 	The abdomen is soft, round, protuberant, and symmetrical. Bowel sounds are present, but may be hypoactive for the first few days. Passage of meconium stool within 48 hours post-birth. The cord is opaque or whitish-blue with two arteries and one vein, and covered with Wharton's jelly. The cord becomes dry and darker in color within 24 hours post-birth and detaches from the body within 2 weeks.	Asymmetrical abdomen indicates a possible abdominal mass. Hernias or diastasis recti are more common in African-American neonates and usually resolve on their own within the first year. One umbilical artery and vein is associated with heart or kidney malformation. Failure to pass meconium stool is often associated with imperforated anus or meconium ileus.
RECTUM	Inspect the anus.	The anus is patent. Passage of stool within 24 hours.	Imperforated anus requires immediate surgery. Anal fissures or fistulas.
GENITOURINARY FEMALE	Place thumbs on either side of the labia and gently separate tissue to visually inspect the genitalia. Assess for the presence and position of clitoris, vagina, and urinary meatus. 	Labia majora covers labia minora and clitoris. Labia majora and minora may be edematous. Blood-tinged vaginal discharge related to the abrupt decrease of maternal hormones (pseudomenstruation). Whitish vaginal discharge in response to maternal hormones. The neonate urinates within 24 hours. The urinary meatus is midline and an uninterrupted stream is noted on voiding.	Prominent clitoris and small labia minora are often present in preterm neonates. Ambiguous genitalia; may require genetic testing to determine sex. No urination in 24 hours may indicate a possible urinary tract obstruction, polycystic disease, or renal failure.
GENITOURINARY MALE	Inspect the penis, noting the position of the urinary meatus. Inspect and palpate the scrotum to assess for testicles. With the thumb and forefinger of one hand, palpate each testis while the other thumb and forefinger are placed over the inguinal canal to prevent the ascent of testes during assessment. Start at the upper	The urinary meatus is at the tip of the penis. The scrotum is large, pendulous, and edematous with rugae (ridges/creases) present. Both testes are palpated in the scrotum. The neonate urinates within 24 hours with an uninterrupted stream.	Hypospadias: The urethral opening is on the ventral surface of penis. Epispadias: The urethral opening is on the dorsal side of penis. Undescended testes are testes not palpated in the scrotum. Hydrocele is enlarged scrotum due to excess fluid.

Continued

TABLE 15–3   NEONATAL ASSESSMENT BY AREA/SYSTEM—cont'd

AREA OR SYSTEM	TECHNIQUE AND ASSESSMENT	EXPECTED FINDINGS FOR TERM NEONATE	DEVIATIONS FROM NORMAL
	aspect of the scrotum and move away from the body.		No urination in 24 hours may indicate possible urinary tract obstruction, polycystic disease, or renal failure. Ambiguous genitalia may require genetic testing to determine sex. Inguinal hernia.
MUSCULOSKELETAL	Inspect extremities, spine, and gluteal folds. Palpate the clavicles. Perform the Barlow–Ortolani maneuver.	Arms are symmetrical in length and equal in strength. Legs are symmetrical in length and equal in strength. 10 fingers and 10 toes. Full range of motion of all extremities. No clicks at joints. Equal gluteal folds. C curve of spine with no dimpling.	Polydactyly: Extra digits may indicate a genetic disorder. Syndactyly: Webbed digits may indicate a genetic disorder. Unequal gluteal folds and/or positive Barlow-Ortolani maneuver are associated with congenital hip dislocation. Decreased range of motion and/or muscle tone indicates possible birth injury, neurological disorder, or prematurity. Swelling, crepitus, and/or neck tenderness indicates possible broken clavicle, which can occur during the birthing process in neonates with large shoulders. Simian creases, short fingers, wide space between big toe and second toe are common with Down's syndrome.
NEUROLOGICAL	Assess posture. Assess tone. Test newborn reflexes (see Table 15-5).	Flexed position Rapid recoil of extremities to the flexed position Positive newborn reflexes	Hypotonia: Floppy, limp extremities indicate possible nerve injury related to birth, depression of CNS related to maternal medication received during labor or to fetal hypoxia during labor, prematurity, or spinal cord injury. Hypertonia: Tightly flexed arms and stiffly extended legs with quivering indicate possible drug withdrawal. Paralysis indicates possible birth trauma or spinal injury. Tremors are possibly due to hypoglycemia, drug withdrawal, cold stress.

Adapted from Dillon, P. (2007). *Nursing health assessment,* chapter 24, an F.A. Davis publication with expected findings supported by AWOHNN sponsored publication, Mattson, S. & Smith, J. (2011). *Core curriculum for maternal-newborn nursing (4th ed.).*

TABLE 15–4   COMMON NEWBORN CHARACTERISTICS

CHARACTERISTIC	APPEARANCE	SIGNIFICANCE
ACROCYANOSIS	Hands and/or feet are blue.	Response to cold environment Immature peripheral circulation
CIRCUMORAL CYANOSIS	A benign localized transient cyanosis around the mouth	Observed during the transitional period; if it persists it may be related to a cardiac anomaly.
MOTTLING	A benign transient pattern of pink and white blotches on the skin	Response to cold environment
HARLEQUIN SIGN	One side of body is pink and the other side is white.	Related to vasomotor instability
MONGOLIAN SPOTS	Flat, bluish discolored area on the lower back and/or buttock. Seen more often in African American, Asian, Hispanic, and Native American infants.	Might be mistaken for bruising. Need to document size and location. Resolves on own by school age.
ERYTHEMA TOXICUM	A rash with red macules and papules (white to yellowish-white papule in center surrounded by reddened skin) that appear in different areas of the body, usually the trunk area Can appear within 24 hours of birth and up to 2 weeks.	Benign Disappears without treatment.
MILIA	White papules on the face; more frequently seen on the bridge of the nose and chin	Exposed sebaceous glands that resolve without treatment. Parents might mistake these for "whiteheads." Inform parents to leave them alone and let them resolve on own.

Continued

TABLE 15–4   COMMON NEWBORN CHARACTERISTICS—cont'd

CHARACTERISTIC	APPEARANCE	SIGNIFICANCE
LANUGO 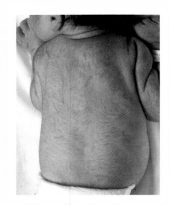	Fine, downy hair that develops after 16 weeks of gestation. The amount of lanugo decreases as the fetus ages. Often seen on the neonate's back, shoulders, and forehead.	Gradually falls out. The presence and amount of lanugo assist in estimating gestational age. Abundant lanugo may be a sign of prematurity or genetic disorder.
VERNIX CASEOSA 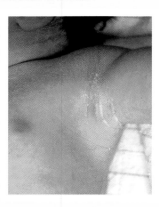	A protective substance secreted from sebaceous glands that covered the fetus during pregnancy It looks like a whitish cheesy substance. May be noted in auxiliary areas and genital areas of full-term neonates.	The presence and amount of vernix assist in estimating gestational age. Full-term neonates usually have none or small amounts of vernix.
JAUNDICE 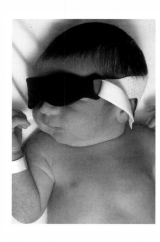	Yellow coloring of skin. First appears on the face and extends to the trunk and eventually the entire body. Best assessed in natural lighting. When jaundice is suspected, the nurse can apply gentle pressure to the skin over a firm surface such as nose, forehead, or sternum. The skin blanches to a yellowish hue.	Jaundice within the first 24 hours is pathological; usually related to problem of the liver (see Chapter 17). Jaundice occurring after 24 hours is referred to as physiological jaundice and is related to increased amount of unconjugated bilirubin in the system (see Chapter 17).

TABLE 15–4 COMMON NEWBORN CHARACTERISTICS—cont'd

CHARACTERISTIC	APPEARANCE	SIGNIFICANCE
MOLDING 	Elongation of the fetal head as it adapts to the birth canal	Resolves within 1 week.
CAPUT SUCCEDANEUM 	A localized soft tissue edema of the scalp It feels "spongy" and can cross suture lines.	Results from prolonged pressure of the head against the maternal cervix during labor. Resolves within the first week of life.
CEPHALHEMATOMA 	Hematoma formation between the periosteum and skull with unilateral swelling. It appears within a few hours of birth and can increase in size over the next few days. It has a well-defined outline. It does not cross suture lines.	Related trauma to the head due to prolonged labor, forceps delivery, or use of vacuum extractor. Can contribute to jaundice due to the large amounts of red blood cells being hemolyzed. Resolves within 3 months.
EPSTEIN'S PEARLS 	White, pearl-like epithelial cysts on gum margins and palate	Benign and usually disappears within a few weeks.

Continued

TABLE 15–4   COMMON NEWBORN CHARACTERISTICS—cont'd

CHARACTERISTIC	APPEARANCE	SIGNIFICANCE
NATAL TEETH 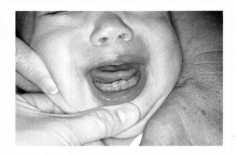	Immature caps of enamel and dentin with poorly developed roots Usually only one or two teeth are present.	They are usually benign, but can be associated with congenital defects. Natal teeth are often loose and need to be removed to decrease the risk of aspiration.

Adapted from Dillon, P. (2007). *Nursing assessment* (pp. 855–867). Philadelphia: F.A. Davis.

TABLE 15–5   NEWBORN REFLEXES

REFLEX	HOW ELICITED	EXPECTED RESPONSE	ABNORMAL RESPONSE
MORO Present at birth; disappears by 6 months.	Jar the crib or hold the baby in a semisitting position and let the head slightly drop back.	Symmetrical abduction and extension of arms and legs, and legs flex up against trunk. The neonate makes a "C" shape with thumb and index finger.	A slow response might occur with preterm infants or sleepy neonates. An asymmetrical response may be related to temporary or permanent birth injury to clavicle, humerus, or brachial plexus.
STARTLE Present at birth; disappears by 4 months	Make a loud sound near the neonate.	Same as Moro response	Slow response when sleeping Possible deafness Possible neurological deficit
TONIC NECK Present between birth and 6 weeks; disappears by 4 to 6 months	With the neonate in a supine position, turn the head to the side so that the chin is over the shoulder.	The neonate assumes a "fencing" position with arms and legs extended in the direction in which the head was turned.	Response after 6 months may indicate cerebral palsy.

TABLE 15–5   NEWBORN REFLEXES—cont'd

REFLEX	HOW ELICITED	EXPECTED RESPONSE	ABNORMAL RESPONSE
ROOTING Present at birth; disappears between 3 and 6 months	Brush the side of a cheek near the corner of the mouth. 	The neonate turns his head toward the direction of the stimulus and opens his mouth. Instruct mothers who are lactating to touch the corner of the neonate's mouth with a nipple and the infant will turn toward the nipple for feeding.	May not respond if recently fed. Prematurity or neurological defects may cause weak or absent response.
SUCKING Present at birth; disappears at 10–12 months	Place a gloved finger or nipple of a bottle in the neonate's mouth. 	Sucking motion occurs.	May not respond if recently fed. Prematurity or neurological defects may cause weak or absent response.
PALMER GRASP Present at birth; disappears at 3–4 months	The examiner places a finger in the palm of the neonate's hand. 	The neonate grasps fingers tightly. If the neonate grasps the examiner's fingers with both hands, the neonate can be pulled to a sitting position.	Absent or weak response indicates a possible CNS defect; or nerve or muscle injury.
PLANTAR GRASP Present at birth; disappears at 3–4 months	Place a thumb firmly against the ball of the infant's foot. 	Toes flex tightly down in a grasping motion	Weak or absent may indicate possible spinal cord injury.
BABINSKI Present at birth; disappears at 1 year	Stroke the lateral surface of the sole in an upward motion. 	Hyperextension and fanning of toes	Absent or weak may indicate a possible neurological defect.

Continued

TABLE 15–5 NEWBORN REFLEXES—cont'd			
REFLEX	HOW ELICITED	EXPECTED RESPONSE	ABNORMAL RESPONSE
STEPPING OR DANCING Present at birth; disappears at 3–4 weeks	Hold the neonate upright with feet touching a flat surface.	The neonate steps up and down in place. 	Diminished response may indicate hypotonia.

Adapted from Dillon, P. (2007). *Nursing assessment* (pp. 868–873). Philadelphia: F.A. Davis.

of gestational age by instruments such as Dubowitz neurological exam or Ballard scale of physical and neuromuscular maturity assists in predicting potential problems and establishing plan of care based on gestational age.

- Most hospital nurseries have written policies on which neonates should routinely be assessed for gestational age. Gestational age assessment is commonly completed on:
  - *Neonates who, based on the maternal menstrual history, are **preterm**, born before 37 weeks; or **post-term**, born after 42 weeks by dates*
  - *Neonates who weigh less than 2,500 grams or more than 4,000 grams*
  - *Neonates of diabetic mothers*
  - *Neonates whose condition requires admission to a neonatal intensive care unit (NICU).*
- The **Dubowitz neurological exam** is a standardized tool that assesses 33 responses in four areas:
  - *Habituation (the response to repetitive light and sound stimuli)*
  - *Movement and muscle tone*
  - *Reflexes*
  - *Neurobehavioral items*
- The **Ballard Maturational Score (BMS)** is calculated by assessing the physical and neuromuscular maturity of the neonate. It can be completed in less time than the Dubowitz neurological exam. It consists of six evaluation areas for neuromuscular maturity and six items of observed physical maturity (**Table 15-6**). The examination determines weeks of gestation and classifies the neonate as preterm (<37 weeks), term (37–42 weeks), or post-term (>42 weeks).
- The scores from these exams provide a gestational age that is graphed based on weight, length, and head circumference to determine if the neonate is average for gestational age (AGA), small for gestational age (SGA), or large for gestational age (LGA) (**Fig. 15-8**).
  - *SGA is a term used for neonates whose weight is below the 10th percentile for gestational age.*
  - *LGA is a term used for neonates whose weight is above the 90th percentile for gestational age.*

Pain Assessment

Neonates are subjected to a variety of painful stimuli during their transition to extrauterine life (e.g., injections, heel sticks for blood samples, and circumcision). In the past, health care providers believed that neonates did not experience the sensation of pain, so little attention was given to assessing and reducing pain in the neonate. In the 1990s, researchers began to address this lack of knowledge by gaining a better understanding of neonatal pain, developing tools that assess for neonatal pain, and determining appropriate and safe pain management for neonates.

- The 1995 National Association of Neonatal Nurses (NANN) position statement on pain management in infants states that "all health care professionals who care for neonates/infants need ongoing education in the assessment and management of neonatal pain and that neonates/infants be protected from the adverse effects of pain" (NANN, 1995).
- The 2001 Joint Commission on Accreditation of Healthcare Organizations (JCAHO) pain management standards states that "every patient has a right to have his or her pain assessed and treated" (JCAHO, 2001), including neonates.

TABLE 15–6   BALLARD MATURATIONAL ASSESSMENT

NEUROMUSCULAR MATURITY	PHYSICAL MATURITY
POSTURE Assess the position the neonate assumes while lying quietly on his back. The more mature, the greater degree of flexion in legs and arms.	**SKIN** The examiner inspects the neonate's chest and abdominal skin areas for texture, transparency, thickness, and for peeling and/or cracking. A preterm neonate's skin is smooth, thin, and translucent (numerous veins visible). A full-term neonate's skin is thicker and more opaque with some degree of peeling.
SQUARE WINDOW Assess the degree of the angle created when the examiner flexes the neonate's hand toward the forearm. The more mature, the greater the flexion.	**LANUGO** The examiner assesses the amount of lanugo on the neonate's back. Lanugo begins to form around the 24th week of gestation. It is abundant in preterm neonates and decreases in amount as the neonate matures.
ARM RECOIL With the neonate in a supine position, the examiner fully flexes the forearm against the neonate's chest for 5 seconds. The examiner extends the arms and releases them. The more mature, the faster the arms return to the flexed position (recoil).	**PLANTAR CREASES** The examiner inspects the bottom of the feet for location of creases. The more creases over the greater proportion of the foot, the more mature the neonate.
POPLITEAL ANGLE With the neonate in a supine position and pelvis flat, the examiner flexes the neonate's thigh to the abdomen. The leg is then extended. The angle at the knee is estimated. The lesser the angle, the greater the maturity.	**BREAST TISSUE** The examiner assesses the degree of nipple formation. The size of the breast bud is measured by gently grasping the tissue with thumb and forefinger and measuring the distance between thumb and forefinger. The greater the degree of nipple formation and size of the breast bud, the greater the maturity.
SCARF SIGN With the neonate in a supine position, the examiner takes the neonate's hand and moves the arm across the chest toward the opposite shoulder. The examiner notes where the elbow is in relationship to the midline of the chest. The more preterm, the more the elbow crosses the midline.	**EAR FORMATION** The examiner assesses the ear for form and firmness. The more defined the ear is and the firmer it is, the more mature the neonate.
HEEL TO EAR With the neonate in a supine position, the examiner takes the neonate's foot and moves it toward the ear. The lesser the flexion (the further the heel is from the ear), the greater the maturity.	**GENITALIA** Male: The examiner palpates the scrotum for the presence of testis and inspects the scrotum for appearance. The greater the descent of the testis and the greater degree of rugae (creases), the greater the maturity. Female: The examiner moves the neonate's hip one half abduction and visually inspects the genitalia. The more the labia majora covers the labia minora and clitoris, the greater the maturity.

Neuromuscular Maturity

	-1	0	1	2	3	4	5
Posture							
Square Window (Wrist)	-90°	90°	60°	45°	30°	0°	
Arm Recoil		180°	140°-180°	110°-140°	90°-110°	<90°	
Popliteal Angle	180°	160°	140°	120°	100°	90°	<90°
Scarf Sign							
Heel To Ear							

Physical Maturity

Skin	sticky friable transparent	gelantinous red translucent	smooth pink visible veins	superficial peeling or rash, few veins	cracking pale areas rare veins	parchment deep cracking no vessels	leathery cracked wrinkled
Lanugo	none	sparse	abundant	thinning	bald areas	mostly bald	
Plantar Surface	heel-toe 40–50 mm:-1 <40 mm:-2	>50 mm no crease	faint red marks	anterior transverse crease only	creases ant. 2/3	creases over entire sole	
Breast	imperceptible	barely perceptible	flat areola no bud	stippled areola 1–2 mm bud	raised areola 3–4 mm bud	full areola 5–10 mm bud	
Eye/ear	lids fused loosely:-1 tightly:-2	lids open pinna flat stays folded	sl. curved pinna; soft; slow recoil	well-curved pinna; soft but ready recoil	formed and firm instant recoil	thick cartilage ear stiff	
Genitals (Male)	scrotum flat, smooth	scrotum empty faint rugae	testes in upper canal rare rugae	testes descending few rugae	testes down good rugae	testes pendulous deep rugae	
Genitals (Female)	clitoris prominent labia flat	prominent clitoris small labia minora	prominent clitoris enlarging minora	majora and minora equally prominent	majora large minora small	majora cover clitoris and minora	

Maturity Rating

Score	Weeks
-10	20
-5	22
0	24
5	26
10	28
15	30
20	32
25	34
30	36
35	38
40	40
45	42
50	44

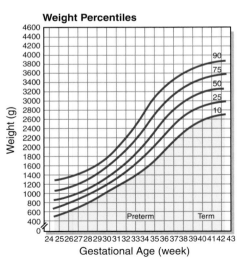

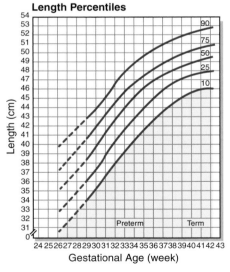

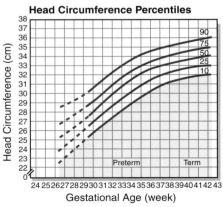

Classification of Infant*

	Weight	Length	Head Circ.
Large for gestational age (LGA) (>90th percentile)			
Appropriate for gestational age (AGA) (10th to 90th percentile)			
Small for gestational age (SGA) (<10th percentile)			

*Place an "X" in the appropriate box (LGA, AGA, or SGA) for weight, for length and for head circumference.

Figure 15–8 Ballard Gestational Age Assessment Tool.

■ Several pain scales, such as Premature Infant Pain Profile (PIPP) and Neonatal Infant Pain Scale (NIPS), have been developed to assess for neonatal pain. Pain assessment tools commonly look at state of arousal, cry, motor activity, respiratory pattern, and facial expressions. Some tools may also include blood pressure and oxygen saturation level.

■ Pain assessment is part of the nursing care of neonates, and the tool used for assessment varies based on hospital policies and procedures (**Box 15-1**)

BEHAVIORAL CHARACTERISTICS

The neonate is a biosocial being with very unique behavioral characteristics that affect parent-infant attachment (see Chapter 13). Temperament can vary from a neonate being an "easy" baby to a "fussy" baby. Most neonates vacillate between the two extremes of temperament. The neonate experiences predictable periods referred to as periods of reactivity.

Periods of Reactivity

During the first 6–8 hours of extrauterine life, the neonate transitions between periods of activity and inactivity. This is often referred to "periods of reactivity." Each of the periods has predictable neonatal behaviors.

Initial Period of Reactivity

■ Occurs in the first 15–30 minutes post-birth
■ The neonate is alert and active.
■ The neonate vigorously responds to external stimuli.
■ Respirations are irregular and rapid (can be as high as 90 breaths per minute).
■ The neonate may exhibit momentary grunting, flaring, and retractions.
■ Brief periods of apnea may occur.
■ The heart rate is rapid and can be as high as 180 beats per minute.
■ Brief period of cyanosis can occur.
■ The amount of oral mucus increases.

Period of Relative Inactivity

■ Begins approximately 30 minutes after birth and lasts 2 hours
■ Sleep state

BOX 15–1 ASPMN POSITION STATEMENT: PAIN ASSESSMENT IN THE PATIENT UNABLE TO SELF-REPORT

"The American Society for Pain Management Nursing (ASPMN) positions that all persons with pain deserve prompt recognition and treatment. Pain should be routinely assessed, reassessed, and documented to facilitate treatment and communication among health care clinicians. In patients who are unable to self-report pain, other strategies must be used to infer pain and evaluate interventions."

Herr et al., 2011.

■ The neonate is unresponsive to external stimuli.
■ The respiratory rate decreases and can fall slightly below normal range.
■ The heart rate decreases and is within normal limits.
■ Oral mucus production decreases.

Second Period of Reactivity

■ Follows the period of relative inactivity and lasts 2–8 hours
■ Varies between active alert and quiet alert state
■ Periods of rapid respiration in response to stimuli and activity
■ Heart rate varies related to activity level and response to stimuli.
■ Increased bowel activity and may pass meconium stool
■ The neonate responds to external stimuli.

The initial period of activity provides an opportunity for the parents and neonate to respond to each other. It is an ideal time to initiate breastfeeding. The neonate is not responsive during the period of inactivity and will not be interested in feeding/sucking. During the second period of reactivity, the neonate is interested in feeding/sucking, and this is another ideal time for breastfeeding.

Brazelton Neonatal Behavioral Assessment Scale

The Brazelton Neonatal Behavioral Assessment Scale (BNBAS) is used to assess the neonate's neurobehavioral system. The BNBAS was originally developed as a research tool and has been adapted for use in the clinical setting. The BNBAS is not routinely preformed on healthy neonates. It is composed of 28 behavior items and 18 reflex items. These behaviors/reflex items are divided into six categories:

■ **Habituation:** The development of decreased sensitivity to a repeated stimulus such as light, sound, or heel stick. It is a protective mechanism against overstimulation. Habituation may not be fully developed in premature neonates or in neonates with CNS abnormalities or injuries.
■ **Orientation:** The ability of the neonate to focus on visual and/or auditory stimuli. The neonate will turn his or her head in the direction of sound or will follow a visual stimulus. This response is diminished in premature neonates.
■ **Motor maturity:** The ability of the neonate to control and coordinate motor activity. Normal findings are smooth, free movement with occasional tremors. Movement is jerky in premature neonates and/or in neonates with CNS abnormalities or injuries.
■ **Self-quieting ability:** The ability of the neonate to quiet and comfort self. It is accomplished by sucking on the fist/hand or attending to external stimuli. The ability is diminished in neonates with neurological injuries or in neonates exposed to drugs in utero.
■ **Social behaviors:** The ability of the neonate to respond to cuddling and holding. These behaviors are diminished or absent in neonates with neurological injuries or in neonates exposed to drugs in utero.

■ **Sleep/awake states:** These are also referred to as infant states or behavior states. There are two sleep states and four awake states.

■ *Deep sleep: During this state, there is no body movement except for an occasional startle reflex. The startle reflex is delayed in response to external stimuli. External stimuli are less likely to cause a change in state. The eyes are closed and there are no eye movements. Breathing is smooth and even.*

■ *Light sleep: During this state, there is random body movement. Rapid eye movement (REM) is present. The neonate responds to external stimuli with a startle reflex and with a possible change of state. Breathing is irregular.*

■ *Drowsy: During this state, there is intermittent body movement. Eyes open and close, and have a dull and heavy-lidded appearance. Breathing is irregular. Response to sensory stimuli is delayed. External stimuli will most likely cause a change in state. Breathing is irregular.*

■ *Alert: During this state the neonate's eyes are wide open with a bright look and focus on the sources of stimuli. There is a delay in response to stimuli and minimal body movement. Respirations are regular.*

■ *Eyes open: During this state, there is a considerable body movement with periods of fussiness. The eyes are open. The neonate responds to external stimuli with increased startle reflexes and motor activity. Breathing is irregular.*

■ *Crying: During this state, there is high motor activity and intense crying. It is difficult to calm the neonate. The eyes are opened or tightly closed. Breathing is irregular (Brazelton & Nugent, 1995).*

NURSING CARE OF THE NEONATE

Nursing care of the neonate during hospitalization is divided into two time frames. The first is the 4th stage of labor, which is from birth through the first 4 hours of extrauterine life. The second is from 4 hours of age to discharge.

Nursing Actions During the 4th Stage of Labor

The changes that occur in the neonate's body during the transition to extrauterine life require frequent assessments and monitoring to identify early signs of physiological compromise (see Critical Component: Danger Signs *and* Critical Component: Hypothermia). Early identification of complications or difficulty with transition allows for earlier initiation of nursing and medical actions to support the neonate in a healthy transition. The following nursing actions occur in the labor/delivery/recovery room and/or nursery depending on hospital policies and health state of the neonate. These actions are supported by the Association of Women's Health, Obstetric and Neonatal Nurses (AWHONN) in its 2011 publication, *Core curriculum for maternal-newborn nursing.*

■ Review prenatal and intrapartal records for factors that place the neonate at risk, such as prolonged rupture of membranes (risk of infection), meconium-stained fluid (risk of respiratory distress), and gestational diabetes (risk of hypoglycemia).

■ Decrease risk of cold stress by:

■ *Drying the neonate immediately after birth to prevent excessive heat loss through evaporation.*

■ *Discarding wet blankets and placing the neonate on dry, warm blankets or sheets.*

■ *Placing a stocking cap on the neonate's head to decrease the risk of heat loss through convection.*

■ *Placing the neonate in the mother's arms with skin-to-skin contact and a warm blanket over mother and baby or placing the neonate under a preheated radiant warmer.*

■ Support respirations by clearing the mouth and nose of excessive mucus with a bulb syringe when indicated.

■ Use universal precautions and wear gloves until after the neonate has been bathed to decrease exposure to blood-borne pathogens from amniotic fluid and maternal blood.

■ Obtain the Apgar score at 1 and 5 minutes and initiate appropriate actions based on the score (see Chapter 8).

■ Assess vital signs.

■ *This is usually done within 30 minutes of birth, 1 hour after birth, and then every hour for the remainder of the recovery period.*

■ The frequency of assessments may vary based on institutional policies and the health of the neonate.

■ Vital signs are assessed every 5–15 minutes for neonates with signs of distress.

■ *Administer O$_2$ per institutional protocol, if the heart rate is below 100 beats per minute, cyanosis is present, and/or apnea occurs. Before administration of O$_2$ the nurse should:*

■ Check the airway and apply suction if indicated.

■ Stimulate the neonate by rubbing his back.

■ Inspect the clamped cord for number of vessels and f⌐ bleeding.

■ Complete and place identifying bands on the ⌐ ⌐ ⌐ ⌐d parents ⌐ ⌐

taker

■ We

■ Cor

■ *E*

pe

■ Com⌐

polici⌐

■ Obtair

■ *This*

hypo⌐

hypo⌐

■ Administ⌐

■ *The A⌐*

for Dis⌐

that op⌐

to all ne⌐

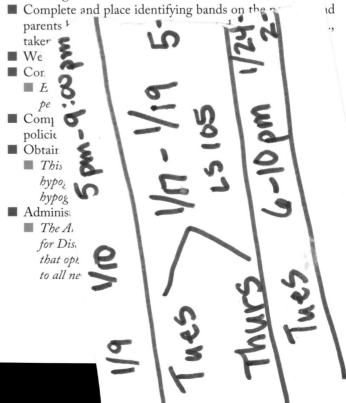

■ *Refer to institutional policies for timing of the application of ointment.*
■ Administer phytonadione IM.
■ Support breastfeeding by providing a relaxing environment for the woman and her newborn (**Fig. 15-9**).
■ Bathe the neonate with neutral pH soap. The initial bath is delayed until the neonate's temperature is stable and within normal limits.
■ Promote parent-infant attachment by creating a relaxing environment:
   ■ *Cluster nursing activities to allow for periods of uninterrupted time for new parents to spend time with their newborn.*
   ■ *Dim lights and close room door.*
■ Notify the neonate's physician or nurse practitioner of the neonate's date and time of birth, and assessment findings.

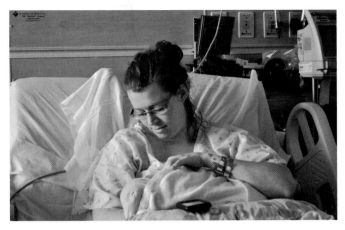

Figure 15-9 Newborn breastfeeding during the fourth stage of labor.

Medication

Erythromycin Ophthalmic Ointment (0.5%)

■ Indication: Prophylaxis treatment for gonococcal or chlamydial eye infections
■ Action: Prevents bacterial growth by inhibiting folic acid synthesis
■ Common side effects: Edema and inflammation of eyelids
■ Route and dose: Apply a ¼-inch bead of ointment to lower eyelid of each eye.
■ Precaution: Prevent the applicator tip from directly touching the eye by holding the application tube ½ inch from the eye.

(Data Vallerand & Sanoski, 2013)

CRITICAL COMPONENT

Promoting Parent-Infant Attachment

The promotion of parent-infant attachment is a critical component of nursing care, and needs to occur as soon as possible after birth. Often nurses allow other nursing actions to take priority over parent-infant attachment or find it is easier to do assessments under the warming unit. Assessments and monitoring of vital signs can be performed in the parent's arms when the neonate is full term, the Apgar score is 8 or higher, and there were no signs of fetal distress during labor or at the time of birth.

Nursing Actions

■ Skin-to-skin contact with a warm blanket over the neonate and parent.
■ Point out and explain expected neonatal characteristics such as molding, milia, and lanugo.
■ Provide alone time for the couple and their newborn by organizing care that allows for uninterrupted time.
■ Delay administration of eye ointment until parents have had an opportunity to hold the baby. Once ointment is administered, the neonate is less likely to open his or her eyes and make eye contact with parents.

CRITICAL COMPONENT

Danger Signs

The following signs may be an indication of an abnormality or complication. Document these signs in the neonatal record and report them to the physician or nurse practitioner:

■ Tachypnea (>60 breaths per minute)
■ Retractions of chest wall
■ Grunting
■ Nasal flaring
■ Abdominal distention
■ Failure to pass meconium stool within 48 hours of birth
■ Failure to void within 24 hours of birth
■ Convulsions
■ Lethargy
■ Jaundice within first 24 hours of birth
■ Abnormal temperature, either abnormally high or low
■ Jitteriness
■ Persistent hypoglycemia
■ Persistent temperature instability

Nursing Actions from 4 Hours of Age to Discharge

The second stage of neonatal care focuses on monitoring the neonate's adaptation to extrauterine life and assisting parents in learning about their newborn and how to care for her (see Critical Component: Promoting Parent-Infant Attachment). The nursing actions listed are for neonates who do not exhibit signs of distress or potential complications.

■ Assess vital signs as per hospital policy.
   ■ *Vital signs for stable neonates are assessed at a minimum of once a shift.*
      ■ The neonate may continue to have difficulty in regulating her body temperature.
      ■ Notify the physician or nurse practitioner if temperature decrease persists.
■ Complete neonatal assessment once per shift. The type of assessment varies based on institutional policies.

■ Promote parent-infant attachment by providing uninterrupted times with the infant.

■ Promote sibling attachment by providing opportunities for interactions with the newborn, such as having older siblings assist with newborn care or listen to the newborn's heart.

■ Prevent infant abduction from the hospital. Each hospital has policies and procedures addressing methods to prevent infant abduction. Common steps that are taken are:

■ *Footprints and photo of infant for identification purposes*

■ *Arm bands on the mother, father, and neonate that contain the same identification number. The bands of the neonate should be checked with the bands of the parents at the beginning of each shift and when taking or returning the neonate from or to the mother's room.*

■ *Personnel working in the maternal–newborn units should have name tags that are specific to that unit. Name tags should have a photo and name of the person.*

■ *Instruct parents and family members to not allow a person to take their newborn if the person does not possess the appropriate identification that is specific to the maternity unit.*

■ *Encourage parents to accompany any person who removes their infant from the mother's room.*

■ *Place the neonate's crib on the far side of the room away from the door leading to the hallway.*

■ *Instruct parents not to leave their newborn in the mother's room unattended. This includes when she is taking a shower.*

■ *The maternal–newborn units should be secure and only visitors with identification allowed to enter.*

■ Assist parents with infant feeding (see Chapter 16).

■ Provide information to parents on newborn care (see Chapter 16).

■ Teach parents about normal newborn characteristics (see Table 15-4).

■ Instruct parents to place their newborn on his back or side to decrease the risk of sudden infant death syndrome (see Chapter 16).

CRITICAL COMPONENT

Hypothermia

Neonates with temperatures below 36.5°C (97.7°F) are at risk for hypothermia.

Nursing actions:

■ Parent-infant skin-to-skin contact with a warm blanket over both the neonate and the parent.

■ Wrap the neonate in warm blankets.

■ If the temperature remains below 36.5°C (97.7°F), place the neonate under a preheated warmer. Unwrap the neonate so that the skin is exposed to the radiant heat. Attach the electronic skin probe. The warmer is set at 1.5°C above the neonate's temperature. Continue to adjust the radiant temperature in relationship to the neonate's temperature.

■ Monitor the blood glucose level as per institutional policies, as hypothermia can lead to hypoglycemia.

■ Notify the physician or nurse practitioner if the neonate's temperature does not return to normal ranges.

■ Document the temperature and actions taken.

SKIN CARE

The skin of a term neonate is smooth, soft, slightly transparent, and has less pigmentation than that of an older child (Blackburn, 2012). The neonate's skin is subjected to a variety of stresses related to the birthing process and transition to extrauterine life. Causes of potential threats to skin integrity are:

■ Pressure exerted on the presenting part of the fetus during the labor and birthing process from maternal structures such as the pelvis, causing edema and hematomas

■ Abrasions, bruising, and edema of the skin related to use of vacuum extractors, forceps, and internal fetal monitoring

■ Exposure to bacteria from the maternal genital tract

■ Use of adhesives

■ *Use stretchy wraps vs adhesives for securing probes and electrodes*

■ Drying out and flacking of skin during the first few weeks of life

■ *This is a natural process in the skin's transition from intrauterine to extrauterine life.*

■ Diaper dermatitis

■ *Actions to decreases risk of diaper dermatitis:*

■ Change diapers with each feeding.

■ Use superabsorbent diapers that contain gelling materials which keep moisture away from skin.

■ Apply barrier products containing petrolatum and/or zinc oxide.

■ Apply antifungal creams when fungal infection is present (Heimall et al., 2012)

Because intact and healthy skin is a first-line defense against infection, the neonate's skin needs to be assessed at each shift and with each diaper change, and care must be provided to maintain healthy skin.

LABORATORY AND DIAGNOSTIC TESTS

Newborn Screening

Newborn screening is a blood test that screens for infections, genetic diseases, and inherited and metabolic disorders and is performed on all babies born in the United States (ACOG, 2003) (**Box 15-2**).

■ Routine newborn screening began in the 1960s when all babies were screened for phenylketonuria (PKU), and over the years technologies advanced and can now screen for approximately 30 disorders.

■ *Phenylketonuria (PKU) is an inborn error of metabolism. Neonates with PKU are unable to metabolize phenylalanine, which is an amino acid commonly found in many foods such as breast milk and formula. This leads to a buildup of phenylpyruvic and phenylacetic acids, which are abnormal metabolites of phenylalanine. The buildup of abnormal metabolites can cause permanent brain damage and death, which can be prevented by early detection and dietary management.*

■ Each state has statutes or regulations on newborn screening, and the degree of screening varies from state to state.

■ *Healthy People 2020* goal is to increase the number of states and the District of Columbia that verify through linkage with vital records that all newborns are screened shortly after birth for conditions mandated by their state-sponsored screening program from 21 states to 45 states including District of Columbia (Healthy People, 2012).

■ The National Newborn Screening and Genetics Resource Center provides a current status report as to which tests

are required for each state. The list can be accessed at http://genes-r-us.uthscsa.edu/nbsdisorders.pdf.

■ Some states screen for human immunodeficiency virus (HIV).

■ Obtaining blood sample:
   ■ *Provide parents with information regarding the screening test. Some states require the parents' written consent.*
   ■ *The blood is obtained from a heel stick and may be collected by nursing or laboratory personnel (see Critical Component: Heel Stick).*
   ■ *The ideal time of collection is at 2–5 days of age, which provides time for the neonate to ingest breast milk or formula. Most are done within the first 24–48 hours because of discharges occurring during that time period. Neonates are usually retested later at a routine newborn check-up.*

Newborn Hearing Screening

The National Institute on Deafness and Other Communication disorders (NIDCD) reports that 2–3 out of every 1,000 infants in the United States are born with a hearing impairment (NIDCD, 2006). The 2012 U.S. screening status report lists 34 states and Washington, DC, that have laws requiring hearing screening of all newborns (NNSGRC, 2012). The hearing screening test is usually done in the hospital before discharge by a member of the nursing staff who has completed special training and education in conducting the test (**Fig. 15-10**).

■ There are two types of screening tests that may be used either alone or together. The screening tests rely

---

CULTURAL AWARENESS: Cultural and Ethical Variations in Infants

African American: Mongolian spots and other birthmarks are more prevalent than in other ethnic groups.

Amish: Babies are seen as gifts from God. Have high birth rates, large families.

Appalachian: Newborns wear bands around the abdomen to prevent umbilical hernias and asafetida bags around the neck to prevent contagious diseases.

Arab American: Children are "dearly loved."

Chinese American: Male circumcision is a religious requirement; children are highly valued; Mongolian spots occur in about 80% of infants; bilirubin levels are higher in Chinese newborns than in others, with the highest levels seen on post-birth day 5 or 6.

Cuban American: Childbirth is a celebration; the family takes care of both the mother and infant for the first 4 weeks; tend to bottle feed rather than breastfeed; if breastfeeding, weaning is early, around 3 months; if bottle feeding, weaning is late, around 4 years.

Egyptian American: Children are very important.

Filipino American: Eyes are almond shaped, low to flat nose bridge with mildly flared nostrils; Mongolian spots common.

French Canadian: Five mutations account for 90% of phenylketonuria (PKU); high incidence of cystic fibrosis and muscular dystrophy.

Greek American: High incidence of two genetic conditions: thalassemia and glucose-6-phosphate dehydrogenase (G6PD) deficiency.

Iranian American: Believe in hot/cold influences, with baby boys "hotter" than baby girls; infants may be confined to the home for the first 40 days; ritual bath between the 10th and 40th post-birth day.

Jewish American: Children are seen as valued treasures; high incidence of Tay-Sachs disease; male circumcision is a religious ritual.

Mexican American: Wear stomach belt (*ombliguero*) to prevent umbilicus from popping out when the infant cries.

Navajo Native American: Infants are kept in cradle boards until they can walk; Mongolian spots are common.

Vietnamese American: Mongolian spots are common.

(Purnell, 2012)

BOX 15–2   AWHONN POSITION STATEMENT: NEWBORN SCREENING

"The Association of Women's Health, Obstetric and Neonatal Nursing (AWHONN) supports national minimum standards for newborn screening programs. Federal oversight is necessary to guarantee that all newborns have equal access to timely identification and interventions for disorders that have been identified for routine screening. In addition, a combination of federal and state funding should be allocated to initiate and sustain programs that limit the effects of these disorders."

"AWHONN recommends that Newborn Screening programs include the following:

■ Health care provider education
■ Parent education
■ Parental notification and consent, even if tests are mandatory
■ Timely screening tests prior to hospital or birthing facility discharge
■ Post discharge follow-up for additional screening tests or other services, when appropriate
■ Resources for appropriate referrals
■ Accurate and consistent systems for data collection
■ Access to interventions and treatments indicated by the diagnosis."

The Association of Women's Health, Obstetric and Neonatal Nursing (AWHONN), 2011.

CRITICAL COMPONENT

Heel Stick

- The heel stick is a common procedure performed on neonates.
- Blood is collected to assess blood glucose and hematocrit and for newborn screening.

Procedure

1. Provide parents with information on the test that has been ordered for their child.
2. Obtain required consents.
3. Warm the neonate's foot for 10 minutes by wrapping in a warm, moist washcloth. This will help facilitate circulation to the peripheral area.
4. Don gloves.
5. With the nondominant hand, hold the neonate's foot in a dorsiflexed position. The nurse or technician should have a firm grasp of the foot, but the foot should not be squeezed.
6. Clean the heel with alcohol.
7. Puncture the skin in the lateral or medial aspect of the heel to decrease the risk of nerve damage.

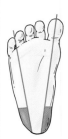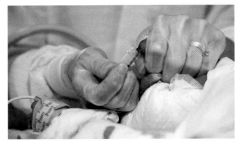

8. Wipe off the first few drops of blood.
9. Allow large drops of blood to form and to fall on the testing material.
10. Clean the puncture area and place a small dressing over it.

Document that blood was collected, type of test, site of puncture, and response of the neonate.

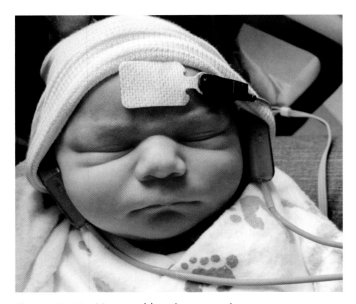

Figure 15–10   Neonatal hearing screening.

BOX 15–3   JCIH POSITION STATEMENT: INFANT HEARING SCREENING

"The Joint Committee on Infant Hearing (JCIH) endorses early detection of and intervention for infants with hearing loss. The goal of early hearing detection and intervention (EHDI) is to maximize linguistic competence and literacy development for children who are deaf or hard of hearing. Without appropriate opportunities to learn language, these children will fall behind their hearing peers in communication, cognition, reading, and social-emotional development. Such delays may result in lower educational and employment levels in adulthood. To maximize the outcome for infants who are deaf or hard of hearing, the hearing of all infants should be screened at no later than 1 month of age. Those who do not pass screening should have a comprehensive audiological evaluation at no later than 3 months of age. Infants with confirmed hearing loss should receive appropriate intervention at no later than 6 months of age from health care and education professionals with expertise in hearing loss and deafness in infants and young children. Regardless of previous hearing-screening outcomes, all infants with or without risk factors should receive ongoing surveillance of communicative development beginning at 2 months of age during well-child visits in the medical home. EHDI systems should guarantee seamless transitions for infants and their families through this process."

Joint Committee on Infant Hearing (JCIH), 2007.

on physiological measures versus behavioral response. The screening tests do not provide information on the type or degree of hearing impairment (**Box 15-3**). These screening tests are:

- *Otoacoustic emissions (OAE) is a painless test that is conducted when the neonate is asleep or lying still. A tiny, flexible ear probe is inserted into the neonate's ear. It records responses of the outer hairs cells of the cochlea to clicking sounds coming from the probe's microphone. A referral is made to a hearing specialist when there is no recorded response from the cochlear hair cells.*
- *Automated auditory brain stem response (AABR) is a painless test conducted when the neonate is asleep or lying still. Disposable electrodes are placed high on the neonate's forehead, on the mastoid, and on the nape of the neck. This screening test assesses electrical activity of the cochlea, auditory nerve, and brain stem in response to sound. A referral to a hearing specialist is recommended for neonates who do not have a positive response to the sound stimuli.*
- Both tests need to be conducted in a quiet room.
- Vernix, blood, and amniotic fluid in the ear can interfere with accurate screening.
- Neonates who fail the initial screening test are rescreened in one month. Diagnostic testing is recommended for neonates who fail the second screening (Delaney & Meyers, 2012).

THERAPEUTIC AND SURGICAL PROCEDURES

Immunizations

Hepatitis B is a disease that is spread through contact with blood of an infected person or by sexual contact with an infected person, and it causes inflammation of the liver.

- The CDC recommends that all neonates be vaccinated for hepatitis B before hospital discharge (see Critical Component: Intramuscular Injections).
- CDC also recommends that neonates who have been or possibly have been exposed to hepatitis B during birth be given both hepatitis B vaccine and hepatitis B immune globulin (HBIg) within 12 hours of birth.
- The second dose of hepatitis B vaccine is given at 1–2 months of age. The third dose is given at 6–18 months of age.

Circumcision

Male circumcision is an elective surgery to remove the foreskin of the penis. It is reported that 55% of newborn males born in the United States in 2009 were circumcised (O'Reilly, 2012). The decision to circumcise the neonate is made by the parents and is based on their cultural, religious, and personal beliefs (**Box 15-4**).

- Contraindications for circumcision include:
  - *Preterm neonates*
  - *Neonates with a genitourinary defect*
  - *Neonates at risk for bleeding problems*
  - *Neonates with compromising disorders such as respiratory distress syndrome*

- Risks related to circumcision:
  - *Hemorrhage*
  - *Infection*
  - *Adhesions*
  - *Pain*
- Benefits related to circumcision:
  - *Decreased incidence of urinary tract infections*
  - *Decreased incidence of sexually transmitted infections*
- The surgical procedure is performed by the physician before discharge or at a well-child check-up.
- Three common circumcision devices used are Gomco clamp, Mogen clamp, and Plastibell (**Fig. 15-11**)
  - *Mogen clamp is commonly used by Mohels when performing ceremonial circumcisions.*

Procedure

- Preoperative
  - *Provide parents with information on the benefits and risks of circumcisions, and the procedure. This is usually done by the neonate's health care provider.*
  - *Obtain written consent from the parents.*
  - *Verify that the neonate has voided.*
    - A lack of voiding may be related to an anatomical abnormality. Circumcisions are contraindicated when there is an anatomical abnormality.
  - *Ensure that the neonate does not eat 2–3 hours before the procedure.*
    - This decreases the risk of vomiting and aspiration during the procedure.
  - *Administer acetaminophen 1 hour before procedure per the physician's order.*
    - Given for pain management (**Box 15-5**).

CRITICAL COMPONENT

Intramuscular Injections

Procedure

1. Review the written orders for the newborn.
2. Inform the parents of the reason for the medication or vaccine.
3. Obtain written consent when required.
4. Follow the five rights of medication administration.
5. Draw up medication or vaccine in a 1-mL syringe with a 25-gauge 5/8 needle.
6. Invite the parents to comfort their infant by stroking the infant's head or hands.
7. Put on gloves.
8. Undo the diaper for full exposure of the leg.
9. Identify the injection site. The preferred site is the vastus lateralis.
10. Clean the area with an alcohol swab and let the area dry. It is extremely important to remove all maternal blood and amniotic fluid from the injection site to prevent transmission of blood-borne pathogens.
11. Stabilize the knee with the heel of hand. Grasp the tissue of the injection site with your thumb and forefinger.
12. Insert the needle at a 90-degree angle.

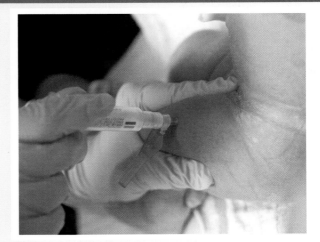

13. Slowly inject medication or a vaccine to decrease the amount of discomfort.
14. Withdraw the needle and rub the site to promote absorption.
15. Place a small dressing over the site.
16. Properly dispose of the needle and syringe
17. Document date, time, and location of injection.

BOX 15–4   STANDARD OF PRACTICE: CIRCUMCISION

The American Academy of Pediatrics conducted an analysis of medical research on circumcisions. The following is a summary of their findings and recommendations:

"Existing scientific evidence demonstrates potential medical benefits of newborn circumcision; however, these data are not sufficient to recommend routine neonatal circumcision. In the case of circumcision, in which there are potential benefits and risks, yet the procedure is not essential to the child's current well-being, parents should determine what is in the best interest of their child. To make an informed choice, parents of all male infants should be given accurate and unbiased information and be provided the opportunity to discuss their decision. It is legitimate for parents to take into account cultural, religious, and ethnic traditions, in addition to the medical factors, when making this decision. Analgesia is safe and effective in reducing procedural pain associated with circumcision; therefore, if a decision for circumcision is made, procedural analgesia should be provided. If circumcision is performed in the newborn period, it should be done on infants who are stable and healthy."

American Academy of Pediatrics (1999).

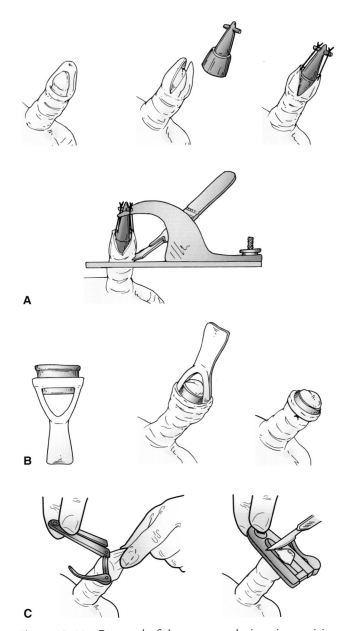

Figure 15–11   Removal of the prepuce during circumcision. *A.* Gomco clamp. *B.* Plastibell. *C.* Mogen clamp.

- Intra-operative
  - *The neonate is positioned and secured on a specially designed plastic board, often referred to as a circumcision board.*
    - The board is padded to promote comfort.
    - The upper part of the neonate is swaddled to promote comfort and reduce heat loss.
  - *An ear bulb is placed near the neonate to use if there is vomiting or increased mucus.*
  - *The penis is cleansed and a sterile drape specially designed for circumcision is placed over the trunk.*
  - *A sucrose-dipped pacifier is offered during the block and procedure for pain management.*
  - *The physician administers a penile nerve block.*
  - *The physician applies a Gomco clamp, Mogen clamp, or Plastibell (see Fig. 15–12).*
  - *The physician surgically removes the foreskin with a scalpel.*
  - *Petroleum-impregnated gauze is wrapped around the end of the penis.*
    - This promotes comfort by reducing the amount of irritation caused by friction with the diaper.
- Postoperative
  - *The penis should be assessed every 15 minutes for the first hour for signs of bleeding, then every 2–3 hours according to hospital policies.*
    - The physician is notified when bleeding is present (larger than the size of a quarter).
  - *Acetaminophen PO is administered every 4–6 hours.*
  - *Voidings are assessed and documented.*
    - The neonate should void within 24 hours after the procedure.

- Parent Education
  - *Instruct parents to watch for bleeding and signs of infection, and to note when their child voids.*
  - *Inform parents that the gauze will fall off on its own and they should not pull it off.*
    - Pulling gauze off can interfere with the healing process.
  - *Instruct parents to fasten diapers loosely.*
    - Loosely fitting diapers promote comfort by decreasing pressure on the surgical site.
  - *Instruct parents to notify the physician when:*
    - Bleeding is present (larger than the size of a quarter),
    - Signs of infection are present, or
    - The neonate has not voided within 24 hours.

Evidence-Based Practice: Sucrose as Analgesia for Procedural Pain Management in Neonates

Copper, S., and Petty, J. (2012). Promoting the use of sucrose as analgesia for procedural pain management in neonates: A review of the current literature. *Journal of Neonatal Nursing, 18,* 121–128.

A literature review was conducted in the area of neonatal pain management. Recommendations for practice were developed based on the literature review. These recommendations include:

■ Develop evidence-based protocols and practice guidelines in the use of sucrose in procedural pain management.
■ Use a combination of strategies in pain management such as breast milk, pacifier, skin-to-skin contact with parents and neonate, with use of sucrose.
■ Use breast milk if sucrose cannot be given.
■ Facilitate the use of pain management techniques for neonates who are undergoing potentially painful procedures.

BOX 15–5 ASPMN POSITION STATEMENT: MALE INFANT CIRCUMCISION PAIN MANAGEMENT

"The American Society for Pain Management Nursing (ASPMN) holds the position that nurses and other health-care professionals must provide optimal pain management throughout the circumcision process for male infants. Parents must be prepared for the procedure and educated about the infant's pain assessment. They must also be informed of pharmacologic and integrative pain management therapies."

   Nursing actions include:

■ Administering acetaminophen 1 hour prior to procedure
■ Applying topical anesthetic cream prior to procedure
■ Positioning newborn in a semi-recumbent position on a padded surface with arms swaddled
■ Administering 24% sucrose or breast milk orally 2 minutes before penile manipulation or offering pacifier for non-nutritive sucking if sucrose or breast milk contraindicated
■ Administrating oral acetaminophen for at least 24 hours post procedure
■ Instructing parents in infant pain assessment and management, and in care of circumcision

The American Society for Pain Management Nursing (ASPMN), 2011.

CONCEPT MAP

Cold Stress

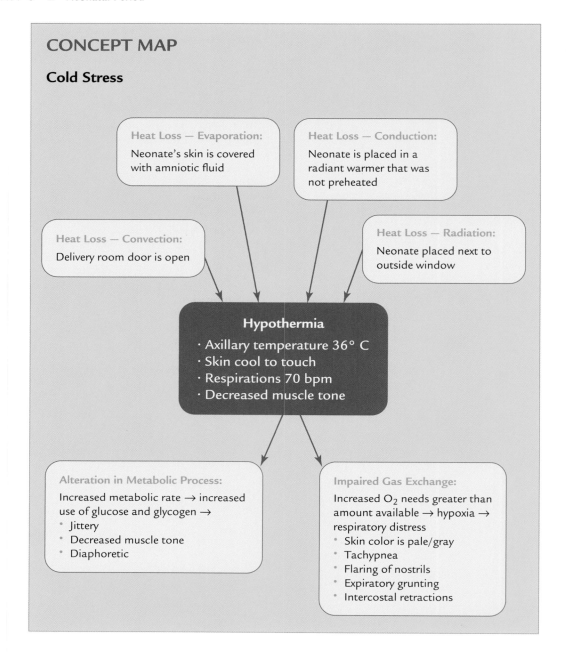

Heat Loss — Evaporation:
Neonate's skin is covered with amniotic fluid

Heat Loss — Conduction:
Neonate is placed in a radiant warmer that was not preheated

Heat Loss — Convection:
Delivery room door is open

Heat Loss — Radiation:
Neonate placed next to outside window

Hypothermia
· Axillary temperature 36° C
· Skin cool to touch
· Respirations 70 bpm
· Decreased muscle tone

Alteration in Metabolic Process:
Increased metabolic rate → increased use of glucose and glycogen →
* Jittery
* Decreased muscle tone
* Diaphoretic

Impaired Gas Exchange:
Increased O_2 needs greater than amount available → hypoxia → respiratory distress
* Skin color is pale/gray
* Tachypnea
* Flaring of nostrils
* Expiratory grunting
* Intercostal retractions

Problem 1: Heat loss due to evaporation
Goal: Maintain a neutral thermal environment (NTE)
Outcome: The neonate's temperature is within normal range.

Nursing Actions

1. Dry neonate's body with warm towel.
2. Remove wet bedding and clothing
3. Monitor vital signs.

Problem 2: Heat loss due to conduction
Goal: Maintain NTE
Outcome: The neonate's temperature is within normal range.

Nursing Actions

1. Skin-to-skin contact with parent with warm blanket over both the neonate and the parent.
2. Preheat warmer prior to use.
3. Use warm blankets.
4. Warm hands prior to touching neonate.
5. Warm equipment prior to contact with neonate.
6. Monitor vital signs.

Problem 3: Heat loss due to convection
Goal: Maintain NTE
Outcome: The neonate's temperature is within normal range.

Nursing Actions

1. Close doors to room.
2. Place the neonate away from air vent, windows, and doors.
3. Place a stocking cap on the neonate's head.
4. Warm O_2 when administering oxygen.
5. Monitor vital signs.

Problem 4: Heat loss due to radiation
Goal: Maintain NTE
Outcome: The neonate's temperature is within normal range.

Nursing Actions

1. Preheat radiant warmer prior to use.
2. Place the neonate away from cold walls and windows.
3. Keep cold objects away from the neonate.
4. Place stocking cap on the neonate's head.
5. Monitor vital signs.

Problem 5: Alteration in metabolic processes: Hypoglycemia
Goal: Manage episode of hypoglycemia.
Outcome: The neonate's glucose level is within normal range.

Nursing Actions

1. Monitor for signs and symptoms of hypoglycemia.
2. Monitor glucose levels.
3. Assist the woman with breastfeeding or feed the neonate with either formula or dextrose water.
   a. Assess glucose levels 30 minutes after feeding.
4. Maintain a NTE.

Problem 6: Impaired gas exchange—Respiratory distress
Goal: Adequate gas exchange
Outcome: PaO_2 is 60–70 mm Hg; $PaCO_2$ is 35–45 mm Hg; skin color is pink; lung sounds are clear; and no signs of retractions, grunting, or nasal flaring.

Nursing Actions

1. Monitor vital signs, oxygen saturation, and arterial blood gases.
2. Maintain patent airway.
3. Suction airway as indicated.
4. Administer oxygen as per orders.
5. Maintain a NTE.

Clinical Pathway for Full-Term Low-Risk Neonate
Delivery Date and Time

Focus of Care	Birth to First Hour	1–4 Hours of Age	4–24 Hours of Age	24 Hours of Age to Discharge
Assessments	Obtain Apgar score at 1 and 5 minutes. Inspect the skin for abrasions or bruises.	Complete neonatal assessment by 2 hours of age. Complete gestational assessment as per hospital policy. Weigh and measure the head, chest, and length.	Assess at the beginning of each shift or per hospital policies. Weigh the newborn each day per hospital policy.	Assess at the beginning of each shift or per hospital policies and before discharge. Weigh the newborn each day per hospital policy.
Thermoregulation	Close the doors to the birthing room. Dry the neonate thoroughly and place in a prewarmed crib or skin-to-skin on the mother's chest with a warm blanket over them. Place a stocking cap over the top of the neonate's head. Assess axillary temperature every 30 minutes or per hospital policy.	Prevent heat loss by maintaining a NTE. Encourage skin-to-skin contact with either the mother or father and with a warm blanket over both the neonate and parent. Wrap the neonate in blankets when in an open crib. Place a stocking cap on the head.	Prevent heat loss by maintaining a NTE. Wrap the neonate in blankets when in an open crib. Place a stocking cap on the neonate's head.	Prevent heat loss by maintaining a NTE. Assist the mother in dressing her infant for discharge in clothing and blankets that help maintain the neonate's normal body temperature.

Continued

Clinical Pathway for Full-Term Low-Risk Neonate—cont'd
Delivery Date and Time

Focus of Care	Birth to First Hour	1–4 Hours of Age	4–24 Hours of Age	24 Hours of Age to Discharge
Respiratory	Clear the nose and mouth of mucus with use of an ear bulb. Assess respirations every 30 minutes. Assess lung sounds. Monitor for signs of respiratory distress: grunting, flaring, retractions.	Keep the nose and mouth free of mucus with use of an ear bulb. Assess respirations every hour. Assess lung sounds. Monitor for signs of respiratory distress: grunting, flaring, retractions.	Assess respirations once per shift. Assess lung sounds once per shift. Monitor for signs of respiratory distress: grunting, flaring, retractions.	Assess respirations once per shift. Assess lung sounds once per shift and before discharge.
Cardiovascular	Assess skin color for cyanosis. Assess heart rate every 30 minutes.	Assess skin color for cyanosis. Assess heart rate every hour.	Assess the heart rate once per shift.	Assess heart rate once per shift and before discharge.
Activity	Assess the level of activity and compare to periods of reactivity. Monitor for signs of hypoglycemia, i.e., jitteriness.	Assess the level of activity and compare to periods of reactivity. Monitor for signs of hypoglycemia, i.e., jitteriness.	Assess the level of activity and compare to periods of reactivity. Monitor for signs of hypoglycemia, i.e., jitteriness.	Assess the level of activity.
Nutrition	Ideal time to introduce breastfeeding is when the neonate is in the first period of reactivity. May need to feed the neonate glucose water or formula if hypoglycemic.	Breastfeed on demand. May need to feed the neonate glucose water or formula if hypoglycemic.	The ideal time for feeding is when the neonate is in the second period of reactivity. Breastfeed or bottle feed on demand; feeding should be every 3–4 hours.	Breastfeed or bottle feed on demand; feeding should be every 3–4 hours.
Elimination	The neonate may or may not void or pass meconium stool.	The neonate may or may not void or pass meconium stool.	The neonate voids within 24 hours. The neonate may or may not pass meconium stool.	The neonate voids a minimum of 2 times on day 2 and 5–6 times on day 3. The neonate passes meconium or transitional stools several times a day.
Medications and Immunizations	Inform the parents which medications are being administered and why. Administer vitamin K injection and instill eye ointment as per physician's order.	Inform parents which medications are being administered and why. Administer vitamin K injection and instill eye ointment if not done during first hour as per physician order.	Provide parents with information on hepatitis B vaccine and obtain written consent if required. Administer hepatitis B vaccine as per physician order. Administer hepatitis B immune globulin vaccine when indicated per physician order.	

Clinical Pathway for Full-Term Low-Risk Neonate—cont'd
Delivery Date and Time

Focus of Care	Birth to First Hour	1–4 Hours of Age	4–24 Hours of Age	24 Hours of Age to Discharge
Special Procedures	Heel stick to assess glucose levels as indicated, i.e., jitteriness, LGA, and SGA.	Heel stick to assess glucose levels as indicated, i.e., jitteriness, LGA, and SGA.		Newborn screening tests: ☐ Blood sample collected. ☐ Newborn hearing screening conducted. Circumcision might be done several hours before discharge.
Family Attachment	Delay eye ointment until parents have had the opportunity to hold their newborn. Provide time for parents to see and touch and/or hold the newborn. Explain to the new father that he can stay with his newborn while assessments are being completed.	Complete necessary assessments as quickly as possible in order to provide uninterrupted time for parents to hold and be with their newborn. Complete assessments at bedside when possible.	Arrange nursing care to provide uninterrupted time for parents and their newborn. Teach parents about normal newborn characteristics and behavior.	Arrange nursing care to provide uninterrupted time for parents and their newborn.
Education	Point out normal newborn characteristics such as molding, lanugo, and vernix. Begin education on breastfeeding (e.g., positioning, latching on, releasing suction).	Teaching is kept to a minimum since parents are usually tired during this period of time or want to call family members to announce the birth.	Ideal time for teaching. Provide information on caring for a newborn (see Chapter 16).	Continue teaching parents about the care of their newborn (see Chapter 16). Complete the appropriate hospital discharge teaching forms. Give parents a copy of written discharge instructions. Explain the importance of follow-up well-child check-ups and the importance of scheduling their first appointment as recommend by their pediatrician or PNP.

Continued

Clinical Pathway for Full-Term Low-Risk Neonate—cont'd
Delivery Date and Time

Focus of Care	Birth to First Hour	1–4 Hours of Age	4–24 Hours of Age	24 Hours of Age to Discharge
Safety	Place completed ID bands on the neonate, mother, and father. Keep the side of warmer up when not at crib side. Teach parents how to support the head and neck of their neonate. Use the five rights when administering medications. Wear gloves until after the first bath.	Teach parents abduction prevention protocol. Place the neonate on his back. Instruct parents not to leave the newborn unattended on a flat surface such as the mother's bed. Teach parents the importance of placing the neonate on his back. Wear gloves if there is the possibility of exposure to body fluids.	Provide education on infant safety (see Chapter 16). Follow hospital policies to prevent infant abduction. Wear gloves if there is the possibility of exposure to body fluids.	Review infant safety before discharge. Follow hospital policies to prevent infant abduction. Wear gloves if there is the possibility of exposure to body fluids. Inform parents that a federally approved car seat will be needed to transport the infant home, and that it will need to be properly placed in the car.

Nursing Care Plan

Problem (Check appropriate line)	Actual or Potential	Action (Initial care provided)	Expected Outcome/ Discharge Criteria (Initial outcomes obtained)
Altered body temperature related to: _____ Decreased subcutaneous fat _____ Large body surface _____ Heat loss due to radiation, convection, conduction, and/or evaporation	Initiate by: RN _____ Date/Time _____ ☐ Actual ☐ Potential Change in status: Date/Time _____ RN _____ ☐ Actual ☐ Potential Resolved: Date/Time _____ RN _____	_____ Maintain NTE by keeping doors closed and adjusting environmental temperature. _____ Keep the neonate dry. _____ Wrap the neonate in warm, dry blankets. _____ Place a stocking cap on the neonate's head. _____ Place the neonate in skin-to-skin contact with the parent and a warm blanket over both. _____ Monitor temperature per institutional protocol. _____ Place in a preheated warmer with a skin probe attached. _____ Notify the physician or nurse practitioner if the neonate's temperature remains low or is elevated.	_____ Neonate's temperature within normal ranges _____ No signs of cold stress _____ No sign of respiratory distress

Nursing Care Plan—cont'd

Problem (Check appropriate line)	Actual or Potential	Action (Initial care provided)	Expected Outcome/ Discharge Criteria (Initial outcomes obtained)
Infection related to: _____ Breakdown of skin _____ Poor hand washing techniques by health care providers, parents, and/or visitors _____ Prematurity	Initiate by: RN _____ Date/Time _____ ☐ Actual ☐ Potential Change in status: Date/Time _____ RN _____ ☐ Actual ☐ Potential Resolved: Date/Time _____ RN _____	_____ Monitor skin for tissue breakdown. _____ Monitor temperature per institutional protocol. _____ Keep the skin clean and dry. _____ Instruct parents and visitors in proper hand washing before touching the neonate. _____ Instruct parents to wash hands after changing diapers. _____ Notify the physician or nurse practitioner if the neonate is lethargic, has elevated temperature or skin lesions, is eating poorly, and/or has signs of respiratory distress.	_____ Temperature within normal ranges _____ Skin intact with no signs of irritation _____ No signs or symptoms of infection
Impaired gas exchange related to: _____ Transition from intrauterine to extrauterine live _____ Cold stress _____ Excessive mucus	Initiate by: RN _____ Date/Time _____ ☐ Actual ☐ Potential Change in status: Date/Time _____ RN _____ ☐ Actual ☐ Potential Resolved: Date/Time _____ RN _____	_____ Monitor respiratory and cardiac function as per institutional protocol. _____ Auscultate breath sounds. _____ Assess for the presence and location of cyanosis. _____ Maintain NTE. _____ Suction the mouth and nose PRN. _____ Position the neonate on his back. _____ Administer oxygen per protocol/orders. _____ Report signs of respiratory distress to the physician or nurse practitioner.	_____ Respiratory rate within normal limits _____ Breath sounds clear _____ Heart rate and rhythm within normal limits _____ Skin pink and warm to touch _____ Airway is clear _____ No signs of respiratory distress

Continued

Nursing Care Plan—cont'd

Problem (Check appropriate line)	Actual or Potential	Action (Initial care provided)	Expected Outcome/ Discharge Criteria (Initial outcomes obtained)
Fluid volume deficit related to: _____ Limited oral intake _____ Insensible water loss	Initiate by: RN _____ Date/Time _____ ☐ Actual ☐ Potential Change in status: Date/Time _____ RN _____ ☐ Actual ☐ Potential Resolved: Date/Time _____ RN _____	_____ Monitor intake and output. _____ Monitor for signs of dehydration, i.e., sunken fontanels, poor skin turgor, dry mucous membranes. _____ Initiate oral feedings. _____ Maintain NTE.	_____ Feeds every 3–4 hours _____ 6–8 wet diapers per day _____ Vital signs within normal limits
Knowledge deficit related to: _____ First time parenting _____ Limited learning resources	Initiate by: RN _____ Date/Time _____ ☐ Actual ☐ Potential Change in status: Date/Time _____ RN _____ ☐ Actual ☐ Potential Resolved: Date/Time _____ RN _____	_____ Assess level of parents' knowledge. _____ Provide information on newborn characteristics and behavior. _____ Provide information on newborn care (see Chapter 16). _____ Assist parents with care of their newborn. _____ Praise parents for their care of their newborn.	_____ Parents feed newborn without difficulty. _____ Parents change newborn's diapers without difficulty. _____ Parents verbalize understanding of newborn characteristics, behaviors, and care.

You are assigned to the mother-baby couplet unit. Your assignment for the day includes the Sanchez family. Margarite is a 28-year-old G3 P2 Hispanic woman who gave birth to a healthy boy, Manuel, at 0839. Margarite experienced an uncomplicated labor of 12 hours. Membranes ruptured 7 hours before delivery. She received 2 doses of Nubain during labor. The last dose was given at 0440.

Manuel weighs 3,800 grams and is 50 cm in length. His 1- and 5-minute Apgar scores were 8 and 9. Manuel is 2 hours old. The Ballard score indicates that Manuel is 39 weeks. Margarite breastfed her son for 15 minutes on each breast immediately after the birth.

Your initial shift assessment findings are:

Vital signs: Axillary temperature, 36.2°C; apical pulse, 100 beats per minute; respirations, 30 breaths per minute.
Skin is warm and pink with acrocyanosis.
Fontanels are soft and flat.
Molding is present.
Lung sounds are clear.
There is mild nasal flaring.
Manuel is in a sleep state and unresponsive to external stimuli.
Based on the above information, discuss the primary nursing diagnoses for baby Manuel.
Discuss the immediate nursing actions for baby Manuel. Provide rationales for your nursing actions.

Thirty minutes later you note that Manuel is jittery and exhibits signs of hypoglycemia.

List the signs and symptoms of hypoglycemia and related nursing actions.

Several hours later, Manuel's father is present and holding Manuel.

List signs of parent-infant bonding.
Discuss nursing actions that will support parent-infant attachment.

■ ■ ■ Review Questions ■ ■ ■

1. The most critical physiological change required of neonates during the transition from intrauterine to extrauterine life is:
   A. Initiation and maintenance of cardiac function
   B. Initiation and maintenance of respiratory function
   C. Initiation and maintenance of metabolic function
   D. Initiation and maintenance of hepatic function

2. You are caring for a newborn girl who weighs 3,800 grams with an estimated gestational age of 41 weeks. During your assessment at 1 hour of age, you note that the newborn is jittery and irritable. Your first nursing action is:
   A. Increase the temperature of the warmer
   B. Feed the infant formula
   C. Transfer the infant to the NICU
   D. Assess the blood glucose level

3. Heat loss through evaporation can be reduced by:
   A. Closing the door to the room
   B. Using warming equipment on the neonate
   C. Drying the neonate
   D. Placing the crib near a warm wall

4. The nurse would expect the stools of a 3-day-old breastfed newborn to be:
   A. Sticky, thick, and black
   B. Greenish-brown to greenish-yellow
   C. Golden yellow and pasty
   D. Loose and green

5. In the birth suite during the initial newborn assessment, the new father seems concerned and asks why his baby girl is so hairy. The best response is:
   A. "Over the next few months the hair on the back will fall out."
   B. "This is a normal characteristic of newborns, so no need to be concerned."
   C. "This is called lanugo, which covered the baby while inside the mother. It will fall out in a few months."
   D. "You seem overly concerned about this. Do you want to talk about your feelings?"

6. Which of the following measurements fall above or below the normal range for a newborn born at 40 weeks gestation? Select all that apply.
   A. Head circumference: 34 cm
   B. Chest circumference: 32 cm
   C. Weight: 4, 250 grams
   D. Length: 43 cm

7. Select all that are true regarding the anterior fontanel of a full term neonate.
   A. Approximately 0.5–1 cm in size
   B. Approximately 2.5–4 cm in size
   C. Diamond shape
   D. Triangle shape

8. The point of maximal impulse (PMI) is located at _____.
   A. the 1st or 2nd intercostal space
   B. the 2nd or 3rd intercostal space
   C. the 3rd or 4th intercostal space
   D. the 4th or 5th intercostal space

9. Which of the following assessment data of a 12 hours of age neonate needs additional evaluation? Select all that apply.
   A. Localized soft tissue edema of the scalp
   B. Transient cyanosis around the mouth
   C. A 10 cm flat bluish area on the buttock
   D. Jaundice that is limited to the face

10. The initial bathing of the neonate should occur _____.
    A. within 30 minutes of the birth
    B. before applying eye ointment
    C. after temperature has stabilized
    D. 3 hours after the birth

References

American College of Obstetricians and Gynecologists (ACOG). (2003). Newborn screening: ACOG committee opinion No. 287. *Obstetrics and Gynecology, 102*, 887–889.

The American Society for Pain Management Nursing (ASPMN). (2011). Position statement: Male infant circumcision pain management. Retrieved from www.aspmn.org/organization/documents/circumcisiom.pdf

Association of Women's Health, Obstetric and Neonatal Nurses (AWHONN). (2006). *The compendium of postpartum care* (2nd ed.). Philadelphia: Medical Broadcasting Company.

Association of Women's Health, Obstetric and Neonatal Nurses (AWHONN). (2011). Newborn screening. *JOGNN, 40,* 136–137.

Ballard, J., Khoury, J., Wedig, K., Wang, L., Eilers-Walsman, B., & Lipp, R. (1991). New Ballard Score, expanded to include extremely premature infants. *Journal of Pediatrics, 119,* 417–423.

Blackburn, S. (2012). *Maternal, fetal, and neonatal physiology* (4th ed.). St. Louis, MO: W. B. Saunders.

Brazelton, T., & Nugent, J. (1995). *Neonatal behavioral assessment scale.* London: MacKeith Press.

CDC. (2012). *2012 recommended immunization for children age 0 through 6 years.* Retrieved from www.cdc.gov/vaccines/parents/downloads

Copper, S., and Petty, J. (2012). Promoting the use of sucrose as analgesia for procedural pain management in neonates: A review of the current literature. *Journal of Neonatal Nursing, 18,* 121–128.

Delaney, A., and Meyers, A. (2012). Newborn hearing screening. *E-Medicine.* Retrieved from www.emedicine.medscape.com/article/836646-overview

DHHS. (2009). *How to know if your baby is getting enough milk.* Retrieved from www.womenshealth.gov/publicatins/diaper_checklist.pdf

Dillon, P. (2007). *Nursing health assessment* (2nd ed.). Philadelphia: F.A. Davis.

Heimall, L., Storey, B., Stellar, J., and Davis, K. (2012). Beginning at the bottom: Evidence-based care of diaper dermatitis. *MCN, 37,* 10–16.

Herr, K., Coyne, P., McCaffery, M., Manworren, R., and Merkel, S. (2011). Pain assessment in the patient unable to self-report: Position statement with clinical practice recommendations. *Pain Management Nursing, 12,* 230–250.

Joint Commission on Accreditation of Healthcare Organizations (JCAHO). (2001). Pain management standard [online]. Retrieved from www.jcaho.org

Matterson, S., & Smith, J. (2011). *Core curriculum for maternal-newborn nursing (4th ed.).* St. Louis, MO: Elsevier Saunders.

National Association of Neonatal Nursing (NANN). (1995). Position statement on pain management in infants. *Neonatal Network, 14,* 54–55.

National Institute on Deafness and Other Communication Disorders. (2006). Has your baby's hearing been screened [online]. Retrieved from www.nidcd.nih.gov

National Newborn Screening and Genetics Resource Center (NNSGRCU). (2012). National newborn screening status report [online]. Retrieved from http:/genes-r-us.uthscsa.edu/nbsdisorders.pdf

O'Reilly, K. (2012). Male newborn circumcision rate falls to lowest level. *Amednews.com.* Retrieved from www.ama-assn.org/amednews/2012/02/27/pres0302.htm

Purnell, L. (2012). *Transcultural health care: A culturally competent approach* (4th ed.). Philadelphia: F.A. Davis.

Scanlon, V., & Sanders, T. (2011). *Essentials of anatomy and physiology* (6th ed.). Philadelphia: F.A. Davis.

Vallerand, A., and Sanoski, C. (2013). *Davis's drug guide for nurses* (13th ed.). Philadelphia: F.A. Davis.

Discharge Planning and Teaching

16

EXPECTED STUDENT OUTCOMES

On completion of this chapter, the student will be able to:

- ☐ Define key terms.
- ☐ Incorporate principles of teaching and learning when providing newborn care information to parents.
- ☐ Discuss the nutritional needs of newborns and infants.
- ☐ Demonstrate awareness of cultural values in care of newborns.
- ☐ Describe the stages of human milk.
- ☐ Describe the process of human milk production.
- ☐ Develop a teaching plan for breastfeeding.
- ☐ Develop a teaching plan for formula feeding.
- ☐ Provide parents with information regarding newborn care that reflects the assessed learning needs of parents.

Nursing Diagnoses

- ☐ Knowledge deficit related to infant feeding due to lack of experience and/or information
- ☐ Knowledge deficit related to newborn care due to lack of experience and/or information
- ☐ Knowledge deficit related to signs of newborn/infant illness related to lack of information

Nursing Outcomes

- ☐ The woman will effectively feed her newborn.
- ☐ The parents will demonstrate proper care of their newborn.
- ☐ The parents will convey they are comfortable with caring for their newborn.
- ☐ The parents will list signs of potential newborn/infant illness that need to be reported to the health care provider.

INTRODUCTION

Caring for a newborn and raising a child are major responsibilities couples take on with minimal formal educational preparation; yet, it is one of the most important roles a person assumes in his or her lifetime. Couples' knowledge pertaining to newborn care varies based on their past experiences with children, their cultural beliefs, information gained from friends and relatives, and what they have read or classes they have attended.

Discharge planning and teaching begins during pregnancy, when couples are encouraged to read about infant care and attend infant care classes in preparation for their emerging role of parent, and as they receive information from their health care provider. Throughout the postpartum hospital stay, teaching is provided in short sessions to the woman, her partner, and other significant people who will be assisting the woman in the care of the newborn. Topics of instruction are reviewed on the day of discharge to ensure that all teaching topics have been covered and parents feel ready to care for their newborn. Most hospitals or birthing centers have standard discharge teaching forms that are completed and signed by the woman and the discharge nurse. A written copy of key points of infant care is given to parents on discharge so that they can refer to the information provided.

PRINCIPLES OF TEACHING AND LEARNING

Teaching plans need to be individualized and reflect the needs of the parents. This is accomplished by incorporating teaching-learning principles in the parents' education regarding the care of their newborn. The five rights of teaching should be included in teaching plans for parents (**Box 16-1**).

Don't have time to read this chapter? Want to reinforce your reading? Need to review for a test? Listen to this chapter on *DavisPlus*.

BOX 16–1   THE FIVE RIGHTS OF TEACHING

When you are making a teaching plan, you can use this as a checklist to ensure that you consider each of the five "rights" of teaching in the plan.

Right Time
- Is the learner ready, free from pain and anxiety, and motivated?
- Do you and the learner have a trusting relationship?
- Have you set aside sufficient time for the teaching session?

Right Context
- Is the environment quiet, free of distractions, and private?
- Is the environment soothing or stimulating, depending on the desired effect?

Right Goal
- Is the learner actively involved in planning the learning objectives?
- Are you and your client both committed to reaching mutually set goals of learning that achieve the desired behavioral changes?
- Are family and friends included in planning so that they can help follow through on behavioral changes?
- Are the learning objectives realistic and valued by the client; do they reflect the client's lifestyle?

Right Content
- Is the content appropriate for the client's needs?
- Is the information new or a reinforcement of information that has already been provided?
- Is the content presented at the learner's level?
- Does the content relate to the learner's life experiences or is it otherwise relevant to the learner?

Right Method
- Do the teaching strategies fit the learning style of the client?
- Do the strategies fit the client's learning ability?
- Are the teaching strategies varied?

Wilkinson & Van Leuven (2007), p. 530, Box 24-1.

BOX 16–2   POSITION STATEMENTS ON BREASTFEEDING

"AWHONN supports breastfeeding as the optimal method of infant nutrition. AWHONN believes that women should be encouraged to breastfeed and receive instruction and support from the entire health care team to successfully initiate and sustain breastfeeding. Discussions with the woman and her significant others concerning breastfeeding should begin during the preconception period and continue through the first year of life or longer" (AWHONN, 2007).

"Breastfeeding is the ideal way of providing young infants with the nutrients they need for healthy growth and development. Virtually all mothers can breastfeed, provided they have accurate information, and the support of their family and health care system" (WHO, 2008).

"The U.S. Surgeon General recommends that babies be fed with breast milk only – no formula – for the first 6 months of life. It is better to breastfeed for 6 months and best to breastfeed for 12 months, or longer ..." (DHHS, 2000).

"From its inception, the American Academy of Pediatrics (AAP) has been a staunch advocate of breastfeeding as the optimal form of nutrition for infants. Although economic, cultural, and political pressures often confound decisions about infant feeding, the AAP firmly adheres to the position that breastfeeding ensures the best possible health as well as development and physiological outcomes of the infant" (AAP, 2008).

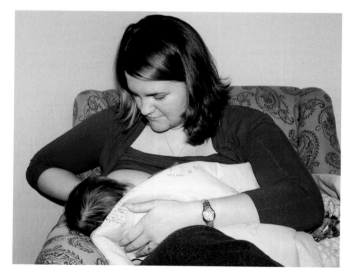

Figure 16–1   Breastfeeding enhances mother-infant attachment.

NEWBORN NUTRITION AND FEEDING

Breastfeeding and bottle feeding are the two basic methods of infant feeding. Neonates who are unable to suck and/or swallow are gavage fed (see Chapter 17). The choice between breastfeeding and bottle feeding is influenced by past infant feeding experiences, cultural beliefs, friends and family, health of the woman and baby, support of the partner, perceived health effects, and discussion during pregnancy with a health care provider.

Breastfeeding

Breastfeeding is the method of infant feeding recommended by the Association of Women's Health, Obstetric and Neonatal Nurses (AWHONN), the American College of Nurse-Midwives (ACNM), American Academy of Pediatrics (AAP), and the American College of Obstetricians and Gynecologists (ACOG) (**Box 16-2** and **Fig. 16-1**). See Critical Component: Primary Care Interventions to Promote Breastfeeding.

An objective of *Healthy People 2020* is an increase in the proportion of infants who are breastfed from 74% to 81.9%. Target goals are that by 2020 there will be an increase in the proportion of:

- Infants breastfed at 6 months from 45.5% to 60.6%.
- Infants breastfed at 1 year from 22.7% to 34.1%.
- Infants who are exclusively breastfed through 3 months from 33.6% to 46.2%.

■ Infants who are exclusively breastfed through 6 months from 14.1% to 25.5%.

■ Employers that have worksite lactation support programs from 25% to 38% (DHHS, 2012)

The decision to breastfeed is influenced by the woman's age, educational level, previous infant feeding method, career obligations, support from her partner, and cultural beliefs.

■ The woman's partner plays a significant role in the woman's choice to breastfeed and to continue breastfeeding.

■ *The partner's knowledge and attitudes regarding breastfeeding are influenced by the partner's culture, past experiences, age, and family and friends.*

■ *The woman's feelings and success at breastfeeding are enhanced when her partner supports breastfeeding, assists in the care of the newborn, and does household tasks, which facilitate the woman's ability to rest and conserve energy.*

CULTURAL AWARENESS: BREASTFEEDING BELIEFS

Cultural Heritage	Beliefs Regarding Breastfeeding
Arab	Breastfeeding is delayed until the second or third postpartum day so that the mother can rest.
Chinese	May use formula until milk comes in.
Filipino	Women from rural areas are more likely to breastfeed for longer periods of time than are women from urban areas. Start supplementing with other fluids as early as 2 months.
Greek	Believe that taking showers in the first few days of breastfeeding can cause diarrhea and milk allergy in the infant.
Hindu	Some believe that colostrum is not suitable for newborns and feed sugar water or formula until milk comes in. Breastfeeding is often supplemented with cow's milk that is diluted with sugar water.
Japanese	The grandmother will feed the infant formula if the mother is sleeping to provide the rest needed for successful breastfeeding.
Mexican	May use a mixture of cornstarch and cow's milk when weaning from the breast.
Navajo	Soon after birth, the newborn is given a mixture with juniper bark to cleanse her insides and remove the mucus. A ceremonial food of corn pollen and water is given.
Vietnamese	Some women will not feed newborn colostrum and will feed the newborn a rice paste or boiled water until milk comes in.

(Purnell & Paulanka, 2008)

Advantages of Breastfeeding

■ Decreased risk of infant diarrhea
■ Decreased risk of respiratory infections
■ Decreased risk of being hospitalized for respiratory syncytial virus
■ Decreased risk of otitis media
■ Decreased risk of necrotizing enterocolitis
■ Decreased risk of childhood obesity
■ Decreased cost (DHHS, 2010)

Contraindications for Breastfeeding

■ Women who are using illicit drugs
■ Women with active and untreated tuberculosis
■ Women who are receiving diagnostic or therapeutic radioactive isotopes
■ Women who are receiving antimetabolites or chemotherapeutic agents
■ Women who have herpes simplex lesions on a breast
■ Women who are HIV positive (AAP, 2005a; DHHS, 2010)

■ *In the developing world, the risks of artificial feedings outweigh the risks of acquiring HIV through breast milk; therefore, women are encouraged to breastfeed (AAP, 2005a).*

■ Infants with galactosemia
■ Infants with phenylketonuria (PKU)

■ *Infants may be partially breastfed (D'Alessandro, 2010).*

CRITICAL COMPONENT

Primary Care Interventions to Promote Breastfeeding

Interventions to promote and support breastfeeding include:

■ Formal breastfeeding education for mother and families
■ Direct support of mothers during breastfeeding
■ Training of primary care staff in breastfeeding and techniques for breastfeeding support
■ Peer support

U.S. Preventive Services Task Force, 2008

Composition of Human Milk

■ Contains proteins, carbohydrates, and fats that are synthesized in alveolar glands of the breast

■ *Protein in human milk is easier to digest than protein in prepared formulas. Proteins account for approximately 6% of the calories in human milk.*

■ *Lactose is the main carbohydrate. Carbohydrates account for approximately 42% of the calories in human milk.*

■ *Cholesterol, which is essential for brain development, is higher in human milk. Fats account for approximately 52% of the calories in human milk.*

■ Contains vitamins and minerals that are transferred to the human milk from the maternal plasma

■ Contains antibodies from the maternal system, which decreases the risk for neonatal infections

Stages of Human Milk

There are three stages of human milk as the body establishes the lactation process.

- Stage 1: **Colostrum** is a yellowish breast fluid that is present for 2–3 days after birth. Colostrum is also excreted during the later part of pregnancy.
  - *It has higher levels of protein and lower levels of fats, carbohydrates, and calories than mature human milk.*
  - *It is high in immunoglobulins G and A.*
  - *It acts as a laxative and assists in the passage of meconium.*
- Stage 2: Transitional milk consists of colostrum and milk.
  - *This stage lasts from day 3 to day 10.*
  - *Decreasing levels of protein and increasing levels of fats, carbohydrates, and calories*
- Stage 3: Mature milk is composed of 20% solids and 80% water.
  - *It contains approximately 22–23 calories per ounce.*
  - *Foremilk is the milk that is produced and stored between feedings and released at the beginning of the feeding session. It has a higher water content.*
  - *Hind milk is the milk produced during the feeding session and released at the end of the session. It has a higher fat content.*

Overview of Milk Production

- **Lactation** is the production of breast milk.
- The woman's body prepares for lactation as the breasts develop during puberty and undergo further changes during pregnancy.
- Milk is produced in the alveolar glands and is transported to the nipple through the lactiferous ducts (**Fig. 16-2**).
- Milk production is influenced by hormones and suckling.
- **Prolactin,** the primary hormone responsible for lactation, is produced during pregnancy, but high levels of estrogen and progesterone suppress lactation.
  - *Estrogen and progesterone levels decrease after childbirth and prolactin levels increase, which results in the stimulation of milk production.*

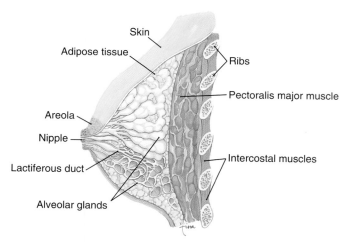

Skin
Adipose tissue
Ribs
Pectoralis major muscle
Areola
Nipple
Lactiferous duct
Intercostal muscles
Alveolar glands

Figure 16–2   Mammary gland shown in midsagittal section.

- Suckling increases prolactin levels and volume of milk production.
  - *Milk production can be viewed as a supply-demand effect. The more milk the infant takes in, the more milk is produced.*
- Extreme malnutrition can lower the fatty acid content of breast milk.

Let-down Reflex

The **let-down reflex** or milk ejection reflex results in milk being ejected into and through the lactiferous duct system.

- Oxytocin causes the myoepithelial cells of the alveoli to contract and force the milk into the duct system.
- Oxytocin is released in response to suckling and/or maternal emotional response to hearing a baby cry or thinking of her baby (see Critical Component: Infant Crying).
- The let-down reflex can occur during sexual arousal or activity due to the natural release of oxytocin in response to an orgasm.
- The let-down reflex can be inhibited by stress, anxiety, pain, and fatigue.
- Let-down occurs multiple times during each feeding.

CRITICAL COMPONENT

Infant Crying
- Crying is a late sign of hunger.
- Newborns whose cry is strong and continuous have difficulty latching onto the breast.
- Newborns who are crying need to be calmed by holding or by other comfort measures before being put to the breast.

Process of Breastfeeding

- Breastfeeding is a natural process, with its success dependent on the woman's desire to breastfeed, proper positioning, latching-on, suckling, and transferring of milk (Mulder, 2006).
- Newborns indicate hunger by being in an awake/alert state, making mouth and tongue movements, making hand-to-mouth movements, and rooting (AWHONN, 2006).
- The woman needs to be in a comfortable position.
  - *Pain and discomfort can prevent or delay the let-down reflex.*
  - *A sitting position in a chair is recommended because it facilitates good body posture.*
    - Other positions are lying on the side or back or sitting in bed.
- The newborn is held in a cradle position, "football" position, or cross-cradle position.
- Pillows are used to support the newborn and/or the woman.
- The front of the newborn is completely facing the breast to prevent the newborn's head from being turned. Another

way to describe this is that the newborn's ear, shoulder, and hip are aligned.

■ The woman supports her breast by placing one hand around the breast several inches behind the areola.
  ■ *Supporting the breast takes the weight of the breast away from the newborn's chin and makes latching on easier (AWHONN, 2006).*
  ■ *The woman should avoid pushing down on the breast, which can tip the nipple upward and increase the risk for sore nipples.*

■ The newborn is brought to the breast, and not the breast to the newborn.
  ■ *The woman brings the newborn to her breast when the newborn's mouth is open wide. This assists with latching on.*
    ■ To encourage the newborn to open wide, take advantage of the rooting reflex by touching the newborn's chin to the breast. This signals the newborn to open the mouth. The newborn then reaches up and over the nipple to achieve an asymmetrical latch with more areola visible at the top of the mouth than on the bottom.

■ *Latching-on refers to the newborn's ability to grasp the breast and to effectively suckle. The newborn's mouth is around the areola with the nipple in the back of the newborn's mouth. The lips create a firm seal around the areola (Fig. 16-3)*

CRITICAL COMPONENT

Signs of Successful Breastfeeding

■ The woman feels a tugging sensation when the newborn begins to suckle.
■ Latch-on pain should last no longer than 10 seconds. Pain beyond this is a sign of poor latch.
■ The newborn's tongue is between the lower gum and breast.
■ Swallowing can be heard (AWHONN, 2006).

■ The newborn rapidly suckles at the beginning of the feeding session. Suckling gradually decreases and the newborn relaxes.

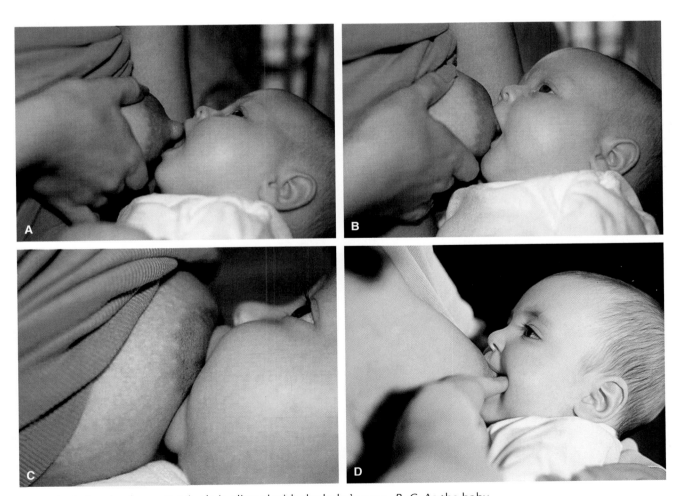

Figure 16–3 Infant latch-on. *A.* Nipple is aligned with the baby's nose. *B, C.* As the baby latches to the nipple, the baby's mouth is placed 1–2 inches beyond the base of the nipple. *D,* To remove the baby from the breast, the woman inserts her finger into the corner of the baby's mouth to break the seal.

■ Signs that the newborn's hunger has been satisfied are that the newborn:
  ■ *Spontaneously releases suction from breast*
  ■ *Does not respond with a rooting reflex when stimulated*
  ■ *Is relaxed and calm (Mulder, 2006)*
■ The newborn should feed completely from one side and then be offered the second breast. Many newborns and infants nurse only from one breast at each feeding. It is recommended to start feeding from the breast that the newborn finished on during the previous feeding. This promotes complete emptying of each breast every 6–8 hours and facilitates adequate milk supply in each breast.
■ Newborns are burped at the end of the feeding session.

Removing the Newborn from the Breast

Proper removal of newborn from the breast is important in decreasing nipple irritation.

■ Place a clean finger in the corner of the newborn's mouth and slide it into the mouth to break suction (**Fig. 16-3**)
■ Once suction is broken, leave the finger in while removing the newborn from the breast.

Teaching Topics

An increasing number of lactation consultants are employed by hospitals to assist women with breastfeeding. Lactation consultants are valuable members of the maternity nursing staff but do not replace the nurse's responsibility in providing proper breastfeeding teaching and support. The nurse and lactation consultant work together to ensure a positive breastfeeding experience. Before discharge, the woman should be given information on lactation consultants and lactation groups she can contact if she has questions or problems.

A primary role of a nurse caring for a woman who is breastfeeding is to facilitate successful breastfeeding by providing information and assisting the woman in her breastfeeding techniques. It is recommended that at least three complete feeding sessions per day during hospitalization be observed by the nurse or lactation consultant to assess the woman's ability to assist her infant with correctly latching-on to the breast (AWHONN, 2007).

■ AWHONN Quick Care Guide to Breastfeeding is a summary of AWHONN's evidence-based clinical guidelines for breastfeeding support that can be used to assist nurses in providing evidence-based nursing care.
■ Maternal and newborn positions
  ■ *Lying down position: The woman lies in bed or on the sofa in a comfortable position. Pillows are used to provide proper support of her head and neck. The newborn lies next to the woman on his side so that his head is directly facing the nipple. A pillow or rolled blanket can be used to support the newborn in this position.*
  ■ *Sitting position: The woman sits in a chair or bed with shoulders and back straight to reduce strain on her back and shoulder. The newborn can be held in several different positions. Three of these positions are:*
    ■ Cross-cradle position: The newborn's head is supported by the woman's hand, and the newborn's back is against the woman's forearm. The abdomen of the newborn is facing/touching the woman's abdomen. This is an ideal position to use when the woman is first learning to breastfeed and it facilitates good head control.
    ■ Football hold position: The newborn's head is cradled in the woman's hand and the body is supported between the woman's arm and her side. The newborn's head is directly facing the nipple (**Fig. 16-4A**).
    ■ Cradle position: The newborn's head is cradled in the crook of the woman's arm. The woman supports the newborn's back with her arm and his buttock with her hand. The abdomen of the newborn is facing/touching the woman's abdomen (**Fig. 16-4B**).
■ Determining effective feeding
  ■ *The woman feels physically and emotionally comfortable when feeding her newborn.*
  ■ *The newborn properly latches on, as indicated by no nipple pain or trauma.*

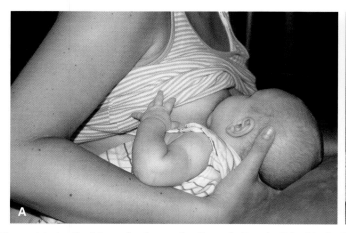
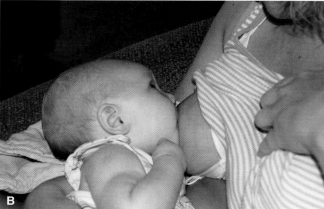

Figure 16–4 Positions for breastfeeding. *A.* Football hold. *B.* Cradle hold.

■ *The newborn suckles and the woman can hear and/or see swallowing, which indicates the transfer of milk.*

■ *The newborn spontaneously releases his grip on the breast when satiated.*

　■ Limiting time is not necessary and can be harmful in the establishment of milk supply (Chantry, Howard, & McCoy, 2003).

■ *Newborn is drowsy and arms and legs are relaxed at the end of the feeding session.*

■ *There are at least eight wet diapers and several stools per day once breast milk has come in and breastfeeding is established.*

■ *The newborn recovers his birth weight by 2 weeks of age.*

■ *A common tool used to assess and document breastfeeding efforts is LATCH (Table 16-1).*

　■ The tool assesses both the woman and her infant and assists in determining the level of support needed and the type of interventions required for the dyad.

　■ The lower the score, the higher the need for support and education.

　■ The score can vary from one feeding to the next feeding.

■ Decreasing the risk of nipple tissue breakdown

　■ *Nipple irritation can lead to tissue breakdown and mastitis.*

　■ *Painful nipples are a major reason that women stop breastfeeding before the 8th week (Lewallen et al., 2006).*

■ *Interventions to decrease irritation include:*

　■ Teach proper technique for latching-on and releasing suction. Problems with latching-on increase the risk for early cessation of breastfeeding (Lewallen et al., 2006).

　■ Apply warm compresses to the breasts/nipples before feeding to enhance the let-down reflex (AWHONN, 2006).

　■ Instruct the woman to express colostrum or milk and rub it on the nipple and areola at the end of the feeding session (AWHONN, 2007).

　■ Teach the woman to inspect her nipples for signs of irritation: redness, bruising, and tissue breakdown. Early interventions can decrease the risk of infection and bleeding.

　■ Change holding positions when feeding (e.g., football to cradle hold) to reduce pressure areas that have signs of irritation, as the pressure exerted on the nipples by the newborn is not uniform.

　■ Begin the feeding session on the less sore breast because suckling is more vigorous at the beginning of the feeding session.

　■ Instruct the woman to wash her breasts with water only. She should avoid use of soaps and alcohol, which cause excessive dryness of the breast/nipple.

　■ Instruct the woman to contact her health care provider if she is experiencing cracked and/or bleeding nipples. The breasts then need to be assessed for signs of possible infection.

TABLE 16–1　LATCH SCORING SYSTEM			
	0	1	2
L Latch	Too sleepy or reluctant No latch achieved	Repeated attempts Hold nipple in mouth Stimulate to suck	Grasps breast Tongue down Lips flanged Rhythmic sucking
A Audible swallowing	None	A few with stimulation	Spontaneous and intermittent <24 hours old Spontaneous and frequent >24 hours old
T Type of nipple	Inverted	Flat	Everted (after stimulation)
C Comfort (Breast/nipple)	Engorged Cracked, bleeding, large blisters, or bruises Severe discomfort	Filling Reddened/small blisters or bruises Mild/moderate pain	Soft Tender
H Hold (Positioning)	Full assist (staff holds infant at breast)	Minimal assist (i.e., elevate head of bed; place pillow for support) Teach one side; mother does the other side Staff holds and then mother takes over	No assist from staff Mother able to position/hold infant

Jensen, Wallace, & Kelsay (1994).

■ Comfort and relaxation

High levels of anxiety and discomfort interfere with successful breastfeeding by preventing or delaying the let-down reflex, which can cause a decrease in milk transfer and a decrease in milk supply (Mulder, 2006). Decreased milk supply is one reason women stop breastfeeding by or before the 8th week (Lewallen et al., 2006).

■ *Assist in lowering the maternal anxiety level*

■ Provide the woman/couple with easily understood breastfeeding information over several teaching sessions so she is not overwhelmed by too much information.

■ Be calm and patient in interactions with the woman/couple during breastfeeding sessions.

■ Explain that it can take time for both the woman and newborn to become comfortable with breastfeeding.

■ Ensure that the newborn is alert and ready to feed before bringing him or her to the breast. Newborns will not feed well when they are asleep/not ready to feed.

■ Praise the woman for her decision to breastfeed her infant.

■ *Provide instructions on methods to reduce pain and to promote comfort:*

■ Explain the relationship of rest, relaxation, and comfort on milk production.

■ Teach the proper use of analgesics that are recommended by the health care provider and are safe for lactating women.

■ Demonstrate the use of pillows to support both the mother's and newborn's body.

■ Teach breathing and relaxation techniques.

Evidence-Based Practice: Breastfeeding Privacy Sign

Albert, J., and Heinrichs-Breen, J. (2011). An evaluation of a breastfeeding privacy sign to prevent interruptions and promote successful breastfeeding. *JOGNN, 40,* 274–280.

The aim of this quasi-experimental study was to determine if using a breastfeeding privacy sign during hospital breastfeeding sessions improves breastfeeding outcomes and maternal satisfaction.

The control group received routine hospital care and was asked to complete a feeding diary and questionnaire. The intervention group received routine hospital care, was asked to complete a feeding diary and questionnaire, and was given a privacy sign and instructed to place it on the outside of their room door during feeding sessions.

The intervention group reported fewer interruptions during feeding sessions than the control. A significantly larger number of women in the intervention group than in the control group reported that their breastfeeding sessions were successful.

Implications for nursing practice: Decreasing the number of interruptions during feeding sessions by alerting nursing staff, hospital personnel, and visitors via a door sign can promote comfort and relaxation during feeding sessions and increase the success of breastfeeding during the hospital stay.

■ Nutrition and fluids

Decreased caloric intake and fluids can decrease milk volume. Lactating women need to consume an additional 500 calories/day over the recommended pre-pregnant requirements due to the increased energy requirement for milk production. They also need to drink a minimum of 2 liters of fluid per day.

■ *Instruct women to develop a food plan based on "My Plate" (www.ChooseMyPlate.gov)*

■ *Instruct women to have a glass of fluid next to them and drink it while they are nursing their infant since it is common to become thirsty while nursing.*

■ Expressing and storing breast milk

Teach women who breastfeed how to express milk and how to store milk properly, as most will need to skip a feeding or feedings when they are away from their infant for more than a few hours or when returning to work (**Box 16-3**). Milk can be expressed by hand or with the use of an electric breast pump.

■ *For manual expression of milk, instruct the woman to:*

1. Wash her hands before touching her breasts.
2. Massage each quadrant of her breast.
3. Place her thumb and forefinger so they form the letter "C" with the thumb at the 12 o'clock position and the forefinger at the 6 o'clock position.
4. Push the thumb and finger toward the chest wall.
5. Lean over and direct the spray of milk into a clean container.
6. Repeat this several times.
7. Occasionally massage the distal area of the breast.
8. Reposition the thumb and forefinger to the 3 and 9 o'clock positions and repeat the above sequence.

■ *Electric breast pumps*

■ A variety of electric and battery-operated breast pumps are available.

■ Electric pumps can be fitted with bilateral accessory kits so that both breasts can be pumped at the same time.

■ Electric pumps closely simulate the suckling of infants.

■ Instruct women to follow the directions provided with the electric pump of choice.

■ *Women can begin expressing and storing milk once they are comfortable with breastfeeding and the milk supply is established.*

■ *Women can express milk at the end of a feeding session and store it for use when they are not present to breastfeed.*

BOX 16–3   AWHONN POSITION STATEMENT: BREASTFEEDING IN THE WORKPLACE

"Recognizing the fact that breastfeeding is the optimal form of infant nutrition, AWHONN supports legislation and initiatives that promote and protect lactation in the workplace. AWHONN believes that employers should provide lactating women with break time that permits adequate frequency and duration of milk expression within the workplace."

Source: AWHONN, 2008.

■ *Women's hands and nails should be washed and all equipment properly cleaned before expressing and storing milk.*
■ *Breast milk can be stored:*
  ■ At room temperature (77°F) for up to 6–8 hours
  ■ In the refrigerator for up to 5 days
  ■ In the freezer that is attached to a refrigerator for 3–6 months
  ■ In a deep freezer for 6–12 months (AABM, 2008; AWHONN, 2006)
■ *Glass, hard BPA-free plastic containers or plastic bags designed for storage of breast milk can be used for milk being stored longer than 72 hours.*
  ■ The storage container needs to be labeled with the date the milk was expressed.
■ *An inch of space should be left between the top of the container and the milk to allow for the expansion of the milk that occurs during the freezing process.*
■ *Frozen milk should be stored in the back of the freezer and not on the freezer door.*
■ *Breast milk is thawed by:*
  ■ Placing the bottle or bag in the refrigerator overnight or
  ■ Placing it under warm running water or
  ■ Setting it in a container of warm water.
■ *Breast milk should not be heated in the microwave oven as it can cause uneven heating or overheating (AWHONN, 2006). Overheating by either microwave or stovetop can destroy antibodies within the breast milk (AABM, 2008).*
■ Medications
  ■ *Instruct the woman to check with her primary care provider and the infant's primary care provider before she takes prescribed and nonprescribed medications, including vitamins and herbal supplements (AWHONN, 2007).*

Bottle Feeding

Breast milk is the recommended form of newborn/infant nutrition, but owing to maternal or newborn health or personal reasons, not every woman breastfeeds (**Fig. 16-5**). Commercially prepared formulas are a nutritious alternative to breast milk.

Advantages of Formula Feeding

The advantages for formula feeding are mainly for the parents in that it:

■ Provides a very pleasurable child caring experience for the partner, as either parent can feed the newborn/infant.
■ Provides the opportunity for the woman to leave the newborn/infant with other people while she goes out or returns to work without the need to pump her breast or plan activities around the newborn/infant's feeding schedule.
■ Decreases the frequency of feedings because digestion of formula is slower than that of human milk.

Disadvantages of Formula Feeding

■ Need for increased time to prepare formula
■ Increased cost compared to breastfeeding

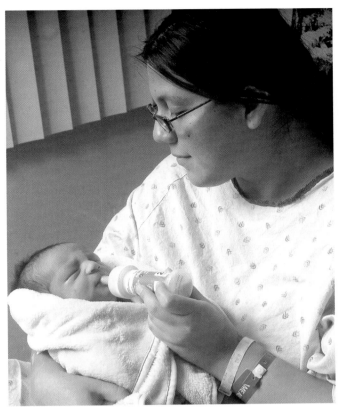

Figure 16-5 Bottle feeding is an alternate method of nourishing a newborn.

■ Increased risk of infection due to lack of antibodies that are naturally present in human milk
■ Increased risk of childhood obesity and insulin-dependent diabetes

Composition of Manufactured Formulas

■ Contains 50% more protein than human milk.
■ Uses vegetable oils, which are easier to digest than animal fat but are devoid of cholesterol
  ■ *Cholesterol is essential for brain development.*

Teaching Topics

■ Bottles
  ■ *There are a variety of bottles. Parents need to select ones that are free of BPA and can be easily cleaned.*
■ Nipples
  ■ *There are both rubber and silicone nipples.*
    ■ Silicone nipples retain fewer odors and last longer
    ■ Rubber nipples are cheaper but tend to break down faster and retain odors
  ■ *There are three types of flow rates:*
    ■ Slow – designed for newborn infants
    ■ Medium – designed for infants under 6 months
    ■ Fast – designed for older infants
  ■ *Flow rates are controlled by either the shape of the hole or the size of the hole.*
  ■ *Nipples need to be washed with soapy warm water and rinsed well.*

■ Formula preparation (see Critical Component: Preparing Infant Formula)

■ *Formulas are available in powder, concentrated, and ready-to-use forms.*

■ *Instruct parents to follow the directions provided by the manufacturer when mixing powder or diluting concentrated forms of formulas. Prolonged overdilution of formulas can cause water intoxication, and prolonged underdilution can cause dehydration.*

■ *Inform parents that once bottles of formula have been prepared, they need to be kept refrigerated and used within 48 hours to decrease risk of bacterial contamination (AAP, 2012).*

■ *Inform parents that opened cans or bottles of ready-to-use formula need to be kept refrigerated and used within 48 hours to decrease risk of bacterial contamination (AAP, 2012).*

■ *Instruct parents to clean bottles, nipples, and can openers in a dishwasher or with hot soapy water.*

■ *Instruct parents to discard unused formula that remains in the bottle at the end of feeding to decrease risk of bacterial contamination.*

CRITICAL COMPONENT

Preparing Infant Formula

- Clean and disinfect the formula preparation area
- Wash hands
- Use bottles and nipples that have been washed in hot, soapy water and rinsed well or have been washed in a dishwasher
- Use boiled non-fluoride water or distilled water to mix with concentrated or powdered formula

  - The water should be cooled (room temperature) before mixing it with the formula.
  - Well water should not be used due to the risk of nitrate poisoning (AAP, 2012).

- Check the expiration date on the formula packaging.
- Wash, rinse, and dry the top of the formula can.
- Follow directions on the formula packaging for proper dilution of concentrate or amount of powder formula per ounce of water.
- Mix the formula by gently shaking or swirling the bottle.
- Store mixed formula in airtight bottles in the refrigerator for up to 48 hours.
- Warm a refrigerated bottle by placing it in a container filled with warm water.
- Store open containers of ready-to-use, concentrated formula, or prepared bottle in the refrigerator and dispose of after 24 hours.

APP, 2012; WHO, 2007.

■ Frequency and amount of feedings

■ *Newborns take in 1/2–1 ounce (15–30 mL) per feeding during the first few days of life. This increases to 2 1/2–3 ounces (75–90 mL) per feeding by day 4 and gradually increases to 32 ounces (950 mL) per day.*

■ *Newborns/infants can be fed on demand or at least every 3–4 hours.*

■ Feeding positions

■ *Newborns/infants should be held during feedings with the head slightly higher than the trunk of the body.*

■ This position can decrease the risk of otitis media.

■ *Newborns/infants are usually fed in a cradle holding position.*

■ Burping

■ *Burp the newborn/infant halfway through feeding and at end of feeding.*

■ *Tap the newborn/infant on the back for a few minutes.*

■ *Some newborns/infants may not need to burp with each feeding (AWHONN, 2006).*

CRITICAL COMPONENT

Bottle Feeding

- Mix the formula as directed by the manufacturer.
- Hold the newborn/infant close to the body, similar to breast-feeding.
- Tilt the bottle so that the nipple is full of milk to decrease the amount of air swallowed by the newborn/infant.
- Do not prop bottles, as propping bottles places infants at higher risk for choking, otitis media, and tooth decay.
- Check the size of the nipple hole.

  - The hole may be too big if the infant has a sudden mouthful of formula and almost chokes; or when you turn the bottle upside down and the milk flows out of the nipple instead of dripping.
  - The hole may be too small if the infant seems to be working hard when sucking; or when the bottle is upside down and it takes longer than a second per drip of formula.

- Discard unused formula from the bottle at the end of the feeding.

Nutritional Needs

During the first year of life, the infant experiences rapid growth. The infant will double his birth weight by 5 months and triple his weight by his first birthday. Caloric needs vary based on size of infant, rate of growth, activity, and metabolic rate.

■ Infants experience growth spurts at 3–5 days, 1 week, 6 weeks, 3 months, and 6 months and require more frequent feedings during these periods of time (AWHONN, 2006).

■ Adequate nutritional intake is determined by plotting the weight and length of the infant at each well-child checkup.

Birth–4 Months

■ The nutritional requirements for infants are ideally met by breast milk. Iron-fortified infant formula is substituted when the woman is not breastfeeding.

■ *Breastfeeding is on demand. Newborns usually feed 8–12 times per day during the first few weeks, gradually decreasing to 6–10 feedings per day. Women produce 500–600 mL of breast milk per day during the first few weeks and 700–800 mL until semisolid foods are introduced. Milk production decreases once semisolid foods are introduced.*

■ *Formula feeding is either on demand or every 3–4 hours. Newborns start with ½–1 ounce (15–30 mL) per feeding and gradually increase to 32 ounces (960 mL) per day.*

4–6 Months

■ Feeding breast milk or formula is continued.
■ Introduction of semisolid foods is determined by the physician or nurse practitioner in collaboration with parents. American Academy of Pediatrics (AAP) and World Health Organization (WHO) guidelines recommend waiting to start solids until 6 months of age to reduce allergy risks.
■ Parents should not introduce semisolid foods until recommended by the health care provider.
■ Infants are ready for semisolid foods when they:
  ■ *Can sit independently*
  ■ *Can draw in the lower lip as a spoon is removed*
  ■ *Indicate hunger by opening the mouth*
  ■ *Refuse food by closing the mouth and turning away*
■ Before 4–6 months, the sucking reflex forces semisolid food out of the mouth versus to the back of the mouth.
■ Pureed fruits and vegetables and single-grain cereal such as rice and oats are the first food to be introduced.
■ Cereal should not be given in bottles because there is an increased risk of choking and aspiration when cereal is given by bottle.

NEWBORN CARE

It is the responsibility of the nursing staff in the postpartum unit to ensure that couples have an adequate knowledge of newborn care to safely care for their child. A teaching plan is developed for all couples based on assessment of their knowledge level. Some couples require a minimal amount of teaching while others require intensive amounts of teaching. The following information on infant care is in alphabetical order for easier reference.

Abusive Head Trauma

Abusive head trauma (AHT), also referred to as shaken baby syndrome, is a traumatic brain injury that occurs when an infant is violently shaken (Christian et al., 2009). Approximately 20% of AHT cases are fatal (National Center on Shaken Baby Syndrome, 2008).

■ Infants are at higher risk for injury related to violent shaking due to:
  ■ *Weak neck muscles*
  ■ *Large and heavy head*
■ When the infant is violently shaken, his or her brain bounces back and forth against the skull, causing bruising, swelling, and bleeding within the brain tissue.

Injuries caused by shaking can cause death or permanent and severe brain damage such as:
■ *Static encephalopathy*
■ *Mental retardation*
■ *Cerebral palsy*
■ *Cortical blindness*
■ *Seizure disorders*
■ *Learning disabilities (Christian et al., 2009)*
■ Symptoms of injury related to AHT are extreme irritability, poor feeding, breathing problems, convulsions, vomiting, and pale or bluish skin (NINDS, 2007).
■ Parents need to be educated regarding AHT and given resources they can seek when their frustrations levels are high and they need assistance in caring for their infant.
  ■ *Inform parents that it is normal for infants to cry for 30–40 minutes*
  ■ *Inform parents it is normal to feel frustrated when efforts to calm a baby are not effective.*
  ■ *Inform parents it is okay to place the baby in its crib and leave the room.*
  ■ *Inform parents to call family, friends, or Parental Stress Line when they are feeling overwhelmed (Meskauskas et al., 2009).*

Bathing

■ The first few bathing experiences can be stressful for the parents, but over time become a very pleasurable experience for both the parents and their child.
■ Daily bathing with soap is not necessary and can cause skin irritation (AWHONN, 2006). Cleansing of genital and rectal areas at each diaper change and washing face and neck areas after feedings with plain water is adequate.
■ Mild soap that has neutral pH and is preservative free is recommended to decrease the risk of skin irritation.
■ Use of soap on the face is not recommended.
■ Bathing is done in a warm room that is free from drafts.
■ Do not leave the newborn/infant unattended in bath water.
■ Gather all items required for bathing (e.g., soap, towels, washcloth, clean clothing, diapers, blankets) before the bath.
■ Bathing is best done before a feeding to decrease the risk of emeses related to jostling during bathing.
■ Use warm water for bathing (100.4°F /38°C) (AWHONN, 2006).
■ Immerse the newborn/infant in warm water deep enough to cover the shoulders (AWHONN, 2006). There is controversy regarding when an infant can be immersed in water. Some believe that it needs to be delayed until the cord has fallen off and the cord site is healed, whereas others do not. Follow the institution's policy on newborn bathing (**Fig. 16-6**).
■ The newborn/infant's head and neck are supported by the parent's forearm.
■ Start from the cleanest area (eyes) and end with the dirtiest area (buttock).

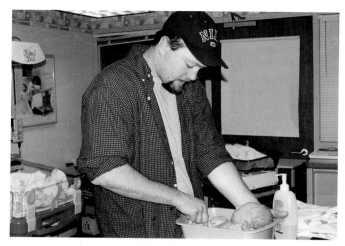

Figure 16-6   Father bathing his newborn.

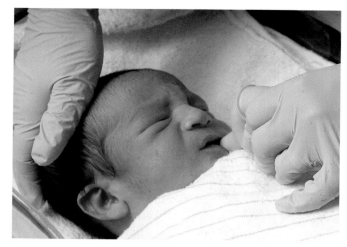

Figure 16-7   A bulb syringe in used to remove mucus.

■ Cleanse eyes from the inner to outer aspects using a clean corner of the washcloth per eye. This helps to reduce the risk of transfer of infection from one eye to the other.

■ Wash hair and massage the scalp.

■ Lift the chin to clean neck folds, where milk often collects.

■ Cleanse the upper body.

■ Cleanse the lower body.

■ Clean female genitals by washing from front to back to decrease the risk of cystitis.

■ Elevate the scrotum and cleanse the area.

■ Dry the newborn/infant and put on a clean diaper and clothes.

Bulb Syringe

■ Instruct parents in the proper use of a bulb syringe for clearing mucus from the newborn/infant's mouth and nose.

　■ *Each newborn should have his or her own bulb syringe and it should be cleaned with soapy water and rinsed after each use.*

　■ *Compress the syringe and insert it into either the nose or the mouth.*

　　■ When using in the mouth, the syringe is placed in each side of the mouth, the roof of the mouth, and the back of the mouth (**Fig. 16-7**).

　　■ When using in the nose, the syringe is placed in each nostril.

　■ *Release pressure from the syringe and allow it to slowly expand.*

　■ *Remove the syringe from the area.*

　■ *Remove drainage from the syringe and into a tissue by compressing it.*

Circumcision Care

■ Gomco or Mogen clamp:

　■ *Apply a protective lubricant over the circumcision site after each diaper change for the first week. The protective*

lubricant helps keep the area clean and keeps the wound from adhering to the diaper.

　■ *The circumcised area heals within 2 weeks.*

■ Plastibell method:

　■ *Applying lubricants on the penis when a Plastibell has been used is not recommended because lubricants can increase the risk of displacement of the plastic ring (AWHONN, 2006).*

　■ *The plastic ring falls off in 7–10 days. Parents should not pull it off.*

■ The **glans penis** (tip of the penis) appears red and forms yellow crusted areas as it heals. Parents should not wash off these areas.

■ Instruct parents to notify the health care provider if the newborn has not voided within 24 hours.

■ Instruct parents to check for bleeding every 4 hours for the first 24 hours and to notify the health care provider if there is bleeding at the circumcised area.

■ Instruct the parents to notify the health care provider if the entire penis is red, warm, and swollen and/or there is drainage from the surgical site (signs of infection).

Clothing

■ The amount of clothing varies based on whether the newborn/infant is inside or outside and on the temperature of the environment.

■ Newborns/infants are usually comfortable wearing a diaper, t-shirt, and loose-fitting outfit when inside.

　■ *100% cotton is the most comfortable clothing for infants. Infants are at greater risk for skin irritation with synthetic clothing.*

■ Avoid overheating/overbundling infant at sleep to decrease risk of sudden infant death syndrome (SIDS). Signs of overheating are:

　■ *Sweating*

　■ *Damp hair*

　■ *Heat rash*

　■ *Rapid breathing*

　■ *Restlessness*

- More clothing or heavier blankets are used when the newborn/infant is outside in cooler weather.
- A hat should be used when the newborn/infant is outside during colder weather.
- The newborn/infant's skin needs to be protected from the sun.
- Newborns/infants can become overheated with too many clothes or blankets.

Colic

- **Colic** is uncontrollable crying in healthy infants younger than the age of 5 months. The cause of colic is unknown.
  - *It is common for newborns to have a steady increase in crying until age 6 weeks, when it gradually decreases. This type of pattern is not necessarily colic.*
- Healthy infants who cry for 3 hours for 3 or more days a week and for at least 3 weeks are considered to be colicky.
- Symptoms:
  - *Infant flexes/curls legs when crying*
  - *Infant has difficult/discomfort with bowel movements*
  - *Infant is more irritable after a feeding*
  - *Infant is more irritable when placed in crib*
  - *Infant appears in pain*
  - *Infant requires frequent cuddling*
  - *Infant suddenly changes from happy to crying (Kvitvaer, B., et al., 2011).*
- Parents of colicky infants become frustrated as it becomes increasingly difficult to calm/comfort their infant. Parents should give each other "breaks" so the partner can rest and "regroup."
- Methods for soothing colicky infants:
  - *Hold the infant and sway from side to side or walk around with the infant.*
  - *Give the infant a pacifier.*
  - *Swaddle the infant.*
  - *Place the infant (abdomen facing down) over the knees and gently rub or pat the infant's back.*
  - *Place the infant in a baby bouncer.*
  - *Place the infant in a car seat and take him or her for a ride in the car.*
  - *Place the infant in a car seat and put on top of a running clothes dryer. Do not leave the infant unattended on the dryer.*
  - *Place the infant in a stroller and go for a walk.*

Cord Care

- The umbilical cord begins to dry once the cord is clamped and cut.
- The cord clamp is removed after 24 hours of life. At this point, the cord is dry, hard, and black.
- The cord falls off and the site heals within 2 weeks.
- The diaper is placed below the cord to facilitate drying of the cord (**Fig. 16-8**).
- Instruct parents to contact the health care provider if there is bleeding from the cord site, foul-smelling drainage, redness in the surrounding skin, or fever.

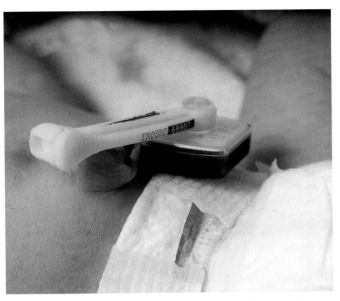

Figure 16–8 When diapering, the cord is left exposed.

Diapering

- Most parents use disposable diapers that come in various sizes based on the weight of the infant; others use cloth diapers such as all-in-one diapers that contain a cotton diaper, nylon cover and Velcro or snap fasteners; other parents use a combination of both—cloth at home and disposable when away from home.
- Change a diaper when it becomes wet or soiled to prevent skin irritation. Parents need to check diapers every few hours to see if they need changing.
- Gather supplies (e.g., clean diaper, clean clothing, and wet washcloth) before placing the infant on a flat surface such as a changing table.
- Unfasten diaper and lower the front of the diaper.
- Lift the infant's bottom using an ankle hold and fold the soiled diaper under the bottom.
- Use water to clean genital and rectal areas, wiping from front to back.
- Lift the bottom of the infant with use of an ankle hold, remove the soiled diaper, and then place a clean diaper under the infant.
- Fasten both sides of the diaper so that there is a snug fit.
- Dress the newborn.
- Properly dispose of the diaper.
- Wash hands.

Elimination

- Instruct parents on the stages of newborn stools (see Chapter 15).
- Explain that newborns pass several stools per day. At 1 month of age, breastfed infants may pass a stool only every other day due to breast milk being more easily

digested, while bottle fed infants continue to pass one or two stools per day.

■ Inform parents that newborns should have at least six wet diapers per day once breastfeeding or bottle feeding has been established.

■ Inform parents that newborn diapers may have a pink stain related to urates, which is a normal occurrence.

■ *Urates persisting in more than two diapers may suggest dehydration and weight loss. Parents need to report a continued presence of urates to the physician or nurse practitioner for further evaluation.*

■ Inform parents that blood may occur on the diaper of newborn girls related to a withdrawal of maternal hormones. This is referred to as **pseudomenstruation.**

■ Instruct parents to notify the health care provider if stools are runny and green and/or if newborn/infant has less than six wet diapers per day.

■ Instruct parents to notify the health care provider if the newborn/infant becomes constipated. Constipation can be a sign of inadequate intake and needs to be evaluated by the health care provider.

Feeding

Review information provided earlier in this chapter.

Follow-up Care

Routine follow-up care of the newborn is an important component of health promotion. The well-child checkups provide an opportunity to:

■ Assess the infant's growth
■ Assess feeding pattern
■ Assess the developmental level
■ Assess for jaundice
■ Provide the appropriate immunizations
■ Do follow-up metabolic screening
■ Continue teaching parents about the care of their child and what to expect at each developmental milestone.

Parents need to understand the importance of the check-ups and how they can promote wellness. The American Academy of Pediatrics recommends the following:

■ First visit within 3–4 days after hospital discharge
■ The second visit is 2 weeks later.
■ Subsequent visits are at 1, 2, 4, 6, 9, and 12 months of age.

Nonnutritive Sucking

Sucking is a pleasurable experience for newborns and infants. There is both nutritive sucking (sucking during breastfeeding or bottle feeding) and nonnutritive sucking. Nonnutritive sucking, using a pacifier or the infant's fist and fingers, is used to soothe or calm an infant.

■ The parents' choice to use a pacifier is influenced by cultural, societal, and community norms.

■ A pacifier should not be used with breastfed infants until 1 month of age. This provides the time needed for infants to establish breastfeeding.

■ *Pacifiers have been linked to shorter breastfeeding duration.*

■ *The mouth motions a newborn uses when breastfeeding, referred to as suckling, are different from the mouth motions (sucking) used with bottle feeding or use of pacifier.*

■ A pacifier should not be used to delay feedings or substitute for parental attention.

■ Do not tie the pacifier around the newborn/infant's neck. A cord around the neck places the infant at risk for strangulation.

■ Wash pacifiers with warm soapy water.

Potential Signs of Illness

Parents should notify the infant's health care provider in the following situations:

■ Rectal temperature >100.4°F (38.0°C) or <96.8°F (36.0°C)
■ Loss of appetite
■ Lethargy (infant is sleepy and not as active as usual)
■ Watery green stools
■ Vomiting
■ Decrease in the number of wet diapers
■ Skin rash
■ Fontanels are sunken or bulging
■ Bleeding from circumcision site and/or cord site
■ Foul odor from the circumcision site and/or cord site

Prevention of Dental Decay

Infants' teeth are susceptible to "baby bottle tooth decay," a condition that occurs when sweetened liquids are given in bottles to infants and allowed to remain in the mouth for a period of time (see Critical Component: Decreasing the Risk of Baby Bottle Tooth Decay). Within 20 minutes, the sugar from the sweetened liquid responds to mouth bacteria and forms acids that cause dental decay (ADA, 2007). Infants who fall sleep with a bottle in their mouth or who receive several bottles of sweetened liquids during the day are at higher risk for tooth decay.

CRITICAL COMPONENT

Decreasing the Risk of Baby Bottle Tooth Decay

The American Dental Association (2007) recommends the following to decrease risk of baby bottle tooth decay:

■ Do not put infants to bed with a bottle of milk, juice, or sugar water.
■ Do not give infants bottles with sugar water or sodas.
■ Clean the infant's gums with a clean gauze after each feeding.
■ Brush teeth once the first tooth erupts.
■ Consult a dentist regarding fluoride treatments if the water supply does not contain fluoride.
■ Begin regular dental appointments by the first birthday.

Safety

Parents are responsible for the safety of their children. Newborns and infants are at risk for injury related to falls, ingestion of harmful products, and accidents.

- Infant car seats
  - *Infant car seats need to be used for all infants when traveling in a motor vehicle, including on the day of discharge from the hospital.*
  - *Infants are safest when secured in the back seat. Rear-facing car seats are used with infants until they are 1 year of age and weigh 20 pounds.*
  - *Parents need to select a car seat that best fits their vehicle and follow the instructions on how to secure the seat to the vehicle's seat and how to properly position and secure the infant into the car seat.*
  - *Parents can contact a certified Child Passenger Safety Technician (CPS) for assistance in the installation and use of infant car seats before bringing the newborn home. Instruct parents to visit www.seatcheck.org to locate a CPS near their home.*
  - *Each state has laws that govern the use of infant and children car seats. Laws for specific states can be viewed at www.seatcheck.org.*
  - *Instruct parents to never leave their child in a car unattended.*
- Prevention of falls
  - *Instruct parents not to leave their newborn/infant on an elevated flat surface without supervision.*
  - *Instruct parents not to leave their newborn/infant in an infant car seat on an elevated surface unattended.*
  - *Install gates at stairwells.*
  - *Select a highchair with a wide base to prevent tipping over.*
- Prevention of ingesting harmful substances
  - *Place all cleaning materials in upper cabinets out of the infant's reach.*
  - *Place all medications, including vitamins, in upper cabinets out of the infant's reach.*
  - *Place safety latches on all lower cabinets and keep the cabinet doors closed.*
  - *Remove lead paint from older cribs and infant furniture and walls.*
  - *Never leave infants unattended in rooms or yards.*
- Prevention of accidents
  - *Keep small objects out of the reach of infants to prevent choking.*
  - *Remove strings and ribbons from bedding, sleepwear, and pacifiers to prevent strangulation.*
  - *Keep plastic bags out of reach.*
  - *Keep all sharp objects in drawers or cabinets out of the infant's reach.*
  - *Check water temperature used for bathing. Water temperature should be 100.4°F (38°C) (AWHONN, 2006).*
    - Set the water heater thermostat at 120°F or lower.
  - *Do not leave the infant in the bathtub unsupervised.*
  - *Keep any guns unloaded and locked and out of the infant's reach.*
  - *Install safety devices around swimming pools.*
  - *Do not cook while holding the infant.*
  - *Supervise infants when pets are in the room.*
  - *Ensure infant crib, highchair, and other furniture or play equipment meet current safety standards, i.e., all four sides of cribs are fixed/unmovable.*
  - *Cover electrical outlets.*

Sibling Rivalry

There will be some degree of sibling rivalry when a new baby is introduced into the family. Older children will feel the shift of attention from them to the new baby and may react to this change in a negative manner. Toddlers may begin wetting themselves or wanting to use diapers or crying to get attention. Others may want to drink from a bottle. Some children may hit or pinch their new sibling.

- Methods to decrease the degree of sibling rivalry:
  - *Start preparing older children during pregnancy for the new family addition by talking to them about becoming an older brother or sister; having them feel the baby kick; and having them around newborn infants (see Chapter 5).*
  - *Have older siblings attend sibling classes that are offered by some hospitals and agencies.*
  - *Bring older children to the postpartum unit to meet their new sibling.*
  - *Give the older children a gift and tell them it is from their new brother or sister.*
  - *Spend quality time with older children such as reading or playing games.*
  - *Take older children on special outings without the new sibling.*
  - *Teach the older sibling about why babies cry and why Mom or Dad needs to attend to the baby's cry.*

Skin Care

The newborn's skin is delicate and can be irritated easily. The skin should be inspected daily for signs of tissue irritation and breakdown (Appendix B).

- General skin care
  - *Avoid daily bathing with soap.*
  - *Use cleansers that have neutral pH.*
  - *Avoid use of adhesives because they can remove the epidermis layer of the skin and lead to a breakdown of the skin barrier.*
  - *Apply petroleum-based ointments sparingly to dry skin and avoid the head and face.*
  - *Avoid use of skin ointments with perfume, dyes, and preservatives (AWHONN, 2001).*
- Diaper dermatitis is common.
  - *Methods to reduce risk of and treat diaper dermatitis:*
    - Changing diapers frequently (8 times a day)

■ Rinsing or wiping infant's bottom during each diaper change

■ Using petroleum-based or zinc oxide ointments during diaper changes (at the first sign of a rash)

■ Avoiding use of powders. Powders increase the risk of bacterial and candidal growth

■ Avoiding use of antibiotic ointments, which can increase the risk of allergic skin reactions

■ Exposing the infant's bottom to the air (done when the infant is sleeping)

■ Adding a ½ cup of vinegar to the rinse cycle of cloth diapers to help remove soap residues and alkaline irritants.

■ *Diaper rash may occur when there is a change in the infant's diet, when the infant is teething, or when the infant is taking medications since these may change the chemistry of the urine or stools.*

Soothing Babies

Newborns and infants cry when they are hungry, uncomfortable, bored, exposed to new experiences, or sick. Parents need to determine the cause of crying. There are various methods to soothe the newborn/infant:

■ Feed if crying is related to hunger.

■ Reposition the newborn/infant to a more comfortable position when it is sleep time.

■ Swaddle the newborn/infant.

■ Hold the newborn/infant close to the body so she can feel the warmth of the parent's body and hear the parent's heartbeat.

■ Hold the newborn/infant and rock back and forth or walk around the house or dance with the infant in the parent's arms.

■ Place the newborn/infant in a stroller and go for a walk.

Sudden Infant Death Syndrome

Sudden infant death syndrome (SIDS) is the sudden death of an infant younger than the age of 1 year (AWHONN, 2006). See Critical Component: Reducing the Risk of SIDS.

■ SIDS is this third leading cause of infant death, with 1,890 infant deaths reported in 2010 (Murphy et al., 2012).

■ There has been a 50% reduction of deaths related to SIDS since parents have been instructed to place their infants on their backs when sleeping (AWHONN, 2006).

■ Objectives of *Healthy People 2020:*

  ■ *A reduction of infant deaths from SIDS by 10% from 0.55 infant deaths per 1,000 in 2006 to 0.50 infant deaths per 1,000 by 2020*

  ■ *An increase in the proportion of infants who are put to sleep on their backs from 69% in 2007 to 75.9% by 2020 (DHHS, 2012)*

CRITICAL COMPONENT

Reducing the Risk of SIDS

To reduce the risk of SIDS, the American Academy of Pediatrics recommends:

■ Placing newborns and infants on their backs when sleeping (**Fig. 16-9**)
■ Placing newborns or infants on a firm mattress for sleeping
■ Keeping pillows or stuffed animals out of the sleeping area
■ Breastfeeding
■ Maintaining a smoke-free environment
■ Preventing overheating of the infant by controlling room temperature and using lightweight clothing (AAP, 2005b)

Swaddling

Swaddling is wrapping the newborn's blanket snugly around him. This provides warmth and a sense of security for the newborn, which can have a calming effect.

1. Place the blanket on a flat surface.
2. Fold the top corner over (**Fig. 16-10**).
3. Place the newborn on the blanket with the neck at the fold line of the blanket.
4. Fold one corner across the newborn's body and tuck under his back (**Fig. 16-11**).
5. Bring the bottom corner up and fold under the neck (**Fig. 16-12**).
6. Pull the remaining corner across the newborn's body and tuck under the back (**Fig. 16-13**).

Temperature Taking

■ Instruct parents to take the infant's temperature before calling the health care provider if they feel that their child is sick.

■ Digital thermometers are recommended over mercury-filled thermometers.

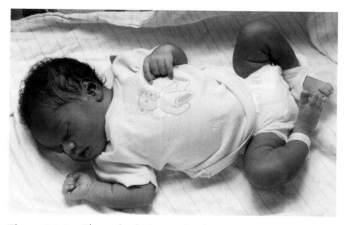

Figure 16–9   Place the baby on his back to sleep.

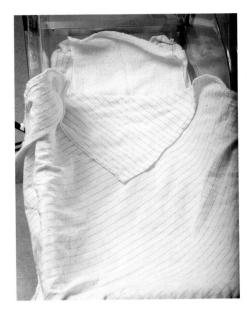

Figure 16–10 Top fold.

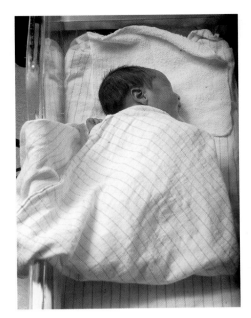

Figure 16–12 Bottom fold.

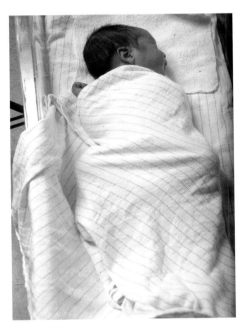

Figure 16–11 Left corner fold.

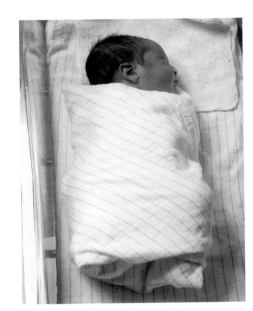

Figure 16–13 Right corner fold.

■ The American Academy of Pediatrics (2012) recommends the following:
  ■ *Rectal temperatures for children 3 years of age and younger*
  ■ *Oral temperatures for children 4 years of age and older*
  ■ *Axillary temperature (although not as accurate) can also be used for children older than 3 months.*
■ Instruct parents to take an axillary temperature by placing thermometer in the axillary region and holding the child's arm against his side until the thermometer beeps (approximately 1 minute) (**Fig. 16-14**).

■ Teach parents how to take a rectal temperature:
  1. Clean the end of the thermometer with alcohol or soapy water and rinse in cold water.
  2. Lubricate the end of the thermometer with a lubricant such as petroleum jelly.
  3. Place the child on his or her back and hold the legs in a flexed position.
  4. Insert the thermometer no further than 0.5 inches into the rectum.

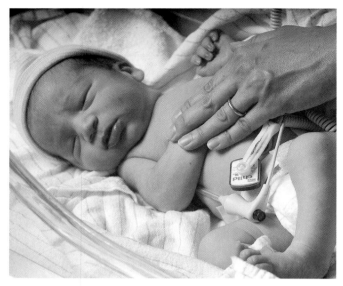

Figure 16–14 Placement of thermometer when taking an axillary temperature.

5. Hold the thermometer in place until it beeps.
6. Remove the thermometer after it has beeped and check the digital reading.
■ Teach parents how to read a thermometer.
   ■ *An elevated temperature might be related to overheating from too many blankets or clothing. Instruct parents to*

decrease the amount of clothing and retake the temperature after 15–20 minutes.
■ *Notify the health care provider if the temperature remains elevated (greater than 99.3°F [37.4°C]).*

Uncircumcised Male

■ Do not force the foreskin over the penis.
   ■ *The foreskin fully retracts on its own around 3 years of age.*
   ■ *Forcing the foreskin over the penis or using cotton swabs to clean under the foreskin can damage the inner layer of the foreskin, which can lead to adhesion formation.*
■ Gently cleanse the penis when bathing the infant and when changing the diaper.
■ Once the foreskin naturally retracts (around age 3), gently clean between the foreskin and glans of the penis when bathing the child.

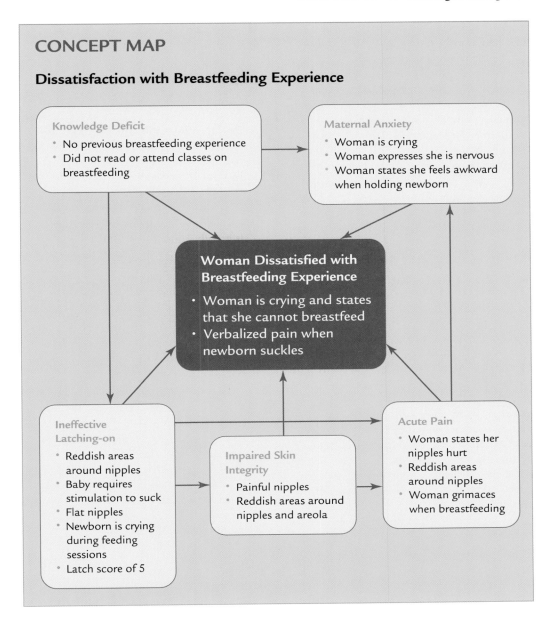

CONCEPT MAP

Dissatisfaction with Breastfeeding Experience

Knowledge Deficit
- No previous breastfeeding experience
- Did not read or attend classes on breastfeeding

Maternal Anxiety
- Woman is crying
- Woman expresses she is nervous
- Woman states she feels awkward when holding newborn

Woman Dissatisfied with Breastfeeding Experience
- Woman is crying and states that she cannot breastfeed
- Verbalized pain when newborn suckles

Ineffective Latching-on
- Reddish areas around nipples
- Baby requires stimulation to suck
- Flat nipples
- Newborn is crying during feeding sessions
- Latch score of 5

Impaired Skin Integrity
- Painful nipples
- Reddish areas around nipples and areola

Acute Pain
- Woman states her nipples hurt
- Reddish areas around nipples
- Woman grimaces when breastfeeding

Problem No. 1: Knowledge deficit

Goal: The woman will demonstrate proper breastfeeding techniques before discharge.

Outcome: Establishment of breastfeeding as evidenced by:
- ■ Proper alignment of the baby and woman
- ■ Proper latch-on
- ■ LATCH score of 8 or greater
- ■ Audible swallowing
- ■ Absence of reddened areas or blisters
- ■ The woman states she feels comfortable with breastfeeding

Nursing Actions

1. Explain that the ideal time to feed is when the baby is in a quiet alert state and demonstrates feeding cues.
2. Provide information on newborn feeding cues, such as sucking movements and sounds, hand-to-mouth movements, and rooting reflects; explain that crying is a late feeding cue (AWHONN, 2007).
3. Demonstrate different positions for holding the baby when breastfeeding: cross-cradle, cradle, and football positions.
4. Provide information on use of pillows in assisting the woman in a comfortable position.
5. Teach the woman how to properly align the baby's body to her body when breastfeeding, by assisting her and the baby in a proper breastfeeding position and explaining how this facilitates effective feeding.
6. Instruct the woman to support her baby's head and neck while the baby nurses.
7. Instruct the woman to bring the baby to her breast and not the breast to the baby.
8. Explain the importance of having the baby's mouth cover most of her areola with her nipple in the back of the baby's mouth.
9. Explain that the woman should feel a tugging sensation as the baby begins to suckle.

10. Explain that she should not experience pain when the baby is suckling. Pain may be an indication that the baby has not properly latched on and needs to be repositioned.

11. Teach the woman that she should hear audible swallowing as a sign that the baby is suckling properly and receiving milk.

12. Instruct the woman to assess her nipples for signs of nipple irritation and provide information on how to decrease the risk of nipple irritation.

13. Demonstrate how to properly remove the baby from her breast by placing a clean finger in the side of the baby's mouth to release the suction.

14. Provide information on lactation consultants and breastfeeding support groups in the community.

Problem No. 2: Maternal anxiety
Goal: Decrease of anxiety level
Outcome: The woman expresses that she feels comfortable with breastfeeding.

Nursing Actions

1. Assess the woman's beliefs, attitudes, concerns, and questions regarding breastfeeding to identify the source of anxiety to assist in identifying areas to address in the action plan.

2. Assess the woman's knowledge of breastfeeding and provide information to increase her knowledge level.

3. Assess the woman's cultural beliefs regarding breastfeeding and incorporate these in the teaching plan.

4. Assess the level of the partner's support for the woman's desire to breastfeed and explain how he/she can assist the woman with breastfeeding.

5. Assess the woman's comfort level and initiate methods to promote comfort such as relaxation techniques, proper positioning for feeding, use of pillows to support the woman and her baby, and ensuring adequate rest and sleep for the woman.

6. Establish an environment that is conducive for the woman to breastfeed, such as a quiet room and privacy.

7. Provide encouragement for the woman by praising her for her decision to breastfeed, for using proper breastfeeding techniques, and for responding to the baby's feeding cues.

8. Reevaluate the woman's level of anxiety by assessing verbal and nonverbal behaviors.

Problem No. 3: Ineffective latching-on
Goal: Effective latching-on
Outcome: The baby will effectively latch-on as evidenced by:
■ The baby's mouth covers the majority of the woman's areola.
■ The woman's nipple is in the back of the baby's mouth.
■ The baby's lips create a firm seal around the areola.
■ Audible swallowing.

■ Absence of reddened areas or blisters.
■ LATCH score of 8 or greater

Nursing Actions

1. Assess the woman's breastfeeding technique.
2. Assess the nipples and areola for signs of irritation.
3. Provide information on latching-on.
4. Assist the woman and her baby with proper positioning that facilitates latching-on.
5. Instruct the woman to bring the baby to her breast when the baby's mouth is wide open.
6. Instruct the woman to delay use of a pacifier until the baby is able to latch-on and breastfeeding is established, which is usually 1 month (AWHONN, 2007).

Problem No. 4: Acute pain
Goal: Absence of pain
Outcome: The baby will properly latch-on and the woman will state that she is not experiencing pain in the breast area when feeding her baby.

Nursing Actions

1. Assess the level of pain using a pain scale.
2. Assess the breast for signs of irritation, such as reddened areas, blisters, or cracking, and provide information on methods to decrease irritation.
3. Assess the breastfeeding technique by observing the woman during a feeding session.
4. Provide information and assistance to facilitate latching-on.
5. Provide information on various positions for holding the baby during feeding sessions.
6. Explain that warm, moist compresses may decrease nipple pain (AWHONN, 2007).
7. Medicate with analgesia PRN.

Problem No. 5: Impaired skin integrity
Goal: Skin will remain intact.
Outcome: The tissue of the nipples and areola will be intact with no redness or blisters.

Nursing Actions

1. Assess nipples and areolas for signs of irritation.
2. Instruct the woman to inspect her nipples and areolas after each feeding.
3. Assess the woman during feeding sessions for proper breastfeeding techniques.
4. Provide information on proper positioning of the baby for breastfeeding.
5. Provide information on latching-on.
6. Instruct the woman to gently rub breast milk around her nipples and areolas after each feeding session (AWHONN, 2007).

TYING IT ALL TOGETHER

As the nurse, you are caring for Margarite Sanchez, a 28-year-old G3 P2 Hispanic woman who delivered a healthy boy, Manuel. Margarite and her husband have a healthy 2½-year-old boy. Margarite informs you that she breastfed her older child, José, for 9 months without problems. Her older son was interested in the pregnancy and being a big brother, but he has been crying and is restless and irritable during hospital visits. He also does not want to hold his baby brother and is demanding to be taken to the toy store.

Margarite's husband tells you that he was very involved in the care of his first child.

A circumcision is planned for Manuel the morning of discharge.

Based on your knowledge of the Sanchez family, list the priority learning needs and state the rationale for your selection of learning needs.

Describe your teaching plan based on the identified priority learning needs. The plan should include:

- *Preparation of the learning environment*
- *Methods to assess their learning needs*
- *Information that will be shared with the couple*
- *Method for evaluating effectiveness of teaching*

■ ■ ■ Review Questions ■ ■ ■

1. Teaching regarding the care of the newborn begins:
   A. During pregnancy
   B. Within a few hours after delivery
   C. Twelve hours after delivery
   D. The day of discharge

2. During a feeding session, your 19-year-old primipara, who is 12 hours post-birth, asks you how she can tell if her baby girl is getting any milk when nursing. Your best response is:
   A. "Your baby is getting colostrum. Your milk will come in around 2–3 days."
   B. "When your baby falls asleep while nursing."
   C. "You will hear swallowing noises from your baby as she suckles."
   D. "Your baby will refuse to latch-on."

3. You are assigned to a 21-year-old primipara, who is 36 hours post-birth and breastfeeding her healthy newborn son. During your assessment, you note that there is a small reddened area on the right side of the left areola. Based on this assessment finding, which of the following is the priority nursing action?
   A. Instruct the woman to change feeding position from cradle hold to football hold.
   B. Instruct the woman to air-dry her nipples for 15 minutes after each feeding.
   C. Instruct the woman to apply a lanolin cream to the area after each feeding.
   D. Instruct the woman to feed from only the right breast for 24 hours.

4. You are assigned a 16-year-old primipara, who is bottle feeding her healthy full-term baby boy. She asks you why the other nurse told her to tilt the baby's bottle when feeding. Your best response is:
   A. "I will go and get the other nurse so she can clarify the instruction she gave you."
   B. "By tilting the bottle, the nipple is in a more comfortable placement in your baby's mouth."
   C. By tilting the bottle, you keep the nipple full of formula and decrease the amount of air your baby swallows."
   D. "The tilted position provides greater pressure coming from the bottle and makes it easier for your baby to take in the formula."

5. You are developing a discharge teaching plan for your patient. The newborn is a girl and is full term and healthy. Both the woman and her partner are college educated and have one other healthy child, a boy who is 2 years old. The woman bottle fed her son and plans to breastfeed her daughter. She plans to return to work when her daughter is 3 months old. Based on this information, the three primary learning needs for this couple are:
   A. Breastfeeding, sibling rivalry, and infant/child safety
   B. Breastfeeding, storage of breast milk, and bathing
   C. Safety, colic, and storage of breast milk
   D. Cord care, breastfeeding, and safety

6. Contraindications for breastfeeding include which of the following? Select all that apply.
   A. Woman is using cocaine.
   B. Woman is being treated for mastitis.
   C. Woman is receiving chemotherapy for lymphoma.
   D. Infant has thrush.

7. Which of the following are true statements regarding let-down reflex? Select all that apply.
   A. Contractions of the myoepithelial cells forces milk into the duct system.
   B. Oxytocin is released in response to infant suckling and woman's emotions.
   C. It can occur during sexual arousal.
   D. It occurs multiple times during feeding session.

8. You observe that a 2-day postpartum woman is having difficulty breastfeeding. Her baby is crying and moving his head from side to side. Your first nursing action is to: _____.
   A. Assist the woman into a comfortable position.
   B. Assist the woman in calming her baby.
   C. Show the woman how to properly position the baby.
   D. Tell the woman that her baby is not hungry and to wait a few hours.

9. Your discharge teaching for a couple with an uncircumcised boy should include which of the following?
   A. Beginning at 1 month of age, gently retract the foreskin each day during the infant's bath.
   B. Beginning at 6 months of age, clean the area between the foreskin and glans each day with a cotton swab.
   C. Gently wash the penis when bathing and with each diaper change.
   D. Retract the foreskin when there is a yellowish discharge.

10. The American Dental Association recommends that parents can decrease the risk of tooth decay in infants by _____. Select all that apply.
   A. Preparing juice bottles with one part juice and two parts water
   B. Cleaning the infant's gums with a wet, clean gauze after feedings
   C. Rinsing the infant's mouth with sterile water after each feeding
   D. Beginning regular dental checkups by 1 year of age

References

Albert, J., and Heinrichs-Breen, J. (2011). An evaluation of a breast-feeding privacy sign to prevent interruptions and promote successful breastfeeding. *JOGGN, 40*, 274–280.

(AAP). (2005a). Breastfeeding and use of human milk. *Pediatrics, 115*, 496–506.

American Academy of Breastfeeding Medicine (AABM). (2008*). Protocol #8: Human milk storage information for home use for healthy full-term infants.* Retrieved from www.bfmed.org

American Academy of Pediatrics (AAP). (2005b). The changing concepts of sudden infant death syndrome: Diagnostic coding shifts, controversies regarding sleep environment and new variables to consider in reducing risk. *Pediatrics, 116*, 1245–1255.

American Academy of Pediatrics (AAP). (2012). How to take a child's temperature? Retrieved from www.healthychildren.org

American Academy of Pediatrics (AAP). (2008). Breastfeeding initiative. Retrieved from www.aap.org/breastfeeding

American Academy of Pediatrics (AAP). (2012). Preparing, sterilizing, and storing formula. Retrieved from www.healthychildren.org/english/ages-stages/baby/feeding-nutrition/pages/sterilization-storing-formula.apx

American Dental Association (ADA). (2007). Early childhood tooth decay. www.ada.org.

Association of Women's Health, Obstetric and Neonatal Nurses (AWHONN). (2001). *Neonatal skin care.* Washington, DC: Author.

Association of Women's Health, Obstetric and Neonatal Nurses (AWHONN). (2006). *The compendium of postpartum care.* Philadelphia: Medical Broadcasting Company.

Association of Women's Health, Obstetric and Neonatal Nurses (AWHONN). (2007). *Breastfeeding support: Prenatal care through the first year. Evidence-based clinical practice guideline* (2nd ed.). Washington, DC: Author.

Association of Women's Health, Obstetric and Neonatal Nurses (AWHONN). (2008). *Breastfeeding and lactation in the workplace (Position Statement).* Washington, DC: Author.

Chantry, C., Howard, C., & McCoy, R. (2003). *Protocol #5: Peripartum breastfeeding management for the healthy mother and infant at term.* The Academy of Breastfeeding Medicine. Retrieved from www.bfmed.org

D'Alessandro, D. (2010). What are significant contraindications for breastfeeding?PediatricEducation.org. Retrieved from www.pediatriceducation.org/2010/09/13/what-are-significant-contraindications-for -breastfeeding/

Kvitvaer, B., Miller, J., and Newell, D. (2011). Improving our understanding of colicky infants: A prospective observation study. *Journal of clinical nursing, 21*, 63–69.

Lewallen, L., Dick, M., Flowers, J., Powell, W., Zickefoose, K., Wall, Y., & Price, Z. (2006). Breastfeeding support and early cessation. *JOGNN, 35*, 166–172.

Meskauskas, L., Beaton, K., and Meservey, M. (2009). Preventing shaken baby syndrome. *Nursing for Women's Health, 13*, 325–330.

Mulder, P. (2006). A concept analysis of effective breastfeeding. *JOGNN, 35*, 332–339.

Murphy, S., Xu, J., and Kochanek, K. (2012). Deaths: Preliminary data for 2010. *National vital statistics report, 60, 4.* Hyattsville, MD: National Center for Health Science.

National Center on Shaken Baby Syndrome. (2008). *What is shaken baby syndrome.* Retrieved from www.dontshake.com

National Institute of Neurological Disorders and Strokes (NINDS). (2007). *NINDS shaken baby syndrome information page.* Retrieved from www.ninds.nih.gov/disorders/shakenbaby/shakenbaby.htm

Purnell, L., & Paulanka, B. (2008). *Guide to culturally competent health care.* Philadelphia: F.A. Davis.

U.S. Department of Health and Human Services (DHHS). (2000). *Breastfeeding: HHS blueprint for action on breastfeeding.* Retrieved from www.womanshealth.gov/breastfeeding/bluprntbk2.pdf

U.S. Department of Health and Human Services (DHHS). (2010). *Breastfeeding.* Retrieved from www.womenshealth.gov/breastfeeding

U.S. Department of Health and Human Services (DHHS). (2012). Healthy people 2020 topics and objectives. Retrieved from www.Healthypeople.gov/2020/topicsobjectives2020/objectives

U.S. Preventative Services Task Force. (2008). *Primary care interventions to promote breastfeeding: Clinical summary.* AHRQ Publication No. 09-05126-EF-3. Retrieved from www.uspreventativeservicestaskforce.org/uspstf08/breatfeeding/brfeedsum.htm

Wilkinson, J., & Van Leuven, K. (2007). *Fundamentals of nursing.* Philadelphia: F.A. Davis.

World Health Organization (WHO). (2007). How to prepare formula for bottle-feeding at home. Retrieved from www.who.int/entity/foodsafety/publications/micro/PFI_Bottle_en.pdf

World Health Organization (WHO). (2008). *Breastfeeding.* Retrieved from www.who.int/topics/breastfeeding

High-Risk Neonatal Nursing Care

17

EXPECTED STUDENT OUTCOMES

On completion of this chapter, the student will be able to:

- ☐ Define key terms.
- ☐ Describe the physiology and pathophysiology associated with selected complications of the neonatal period.
- ☐ Identify critical elements of assessment and nursing care of the high-risk neonate.
- ☐ Develop a discharge plan for high-risk neonates.
- ☐ Describe the loss and grief process experienced by parents whose infant has died.

Nursing Diagnoses

- Impaired gas exchange related to inadequate surfactant and immature lung tissue
- Risk for ineffective airway clearance related to meconium aspiration
- Ineffective thermoregulation related to prematurity, lack of subcutaneous fat, and environmental temperature
- Imbalanced nutrition related to prematurity; inability to absorb nutrients; decreased perfusion to gastrointestinal tract; postnatal change from high glucose exposure to low glucose exposure and hyperinsulinism; cleft lip/cleft palate
- Risk for infection related to prematurity, exposure to infectious agents, and maternal chorioamnionitis
- Pain related to procedures; birth trauma
- Risk for injury related to lack of oxygen to the brain; prolonged ventilation and oxygen administration; effects of drugs on fetal/neonatal growth and development; birth trauma; hypoglycemia; asphyxia; meconium aspiration; kernicterus
- Risk for ineffective parent/family coping related to infant illness or death
- Grieving related to the infant with a high-risk condition; loss of the dream of the perfect infant; death of the infant
- Risk for impaired parent-infant attachment related to separation

Nursing Outcomes

- The infant exhibits a breathing pattern within normal limits with respiratory rate between 30 and 60 breaths per minute with no signs of respiratory distress.
- The infant maintains temperature within normal limits.
- The infant gains weight, consumes adequate nutritional intake, has adequate output, and is free of signs of hypoglycemia or malnutrition.
- The infant remains free of signs of infection; the white blood cell count is within normal limits and the blood, urine, and CSF cultures are negative.
- The infant exhibits decreased signs of pain after receiving nonpharmacological or pharmacological pain reduction interventions.
- The infant is free of signs of injury.
- Parents communicate needs, state ability to cope, identify a support system, and ask for help and information when needed.
- Parents identify what to expect during the grieving process.
- Parents visit the infant in the intensive care nursery, demonstrate caregiving behaviors, express interest in the newborn, and respond to the infant's behavioral cues.

Don't have time to read this chapter? Want to reinforce your reading? Need to review for a test? Listen to this chapter on DavisPlus.

INTRODUCTION

Infant mortality rates in the United States have significantly decreased from 47.0 per 1000 live births in 1940 to 6.05 per 1000 in 2011 (Hoyert & Jiaquin, 2012). Although this is a significant decrease, the infant mortality rate, which indicates that 23,907 infants died in 2011, is too high for a nation with the amount of available wealth and resources that the United States possesses. One of the primary causes of illness and death in the neonate is complications related to prematurity.

This chapter provides an overview of the critical components of care of the high-risk neonate, which is a subspecialty of maternity nursing. Nurses who elect to work in a neonatal intensive care nursery will need to gain an in-depth knowledge of high-risk neonates through additional readings and classes that focus on the unique needs of high-risk neonates and their parents.

PRETERM NEONATES

Period of gestation and birth weight are the two most important predictors of an infant's health and survival. Prematurity and low birth weight are the second leading causes of infant death in the United States, the first being congenital malformations and chromosomal anomalies. (Hoyert & Jiaquin, 2012). Prematurity is classified as:

■ **Very premature:** Neonates born at less than 32 weeks' gestation (**Fig. 17-1**)
■ **Premature:** Neonates born between 32 and 34 weeks' gestation
■ **Late premature:** Neonates born between 34 and 37 weeks' gestation

The number of premature births has risen from 10.6% of live births in 1990 to 11.72% in 2011 (Hamilton et al., 2012).

■ The greatest increase is in late premature births (**Table 17-1**).

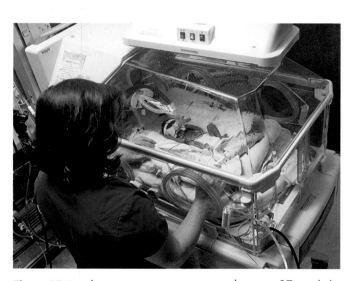

Figure 17–1   A very premature neonate born at 27 weeks' gestation.

TABLE 17–1 PERCENTAGE OF PRETERM BIRTHS		
	1990	2011
VERY PRETERM	1.9	1.92
PRETERM	1.4	1.51
LATE PRETERM	7.3	8.28
Hamilton, Martin, & Ventura (2012).		

■ The percentage of premature births based on the race of the mother are:
  ■ *Non-Hispanic black: 16.75%*
  ■ *American Indian or Alaska Native: 13.5%*
  ■ *Hispanic: 11.66%*
  ■ *Non-Hispanic white: 10.49%*
  ■ *Asian or Pacific Islander: 10.4% (Hamilton et al., 2012)*
■ Prematurity is a primary reason for low birth weight. Classification of birth weight (regardless of gestational age) is as follows:
  ■ *Low birth weight: Less than 2500 grams at birth*
  ■ *Very low birth weight: Less than 1500 grams at birth*
  ■ *Extremely low birth weight: Less than 1000 grams at birth*

Multiple factors place a woman at risk for preterm labor and birth. Many are modifiable, and many are not (**Table 17-2**). Common complications related to prematurity are respiratory distress syndrome, retinopathy of prematurity, bronchopulmonary dysplasia, patent ductus arteriosus, periventricular-intraventricular hemorrhage, and necrotizing enterocolitis (NEC).

Assessment Findings

■ Gestational age by Ballard score is at or below 37 weeks.
■ Physical characteristics vary based on gestational age (**Fig. 17-2**)
  ■ *Tone and flexion increase with greater gestational age. Early in gestation, resting tone and posture are hypotonic and extended.*
  ■ *The skin is translucent, transparent, and red.*
  ■ *Subcutaneous fat is decreased.*
  ■ *Lanugo is present between 20 and 28 weeks' gestation. At 28 weeks' gestation, lanugo begins to disappear on the face and the front of the trunk.*
  ■ *Creases on the anterior part of the foot are not present until 28–30 weeks. As gestation increases, plantar creases increase and spread toward the heel of the foot.*
  ■ *Eyelids are fused in very preterm neonates. Eyelids open between 26 and 30 weeks' gestation.*
  ■ *Overriding sutures are common among premature, low birth weight neonates.*
  ■ *The pinna of the ear is thin, soft, flat, and folded.*
  ■ *The testes are normally not descended, and are found in the inguinal canal.*
  ■ *Tremors and jittery movement may be noted.*

TABLE 17–2   RISK FACTORS FOR PRETERM LABOR AND BIRTH

NONMODIFIABLE RISK FACTORS	TREATABLE/MODIFIABLE RISK FACTORS
Previous preterm birth	Age at pregnancy <17 or >34 years
Multiple abortions	Unplanned pregnancy
Race/ethnic group	Single
Uterine/cervical anomaly	Low educational level
Multiple gestation	Poverty, unsafe environment
Polyhydramnios	Domestic violence
Oligohydramnios	Life stress
Pregnancy induced hypertension	Number of implanted embryos in assisted reproduction
Placenta previa (after 22 weeks)	Low pre-pregnancy weight
DES exposure	Obesity
Short interval between pregnancies	Health problems that can be treated: hypertension, diabetes, clotting problems, anemia.
Abruptio placenta	Incompetent cervix
Parity (0 or >4)	Genitourinary infection
Premature rupture of membranes	Infection
Bleeding in first trimester	Periodontal disease
	Substance/alcohol use
	Cigarette smoking
	Long hours of employment/standing
	Late or no prenatal care
	Air pollution

March of Dimes (2012).

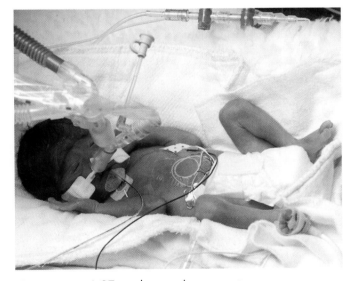

Figure 17–2   A 27-week gestation neonate.

■ *The cry is weak.*
■ *Reflexes may be diminished or absent.*
■ *Immature suck, swallow, and breathing patterns are observed in very premature infants. These neonates may not be able to take adequate oral feedings.*

■ **Apnea,** cessation of breathing for at least 10–15 seconds, and **bradycardia,** heart rate less than 100 beats per minute, are commonly observed (Goodwin, 2010).
■ Hypotension may occur among extremely low birth weight infants.
■ Heart murmur may be present related to patent ductus arteriosus.
■ Anemia is common, especially among very low birth weight babies (Sallmon & Sola-Visner, 2012).

Medical Management

■ Lung maturity is determined with lecithin/sphingomyelin (L/S) ratio or phosphatidylglycerol (PG) before elective induction or cesarean birth, and for women in preterm labor.
■ Corticosteroids, betamethasone or dexamethasone, are administered to the pregnant woman if the woman presents in preterm labor, or if preterm birth is anticipated. Evidence suggests that corticosteroid administration results in reduced respiratory distress syndrome, NEC, cerebroventricular hemorrhage, need for respiratory support, systemic infections, admission to the NICU, and neonatal death (Surbeck, Drack, Irion, Nelle, Huang, & Hoesli, 2012).

■ Continuous pulse oximetry
■ Cardiac monitoring, oxygen saturation, blood gases, and end CO_2
■ Respiratory support
 ■ *Nasal continuous positive airway pressure (NCPAP) or intubation*
■ Laboratory tests
 ■ *Bilirubin levels for neonates who are jaundiced*
 ■ *Blood cultures for neonates with signs of infection*
 ■ *Complete blood count with differential*
 ■ *Electrolytes*
 ■ *Blood glucose*
 ■ *Calcium, blood urea nitrogen (BUN), creatinine, phosphorus, magnesium, albumin, liver function tests, and acid-base status for neonates on total parenteral nutrition (Ditzenberger, 2010).*
■ Medications
 ■ *Sodium bicarbonate to treat metabolic acidosis if present*
 ■ *Dopamine or dobutamine for treatment of hypotension*
 ■ *Erythropoietin administration to stimulate production of red blood cells if indicated*
  ■ Evidence suggests that erythropoietin administration may reduce the need for red blood cell transfusions among preterm/low birth weight infants (Sallmon & Sola-Visner, 2012).
 ■ *Antibiotic therapy as indicated to decrease risk of infection or treatment of infection*
 ■ *Opioids to treat pain associated with procedures that cause moderate to severe pain, such as with surgical procedures*
■ Blood transfusion if the neonate is anemic, or to replace blood loss due to laboratory tests, or blood loss during birth (Charsha, 2010)
■ Intravenous fluids as indicated
■ Parenteral (intravenous) nutrition if indicated by the neonate's gestational age and/or clinical condition
■ Central line if long-term parenteral nutrition is required
■ Umbilical artery and umbilical vein catheters
■ Information about the neonate's condition, treatment plan, and follow-up care is provided to the parents.

Nursing Actions

■ Review prenatal, intrapartal, and neonatal histories for any known risk factors that would potentially impact the neonate.
■ Participate in resuscitation of the neonate as indicated.
 ■ *The NICU nurse, neonatologist, and/or neonatal nurse practitioner should be present at high-risk births.*
■ Transfer the neonate to the neonatal intensive care unit in order to stabilize and provide ongoing specialized care.
■ Perform gestational assessment to determine age and size of neonate.
 ■ *Protocols of care differ with gestational age.*
■ Perform a physical assessment, evaluating for problems associated with prematurity.
 ■ *Nursing care includes the immediate recognition and prioritizing of problems in order to decrease neonatal morbidity and mortality.*

■ Assess for signs of respiratory distress:
 ■ *Grunting*
 ■ *Flaring*
 ■ *Retracting*
 ■ *Cyanosis*
■ Provide respiratory support.
 ■ *Maintain a patent airway.*
 ■ *Administer oxygen to maintain oxygen saturation within ordered parameters.*
  ■ Short-term oxygen administration may be given using a mask.
  ■ Long-term oxygen administration may be given using nasal cannula, oxygen hood, NCPAP, or ventilator.
  ■ Oxygen is humidified and warmed to prevent drying of mucous membranes and dropping of body temperature. A decrease in body temperature increases the body metabolism and increases calorie consumption.
 ■ *Suction airway as needed for removal of secretions as neonates have a smaller airway diameter, which increases the risk of obstruction.*
■ Maintain neutral thermal environment by:
 ■ *Drying the infant gently immediately after birth to prevent heat loss from evaporation*
 ■ *Keeping the head covered to prevent heat loss due to radiation and convection*
 ■ *Using plastic barriers made of polyethylene to cover preterm neonates after birth to prevent heat loss and transepidermal water loss*
 ■ *Using a chemical warming mattress during resuscitation and transport to the neonatal intensive care unit*
  ■ Extremely low birth weight (ELBW) neonates are at high risk for cold stress during the period immediately after birth. Neonates placed in plastic barriers and/or on chemical mattresses immediately after birth have higher admission temperatures upon admission to the NICU (Lewis, Sanders & Brockopp, 2011).
 ■ *Prewarming radiant warmers, incubators, and linens*
 ■ *Controlling environmental temperature with use of servo control. A temperature control probe should be placed on the neonate's abdomen to assist in maintaining the neonate's temperature within the normal range (axillary 97.4°–98.4°F [36.3°–36.9°C] for premature neonates)*
 ■ *Placing the neonate in a double-walled incubator to prevent transepidermal water loss and heat loss*
 ■ *Encouraging kangaroo care (skin-to-skin care) in stable neonates*
 ■ *Weaning infants gradually from incubator to an open crib (Brand & Boyd, 2010)*
■ Assess cardiovascular system:
 ■ *Signs of patent ductus arteriosus*
 ■ *Murmurs*
 ■ *Pulses*
 ■ *Capillary refill*
■ Provide cardiovascular support.
 ■ *Monitor blood pressure, oxygen saturation, and blood gases.*
 ■ *Obtain and monitor hemoglobin and hematocrit as per order.*
 ■ *Administer blood transfusion as per order.*

- Apply transcutaneous monitor or pulse oximeter to monitor O_2 levels.
- Monitor vital signs, oxygen saturation, arterial blood gases, and end CO_2 as per orders.
- Assess responses to interventions. These responses may be changes in breathing, oxygen saturation, vital signs, and neonatal behavior.
- Maintain fluid and electrolyte balance.
  - *Monitor input and output by:*
    - Weighing diapers to determine output
    - Assessing frequency, color, amount, and specific gravity of urine to determine hydration status
    - Recording fluid intake and output: nasal and oral gastric tubes, chest tubes, Foley catheter, stomas
  - *Restrict fluid intake as per order.*
    - Fluid restriction is commonly ordered for neonates with bronchopulmonary dysplasia (BPD) and patent ductus arteriosus (PDA) or other complications that can lead to pulmonary edema.
  - *Monitor electrolyte levels as per order.*
    - Hyperkalemia (elevated potassium levels), hyponatremia (low sodium level), and hypernatremia (high sodium level) may occur among low birth weight infants (Charsha, 2010).
  - *Administer intravenous fluids as per order.*
    - Monitor the site of intravenous access for signs of infection, skin breakdown, and infiltration.
  - *Add humidity to the neonate's environment to decrease water loss that can occur through the neonate's immature skin, known as transepidermal water loss (TEWL).*
    - Humidity added to the environment prevents heat loss, improves skin integrity, decreases TEWL, and promotes electrolyte balance. (Charsha, 2010).
- Meet the neonate's nutrition requirements.
  - *Obtain and monitor blood glucose levels as per order.*
  - *Administer parenteral nutrition (intravenous) if the neonate is unable to receive enteral (via gastrointestinal tract) feedings or is advancing slowly on feeding volumes.*
    - Extremely low birth weight neonates (<1,500 grams) or neonates less than 32 weeks' gestation:
      - *May lack the ability to digest and absorb feedings*
      - *May have an inability to suck, swallow, and breathe*
      - *Will most likely require parenteral nutrition (Charsha, 2010).*
    - The dextrose content is titrated based on the serum glucose level (Charsha, 2010).
  - *Administer **trophic feedings** (small volume enteral feedings) as per order. They are often given while neonates are receiving parenteral feedings to ease the transition to full enteral feedings, and enhance gastrointestinal functioning (Charsha, 2010).*
  - *Administer enteral feedings orally or by gastric tube (gavage feedings) depending on the infant's gestational age and clinical condition. Most neonates who are older than 34 weeks' gestation usually receive oral feedings soon after birth.*
    - Human milk is preferred for enteral feeding.
    - Human milk requires fortification because it does not provide the calories, protein, fat, carbohydrate,

potassium, calcium, sodium, and phosphorus that the premature infant needs (Ditzenberger, 2010).
    - Formulas developed specifically for preterm infants are available. These formulas are modified to promote absorption and digestion for babies with immature gastrointestinal functioning, and contain the extra calories, protein, minerals, and vitamins required by preterm babies (Ditzenberger, 2010).
- Use proper technique for gavage feedings (see Critical Component: Procedure for Gavage Feeding).
  - *When feedings are initiated and before each feeding, assess for signs of feeding tolerance as follows (Ditzenberger, 2010):*
    - Check for the presence of bowel sounds.
    - Assess the abdomen for bowel loops and discoloration.
    - Measure abdominal girth.
    - Check for gastric residuals by aspirating stomach contents with the syringe. Note the amount, color, and consistency of the contents.
    - Assess for emesis.
    - Check stools for occult blood as per order.
    - Check stools for reducing substances as per order.
    - Assess stools for consistency, amount, and frequency.
  - *Use nonnutritive sucking with a pacifier during gavage feedings (Pinelli & Symington, 2010). Nonnutritive sucking eases the transition from gavage feeding to bottle feeding, and results in decreased length of hospital stay for preterm neonates (Pinelli & Symington, 2010).*
  - *Monitor weight daily. Weight gain of 10 to 20 grams per kilogram per day indicates appropriate growth and caloric intake for a preterm neonate (Ditzenberger, 2010).*
  - *Monitor length and head circumference weekly.*
  - *Calculate and monitor intake of fluids, calories, and protein daily (Ditzenberger, 2010). Preterm infants require between 105 and 130 kcal/kg/day.*
- Administer medications as per order.
- Provide skin care:
  - *The skin of the preterm neonate is predisposed to injury related to it being thin and fragile. It is important to carefully assess for skin breakdown and signs of infection (**Fig. 17-3**) (AWHONN & NANN, 2007).*
    - Refer to Figure 17-3, a skin assessment tool developed by Association of Women's Health, Obstetric and Neonatal Nurses (AWHONNs).
  - *Use a neutral pH cleanser and sterile water when bathing and only bathe the soiled areas.*
  - *Use adhesives sparingly*
  - *Change diapers frequently*
  - *Change positions frequently*
  - *Apply emollients to dry areas*
  - *Use water, air, or gel mattresses*
- Obtain laboratory test as per orders.
- Assess for signs of jaundice.
- Assess for signs of NEC such as abnormal vital signs, abdominal distention (increase in abdominal circumference), abdominal discoloration, bowel loops, feeding intolerance, emesis, residuals, bloody stools, and behavioral changes.

■ Transition the neonate from tube feedings to oral feedings (see Critical Component: Oral Feeding Readiness).
- *Transitioning to oral feedings occurs when the neonate:*
  - Has cardiorespiratory regulation
  - Demonstrates a coordinated suck, swallow, and breathe
  - Demonstrates hunger cues such as bringing hand to the mouth, sucking on fingers
  - Maintains a quiet alert state

CRITICAL COMPONENT

Oral Feeding Readiness

The decision to initial oral feedings should not be solely based on the infant's post-conceptual age. Feeding initiation should be based on nursing observation of individual feeding readiness behaviors. Feeding skills develop at different rates, and infants of the same gestational age may not reach full oral feedings in the same time interval. Infants mature at their own pace and are influenced by the severity of their illness.

(Jones, 2012)

- *Properly position the neonate for bottle feeding by holding the swaddled baby in a semi-upright or upright position.*
- *Observe the neonate for respiratory status, apnea, bradycardia, oxygenation, and feeding tolerance.*
- *Pace feeding and allow for breathing breaks since preterm neonates may become fatigued during feedings.*
■ Support breastfeeding.
- *Evidence suggests that breast milk decreases the incidence of NEC (Caplin, 2011).*
- *During the period of time that the neonate is unable to breastfeed, instruct the mother in the use of a breast pump and storage of breast milk.*
- *Encourage the mother to bring breast milk to the NICU so that it can be used for enteral feedings for her infant.*
- *Teach the mother about feeding cues, breastfeeding positions, correct latch, and evaluating the feeding.*
- *Weigh the neonate before and after breastfeeding to monitor intake.*
- *See Appendix A for additional nursing actions.*
■ Manage pain to prevent potential long-term sensory disturbances and altered pain responses that may last into adulthood.
- *Assess the neonate for signs of pain frequently, and especially during painful procedures. Instruments to measure neonatal pain among preterm neonates are available and should be integrated into routine care.*
- *Administer sucrose and promote nonnutritive sucking during painful procedures.*
- *Administer opioids as per orders to treat pain associated with procedures that cause moderate to severe pain.*

CRITICAL COMPONENT

Procedure for Gavage Feeding

Gavage feedings are appropriate for neonates who are <32 weeks' gestation or who cannot safely receive oral feedings.

1. Use a size 5–8 french feeding tube.
2. Measure the tube (used for orogastric route) from the mouth to the ear, and from the ear to the lower end of the sternum.
3. Check for proper placement of the tube after each insertion and before each feeding by:
   - Placing syringe on end of tube and pulling to remove stomach contents, and/or
   - Injecting a small amount of air into the tube with a syringe while listening for a whooshing/gurgling sound with a stethoscope placed on the neonate's abdomen.
4. Use tape to ensure that the tube is secured.

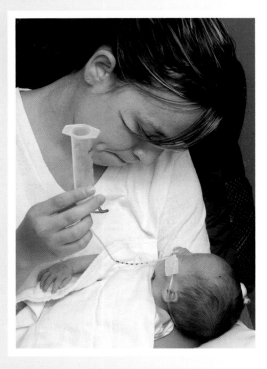

5. Check for residuals before starting the feeding by aspirating stomach contents with the syringe. Note the amount, color, and consistency of the contents.
6. Feedings may be given by gravity or pump over 15–30 minutes.
7. In some cases continuous tube feedings may be ordered.
8. To remove the tube after the feeding, pinch it closed and remove it swiftly.
9. Assess the neonate for feeding intolerance throughout feeding.

(Ditzenberger, 2010)

- *Use nonpharmacological interventions such as swaddling, positioning, kangaroo care, and therapeutic touch, and decrease environmental stimulus.*
- *Evaluate the effectiveness of nonpharmacological and pharmacological interventions.*

Evidence-Based Practice: Sucrose for Analgesia

Hatfield, L., Chang, K., Bittle, M., Deluca, J., & Polomano, R. (2011). The Analgesic Properties of Intraoral Sucrose. *An Integrative Review.*

An integrative review of published randomized control trials was conducted to determine the effective use of oral sucrose as a preprocedural intervention for mild to moderate procedural pain in infants. Conclusion of the review indicates that oral sucrose is an effective, safe, and immediate-acting analgesic for reducing crying time and significantly decreases biobehavioral pain response following painful procedures.

■ Provide developmentally appropriate care to decrease stress and enhance neurodevelopment by:
  ■ *Maintaining a quiet setting to decrease negative physiological responses such as apnea and fluctuations in heart rate, blood pressure, and oxygen saturation*
  ■ *Keeping lighting dim and changing lighting in NICU to simulate night and day*
  ■ *Clustering nursing activities to provide for extended periods of sleep*
  ■ *Avoiding clustering painful interventions together*
  ■ *Providing care when the neonate is awake*
  ■ *Providing individualized care based on the neonate's responses and needs*
  ■ *Allowing a break in care/stimulation if neonate becomes stressed*
  ■ *Minimizing handling for neonates who are in an unstable condition*
  ■ *Positioning and swaddling*
    ■ Change the neonate's position slowly and gently.
    ■ Reposition every 2–3 hours. Assess the infant's response to repositioning.
    ■ Position neonate in the side lying or prone position (enhances oxygenation and gastric emptying).
    ■ The head of the bed may be elevated 15 degrees.
    ■ Swaddle in flexion with arms and hands placed toward the infant's midline.
    ■ Create a nest with blankets to enhance containment. Avoid swaddling or nesting that is overly restrictive to neonatal movement (Carrier, 2010; Goodwin, 2010; Charsha, 2010).
■ Encourage kangaroo care (skin-to-skin contact with the parents) for medically stable neonates. Benefits of kangaroo care are:
  ■ *Decreases risk of low body temperature.*
  ■ *Reduces illness, infection, and pain perception.*
  ■ *Improves daily weight gain and mother-infant attachment.*
  ■ *Decreases the length of hospital stay (Ludington-Hoe, 2011).*
■ Provide emotional support to parents and family members.
■ Involve parents and family in all aspects of the infant's care. This helps to decrease anxiety and fears, thus allowing for an increase in parent-infant bonding.
  ■ *Teach parents what to expect from their preterm infant and how to interpret behavioral cues.*
  ■ *Teach parents how to provide care for their infant (Fig. 17-4).*

  ■ *Encourage parent-infant bonding by welcoming parents to the NICU and praising them for their involvement with their infant.*
  ■ *Teach parents about the infant's condition and involve parents in the plan of care.*
■ Discharge teaching is essential for a safe transition from the NICU to home. Prepare the family for the neonate's discharge by:
  ■ *Teaching parents about infant feeding*
  ■ *Teaching about use of any equipment, such as apnea monitors that may be needed to care for their infant at home*
  ■ *Teaching parents how to perform treatments such as dressing changes, suctioning, and oxygen administration*
  ■ *Teaching parents about medication administration*
  ■ *Teaching parents about safety issues such as car seat use, and positioning the infant on his or her back during sleep*
  ■ *Encouraging parents to learn infant CPR*
  ■ *Teaching parents about basic newborn care*
  ■ *Educating parents on what to expect after discharge, such as sleep patterns, feeding, infant behavior, and developmental milestones*
  ■ *Discussing follow-up care such as physician's visits, immunization schedules, and appointments for developmental care*

Respiratory Distress Syndrome

Respiratory distress syndrome (RDS) is a life-threatening lung disorder that results from underdeveloped and small alveoli and insufficient levels of pulmonary surfactant. These two combined factors can cause an alteration in alveoli surface

AWHONN/NANN RBP4 NEONATAL SKIN CONDITION SCORE (NSCS)
Dryness
1 = Normal, no sign of dry skin 2 = Dry skin, visible scaling 3 = Very dry skin, cracking/fissures
Erythema
1 = No evidence of erythema 2 = Visible erythema, <50% body surface 3 = Visible erythema, ≥50% body surface
Breakdown/excoriation
1 = None evident 2 = Small, localized areas 3 = Extensive
Note: Perfect score = 3, worst score = 9
This scoring system, developed for the AWHONN/NANN Neonatal Skin Care Project (RBP4) was adapted from a visual scoring system used in a previous study (Lane and Drost, 1993). It can facilitate assessment of neonatal skin condition. This tool continues to undergo reliability and validity testing.

Figure 17-3 Neonatal Skin Condition Score.

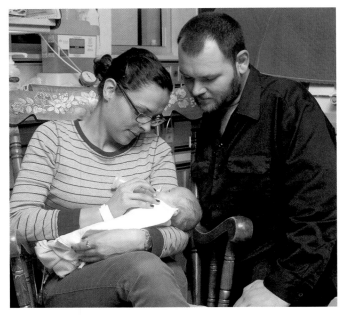

Figure 17–4 Parents bottle feeding their baby.

tension that eventually results in atelectasis. The effects of atelectasis are:

■ Hypoxemia and hypercarbia
■ Pulmonary artery vasoconstriction
■ Right-to-left shunting through the ductus arteriosus and foramen ovale as the neonate's body attempts to counteract the compromised pulmonary perfusion
■ Metabolic acidosis that occurs from a buildup of lactic acid that results from prolonged periods of hypoxemia
■ Respiratory acidosis that occurs from the collapsed alveoli being unable to rid the body of excess carbon dioxide

The incidence of RDS decreases with increasing gestational age. It affects 10% of all premature infants, the majority of these born at less than 28 weeks' gestation (Askin, 2010).

Pulmonary surfactant is a substance that is composed of 90% phospholipids and 10% proteins.

■ It is produced by type II alveolar cells within the lungs.
■ The alveolar cells begin to produce pulmonary surfactant around 24–28 weeks and continue to term.
■ It reduces the surface tension within the lungs and increases the pulmonary compliance which prevents the alveoli from collapsing at the end of expiration. Surfactant replacement therapy is discussed later in this chapter.

Tests used to evaluate fetal lung maturity are:

■ Phosphatidylglycerol (PG):
  ■ *PG is synthesized from mature lung alveolar cells.*
  ■ *It is present in the amniotic fluid within 2–6 weeks of full-term gestation.*
  ■ *The presence of PG indicates lung maturity and a decrease indicates risk of respiratory distress syndrome.*

■ Lecithin/sphingomyelin (L/S) ratio:
  ■ *Lecithin and sphingomyelin are two phospholipids that are detected in the amniotic fluid.*
  ■ *The ratio between the two phospholipids provides information on the level of surfactant.*
  ■ *A L/S ratio greater than 2:1 in a nondiabetic woman indicates the fetus's lungs are mature.*
  ■ *A L/S ratio of 3:1 in a diabetic woman indicates the fetus's lungs are mature.*

Complications of respiratory distress syndrome (RDS) include:

■ Patent ductus arteriosus
■ Pneumothorax
■ Bronchopulmonary hypertension
■ Pulmonary edema
■ Hypotension
■ Anemia
■ Oliguria
■ Hypoglycemia and altered calcium and sodium levels
■ Retinopathy of prematurity
■ Seizures
■ Intraventricular hemorrhage

Assessment Findings

■ Respiratory distress varies based on degree of prematurity.
■ Respiratory difficulty begins shortly after delivery and the neonate must work progressively harder at breathing to maintain open terminal airways (Askin, 2010).
■ Tachypnea is present.
■ Intercostal retractions; seesaw breathing patterns occur.
■ Expiratory grunting.
■ Nasal flaring is present.
■ Increased oxygen requirements are increased to maintain a PaO_2 and $PaCO_2$ within normal limits.
  ■ *The normal range of PaO_2 is 60–70 mm Hg.*
  ■ *The normal range of $PaCO_2$ is 35–45 mm Hg.*
■ Skin color is gray or dusky.
■ Breath sounds on auscultation are decreased. Rales are present as RDS progresses.
■ The neonate is lethargic and hypotonic.
■ X-ray exam shows a reticulogranular pattern of the peripheral lung fields and air bronchograms (Ghodrat, 2006).
■ Hypoxemia may occur (PaO_2 <50 mm Hg).
■ Acidosis may result from sustained hypoxemia.

Medical Management

■ Continuous pulse oximetry
■ Cardiac monitoring, oxygen saturation, arterial blood gases, and end CO_2
■ Endotracheal tube when clinically indicated
■ Exogenous surfactant as indicated for neonates at risk for RDS or with RDS (see Critical Component: Surfactant Replacement Therapy Administration)

■ Respiratory support as indicated. The mode of ventilation and settings are based on the neonate's condition and arterial blood gas results. Methods of respiratory support include:

■ *Oxygen therapy by mask, hood, or cannula for neonates requiring short-term oxygen support*

■ *Continuous positive airway pressure (CPAP) used for neonates who are at risk for RDS or with RDS. It can be administered by mask, nasal prongs, endotracheal tube, or nasopharyngeal route.*

■ *Mechanical ventilation used when CPAP is not effective (use judiciously to avoid damage to lung tissue)*

■ *High-frequency oscillatory ventilation used when mechanical ventilation has proven unsuccessful*

■ Delivers small volumes of gas at a high rate (>300 breaths/minute)

■ Less traumatic on fragile lung tissue

■ *Extracorporeal membrane oxygenation therapy (ECMO) is a cardiopulmonary bypass machine with a membrane oxygenator that is used when the neonate does not respond to conventional ventilator therapy. Blood shunts from the right atrium and is returned to the aorta, allowing time for the lungs to heal and mature.*

■ Diagnostic tests

■ *Chest x-ray exam to assist in evaluation of RDS*

■ Laboratory tests

■ *Arterial, venous, or capillary blood gases*

■ *Blood cultures if infection is suspected*

■ Medications

■ *Antibiotics as indicated*

Nursing Actions

Nursing actions for neonates with RDS are similar to actions for preterm neonates, with additional emphasis on the following:

■ Provide respiratory support.

■ *Maintain a patent airway.*

■ *Assess for correct placement of endotracheal tube.*

■ Listen for equal breath sounds bilaterally, assess for equal chest rise, use commercial end tidal CO_2 detector.

■ *Administer oxygen as ordered to maintain oxygen saturation within ordered parameters.*

■ Hypoxemia and acidosis may further decrease surfactant production.

■ Short-term oxygen administration may be given using a mask or tubing.

■ Long-term oxygen administration may be given using a nasal cannula or oxygen hood.

■ Oxygen is humidified and warmed.

■ *Warmed oxygen aids in thermoregulation for the infant.*

■ *Administer and monitor continuous positive airway pressure (CPAP), mechanical ventilation, high-frequency oscillatory ventilation, and/or ECMO as per order.*

■ *Minimize oxygen demand by maintaining a neutral thermal environment, clustering care to decrease stress, and treating acidosis as clinically indicated and ordered.*

■ *Suction airway as needed for removal of secretions as neonates have a smaller airway diameter, which increases the risk of obstruction.*

■ Suctioning may stimulate the vagus nerve, causing bradycardia, hypoxemia, or bronchospasm.

CRITICAL COMPONENT

Surfactant Replacement Therapy Administration

Natural Surfactant

■ Composed of calf, pig, or cow lung (minced) combined with lipids

■ Examples: Survanta, Curosurf, Infasurf

Synthetic Surfactant

■ Example: Exosurf

Action

■ Reduces surface tension of the alveoli, thus preventing collapse during expiration

■ Enhances lung compliance, allowing easier inflation, which decreases the work of breathing

Indications

■ Respiratory distress, meconium aspiration syndrome, persistent pulmonary hypertension

Route

■ Administered via endotracheal tube

Dosing Regimen (dose and technique vary by product)

■ Prophylaxis: Initiated within 15 minutes of birth, based on risk factors of RDS such as gestational age less than 27–30 weeks. Multiple doses can be given if indicated.

■ Rescue therapy: Treatment of confirmed RDS. Treatment is typically initiated within 8 hours of birth for infants who have increased oxygen demands and need mechanical ventilation.

Adverse Effects

■ Bradycardia, decreased oxygen saturation, tachycardia, reflux, gagging, cyanosis, blockage of the endotracheal tube, hypotension

Benefits of Surfactant Therapy

■ Prophylactic therapy decreases the occurrence of RDS and mortality in preterm neonates.

■ Decreased risk of pneumothorax

■ Decreased risk of intraventricular hemorrhage

■ Decreased risk of bronchopulmonary dysplasia

■ Decreased risk of pulmonary interstitial emphysema

(Askin, 2010; Young & Magnum, 2010)

■ Monitor vital signs, oxygen saturation, blood gases, and end CO_2 as per orders.

■ Maintain neutral thermal environment to decrease risk of cold stress.

   ■ *Cold stress increases oxygen consumption, may promote acidosis, and may further impair surfactant production.*

■ Monitor intake and output and daily weights.

   ■ *Dehydration impairs ability to clear airways because mucus becomes thickened.*

   ■ *Overhydration may contribute to alveolar infiltrates or pulmonary edema.*

   ■ *Weight loss and increased urine output may indicate diuretic phase of RDS.*

■ Promote rest by implementing calming measures or administering ordered sedation.

   ■ *Minimizing stimulation and energy expenditure reduces metabolic rate and oxygen consumption.*

Bronchopulmonary Dysplasia

Bronchopulmonary dysplasia (BPD) is a chronic lung problem that affects neonates who have been treated with mechanical ventilation and oxygen for problems such as RDS (see Critical Component: Bronchopulmonary Dysplasia). Neonates who are dependent on oxygen beyond 28 days of life and/or have been on mechanical ventilation are at risk for BPD. BPD leads to decreased lung compliance and pulmonary function secondary to fibrosis, atelectasis, increased pulmonary resistance, and overdistention of the lungs (Bancalari & Walsh, 2011; Askin, 2010) (**Fig. 17-5**). Pulmonary edema results from the increased pulmonary vascular resistance. The prognosis for infants with BPD is dependent on the severity of the disease and the infant's overall health status. Long-term outcomes may include prolonged hospitalization, long-term oxygen therapy that may be required after discharge, cerebral palsy, retinopathy of prematurity, and hearing loss. The mortality rate once discharged is less than 10% (Askin, 2010).

■ Risk factors for BPD

   ■ *Prematurity*

   ■ *RDS*

   ■ *Oxygen toxicity*

   ■ *Intubation*

   ■ *Assisted ventilation with positive pressure*

   ■ *Lower gestational age and birth weight (<32 weeks)*

   ■ *Infection*

   ■ *Pulmonary vascular damage secondary to excessive fluid administration, right-to-left shunting associated with*

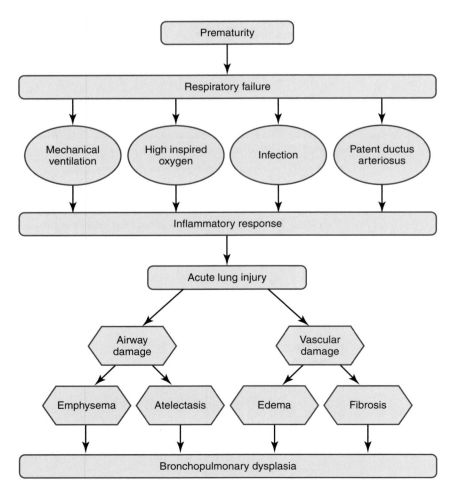

Figure 17–5 Bronchopulmonary dysplasia.

patent ductus arteriosus, and increased airway resistance (Bancalari & Walsh, 2011).
- Complications of BPD:
  - *Pneumonia, upper respiratory infection*
  - *Ear infections*
  - *Congestive heart failure*
  - *Developmental delays*
  - *Cerebral palsy*
  - *Hearing loss*
  - *Retinopathy of prematurity*
  - *Sudden death*

Assessment Findings

- Chest retractions
- Audible wheezing, rales, and rhonchi
- Hypoxia
- Respiratory acidosis
- Bronchospasm
- Difficulty weaning from ventilator or increased requirements for ventilator
- Intolerance to fluids: edema, decreased urinary output, and weight gain
- Chest x-ray exam results exhibit cardiomegaly, lung hyperinflation, and infiltrates (Askin, 2010).

Medical Management

- Diagnostic tests
  - *Chest x-ray exam to assess for cardiomegaly, lung hyperinflation, and infiltrates*
  - *Echocardiogram if cardiac complications are suspected*
- Laboratory tests
  - *Electrolytes*
  - *Arterial blood gases*
- Medications
  - *Bronchodilators: Administered to reduce bronchoconstriction*
  - *Corticosteroids: Administered to reduce bronchospasm, edema, and inflammation of pulmonary tissue*
  - *Diuretics: Administered to treat fluid retention and decrease risk for pulmonary edema*
- Prophylaxes against respiratory syncytial virus, as infants with BPD are predisposed to this infection
- Chest physiotherapy
- Respiratory assistance and oxygen therapy
- Monitor intake and output
- Determine the amount of fluid intake
- Determine the method of feeding to meet the neonate's nutritional and caloric needs

---

CRITICAL COMPONENT

Bronchopulmonary Dysplasia

Treatment for BPH is a regimen of support and time: time for the normal repair process within the lungs to improve functioning and time for the infant to grow and thrive.

Nursing Actions

Nursing actions for neonates with BPD are similar to actions for preterm neonates with additional emphasis on the following:

- Provide mechanical ventilation and oxygen administration as per orders.
  - *Gradually wean neonate from mechanical ventilation as per orders.*
- Provide chest physiotherapy as per order.
- Restrict fluid intake as per orders.
  - *Provide maximum calories with minimal fluid. Fortification of formula or breast milk may be needed to obtain optimal growth.*
    - Infants with BPD have a higher metabolic rate at rest (Bancalari & Walsh, 2011).
- Administer medications as per orders.
- Monitor intake and output.
  - *Infants with BPD are at risk for fluid overload and pulmonary edema.*

Patent Ductus Arteriosus

Patent ductus arteriosus (PDA) occurs when the ductus arteriosus remains open after birth (**Fig. 17-6**). Normally, the ductus arteriosus closes shortly after birth, but prematurity may lead to delayed closure. The incidence of PDA among term neonates is 1:2000 live births (Sadowski, 2010).

- Risk factors for PDA
  - *Prematurity. The occurrence of PDA is greater among neonates of lower gestational age and birth weight.*
    - 45% of neonates who weigh less than 1,750 grams
    - 80% of neonates who weigh less than 1,200 grams at birth (Sadowski, 2010)
- Complications
  - *Congestive heart failure in preterm neonates*
  - *Chronic lung disease*
  - *Renal failure*
  - *NEC*
  - *Intraventricular hemorrhage (Hammerman, Bin-Nun, & Kaplan, 2012)*

Assessment Findings

- Heart murmur heard at the upper left sternal border (some neonates with PDA may not have an audible murmur)
- Active precordium
- Widened pulse pressure with decreased diastolic blood pressure
- Tachycardia and tachypnea
- Recurrent apnea
- Increased work of breathing
- Bounding pulses
- Difficulty weaning from ventilator support
- Increased demand for oxygen or ventilation
- The presence of a patent ductus arteriosus confirmed by echocardiogram
- Chest x-ray exam may show increased pulmonary vasculature, pulmonary edema, and mild enlargement of the heart (Sadwoski, 2010).

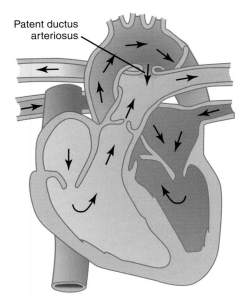

Patent ductus arteriosus

Figure 17–6 Patent ductus arteriosus.

Medical Management

■ Diagnostic tests
  ■ *Echocardiogram to assist in evaluation of PDA*
■ Medications
  ■ *Indomethacin, a prostaglandin inhibitor, is administered to facilitate the closure and reduces the risk for surgical intervention. It is also administered to decrease the risk of severe intraventricular hemorrhage (Johnston, Gilliam-Krakauer, Fuller, & Reese, 2012).*
  ■ *Diuretics*
■ Cardiology consultant to determine the method of treatment and need for surgical intervention
  ■ *Medical treatment may first be fluid restriction and diuretics.*
■ Surgical ligation (suture, clip, or coil) of PDA is indicated for neonates with a hemodynamically significant PDA who do not respond to medical management or indomethacin.

Nursing Actions

Nursing actions for neonates with PDA are similar to actions for preterm neonates with additional emphasis on the following:

■ Administer oxygen and mechanical ventilation as per orders.
■ Restrict fluids as per orders.
■ Administer medications as per orders.
■ Monitor intake and output for signs of fluid overload.
■ Prepare the neonate and family for surgery.

Periventricular–Intraventricular Hemorrhage

Periventricular/Intraventricular hemorrhages (PVH/IVH) are common forms of intracranial hemorrhage in the neonate. They occur among premature neonates, neonates who experience RDS, and those who experience complications associated with ventilation such as pneumothorax, hypercarbia, and acidosis (deVries, 2011).

PVH/IVH occurs in 30%–40% of infants weighing less than 1,500 grams and less than 32 weeks' gestation. Very few full-term neonates (2%–3%) have PVH/IVH (Lynam & Verklan, 2010). The majority of hemorrhages occur within the first week of life, with 90% occurring within 72 hours after birth (Lynam & Verklan, 2010; Malusky & Donze, 2012).

There are four grades of intraventricular hemorrhage based on the extent of involvement; the higher the grade, the higher the risk for long-term sequelae.

■ Grade I: Hemorrhage in germinal matrix
■ Grade II: Intraventricular hemorrhage without ventricular dilatation
■ Grade III: Intraventricular hemorrhage with ventricular dilatation; clots fill more than 50% of the ventricle
■ Grade IV: Extension of blood into cerebral tissue or parenchymal involvement
■ Risk factors for PVH/IVH:
  ■ *Prematurity, birth at less than 34 weeks' gestation*
  ■ *Amniotic fluid infection*
  ■ *Perinatal asphyxia*
  ■ *RDS, or respiratory failure necessitating ventilatory support*
  ■ *Increased arterial pressure*
  ■ *Low 5-minute Apgar score*
  ■ *Maternal general anesthesia*
  ■ *Low birth weight*
  ■ *Alteration of blood pressure, either hypotension or hypertension*
  ■ *Acidosis, hypercarbia*
  ■ *Low hematocrit*
  ■ *Pneumothorax (Lynam & Verklan, 2010)*
■ The long-term prognosis often depends on the severity of the hemorrhage and includes:
  ■ *A death rate of 5% for small hemorrhage, 15% for moderate hemorrhage, and 50% for severe hemorrhage*
  ■ *10% of neonates with a small hemorrhage, 40% with a moderate hemorrhage, and 80% with a severe hemorrhage will exhibit neurodevelopment problems such as cerebral palsy and delayed mental development.*
  ■ *Approximately 50% of premature infants do not experience neurological problems, and 25%–30% of very low birth weight neonates who had PVH/IVH do not exhibit neurodevelopment problems (Lynam & Verklan, 2010).*

Assessment Findings

■ Sudden change in condition
■ Bradycardia
■ Oxygen desaturation
■ Hypotonia
■ Metabolic acidosis
■ Shock
■ Decreased hematocrit
■ Full and/or tense anterior fontanel

■ Hyperglycemia (Lynam & Verklan, 2010)
■ Signs that bleeding is worsening include:
  ■ *Apnea*
  ■ *Increased need for ventilator support*
  ■ *Drop in blood pressure*
  ■ *Acidosis*
  ■ *Seizures*
  ■ *Full and tense fontanels and rapid increase in head size*
  ■ *Diminished activity or level of consciousness (Lynam & Verlan, 2010)*

Medical Management

■ Assessments for signs of hemodynamic, neurological, and behavior changes
■ Diagnostic tests
  ■ *Cranial ultrasounds for all high-risk neonates within the first week of life to assess for PVH/IVH*
  ■ *Lumbar puncture to assist in evaluation of PVH/IVH. Cerebrospinal fluid is analyzed for red blood cells, xanthochromia, decreased glucose, and increased protein (Lynam & Verklan, 2010).*
  ■ *Electroencephalogram (EEG) to evaluate seizure activity*
■ Laboratory tests
  ■ *Hemoglobin and hematocrit to evaluate extent of bleeding*
■ Blood transfusions as indicated

Nursing Actions

Nursing actions for neonates with PVN/IVH are similar to actions for preterm neonates, with additional emphasis on the following:

■ Assess for changes in vital signs, behavior, and neurological status, which may indicate increase intracranial bleeding.
■ Reduce stress to neonate by maintaining a quiet and dark environment.
■ Administer fluid volume replacement slowly to minimize fluctuation in blood pressure.

Evidence-Based Practice: Neutral Head Positioning to Prevent IVH

Malusky, S., & Donze, A. (2011). Neutral head positioning in premature infants for intraventricular hemorrhage prevention: An evidence-based review. *Neonatal Network, 30,* 381-396.

Shifts in cerebral perfusion have been linked to the development of IVH, and many seemingly benign care activities, such as head positioning, have been linked to changes in cerebral blood flow patterns. Articles reviewed examined the connection between the effects of head tilting on brain hemodynamics and changes in the infant's potential ability to autoregulate cerebral blood flow adequately.

Based on the physiological data and the views of experts in the field, implementing midline or neutral head positioning at a 30-degree elevation in the head of bed in infants less than 32 weeks' gestation for the first 72 hours of life is recommended to reduce the incidence of IVH.

Necrotizing Enterocolitis

Necrotizing enterocolitis (NEC) is a gastrointestinal disease that affects neonates. This disease results in inflammation and necrosis of the bowel, usually the proximal colon or terminal ileum (Bradshaw, 2010). Preterm neonates are predisposed to NEC because of multiple factors, including:

■ Altered blood flow regulation, particularly to the intestines
■ Impaired gastrointestinal host defense when faced with stress/injury to the intestinal tissue
■ Alterations in the inflammatory response (Caplan, 2011)

The majority (90%) of NEC cases are among preterm neonates; 5%–10% of cases occur in neonates who were born at 37 weeks or more gestation (Bradshaw, 2010). In term neonates NEC is usually associated with a particular problem (e.g., asphyxia, intrauterine growth restriction) resulting in an ischemic episode in the bowel (Caplan, 2011).

■ Causes of intestinal ischemia/asphyxia include:
  ■ *Hypotension*
  ■ *Hypoxia*
  ■ *Stress*
  ■ *Low body temperature*
  ■ *Hypovolemia*
  ■ *Polycythemia*
  ■ *Patent ductus arteriosus (Bradshaw, 2010).*
■ Risk factors for NEC
  ■ *Prematurity is the most common risk factor for NEC. Roughly 90% of cases occur among premature neonates.*
  ■ *Bacterial colonization can occur from contaminated nasogastric feeding tubes among premature neonates receiving formula.*
  ■ *Umbilical catheter placement (Bradshaw, 2010)*
■ Long-term outcomes include:
  ■ *Approximately 30% of neonates with NEC will die.*
  ■ *30% will have mild NEC and recover with medical management.*
  ■ *An estimated 25% of neonates with NEC will develop bowel obstruction.*
  ■ *Short bowel syndrome may occur in neonates who have had surgical treatment.*
  ■ *Neurodevelopmental problems such as cerebral palsy may develop (Caplan, 2011).*

Assessment Findings

Symptoms typically begin between 3 and 10 days after birth.

■ Apnea, bradycardia, and tachycardia
■ Respiratory failure
■ Hypoxemia
■ Unstable temperature
■ Hypotension, shock
■ Abdominal distention, bloody stools, abdominal tenderness, vomiting, increased gastric residuals, discoloration of abdomen, visible bowel loops
■ Lethargy
■ Abnormally high or low white blood cell count, thrombocytopenia

■ Abnormal electrolyte levels
■ Metabolic acidosis
■ Abdominal x-ray films of neonates with NEC may show distention of the intestines with gas; gas in one part of the intestine, and lack of gas in other parts; air in the wall of the intestine and/or the portal venous system; dilated loops of bowel; and air in abdomen (Bradshaw, 2010).

Medical Management

■ Diagnostic tests
  ■ *Abdominal x-ray exam to assist in evaluation of NEC*
■ Laboratory tests
  ■ *Blood cultures to assess for infection related to perforation of bowel*
■ Medications
  ■ *Antibiotics*
  ■ *Analgesia*
  ■ *Antihypertensives*
■ Discontinuation of feedings and starting gastric decompression
■ Intravenous fluids
■ Surgical intervention for the removal of necrotic bowel, resection of bowel, or for perforation of bowel related to NEC. A temporary colostomy may be performed.

Nursing Actions

Nursing actions for neonates with NEC are similar to actions for preterm neonates with additional emphasis on the following:

■ Assess for abdominal distention, visible bowel loops, emesis, and bloody stools.
  ■ *Early recognition and prompt treatment increase the chances for medical management.*
■ Withhold feedings as per orders and obtain intravenous access.
■ Perform gastric decompression as per orders by placing an orogastric tube and connecting it to low suction.
■ Monitor intake and output.
  ■ *Maintain circulating blood volume*
■ Prepare the neonate and family for surgery when indicated.

Retinopathy of Prematurity

Retinopathy of prematurity (ROP) occurs in premature neonates who are less than 28 weeks' gestation. Before this age, the retina is not completely vascularized and is susceptible to stress or injury (Phelps, 2011). If injury or exposure to a stressor occurs, the normal vascularization of the retina may be interrupted. Vasoproliferation, an abnormal growth of vasculature, occurs when tissue grows within the retina, or extends into the vitreous body. Ultimately, abnormal vascularization and associated bleeding, and fluid leakage, cause scar tissue that pulls and distorts the retina and displaces the macula (Phelps, 2011). It also causes retinal folds and can lead to retinal detachment (Phelps, 2011).

The incidence of ROP is related to gestational age and birth weight. ROP occurs primarily in neonates less than 28 weeks' gestation and in up to 82% of neonates weighing less than 1000 grams *(Askin & Deihl-Jones, 2010b)*. Long-term outcome for this disease depends on the extent of its progression, and ranges from full recovery to blindness (Phelps, 2011).

■ Risk factors for ROP
  ■ *Prematurity and low birth weight are primary problems associated with ROP; the risk of ROP increases as gestational age and birth weight decrease.*
  ■ *Prolonged hyperoxia (exposure to high levels of oxygen), and duration of mechanical ventilation*
  ■ *Hypoxia, hypercapnia, hypocapnia, and acidosis*
  ■ *Shock; vitamin E deficiency*
  ■ *Infection/sepsis*
  ■ *Patent ductus arteriosus*
  ■ *Multiple gestation*
  ■ *Intraventricular hemorrhage*
  ■ *Blood transfusion*
  ■ *Maternal diabetes, bleeding, smoking, and hypertension (Askin & Deihl-Jones, 2010b; Phelps, 2011)*

Manifestations of ROP are primarily observed during an eye examination performed by a pediatric ophthalmologist. The International Classification of Retinopathy of Prematurity provides a system of five stages to classify ROP based on the severity of the disease. Stage 4 is partial retinal detachment, and stage 5, the most severe, is complete retinal detachment. The progression of ROP is variable. An aggressive type of ROP, termed Rush disease, can manifest at 3–5 weeks post-delivery and progress quickly to complete detachment of the retina. In many cases, ROP evolves slowly and may take a year to become stable (Phelps, 2011).

■ Decreasing risk of ROP includes:
  ■ *Proper use of oxygen to maintain prescribed pulse oximetry parameters*
  ■ *Continuous monitoring and assessments of preterm neonates on continuous oxygen therapy*
  ■ *Careful use of oxygen during procedures such as suctioning*
  ■ *Use of equipment such as oxygen blenders to ensure the exact concentration of oxygen*
  ■ *Properly maintaining and calibrating oxygen systems (Askin & Diehl-Jones, 2010b)*
■ Long-term outcomes include:
  ■ *90% of neonates with ROP experience recovery with no or minimal loss of vision.*
  ■ *Treatment modalities such as cryotherapy and laser therapy have decreased the risk of complications leading to blindness.*
  ■ *Complications such as glaucoma, strabismus, cataracts, amblyopia, retinal detachment, and blindness may occur.*
  ■ *Corrective glasses may be needed to treat visual acuity deficits (Askin & Diehl-Jones, 2010b; Phelps, 2011).*

Assessment Findings

■ Retinal changes noted on ophthalmic examination

Medical Management

- Eye evaluation for possible ROP completed by the pediatric ophthalmologist for all neonates born before 29 weeks' gestation, or with a birth weight less than 1,500 grams at birth. Neonates who weigh between 1500 grams and 2000 grams at birth with medical complications should also receive an eye exam. The eye examination should occur at 4–6 weeks after birth (Phelps, 2011). Neonates with immature or abnormal vessel development should have repeated eye exams to monitor progression of the disease (Askin & Diehl-Jones, 2010b).
- Treatment for ROP is determined by the extent of abnormal vessel development and may include (Askin & Diehl-Jones, 2010b):
  - *Laser photocoagulation; laser is used to coagulate the avascular periphery of the retina to prevent vessel proliferation*
  - *Cryotherapy; a supercooled probe is used to prevent vessel proliferation by freezing the avascular retina.*
  - *Vitreoretinal surgery to reattach the retina if the retina becomes detached*

Nursing Actions

- Reduce the risk for ROP.
  - *Administer oxygen to maintain prescribed pulse oximetry parameters.*
  - *Use oxygen blenders and oxygen calibrating systems to ensure exact concentration of oxygen.*
  - *Avoid bright lights by keeping lighting in the nursery at a low level and by covering isolettes and cribs with blankets.*

Evidence-Based Practice: Risk Reduction of Retinopathy of Prematurity

Bellini, S. (2010). Retinopathy of prematurity. *Improving outcomes through evidence-based practice. Nursing for Women's Health, 14,* 382–389.

As ROP is a known cause of childhood blindness, it is critical that nurses working with premature infants understand current treatment and prevention. Retinopathy of prematurity is caused by high concentrations of oxygen therapy. Evidence-based practice guidelines pertain to the management of supplemental oxygen, specifically lower oxygen saturation ranges for premature infants. Oxygen saturation target ranges in the mid 80s to lower-mid 90s are safe and can reduce the severity of ROP in infants less than 32 weeks' gestation.

POSTMATURE NEONATES

A **post-term neonate** is a neonate who is delivered after the completion of 41 weeks' gestation. Postmaturity is related to a higher risk of morbidity and mortality (Furdon & Benjamin, 2010). The cause of postterm pregnancies is unknown. Placental insufficiency related to the aging of the placenta may result in **postmaturity syndrome,** in which the fetus begins to use its subcutaneous fat stores and glycemic stores (McGrath & Hardy, 2011). Placental function decreases, resulting in altered oxygenation and nutrient transport, which increases the risk for hypoxia and hypoglycemia at the onset of labor. If the placenta continues to function well after term, the result may be a newborn who is large for gestational age (LGA). The risk of **macrosomia,** or a birth weight above 4000 to 4500 grams, increases when pregnancy is prolonged.

- Risk factors
  - *Anencephaly*
  - *History of postterm pregnancies*
  - *First pregnancy*
  - *Grand multiparous women*
- Postmature neonates are at risk for:
  - *Meconium aspiration: The presence of meconium in the amniotic fluid related to fetal hypoxia places the neonate at risk for meconium aspiration syndrome (discussed later in this chapter).*
  - *Fetal hypoxia related to placental insufficiency and a decrease in amniotic fluid, which increases the risk of cord compression*
  - *Neurological complications such as seizures related to fetal asphyxia during labor and birth due to alteration in oxygenation*
  - *Hypoglycemia related to alteration in nutrient transport due to decreased placental functioning*
  - *Hypothermia related to:*
    - A lack of development of subcutaneous fat
    - Loss of subcutaneous fat related to insufficient nutrient transport through the placenta
  - *Polycythemia, a compensatory response, is caused by an alteration in oxygenation associated with placental insufficiency; hematocrit greater than 65% is considered polycythemia in a neonate (Diehl-Jones & Askin, 2010).*
  - *Birth trauma related to macrosomia*

Assessment Findings

- Dry, peeling, cracked skin
- Lack of vernix
- Profuse hair
- Long fingernails
- Thin, wasted appearance
- Meconium staining (green or yellow staining on the infant's skin, nail beds, or umbilical cord)
- Hypoglycemia
- Poor feeding behavior

Medical Management

- Oxygen therapy administered for perinatal depression or respiratory distress
- Hematocrit to assess for polycythemia
- Blood glucose monitoring for hypoglycemia

Nursing Actions

- Assess the prenatal record and intrapartum history, including Apgar scores, for risk factors.
- Assess the neonate for:
  - *Gestational age with use of gestational age scoring system*
  - *Birth trauma if neonate is macrosomic*

- *Respiratory distress (e.g., grunting, nasal flaring, chest retractions, tachypnea)*
- *Cyanosis*
- *Oxygen saturation if respiratory distress or cyanosis is present*
- *Signs of meconium staining*
- *Blood glucose levels*
- *Vital signs*
- *Weight*
- *Gross anomalies*
- Monitor for signs of hypoglycemia.
  - *Jitteriness, irritability, poor feeding, apnea, grunting, lethargy*
- Provide early and frequent feedings if respiratory status is stable.
  - *Early and frequent feedings reduce the risk of hypoglycemia.*
- Monitor intake and output.
  - *Postterm infants may be poor feeders and thus are at risk for inadequate fluid intake*

MECONIUM ASPIRATION SYNDROME

Meconium aspiration syndrome (MAS) is a cause of respiratory failure in term and postterm neonates. The fetus may pass meconium stool into the amniotic fluid. This occurs when there is a relaxation of the fetal anal sphincter, usually due to fetal asphyxia in utero, but can also occur with breech presentations and in cephalic presentations without evidence of asphyxia (Blackburn, 2013). Meconium is released into the amniotic fluid in roughly 4%–14% of deliveries and in about 5%–11% of these cases, meconium aspiration syndrome occurs (Blackburn, 2013; Askin, 2010).

There is a risk that the fetus can aspirate the meconium-stained fluid at the time of delivery. The presence of meconium fluid in the neonate's lungs can cause a partial obstruction of the lower airways that leads to a trapping of air and a hyperinflation of the airway distal to the obstruction, causing uneven ventilation (Blackburn, 2013). The presence of meconium in the lungs can also cause a chemical pneumonitis and inhibit surfactant action (Blackburn, 2013). These changes place the neonate at risk for atelectasis.

- Complications related to meconium aspiration:
  - *Obstruction of the airway*
  - *Hyperinflation of the alveoli due to the trapping of air*
  - *Chemical pneumonia*
  - *Decreased surfactant proteins*
  - *Hemorrhagic pulmonary edema that interferes with surfactant production (Askin, 2010).*

Assessment Findings

- Meconium-stained amniotic fluid
- Meconium visualized below the vocal cords
- Greenish or yellowish discoloration of the skin, nail beds, and umbilical cord

- Respiratory depression at the time of birth or within a few hours after birth
- Low Apgar scores
- Need for resuscitation after delivery due to perinatal depression
- Signs of respiratory distress such as nasal flaring, grunting, chest retractions
- Chest may appear barrel shaped and overdistended.
- The expiration phase of breathing may be extended.
- Diminished air movement, and the presence of rales and rhonchi assessed on auscultation
- Atelectasis and hyperinflated areas through the lungs noted on chest x-ray film
- Arterial blood gas findings may include low PaO_2 despite administration of 100% oxygen, and respiratory and metabolic acidosis in serious cases *(Askin, 2010).*

Medical Management

- Suctioning of the oropharynx and the nasopharynx to remove meconium immediately after the delivery of the neonate's head and before the first breath is a common practice. Evidence does not support this practice as effective in preventing meconium aspiration (Blackburn, 2013).
- Direct tracheal suctioning using a tracheal tube in cases in which the infant has a heart rate less than 100 beats per minute, absent respirations, or poor muscle tone
- Arterial blood gases to determine respiratory status and to guide treatment *(Askin, 2010).*
- Chest x-ray exam
- Blood glucose monitoring
- Oxygen with or without assisted ventilation depending on the neonate's condition.
- Surfactant therapy to decrease risk of need for ECMO (Dargaville, Copnell, Mills, & Haron, 2011).
- Sedatives or paralytic agents to relax neonates who are receiving ventilation *(Askin, 2010).*
- Antibiotics to treat pneumonia

Nursing Actions

- Assist with suctioning and resuscitation at the time of delivery.
- Perform a physical assessment to evaluate neonate for:
  - *Respiratory distress*
  - *Cyanosis*
  - *Complications of meconium aspiration syndrome, such as acidosis, hypoglycemia, hypocalcemia, pneumonia, pneumothorax, bronchopulmonary dysplasia, and persistent pulmonary hypertension*
  - *Neurological problems secondary to asphyxia (Askin, 2010).*
- Administer oxygen and/or assisted ventilation as per order.
- Monitor blood glucose as per order.
  - *Complication of respiratory distress is an increased metabolic rate and thus a higher incidence of hypoglycemia.*
- Manage ECMO as per order.

PERSISTENT PULMONARY HYPERTENSION OF THE NEWBORN

Normally after birth there is relaxation of the pulmonary vascular bed, allowing blood circulation to the lungs. **Persistent pulmonary hypertension (PPHN)** results when the normal vasodilation and relaxation of the pulmonary vascular bed do not occur. This leads to elevated pulmonary vascular resistance, right ventricular hypertension, and right-to-left shunting of blood through the foramen ovale and ductus arteriosus (Askin, 2010). PPHN is predominantly a problem among term or near-term neonates who experience hypoxia/asphyxia, RDS, meconium aspiration, sepsis, or congenital lung anomalies such as diaphragmatic hernia (Steinhorn, 2011). Even after the precipitating factor is treated, vasoconstriction and increased vascular resistance may persist, causing decreased pulmonary blood circulation, hypoxemia, lactic acidosis, and acidemia (Askin, 2010).

- Risk factors for PPHN
  - *Hypoxia and asphyxia are the most common risk factors for PPHN.*
  - *RDS, meconium aspiration, pneumonia*
  - *Bacterial sepsis*
  - *Delayed circulatory transition at birth caused by factors such as delayed resuscitation, central nervous system depression, hypothermia*
  - *Hypothermia or hypoglycemia leading to acidosis*
  - *Polycythemia or hyperviscosity of the blood, which could cause blockages in the pulmonary vascular bed*
  - *Prenatal pulmonary hypertension associated with premature closure of the ductus arteriosus, or fetal systemic hypertension*
  - *Underdevelopment of pulmonary vessels associated with congenital anomalies of the lung or heart*
  - *Abnormal development of pulmonary vessels associated with intrauterine asphyxia or intrauterine meconium aspiration, which leads to increased muscularization of pulmonary vessels that causes increased vascular resistance (Askin, 2010)*

Assessment Findings

- Term or near-term neonate
- Low Apgar scores
- Symptoms evident within 12 hours of birth
- Hypoxia and/or asphyxia at the time of birth
- Neonate depressed at birth, slow to breathe, difficulty with administering ventilation
- Tachypnea
- Chest retractions, grunting
- Low PaO_2, even with administration of high levels of oxygen
- Cyanosis
- Hypotension
- Heart murmur
- Pulmonary disorders such as air leaks, and bronchopulmonary dysplasia are possible complications of PPHN.

- Echocardiogram shows pulmonary hypertension, and enlarged right side of the heart.
- Congestive heart failure may occur.
- Hypoglycemia, hypocalcemia
- Metabolic acidosis
- Possible kidney damage, leading to decreased urine output, proteinuria, and hematuria
- Liver damage that may lead to blood clotting problems
- Hematological problems such as hemorrhage, disseminated intravascular coagulation (DIC), and thrombocytopenia may occur as complications of PPHN.
- Long-term outcomes after PPHN include:
  - *Hearing loss (sensorineural)*
  - *Neurological deficits*
  - *Chronic lung disease*
  - *Death (Askin, 2010)*

Medical Management

- Rapid and efficient resuscitation at birth to prevent hypoxia and acidosis
- Treat acidosis if present.
- Preductal and postductal blood gas to distinguish structural heart problems from PPHN.
  - *Right to left shunting is suspected when there is a difference of 10 mm Hg or more between the preductal and postductal PaO_2 (Askin, 2010).*
- Chest x-ray
- Echocardiogram to evaluate for cardiac anomalies, right to left shunting of blood, pulmonary resistance, and pulmonary artery pressures.
- Oxygen and conventional mechanical ventilation
  - *Hyperoxygenation is often used to keep PaO_2 levels above 90 mm Hg, and hyperventilation is used to keep $PaCO_2$ levels in the low normal range, to prevent acidosis, and promote decreased pulmonary artery pressure. Hyperventilation causes alkalosis, which has been found to lower pulmonary resistance (Askin, 2010).*
  - *If conventional mechanical ventilation is ineffective, high-frequency oscillatory ventilation may be instituted.*
  - *ECMO if other treatments are not effective*
- Intravenous fluids
- Laboratory tests (complete blood count, glucose, electrolytes, calcium, arterial blood gases, blood cultures)
- Umbilical catheter for arterial and venous pressure monitoring, blood gas monitoring, and to administer vasopressors as indicated
- Transcutaneous pulse oximetry monitoring
- Surfactant therapy
- Nitric oxide therapy
  - *Nitric oxide induces vasodilation and reduces pulmonary resistance.*
  - *Use of nitric oxide has reduced the percentage of neonates with PPHN being placed on ECMO.*
- Medications
  - *Vasopressors, such as dopamine and nitroprusside, to decrease right to left shunting by maintaining systemic vascular pressure above pulmonary vascular pressure*

■ *Vasodilators, such as prostaglandins and isoproterenol, to promote pulmonary artery dilation*
■ *Muscle relaxants, such as Pavulon, to induce paralysis among neonates who resist ventilation*
■ *Sedatives and analgesics, such as morphine and Versed (midazolam)*
■ *Antibiotic therapy to decrease risk of and/or treat infection*

Nursing Actions

■ Review maternal prenatal, intrapartal, and neonatal histories.
■ Assess the neonate for respiratory distress, meconium aspiration, and clinical manifestations of PPHN.
■ Administer oxygen and mechanical ventilation as ordered.
■ Monitor vital signs and pulse oximetry.
■ Anticipate the placement of umbilical catheters.
　■ *Vasoconstriction makes peripheral intravenous access difficult.*
　■ *Arterial blood gases and lab values are easily accessed via an umbilical catheter, thus preventing the infant from receiving painful heelsticks and venipunctures.*
　■ *Multiple intravenous fluids and medications can be administered simultaneously via umbilical catheters.*
■ Administer IV fluids as per order.
■ Administer medications as per order.
■ Obtain and monitor results of laboratory tests.
　■ *Immediate intervention is required for abnormal lab results.*
■ Keep handling, treatments, suctioning, and stimulation to a minimum, as these can result in decreased PaO_2 levels, and vasoconstriction.
■ Provide emotional support for parents, incorporate them in care of their infant, and keep them informed of their infant's condition.

SMALL FOR GESTATIONAL AGE AND INTRAUTERINE GROWTH RESTRICTION

A **small for gestational age (SGA)** infant is one whose weight is less than the 10th percentile for his or her gestational age. Neonates whose growth is not consistent with gestational age may be affected by **intrauterine growth restriction (IUGR)**. IUGR is due to a decrease in cell production related to chronic malnutrition. There are two types of IUGR:

■ **Symmetric IUGR,** a generalized proportional reduction in the size of all structures and organs except for heart and brain, is the result of a condition that occurs early in pregnancy and affects general growth. When a complication occurs very early in pregnancy, fewer cells develop, leading to smaller organ size (Furdon & Benjamin, 2010).
　■ *Conditions that may result in symmetric IUGR include exposure to teratogenic substances, congenital infections, and genetic problems (Furdon & Benjamin, 2010).*
　■ *Symmetric IUGR can be identified by ultrasound in the early part of the second trimester.*

■ **Asymmetric IUGR,** a disproportional reduction in the size of structures and organs, results from maternal or placental conditions that occur later in pregnancy and impede placental blood flow.
　■ *Examples of conditions that may result in asymmetric IUGR include preeclampsia, placental infarcts, or severe maternal malnutrition (Furdon & Benjamin, 2010).*
■ Risk factors
　■ *Include maternal, fetal, and placental factors* (**Table 17–3**).
■ Neonates with IUGR are at risk for:
　■ *Labor intolerance related to placental insufficiency and inadequate nutritional and oxygen reserves*
　■ *Meconium aspiration related to asphyxia during labor (Askin, 2010)*
　■ *Hypoglycemia related to inadequate glycogen stores and reduced gluconeogenesis, and an increase in metabolic demands from heat loss which diminishes glucose stores (Armentrout, 2010)*
　■ *Hypocalcemia, defined as serum calcium levels less than 7.5 mg/dL, related to birth asphyxia (Halbardier, 2010)*
　　■ Signs of hypocalcemia are often similar to those of hypoglycemia and include jitteriness, tetany, and seizures.

Assessment Findings

■ Physical characteristics of the IUGR neonate include:
　■ *Large head in relationship to the body*
　■ *Long nails*
　■ *Large anterior fontanel*
　■ *Decreased amounts of Wharton's jelly present in the umbilical cord*
　■ *Thin extremities and trunk*
　■ *Loose skin due to a lack of subcutaneous fat*
　■ *Skin that may be dry, flaky, and meconium stained*
■ Weight, head circumference, and length are all below the 10th percentile for gestational age in symmetric IUGR (Furdon & Benjamin, 2010).
■ Head circumference and length are appropriate for gestational age; however, the weight is below the 10th percentile for the baby's gestational age in asymmetric IUGR (Furdon & Benjamin, 2010).
■ RDS may occur in SGA neonates who are born prematurely or have aspirated meconium-stained amniotic fluid (Askin, 2010).
■ Hypothermia related to decreased subcutaneous fat and glucose supply, impaired lipid metabolism, and depleted brown fat stores (Furdon & Benjamin, 2010).
■ Polycythemia

Medical Management

■ Identify IUGR during pregnancy and intervene based on the cause.
■ Assessments for congenital anomalies
■ Oxygen therapy for perinatal depression and respiratory distress
■ Laboratory tests
　■ *Blood glucose monitoring*
　■ *Hematocrit if polycythemia is suspected*
　■ *Serum calcium levels*

TABLE 17–3 FACTORS CONTRIBUTING TO INTRAUTERINE GROWTH RESTRICTION

MATERNAL	FETAL	PLACENTAL	ENVIRONMENTAL
Multiple gestation	Female sex	Small placenta	High altitude
Primiparity	Discordant twins	Abnormal cord insertion	Excessive exercise
Grand multiparity	Congenital anomalies	Placenta previa	Exposure to x-ray
Age <15 years	Chromosomal syndromes	Chronic abruptio placenta	Exposure to toxins
Age >45 years	Congenital infections	Placental hemangiomas	
No prenatal care	Rubella		
Low socioeconomic status	Toxoplasmosis		
Nutritional status	Cytomegalovirus		
Low pre-pregnancy weight	Inborn errors of metabolism		
Low weight gain			
Substance abuse			
Smoking			
Vascular disease			
Renal disease			
Cardiac disease			
Preeclampsia			
Chronic hypertension			
Advanced diabetes			
Sickle cell anemia			
Phenylketonuria			
Medications			
Anticonvulsants			
History of stillbirth			
History of preterm birth			
History of IUGR/LBW baby			
Maternal short stature			

McGrath & Hardy (2011).

Nursing Actions

- Review prenatal and intrapartal records for risk factors.
- Perform a gestational age assessment.
  - *To determine if SGA or preterm*
- Assess for respiratory distress.
- Assess the neonate for gross anomalies.
- Assess the skin for color and signs of meconium staining.
  - *Infants with meconium staining have an increased risk of respiratory distress.*
- Maintain a neutral thermal environment.
  - *SGA infants have decreased subcutaneous fat and are thus are more susceptible to hypothermia.*
- Decrease risk of hypoglycemia.
  - *SGA infants are at high risk for hypoglycemia due to their decreased amount of subcutaneous fat and thus their increased chance of cold stress.*

- *Assess for signs of hypoglycemia.*
- *Monitor blood glucose.*
- *Provide early and frequent feedings.*
  - SGA infants may need gavage feedings due to poor suck or inability to finish feedings due to lack of stamina.
- Monitor for hypocalcemia.
- Daily weights.
  - *SGA infants may require higher caloric intake.*
- Monitor vital signs.
- Monitor for feeding intolerance.
  - *SGA infants are susceptible to NEC due to placental insufficiency.*
- Obtain laboratory tests as per orders.
- Teach parents the importance of keeping the baby warm and providing frequent feedings.

LARGE FOR GESTATIONAL AGE

A large for gestational age (LGA) infant is a neonate whose weight is above the 90th percentile for his or her gestational age. Characteristically LGA infants are macrosomic and have greater body length and head circumference compared to infants who are appropriate for gestational age (AGA) (**Fig. 17-7**).

- Risk factors for LGA
  - *Maternal diabetes*
  - *Multiparity*
  - *Previous macrosomic baby*
  - *Prolonged pregnancy (McGrath & Hardy, 2011).*
- LGA fetuses and neonates are at risk for:
  - *Cesarean births*
  - *Operative vaginal delivery*
  - *Shoulder dystocia*
  - *Breech presentation*
  - *Birth trauma*
  - *Cephalopelvic disproportion*
  - *Hypoglycemia*
  - *Hyperbilirubinemia*

Assessment Findings

- Birth trauma related to shoulder dystocia or breech presentation. These birth traumas include:
  - *Fractured clavicle*
  - *Brachial nerve damage*
  - *Facial nerve damage*
  - *Depressed skull fractures*
  - *Cephalohematoma*
  - *Intracranial hemorrhage*
  - *Asphyxia (McGrath & Hardy, 2011).*
- Poor feeding behavior
- Hypoglycemia
- Polycythemia in neonates of diabetic mothers related to a decrease in extracellular fluid and/or fetal hypoxia

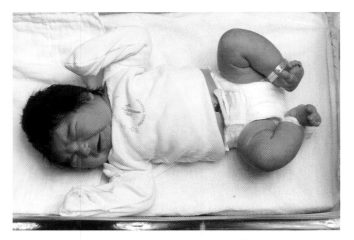

Figure 17–7 Large for gestational age (LGA) neonate.

- Hyperbilirubinemia that occurs 48–72 hours after delivery related to polycythemia, decreased extracellular fluid, or bruising or hemorrhage from birth trauma

Medical Management

- Assessments for birth trauma, hypoglycemia, and respiratory distress
- Laboratory tests:
  - *Blood glucose*
  - *Hematocrit*
  - *Bilirubin levels when indicated for jaundice*

Nursing Actions

- Review prenatal and intrapartal records for risk factors.
- Assess respiratory status.
- Assess neonates for birth traumas such as fractured clavicles, brachial nerve damage, facial nerve damage, and cephalohematoma.
- Obtain and monitor blood glucose per agency protocol.
- Observe for signs of hypoglycemia.
  - *LGA infants are at increased risk for hypoglycemia due to depletion of glycogen stores.*
- Provide frequent feedings to decrease risk for hypoglycemia.
  - *LGA infant may feed poorly and require gavage feedings.*
- Obtain and monitor hematocrit as per orders.
  - *High hematocrit increases the risk for jaundice.*
- Assess skin color for signs of polycythemia, which appears as a red, ruddy skin color.
  - *Infants of diabetic mothers are at risk for polycythemia.*
- Perform a gestational age assessment.
- Observe for jaundice.
  - *LGA infants are at higher risk for jaundice due to polycythemia.*

HYPERBILIRUBINEMIA

Hyperbilirubinemia, high levels of bilirubin in the blood, is common among neonates *(McGrath & Hardy, 2011).* When serum bilirubin levels are greater than 5 mg/dL, neonates will exhibit visible signs of jaundice (Schwartz, Haberman, & Ruddy, 2011). The clinical significance of jaundice is based on the age of the neonate in hours and the total serum bilirubin level (Bradshaw, 2010). Prematurity may result in greater severity of physiological jaundice, and any jaundice among preterm neonates must be evaluated.

A complication of hyperbilirubinemia is kernicterus. **Kernicterus** is an abnormal accumulation of unconjugated bilirubin in the brain cells. Bilirubin accumulates within the brain and becomes toxic to the brain tissue, which causes neurological disorders such as deafness, delayed motor skills, hypotonia, and intellectual deficits (Kaplan, Wong, Sibley, & Stevenson, 2011). A goal of medical and nursing actions is to prevent kernicterus through early identification and treatment of hyperbilirubinemia.

Hyperbilirubinemia is categorized into physiological jaundice and pathological jaundice.

Physiological Jaundice

Physiological jaundice results from hyperbilirubinemia that commonly occurs after the first 24 hours of birth and during the first week of life (Schwartz, Haberman, & Ruddy, 2011). Common physiological characteristics of the neonate place the neonate at risk for physiological jaundice:

■ Neonates have an increased red blood cell volume.
■ Neonatal red blood cells have a life span of 70–90 days, compared to 120 days in adults.
■ Neonates produce more bilirubin (6–8 mg/kg/day) than adults.
■ Neonates reabsorb increased amounts of unconjugated bilirubin in the intestine due to lack of intestinal bacteria, decreased gastrointestinal motility, and increased β-glucuronidase (a deconjugating enzyme).
■ Neonates have a decreased hepatic uptake of bilirubin from the plasma due to a deficiency of ligandin, the primary bilirubin binding protein in hepatocytes.
■ Neonates have a diminished conjugation of bilirubin in the liver due to decreased glucuronyl transferase activity (Bradshaw, 2010).

Risk Factors for Physiological Jaundice

■ Asian, Native American, and Greek ethnicity
■ Fetal hypoxia
■ ABO incompatibility (the woman is blood type O and the neonate is blood type A or B)
■ Rh incompatibility (the woman is Rh negative and the neonate is Rh positive)
■ Use of oxytocin during labor
■ Delayed cord clamping, which increases red blood cell volume
■ Breastfeeding (**Table 17-4**)
■ Delayed feedings, caloric deprivation, or large weight loss
■ Bruising or cephalohematoma
■ Gestational age of 35–38 weeks
■ Maternal diabetes with macrosomia
■ Epidural bupivacaine
■ Asphyxia
■ Older sibling with jaundice

Assessment Findings

■ Physiological jaundice is typically visible after 24 hours of life (Schwartz, Haberman, & Ruddy, 2011)
■ Jaundice is characterized by a yellowish tint to the skin and sclera of the eyes.
  ■ *As total serum bilirubin levels rise, jaundice will progress from the newborn's head downward toward the trunk and lower extremities.*
■ Mean peak total serum bilirubin level is 5–6 mg/dL of full-term neonates between 48 and 120 hours of life among white and African American neonates, and 10–14 mg/dL between 72 and 120 hours among Asian American newborns (Kaplan, Wong, Sibley, & Stevenson, 2011).
■ Declines to 3 mg/dL by the 5th day of life for white and African American babies, and by 7–10 days of life for Asian American neonates (Kaplan, Wong, Sibley, & Stevenson, 2011).

Pathological Jaundice

Pathological jaundice results when various disorders exacerbate physiological processes that lead to hyperbilirubinemia of the newborn. Such disorders can result in pathological unconjugated or conjugated hyperbilirubinemia (**Table 17-5**).

Assessment Findings

■ Jaundice that occurs within the first 24 hours of life
■ Total serum bilirubin levels above 12.9 mg/dL in a term neonate or 15 mg/dL in a preterm baby (Kaplan, Wong, Sibley, & Stevenson, 2011).
■ Total serum bilirubin levels that increase by more than 5 mg/dL per day (Kaplan, Wong, Sibley, & Stevenson, 2011)
■ Jaundice lasting more than 1 week in a term newborn, or more than 2 weeks in a premature neonate (Kaplan, Wong, Sibley, & Stevenson, 2011)

TABLE 17–4 HYPERBILIRUBINEMIA ASSOCIATED WITH BREASTFEEDING: A COMPARISON OF BREASTFEEDING VERSUS BREAST MILK JAUNDICE	
BREASTFEEDING JAUNDICE	**BREAST MILK JAUNDICE**
Early onset of jaundice (within the first few days of life)	Late onset (after 3–5 days)
Associated with ineffective breastfeeding	Gradual increase in bilirubin that peaks at 2 weeks of age
Dehydration can occur.	Associated with breast milk composition in some women that increases the enterohepatic circulation of bilirubin
Delayed passage of meconium stool promotes reabsorption of bilirubin in the gut.	Treatment: Continued breastfeeding in most infants. In some cases where bilirubin levels are excessively high, breastfeeding may be interrupted and formula feedings are given for several days. This typically results in a decline of the bilirubin level. Breastfeeding is resumed when bilirubin levels decline.
Treatment: Encourage early effective breastfeeding without supplementation of glucose water or other fluids.	
Blackburn (2013).	

TABLE 17–5   CAUSES OF PATHOLOGICAL HYPERBILIRUBINEMIA

CAUSES OF PATHOLOGICAL UNCONJUGATED HYPERBILIRUBINEMIA	CAUSES OF CONJUGATED HYPERBILIRUBINEMIA (ALWAYS PATHOLOGIC)
HEMOLYSIS OF RBCs	HEPATITIS
Rh/ABO incompatibilities	Neonatal idiopathic hepatitis
Bacterial and viral infections	Infectious hepatitis
Inherited disorders of red blood cell/bilirubin metabolism	Toxic hepatitis
	Intestinal obstruction
Glucose-6-phospate dehydrogenase deficiency	Ischemic necrosis
	Parenteral alimentation
SEQUESTERED BLOOD:	Metabolic disorders
Cephalohematoma	Hematological disorders
Bruising	Ductal disturbances in bilirubin excretion:
Hemangiomas	• Extrahepatic biliary atresia
Cerebral, pulmonary, retroperitoneal bleeding	• Intrahepatic biliary atresia
Decreased hepatic uptake of bilirubin	• Bile plug syndrome
Decreased hepatic function/perfusion	• Tumors of the liver and biliary tract
• Hypoxia	
• Asphyxia	
• Sepsis	
Increased enterohepatic circulation	
• Delayed feedings	
• Breastfeeding jaundice	
• Breast milk jaundice	
• Intestinal obstructions	
Polycythemia	
Swallowed blood	
Hypothyroidism	
Hypopituitarism	

Kaplan, Wong, Sibley, & Stevenson (2011).

Medical Management for Hyperbilirubinemia

- ■ Diagnostic tests
  - ■ *Total serum bilirubin, with fractionation of serum bilirubin into direct (conjugated bilirubin) and indirect (unconjugated bilirubin) reacting pigments (Kaplan, Wong, Sibley, & Stevenson, 2011).*
  - ■ *Antiglobulin (Coombs') test: Test used to determine hemolytic disease of the newborn related to Rh or ABO incompatibility*
    - ■ Direct antiglobulin (Coombs') test is used to detect abnormal in vivo coating of the neonate's red blood

cells with antibody globulin (maternal antibodies); when present, the test is considered positive.

- ■ *Transcutaneous bilirubinometry, a noninvasive method to estimate total serum bilirubin levels among term and near-term neonates, is used to identify neonates at risk for developing hyperbilirubinemia (McGrath & Hardy, 2011).*
- ■ *Complete blood count assists in management of pathological jaundice.*
- ■ Treatment is determined by the level of bilirubin and the age of the neonate in hours (**Table 17-6**).
- ■ Phototherapy
  - ■ *Phototherapy is the most widely used and effective treatment for hyperbilirubinemia.*
  - ■ *Various types of phototherapy delivery systems are available, including blue lights, white lamps, halogen lamps, fiberoptic blankets, and blue light emitting diodes (LED).*
    - ■ Evidence suggests that the most effective lights are those in the blue-green spectrum. (Schwartz, Haberman, & Ruddy, 2011).
  - ■ *Phototherapy results in photoconverting bilirubin molecules to water-soluble isomers that can be excreted in the urine and stool without conjugation in the liver (Swartz, Haberman, & Ruddy, 2011).*
  - ■ *Total serum bilirubin levels should drop 1–2 mg/dL within 4–6 hours after the initiation of phototherapy.*
  - ■ *Phototherapy should be administered continuously, except during feeding times or parental visits, when eye patches are removed to allow for bonding.*
- ■ Exchange transfusion is used in cases where phototherapy is not effective or severe hemolytic disease is present *(McGrath & Hardy, 2011).*
  - ■ *In this procedure, approximately 85% of the neonate's red blood cells are replaced with donor cells.*
  - ■ *This procedure reduces bilirubin, removes red blood cells coated with maternal antibody, corrects anemia, and removes other toxins associated with hemolysis (McGrath & Hardy, 2011).*
  - ■ *Efforts to prevent Rh hemolytic disease with Rh immunoglobulin (RhoGam) administered to Rh-negative women, and the use of phototherapy, have diminished the need for exchange transfusion (McGrath & Hardy, 2011).*

TABLE 17–6   MANAGEMENT OF HYPERBILIRUBINEMIA IN THE HEALTHY TERM AND NEAR-TERM NEONATE

AGE (HR)	CONSIDER PHOTOTHERAPY	PHOTOTHERAPY
≤24		
25–48	≥12	≥15
49–72	≥15	≥18
>72	≥17	≥20

American Academy of Pediatrics (2004).

■ Infants discharged before 72 hours of life should be seen for follow-up by a health care provider within 1–2 days to assess the neonate's health status and to assess for jaundice.
  ■ *Timely identification of significant hyperbilirubinemia is key to preventing acute bilirubin encephalopathy (Kaplan, Wong, Sibley, & Stevenson, 2011)*

Nursing Actions for Hyperbilirubinemia

■ Review maternal and neonatal record for risk factors.
■ Review laboratory findings, such as neonatal blood type; Rh factor; and indirect and direct Coombs'.
■ Assess degree of jaundice every shift with the use of a transcutaneous meter (McGrath & Hardy, 2011).
  ■ *When meter is not available, in a well-lit area, use your fingers to blanch the neonate's skin on the face, upper trunk, abdomen, thigh, and lower leg and feet. The skin will appear yellow after the pressure is released and before return of normal skin color.*
■ Document the assessment findings.
  ■ *How rapidly the degree of jaundice progresses guides the method of treatment*
■ Notify the physician if jaundice is present.
  ■ Prompt treatment is essential to preventing bilirubin toxicity.
■ Obtain serum bilirubin levels.
  ■ *The rate of rise of the bilirubin level is critical in determining the treatment needed.*
■ Ensure adequate hydration by feeding neonate every 2–3 hours to promote excretion of bilirubin in the urine and stool, and to compensate for insensible water loss due to phototherapy (McGrath & Hardy, 2011).
  ■ *Early feedings decrease the enterohepatic circulation of bilirubin, which decreases bilirubin levels (McGrath & Hardy, 2011).*
■ Implement phototherapy as ordered and provide related nursing care (see Critical Component: Care of the Neonate Receiving Phototherapy).
  ■ *Proper nursing care enhances the effectiveness of phototherapy and minimizes complications.*
■ Assess for side effects of phototherapy:
  ■ *Eye damage*
  ■ *Loose stools*
  ■ *Dehydration*
  ■ *Hyperthermia*
  ■ *Lethargy*
  ■ *Skin rashes*
  ■ *Abdominal distention*
  ■ *Hypocalcemia*
  ■ *Lactose intolerance*
  ■ *Thrombocytopenia*
  ■ *Bronze baby syndrome*
■ Provide verbal and written discharge instructions about how to identify signs of jaundice in an infant and when to notify the physician.
  ■ *For those infants discharged with mild jaundice, teaching should include measures to assess hydration, excretion of bilirubin, and home management of phototherapy lights if applicable.*

CRITICAL COMPONENT

Care of the Neonate Receiving Phototherapy

■ Fluorescent "bili lights" should be positioned 18–20 inches from the infant.
■ Fluorescent lights should be positioned 2 inches from the top of an incubator.
■ A photometer should be used to measure irradiance of lamps to facilitate optimal treatment.
■ Banks of lights should be covered by Plexiglas.
■ The neonate should be placed under lights with only a diaper in place, for maximal exposure to light.
■ Eye patches are placed on infant to protect eyes from the effects of the light.
■ During feedings, eye patches are removed and the neonate should be held by a parent or the nurse.
■ Change the neonate's position frequently to facilitate increased exposure to the light.
■ Vital signs including temperature monitoring should be done per agency protocol.
■ Monitor intake and output. Phototherapy results in increased insensible fluid loss.
■ Feedings every 2–3 hours are important to provide adequate fluids to compensate for insensible fluid loss, and promote excretion of bilirubin.
■ Monitor newborn for side effects of phototherapy.

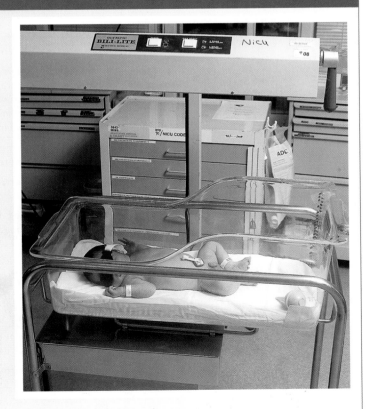

(McGrath & Hardy, 2011)

CENTRAL NERVOUS SYSTEM INJURIES

Various types of central nervous system (CNS) injuries can occur among term and premature neonates. Injury can be the result of intracranial hemorrhage (**Table 17-7**); hypoxia and ischemia during the prenatal and intrapartal periods, and post-birth; systemic chronic fetal compromise such as IUGR; or hypotension that leads to a decreased cerebral perfusion resulting in preventricular leukomalacia (**Table 17-8**).

Depending on the extent and location of the injury, CNS injuries may result in normal outcomes or serious long-term problems such as seizures, neurological deficits, developmental disability, motor deficits, visual impairments, or death (Lynam & Verklan, 2010).

■ Risk factors for CNS injuries
   ■ *Prematurity*
■ *Birth trauma*
■ *Breech delivery or other malpresentations*
■ *Precipitous labor*
■ *Difficult labor, traumatic delivery, and use of forceps*
■ *Hypoxia, asphyxia, hypotension, ischemia, respiratory distress. Hypoxic events may be related to:*
   ■ Maternal causes such as cardiac arrest and hypovolemic shock
   ■ Uteroplacental causes such as placental abruption, cord prolapse, and uterine hyperstimulation
   ■ Fetal causes such as cardiac arrhythmia (Levene & de Vries, 2011)

Assessment Findings

■ Clinical manifestations are specific to the type and extent of the CNS injury (see Tables 17-7 and 17-8).

TABLE 17–7   TYPES OF CENTRAL NERVOUS SYSTEM INJURIES: HEMORRHAGES

	SUBDURAL HEMORRHAGE	SUBARACHNOID HEMORRHAGE	INTRACEREBELLAR HEMORRHAGE
DEFINITION	Tear of the dura overlying the cerebellum or cerebral hemispheres.	Intracranial hemorrhage into the cerebrospinal fluid filled space between the pial and arachnoid membranes on the surface of the brain. Most common neonatal intracranial hemorrhage.	Hemorrhage in the cerebellum from primary bleeding or from extension of intraventricular or subarachnoid hemorrhage into the cerebellum. Occurs more commonly in preterm, low birth weight neonates.
PATHOPHYSIOLOGY	Excessive molding, stretching, or tearing of the falx and tentorium. Stretching or tearing of the vein of Galen or cerebellar bridging veins	May occur because of trauma in a term neonate or hypoxia in a preterm neonate. Venous bleeding in the subarachnoid space related to ruptured small vessels in the leptomeningeal plexus or bridging veins in the subarachnoid space.	Breech presentation, difficult forceps delivery, external pressure over the occiput. History of a hypoxic–ischemic insult. Vitamin K deficiency. Vascular factors.
MANIFESTATIONS	Symptoms may be delayed for first 24 hours, then: Seizures Decreased level of consciousness Asymmetrical motor function Full fontanel Irritability Lethargy Respiratory abnormalities Facial paralysis	Commonly there are no symptoms. Seizures may occur, starting on day 2 of life. Apnea may occur in preterm neonates.	Manifestations occur within the first 2 days to 3 weeks of life. Apnea Bradycardia Decreasing hematocrit. Bloody cerebrospinal fluid
PROGNOSIS	Hydrocephalus Mortality rate 45% Hypoxic–ischemic injury	90% of babies with seizures will have normal follow-up. Abnormal outcome is rare.	Poorer outcome in preterm neonates than in term newborns. Neurological deficits probable.

Lynam & Verklan (2010).

TABLE 17–8   TYPES OF CENTRAL NERVOUS SYSTEM INJURY: HYPOXIC-ISCHEMIC ENCEPHALOPATHY

	HYPOXIC–ISCHEMIC ENCEPHALOPATHY	PERIVENTRICULAR LEUKOMALACIA
DEFINITION	Abnormal neonatal neurological behavior resulting from a hypoxic–ischemic event. Brain edema and massive cellular necrosis. Intraventricular, subdural, or intracerebral hemorrhage.	Necrosis of periventricular white matter resulting from ischemia. Ischemic lesion of arterial origin. Multicystic encephalomalacia with/without hemorrhage into ischemic area.
RISK FACTORS	Hypoxia, anoxia, decreased blood supply to the brain (ischemia). Acute birth asphyxia (e.g., cord compression). Chronic subacute asphyxia (prenatal or intrapartum). Systemic hypotension. Multiorgan system failure may occur.	Systemic hypotension leading to decreased cerebral blood flow. Apnea and bradycardia, secondary to poor cerebral perfusion. Chorioamnionitis
CLINICAL MANIFESTATIONS	Clinical manifestations depend on extent of encephalopathy. Stage I: Mild encephalopathy Hyperalert state Hyper-responsiveness Normal muscle tone and reflexes Increased tendon reflexes Myoclonus present Tachycardia Dilated pupils EEG normal Usually no seizure activity Stage II: Moderate encephalopathy Lethargy and hypotonia Increased tendon reflexes Myoclonus Weak suck Strong grasp Incomplete Moro reflex Seizures Pupils constrict and reactive Abnormal EEG findings Stage III: Severe encephalopathy Level of consciousness deteriorates to comatose. Apnea, bradycardia Mechanical ventilation needed. Seizures occur within 12 hours of life.	Acute phase: Lethargy, central nervous system depression, and hypotension. After 6-10 weeks: Frequent tremors, and startle reflex. Abnormal Moro reflex. Hypertonia, irritability, extension of legs, increased flexion of arms.

Continued

	HYPOXIC–ISCHEMIC ENCEPHALOPATHY	PERIVENTRICULAR LEUKOMALACIA
TABLE 17–8 TYPES OF CENTRAL NERVOUS SYSTEM INJURY: HYPOXIC-ISCHEMIC ENCEPHALOPATHY—cont'd		
	Severe hypotonia, absent Moro, grasp, and suck reflexes. Pupils unequal; poor light reflex and variable reactivity. Deterioration may occur within 24–72 hours. Death may follow.	
PROGNOSIS	Outcome depends on severity of encephalopathy. 20%–50% of asphyxiated babies with hypoxic-ischemic encephalopathy (HIE) will die. Early seizure activity associated with poorer outcome. Less severe HIE associated with hyperactivity and attention deficit problems. Normal outcome may occur.	Outcome depends on location and extent of injury. Motor deficits Spastic diplegia Visual impairments Lower limb weakness Intellectual deficits more common when there is upper arm involvement.

Lynam & Verklan (2010).

Medical Management

- Decrease risk for hypoxia, ischemia, and asphyxia during the perinatal and intrapartal periods.
  - *Identification and treatment of a compromised fetus may prevent asphyxiation and multiorgan damage (Lynam & Verklan, 2010).*
- Neurological and behavioral evaluation
- Laboratory tests
  - *Serum glucose level*
  - *Electrolyte levels*
  - *Arterial blood gas analysis*
  - *Blood, urine, cerebrospinal fluid (CSF) cultures*
  - *Complete blood count with differential*
- Computed tomography (CT) scan, ultrasonography, magnetic resonance image (MRI), and skull radiographs as indicated
- Lumbar puncture for CSF analysis if clinically indicated
- Electroencephalography to confirm occurrence of seizures, and to identify presence and severity of brain damage if clinically indicated
  - *Evoked potentials to predict neurodevelopmental outcomes in cases of hypoxic–ischemic encephalopathy (Levene & de Vries, 2011)*
- Neurology consultant as indicated
- Medications to treat seizure activity
- Infants with hypoxic-ischemic encephalopathy may require the following medical management and treatment (Lynam & Verklan, 2010):
  - *Resuscitation at the time of delivery*
  - *Oxygen and ventilator support*
  - *Monitoring of fluids, electrolytes, and acid-base balance*
  - *Monitoring of blood volume and blood pressure*
  - *Maintaining perfusion and preventing/treating hypotension*
  - *Evaluating and supporting the renal, hepatic, gastrointestinal, pulmonary, and cardiovascular systems*
  - *Total body cooling or selective head cooling for infants with moderate to severe hypoxic–ischemic encephalopathy to improve survival and neurodevelopment (Tagin, Woolcott, Vincer, Whyte, & Stinson, 2012)*

Nursing Actions

- Review maternal prenatal and intrapartal histories for risk factors.
- Perform physical assessment of the neonate, including evaluation of tone, reflexes, and behavior.
- Notify physician of abnormal findings.
- Administer oxygen as per order.
- Obtain laboratory tests as per order.
- Ensure that ordered diagnostic tests are completed.
- Assist with diagnostic procedures such as lumbar puncture.
- Administer medications as per order.
- Monitor temperature closely of infants undergoing cooling therapy.
- Provide the family with support and information about their infant's status, treatment, and follow-up.

INFANTS OF MOTHERS WITH TYPE 1 DIABETES

Diabetes is the most common chronic medical problem affecting pregnant women (Hay, 2012). Maternal diabetes during pregnancy is associated with poor outcomes for the fetus and neonate (Armentrout, 2010). Complications of high maternal levels of glucose during pregnancy are:

■ Congenital anomalies:
  ■ *Cardiac anomalies, such as transposition of the great vessels, ventricular septal defect, and left to right ventricular wall hypertrophy*
  ■ *Skeletal defects, such as sacral agenesis and neural tube defects*
  ■ *Small left colon syndrome and renal anomalies (Hay, 2012)*
■ IUGR, perinatal asphyxia, and SGA neonates due to placental insufficiency related to maternal vascular disease in woman with type 1 diabetes of long duration (Armentrout, 2010)
■ Risk for RDS due to delay in surfactant production related to the high maternal glucose levels and fetal hyperstimulation (Armentrout, 2010)
■ Risk of hypoglycemia during the first few hours of life due to increased levels of fetal and neonatal insulin and decreased circulating glucose after delivery
■ Neurological damage and seizures related to inadequate glucose supply to the brain due to neonatal hyperinsulinism
■ Risk for hyperbilirubinemia related to polycythemia due to insulin-induced increases in metabolism that leads to hypoxia (Armentrout, 2010).
■ Risk of shoulder dystocia during the birthing process related to macrosomia
■ Risk of childhood obesity and type 2 diabetes (Hay, 2012).

Assessment Findings

■ Macrosomia due to fetal exposure to elevated maternal glucose levels. In response to high glucose levels, the fetal pancreas produces insulin. Hyperinsulinemia results in increased fat production and growth (Hay, 2012).
■ Fractured clavicle and brachial nerve damage related to shoulder dystocia (Armentrout, 2010)
■ Hypoglycemia
■ Hypocalcemia and hypomagnesemia
■ Polycythemia
■ Hyperbilirubinemia
■ Low muscle tone
■ Poor feeding abilities

Medical Management

■ Assess for complications associated with maternal diabetes.
■ Laboratory tests such as hematocrit and calcium and magnesium levels.
■ X-ray exams if clinically indicated for birth trauma related to shoulder dystocia.
■ Consult the cardiologist if cardiac anomalies are suspected.
■ Monitor blood glucose. Abnormal results are confirmed by laboratory analysis of plasma glucose (Armentrout, 2010). If the neonate is hypoglycemic, blood glucose levels should be monitored 30 minutes after feeding to evaluate response to treatment *(Miller & Morris, 2011).*
■ Early (by 1–2 hours of age) and frequent oral feedings of breast milk or formula unless the neonate feeds

poorly or is too sick to be fed orally. If oral feedings are contraindicated and/or the neonate is hypoglycemic, 10% dextrose and water is administered intravenously *(Miller & Morris, 2011).*

Nursing Actions

■ Assess neonate for signs of respiratory distress, birth trauma, congenital anomalies, hypoglycemia, hypocalcemia, polycythemia, and hyperbilirubinemia.
■ Monitor blood glucose per agency protocol.
  ■ *May require intravenous fluids along with feedings to maintain adequate blood glucose levels*
■ Provide early and frequent feedings to treat and prevent hypoglycemia.
  ■ *May be passive, lethargic, and difficult to arouse (Miller & Morris, 2011)*
  ■ *Oral feeding skills must be assessed and supported.*
  ■ *Gavage feedings may be indicated.*
■ Obtain laboratory tests as per orders.
■ Maintain a neutral thermal environment to reduce energy needs *(Miller & Morris, 2011).*

NEONATAL INFECTION

Infections among neonates are a leading cause of morbidity and mortality. The immune system of a neonate is immature, placing the newborn at risk for infection during the first several months of life. Neonates can be exposed to infection via vertical or horizontal transmission (Lott, 2010). **Vertical transmission** of infection, the passing of infection from the mother to the baby, can occur in several ways:

■ Transplacental transfer: Infection, such as syphilis, is transmitted to the fetus through the placenta.
■ Ascending infection: Infection ascends into the uterus related to prolonged rupture of membranes.
■ Intrapartal exposure: The neonate is exposed to infection during the birth process (e.g., herpes virus).

Horizontal transmission (nosocomial infection) is an infection that is transmitted from hospital equipment or staff to the neonate (Lott, 2010).

Infections may be caused by bacteria, viruses, fungus, yeast, spirochetes (syphilis), and protozoa (**Table 17-9**).

Infections may affect specific organ systems such as respiratory, urinary tract, brain, gastrointestinal tract, and skin; or local sites such as the umbilical stump and eyes. Neonates may develop systemic infections (sepsis) (Edwards, 2011).

■ Early-onset sepsis occurs within the first 7 days of life. It is a serious, overwhelming infection that is typically acquired through vertical transmission from the mother (Edwards, 2011).
■ Late-onset sepsis occurs after 7 days of life and is associated with a lower mortality rate than early-onset sepsis.
■ Very late onset sepsis affects premature, very low birth weight babies, after 3 months of age. This sepsis is related

TABLE 17–9   CAUSES OF NEONATAL INFECTION

BACTERIAL	VIRAL	FUNGAL	OTHER
Group B *Streptococcus*	Rubella	*Candida albicans*	Syphilis
Escherichia coli	Cytomegalovirus (CMV)	Candidiasis	*Treponema pallidum* (spirochete)
Coagulase-negative	Respiratory syncytial virus (RSV)		Toxoplasmosis
Staphylococcus	Herpes simplex (HSV)		Protozoan parasite
Staphylococcus aureus	Hepatitis B		
Viridans streptococci	Human immunodeficiency virus (HIV)		
Enterococcus species	Varicella-zoster (Chickenpox)		
Group D *Streptococcus*			
Pseudomonas species			
Klebsiella			
Listeria monocytogenes			
Hemophilus influenzae			
Neisseria gonorrhoeae			
C. trachomatis			
Chlamydia			
Mycobacterium tuberculosis			

to long-term use of equipment such as indwelling catheters and endotracheal tubes (Edwards, 2011).
■ Risk factors
   ■ *There are several maternal, neonatal, and environmental factors that predispose a neonate to infection (**Table 17-10**).*

Group B Streptococcus

Group B *Streptococcus* (GBS) is the primary cause of neonatal meningitis and sepsis in the United States (Field, 2011). Approximately 15%–40% of all pregnant women are asymptomatic carriers of GBS, which is found in the urogenital and lower gastrointestinal tract (Field, 2011). Evidence supports the use of antibiotics during labor among women who have positive cultures for GBS during pregnancy in reducing vertical transmission of GBS, and early-onset GBS sepsis (Edwards, 2011). The following are recommendations established by the Centers for Disease Control and Prevention (CDC, 2010) to prevent perinatal Group B streptococcal disease:

■ All pregnant women should be routinely screened for vaginal and rectal GBS colonization at 35–37 weeks' gestation. Women who are positive for GBS should be given prophylactic antibiotics at the time of labor or rupture of membranes.
■ Women who were GBS positive during pregnancy, or have delivered a previous baby with GBS infection, or women with membranes rupture before 37 weeks' gestation, should be given penicillin during the intrapartum period without obtaining a GBS culture.
■ If GBS status is not known at the time of rupture of membranes or labor onset, prophylactic antibiotics

should be administered if: (a) membranes have been ruptured for 18 hours or more, (b) gestational age is less than 37 weeks, or (c) maternal temperature is 100.4°F (38°C) or higher.
■ Women with positive GBS cultures who have a planned cesarean section before rupture of membranes or the onset of labor should not receive routine prophylaxis for perinatal GBS prevention.
■ For intrapartum chemoprophylaxis, penicillin G is recommended at an initial dose of 5 million units intravenously (IV), followed by 2.5 million units every 4 hours until delivery. Ampicillin can be used as an alternative and is given at an initial dose of 2 g IV followed by 1 g IV every 4 hours until delivery. Women who are allergic to penicillin but are not at high risk for anaphylaxis are given cefazolin IV. Erythromycin or clindamycin IV may also be used if the GBS isolate is not resistant to these medications.
■ Neonates of women who received intrapartum chemoprophylaxis do not require routine antibiotic administration, unless they exhibit signs of sepsis.
■ Asymptomatic infants of mothers who received prophylactic antibiotics and who are less than 35 weeks' gestation at the time of delivery should be evaluated with a complete blood count with differential, and blood cultures. These neonates should be observed in the hospital for at least 48 hours.
■ Infants at any gestational age who exhibit signs of infection should have a complete blood count (CBC) with a differential, blood cultures, and a chest x-ray exam if respiratory symptoms are present (Edwards, 2011).

TABLE 17–10 RISK FACTORS FOR NEONATAL INFECTION

MATERNAL FACTORS	NEONATAL FACTORS	ENVIRONMENTAL FACTORS
Poor prenatal nutrition	Prematurity	Length of stay in hospital
Low socioeconomic status	Birth weight <2,500 g	Invasive procedures
Substance abuse	Difficult delivery	Use of humidification in incubator or ventilatory care
History of sexually transmitted infection	Birth asphyxia	Routine use of broad-spectrum antibiotics
Recurrent abortion	Meconium staining	
Lack of prenatal care	Need for resuscitation	
Prolonged rupture of membranes (>12–18 hours)	Congenital anomalies	
Vaginal Group B *Streptococcus* colonization	Black neonates	
Chorioamnionitis	Male neonates	
Maternal temperature during labor and delivery	Multiple gestation	
Premature labor		
Difficult or prolonged labor		
Maternal urinary tract infection		
Invasive procedures during labor and delivery		
Maternal and/or fetal tachycardia		
Fetal scalp electrode use		

Lott (2010).

Antibiotics (ampicillin and gentamicin) should be started immediately after blood cultures are obtained.

■ Neonates who are term, who appear to be healthy, and whose mothers received 4 or more hours of antibiotic prophylaxis can be discharged after 24 hours if they meet all other discharge criteria.

Assessment Findings for Neonatal Infections

■ Signs of infection in a newborn are often nonspecific and subtle (**Table 17-11**).
■ Laboratory findings suggestive of infection include:
  ■ *Leukocytosis: An elevated white blood cell count (WBC >25,000/mm³)*
  ■ *Leukopenia: A low white blood cell count (WBC <1,750/mm³)*
  ■ *Neutrophilia: Increased neutrophil count*
  ■ *Neutropenia: Decreased neutrophil count (<1,500/mm³) is strongly predictive of infection.*
  ■ *An immature to total neutrophil ratio greater than 0.20 is suggestive of infection.*
  ■ *Thrombocytopenia: Platelet count <100,000/mm³ can be related to viral infection or bacterial sepsis (Lott, 2010).*

Medical Management

■ Monitor for clinical signs of infection.
■ Laboratory tests if the neonate exhibits manifestations of infection or is at risk for infection:
  ■ *CBC including a differential to evaluate white blood cell counts*

■ *Microbial cultures of the blood, urine, and CSF*
  ■ Neonatal sepsis can be diagnosed definitively only with a positive blood culture (Edwards, 2011). Urine and CSF cultures may also be obtained when sepsis is suspected. Other cultures are obtained as clinically indicated (e.g., skin).
■ *C-reactive protein levels (CRP) may be measured every 12 hours to detect inflammation associated with infection (Lott, 2010).*
■ *Polymerase chain reaction (PCR) testing for bacterial or viral DNA allows for identification of a specific bacterial or viral gene segment (Lott, 2010).*
■ Antibiotic therapy, if indicated for suspected sepsis after cultures are obtained (Lott, 2010).
  ■ *Antibiotics, such as ampicillin and aminoglycosides, that provide broad-spectrum coverage are often started initially (Lott, 2010).*
  ■ *If culture results are negative, antibiotics will be stopped after 48–72 hours.*
  ■ *If sepsis is confirmed, antibiotics continue for 10–14 days, and 21 days for meningitis (Lott, 2010).*
  ■ *If it is determined the infection is not bacterial in nature, appropriate antiviral or antifungal medications are ordered (Edwards, 2011).*
  ■ *The dosage and frequency of medication administration are dependent on the neonate's weight, gestational age, postnatal age, and liver and kidney function (Edwards, 2011).*
■ Intravenous fluid and parenteral nutrition
■ Monitor glucose and electrolytes.
■ Ventilation as indicated (Edwards, 2011)

TABLE 17–11   SIGNS OF NEONATAL INFECTION

RESPIRATORY	THERMO-REGULATION	CARDIO-VASCULAR	NEUROLOGICAL	GASTROINTESTINAL	SKIN	METABOLIC
Apnea	Hypothermia	Bradycardia	Tremors	Poor feeding	Rash	Glucose instability
Grunting	Fever	Tachycardia	Lethargy	Vomiting	Pustules	Metabolic acidosis
Retractions	Temperature instability	Arrhythmias	Irritability	Diarrhea	Vesicles	
Tachypnea		Hypotension	High-pitched cry	Abdominal distention	Pallor	
Cyanosis		Hypertension	Hypertonia	Enlarged liver/spleen	Jaundice	
		Decreased perfusion	Hypotonia		Petechiae	
			Seizures		Vasomotor instability	
			Bulging fontanelles			

Lott (2010).

Nursing Actions

■ Assess maternal and neonatal histories for factors that may place a neonate at risk for infection, such as maternal Group B *Streptococcus* status.

■ Assess vital signs and adequacy of feedings, and monitor intake and output and weight, per agency protocol.

■ Assess neonate for signs of infection (see Table 17-11).

■ Notify the physician if the neonate demonstrates signs of infection. Early recognition and treatment of neonatal infection is important in preventing morbidity and mortality.

■ Provide respiratory support as per orders.

■ Monitor glucose and electrolytes.

■ Obtain laboratory tests as per order.

■ Assist with diagnostic tests such as lumbar puncture for CSF.
  ■ *CSF is obtained and sent to lab for a Gram stain and culture.*
  ■ *Holding the infant still in a flexed position is imperative for a successful lumbar puncture.*

■ Administer antibiotics as per orders.

■ Administer intravenous fluid and parenteral nutrition as per orders.

■ Wash hands before handling equipment and caring for the neonate.

■ Provide parents with information about the neonate's status, infection prevention strategies such as handwashing before contact with the baby, and diagnostic tests and treatments as appropriate.

■ Include the following in discharge teaching for parents: identification of signs and symptoms of infection, what signs/symptoms should be reported to the physician, how to prevent infection, and scheduling a follow-up appointment before discharge.

SUBSTANCE ABUSE EXPOSURE

In the United States, 4.4% of pregnant women report use of illicit drugs, 10.8% report use of alcohol, and 16.3% report use of tobacco (SAMHSA, 2010). Perinatal use of illicit drugs, alcohol, and tobacco has both short-term and long-term effects on the developing fetus (**Table 17-12**).

Women who use illicit drugs, alcohol, and tobacco are at higher risk for:

■ No or inadequate prenatal care

■ Inadequate prenatal weight gain

■ Sexually transmitted infections

■ Obstetrical complications (e.g., preterm labor and abruptio placentae)

■ Severe mood swings

Assessment Findings

■ Effects of perinatal maternal substance use on the neonate are specific to the substance that has been used (see Table 17-12).

■ Younger gestational age correlates with a lower risk for neonatal withdrawal.

■ **Neonatal abstinence syndrome** (neonatal withdrawal) may result from intrauterine exposure to various substances, including opioids such as heroin, methadone, oxycodone, and Demerol; alcohol; Valium; caffeine; and barbiturates (AAP, 2012). See Critical Component: Signs of Neonatal Withdrawal.
  ■ *The extent to which a newborn exhibits drug withdrawal is dependent on several factors (e.g., timing of the last exposure, type of substance, and the half life of the substance; AAP, 2012).*
  ■ *Neonates exposed to alcohol in utero may demonstrate withdrawal symptoms within 3–12 hours after birth (AAP, 2012).*
  ■ *Neonates exposed to narcotics in utero exhibit withdrawal within 48–72 hours after birth.*
  ■ *Neonates exposed to barbiturates in utero exhibit withdrawal between days 1 and 14 (AAP, 2012).*

■ Alcohol use during pregnancy can cause a wide range of problems from no effect to major long-term

CRITICAL COMPONENT

Signs of Neonatal Withdrawal

- Apnea
- Behavior irregularities
- Diarrhea
- Dysmature swallowing
- Excessive crying
- Excessive/frantic sucking
- Excoriated skin
- Fever
- High-pitched cry
- Hyperreflexia
- Hypertonia
- Irritability/restlessness
- Lacrimation
- Nasal congestion
- Poor feeding
- Seizures
- Skin mottling
- Sleep problems
- Sneezing
- Sweating
- Tachypnea
- Tremors
- Vomiting
- Wakefulness
- Weight loss or failure to gain weight
- Yawning

(Pitts, 2010)

disabilities (Pitts, 2010). The following are conditions resulting from alcohol exposure during pregnancy:

- *Fetal alcohol syndrome (FAS): A wide array and spectrum of physical, cognitive, and behavioral abnormalities associated with maternal alcohol use during pregnancy (Bandstra & Accornero, 2011). Signs of FAS include:*
  - Distinctive facial features: small eyes, thin upper lip, and short nose
  - Heart defects
  - Joint, limb, and finger deformities
  - Delayed physical growth, both intrauterine and post-birth
  - Vision problems
  - Hearing problems
  - Mental retardation
  - Behavior disturbances, such as short attention span, hyperactivity, and poor impulse control *(Bandstra & Accornero, 2011)*
- *Alcohol related birth defects (ARBD): Congenital anomalies associated with alcohol use during pregnancy that may affect the heart, skeleton, kidneys, eyes, and ears*
- *Alcohol related neurodevelopmental disorder (ARND): Abnormalities of the central nervous system that are associated with prenatal alcohol exposure:*
  - Neurological problems (e.g., poor hand-eye coordination and fine motor skills, and neurosensory hearing loss)
  - Decreased cranial size, brain abnormalities
  - Cognitive and behavioral problems (Pitts, 2010)

TABLE 17–12 SUBSTANCES COMMONLY USED DURING PREGNANCY: SIGNS OF WITHDRAWAL AND SHORT- AND LONG-TERM EFFECTS

SUBSTANCE	POST-BIRTH EFFECTS/ SIGNS OF WITHDRAWAL	SHORT- AND LONG-TERM EFFECTS
TOBACCO	None known	Low birth weight Intrauterine growth restriction Smaller head circumference Increased stillbirth Cleft palate/lip Childhood cancer Lower IQ Learning difficulties Attention deficit disorder Increased risk for sudden infant death syndrome Increased risk for asthma/respiratory infections Inner ear infections
ALCOHOL	Onset of withdrawal 12 hours after birth Hypertonia Tremors Weak suck	Facial anomalies: Flat upper lip Flat philtrum Short eye openings

Continued

TABLE 17–12   SUBSTANCES COMMONLY USED DURING PREGNANCY: SIGNS OF WITHDRAWAL AND SHORT- AND LONG-TERM EFFECTS—cont'd

SUBSTANCE	POST-BIRTH EFFECTS/ SIGNS OF WITHDRAWAL	SHORT- AND LONG-TERM EFFECTS
	Poor feeding Crying Increased wakefulness Increased mouthing behavior	Low birth weight Failure to thrive Microcephaly Mental retardation Poor fine motor skills Aggressiveness Attention deficit disorder Poor short-term memory Problem solving difficulties Neurosensory hearing losses Gait problems Hand-eye coordination problems Increased risk of infection Lack of understanding of consequences Impulsive behavior Poor judgment Short attention span
MARIJUANA	Tremors Altered sleep patterns High-pitched cry Exaggerated startle reflex	Social interaction problems Low birth weight Preterm birth Intrauterine growth restriction Attention deficit disorder Impulsiveness Poor self-directed responses Lower scores on verbal and memory assessments Increased risk for sudden infant death syndrome with paternal use Congenital anomalies
COCAINE	Tremors Hyperreflexia Hypotonia Abnormal state patterns—Prolonged periods of being awake/crying Extreme sensitivity to stimuli/easily distressed Depressed interactive behaviors Poor response to comforting Short attention to stimuli Poor suck leading to feeding problems	Prematurity Intrauterine growth restriction Decreased head circumference Low birth weight Congenital anomalies Fetal distress during labor may lead to meconium aspiration Cerebrovascular accident, intraventricular hemorrhage Increased risk for sudden infant death syndrome Attention deficit and behavioral problems Cognitive delays

TABLE 17–12 SUBSTANCES COMMONLY USED DURING PREGNANCY: SIGNS OF WITHDRAWAL AND SHORT- AND LONG-TERM EFFECTS—cont'd

SUBSTANCE	POST-BIRTH EFFECTS/ SIGNS OF WITHDRAWAL	SHORT- AND LONG-TERM EFFECTS
METHAMPHETAMINES	Abnormal sleep patterns Tremors Poor feeding State disorganization Agitation/lethargy Weight gain problems Sweating Vomiting With methamphetamine and cocaine use: Frantic first sucking High-pitched cry Loose stools Yawning Fever Hyperreflexia Excoriation	Intrauterine growth restriction Reduced brain growth Developmental effects Congenital anomalies Increased risk for sudden infant death syndrome
NARCOTICS/OPIOIDS Heroin Methadone Morphine OxyContin	Hypertonia Tremors Hyperreflexia Seizures Irritability/restlessness High-pitched cry Excessive crying Sleep problems Wakefulness Yawning Nasal congestion Sneezing Lacrimation Sweating Fever Skin mottling Diarrhea Vomiting Poor feeding Dysmature swallowing Excessive/frantic sucking Tachypnea Apnea Excoriated skin Behavior irregularities Weight loss or failure to gain weight	Prematurity Hypoxia/low Apgar scores Intrauterine growth restriction Low birth weight Microcephaly Increased risk for meconium stained fluid/meconium aspiration Congenital infections Increased risk for sudden infant death syndrome Increased chromosomal abnormalities (heroin exposure)

Continued

TABLE 17–12　SUBSTANCES COMMONLY USED DURING PREGNANCY: SIGNS OF WITHDRAWAL AND SHORT- AND LONG-TERM EFFECTS—cont'd

SUBSTANCE	POST-BIRTH EFFECTS/ SIGNS OF WITHDRAWAL	SHORT- AND LONG-TERM EFFECTS
INHALANTS	Fetal dysmorphogenesis syndrome - similar to fetal alcohol syndrome Small for gestational age Microcephaly Deep-set eyes Small face Low-set ears Micrognathia Spoon shaped fingertips/small fingernails	Developmental delay Language problems Cerebellar dysfunction Hyperactivity

Edwards (2011); Pitts (2010).

Medical Management

- Review of the maternal history for substance use, prescription drug use, and risk factors for substance use.
- Physical assessment of the neonate, including observation for physical and behavioral effects of prenatal substance use.
- Toxicology screening of the neonate's urine and/or meconium.
- Diagnostic tests such as cranial ultrasound and EEG, if indicated by clinical manifestations of withdrawal symptoms
  - *Problems such as infection and hypoglycemia may manifest symptoms similar to those of neonatal withdrawal and should be ruled out by the appropriate diagnostic tests (AAP, 2012).*
- Use of an assessment tool to determine signs of neonatal abstinence syndrome
  - *Use of the tool should be initiated within 2 hours of birth, and neonates should be assessed for signs of withdrawal every 4 hours (Pitts, 2010).*
  - *Use tool to guide decisions about when a neonate should be evaluated for treatment with medication (Pitts, 2010).*
- Pharmacological therapy is considered if seizures, excessive weight loss, dehydration, poor feeding, diarrhea, vomiting, fever, and inability to sleep occur (AAP, 2012).
- Medications to treat withdrawal in neonates include:
  - *Methadone, morphine, paregoric, tincture of opium, clonidine, and diazepam, for opioid withdrawal*
  - *Benzodiazepines to treat withdrawal from alcohol*
  - *Phenobarbital for hyperactive behavior associated with narcotic withdrawal; also used for withdrawal from non-narcotic agents*
  - *Chlorpromazine for babies exhibiting gastrointestinal and CNS effects of narcotic withdrawal (AAP, 2012; Pitts, 2010)*
- Frequent, small feedings with a high calorie formula (22–24 calories/oz.).

- Monitor feedings, output, and weight daily.
- Patient education regarding substance use and breastfeeding
  - *Breastfeeding is contraindicated if a woman is actively using any of the following substances: cocaine, methamphetamines, alcohol, heroin, and/or marijuana (Pitts, 2010).*
  - *Breastfeeding is not contraindicated with methadone use (AAP, 2012). Infants of mothers on methadone must be weaned gradually to avoid withdrawal (Pitts, 2010).*
  - *Women who smoke cigarettes should be advised to quit and be given information about cessation resources. Women who choose to continue to smoke should be taught to avoid smoking around the baby, to smoke immediately after breastfeeding and not before, and to cut down on the number of cigarettes that they smoke (Pitts, 2010).*
- Comprehensive follow-up care for the mother of the baby or the foster mother before discharge. Infants exposed to substances prenatally often need long-term interdisciplinary physical and developmental care (Pitts, 2010).
  - *Referrals must be made to the appropriate departments and agencies (Pitts, 2010). In many health care settings, health care providers obtain a social service consult for women who have a history of substance use. Notification of agencies such as Child Protective Services is dependent on laws of each state. In some states, neonates who are positive for prenatal substance exposure are placed in foster care.*

Nursing Actions

- Review maternal history, including risk factors of substance use and history of current or past substance use.
- Assess the neonate, including gestational age.
- Assess for congenital anomalies and physical and behavioral signs of withdrawal/neonatal abstinence syndrome.

- Monitor vital signs.
- Obtain toxicology screening as per order.
  - *A clean catch urine or meconium sample may be ordered.*
- Use a scoring tool to assess for signs of withdrawal on neonates who are at high risk for neonatal abstinence syndrome (**Fig. 17-8**).
  - *Notify the physician if the score is outside of what is considered normal.*
  - *The decision to treat with medication is based on the infant's score.*
- Care for neonates experiencing neonatal abstinence syndrome:
  - *Assess feedings and daily weights: Increased activity, decreased sleep, irritability, loose stools, vomiting, and poor feeding behavior may all result in increased caloric needs.*
  - *Provide frequent and small feedings: A higher calorie formula (22–24 cal/oz.) can be used to support increased caloric needs.*
    - Allow the neonate to rest during feedings.
    - Position the neonate upright during feedings.
    - Utilize nipples that have a slower flow if the infant has a strong, frantic suck.
  - *Provide a pacifier to the neonate.*
  - *Bathe the baby in warm water to treat increased tone and irritability.*
  - *Swaddle neonate with arms close to the body.*
  - *Provide a quiet environment, with lights dimmed, and minimize stimuli.*
  - *Be sensitive to infant cues that indicate stress; minimize stress-inducing activities.*
  - *Rock the neonate gently (AAP, 2012; Pitts, 2010).*
- Care for the mother of a neonate with neonatal abstinence syndrome:
  - *Provide nonjudgmental, honest, supportive care.*
  - *Teach what to expect in regard to the neonate's behavior. Educate about strategies that will provide comfort to her infant during withdrawal.*
  - *Teach her how to feed her infant.*
  - *Observe maternal-newborn interactions and involve the mother in the care of her newborn.*
    - Neonates who have been exposed to substances during the prenatal period often exhibit behaviors that interfere with the maternal-newborn relationship, such as irritability, resistance to being comforted, arching while being held, altered sleep states, poor feeding behavior, easily agitated when stimulated, and difficult transitions from one state to another.
    - Characteristics of mothers with a history of substance abuse that may impair the maternal-newborn relationship include lack of sensitivity to infant cues, lack of emotional stability, lack of communication with the infant, and inconsistent/unavailable caregiving.
    - Document all assessments and observations in the medical record per agency protocol (Pitts, 2010).

CONGENITAL ABNORMALITIES

Congenital anomalies or birth defects occur in approximately 20% of infant deaths in the United States (Sterk, 2010). Abnormalities range from being undetectable at birth to major and life threatening.

- Risk factors
  - *Chromosomal abnormalities*
- Environmental factors: Teratogens such as radiation, illicit substances, alcohol, diseases (diabetes), medications, and infections such as TORCH (Toxoplasmosis, Other infections, Rubella, Cytomegalovirus, Herpes simplex virus)
- Multifactorial disorders: Abnormalities that result in a combination of environmental and genetic factors (Sterk, 2010)

Assessment Findings

- See **Table 17-13** for common congenital anomalies.
- See **Table 17-14** for common cardiac anomalies.
- See **Table 17-15** for common metabolic disorders.

Nursing Actions

- Nursing care is determined by the type and severity of anomaly.
- Genetic disease screening is obtained before discharge of the neonate.
- Provide emotional support for parents and family.
- Provide information on support groups.
- Provide information on need for follow-up care.

REGIONAL CENTERS

Women experiencing a high-risk pregnancy may require transfer to a facility that can provide the appropriate level of care to them and their neonate after delivery. Many facilities/communities lack the resources to provide care to high-risk mothers and high-risk neonates; thus, regional centers were developed to provide services such as high-risk perinatal care and neonatal intensive care. Transport of a high-risk neonate to a center with a neonatal intensive care unit (NICU) requires coordination between the transferring and receiving hospitals, appropriate preparation, a highly skilled team, and the appropriate equipment (**Fig. 17-9**). Key considerations of neonatal transport are:

- During the transport process, the transport team provides care that is an extension of the NICU. The aim is to provide the appropriate amount of support to the neonate to maintain stable condition. The transport process should minimize adverse effects of transfer on the neonate, and be carried out in a way that protects the safety of the neonate and the transport team (Bowen, 2010).
- The transport team must be knowledgeable about high-risk neonatal care and assessment. Members of the team may include a neonatal nurse practitioner, neonatologist,

System	Signs and symptoms	Date Time							Comments
CENTRAL NERVOUS SYSTEM DISTURBANCES		Score							
	Crying: Excessive high-pitched	2							
	Crying: Continuous high-pitched	3							
	Sleeps less than 1 hour after feeding	3							
	Sleeps less than 2 hours after feeding	2							
	Sleeps less than 3 hours after feeding	1							
	Hyperactive Moro reflex	2							
	Markedly hyperactive Moro reflex	3							
	Mild tremors: Disturbed	1							
	Moderate-severe tremors: Disturbed	2							
	Mild tremors: Undisturbed	3							
	Moderate-severe tremors: Undisturbed	4							
	Increased muscle tone	2							
	Excoriation (specify area)	1							
	Myoclonic jerks	3							
	Generalized convulsions	5							
METABOLIC, VASOMOTOR, AND RESPIRATORY DISTURBANCES	Sweating	1							
	Fever less than or equal to 101°F (37.2–38.3°C)	1							
	Fever greater than 101°F (38.4°C)	2							
	Frequent yawning (greater than 3)	1							
	Mottling	1							
	Nasal stuffiness	1							
	Sneezing (greater than 3)	1							
	Nasal flaring	2							
	Respiratory rate (greater than 60/min)	1							
	Respiratory rate (greater than 60/min with retractions)	2							
GASTROINTESTINAL DISTURBANCES	Excessive sucking	1							
	Poor feeding	2							
	Regurgitation	2							
	Projectile vomiting	3							
	Loose stools	2							
	Watery stools	3							
	TOTAL SCORE								

Figure 17–8 Neonatal Abstinence Scoring Tool.

resident, fellow, registered nurse, respiratory therapist, and a paramedic or emergency medical technician (Bowen, 2010).

■ The transport process includes the following:
  ■ *Once the need for NICU care is identified, arrangements are made to transfer the high-risk neonate.*
  ■ *Information pertaining to maternal and neonatal histories is communicated during the referral call.*
  ■ *The appropriate team is dispatched with supplies and equipment needed to care for the neonate.*
  ■ *The neonate is stabilized before transport.*
  ■ *During transport the infant is kept in an incubator, thermoregulation is maintained, respiratory support and IV therapy are provided, and the following are monitored:*

  ■ Vital signs, oxygen saturation, blood glucose, the neonate's condition, pain status, and response to transport
  ■ *Strategies should be used to provide developmental care during transfer, such as protecting the neonate's eyes from bright lights, using ear protection in noisy vehicles such as helicopters, using a gel mattress to prevent jarring, and using blankets to promote containment.*
  ■ *Notify parents when the infant arrives at the receiving facility (Bowen, 2010).*

Various vehicles may be used for transport, such as ambulance, helicopter, or fixed wing aircraft. The type of vehicle that is used will be determined by factors such as the neonate's condition and diagnosis, distance of transport, weather, and cost.

TABLE 17–13   COMMON CONGENITAL ANOMALIES

TYPE OF ANOMALY	INCIDENCE	DESCRIPTION	TREATMENT
TRACHEOESOPHAGEAL FISTULA	1 in 4,500 live births	Abnormal opening between the trachea and esophagus	Surgical repair
CHOANAL ATRESIA	2–4 in 10,000 live births	Obstruction of the nasal passages	Surgical repair
DIAPHRAGMATIC HERNIA	1 in 1000–6000 live births	Herniation of abdominal organs through a hole in the diaphragm into the thoracic cavity	Gastric decompression Stabilization Surgical repair
OMPHALOCELE	1 in 5000–6000 live births	Herniation of abdominal contents through the umbilicus which is covered by the peritoneal sac	Surgical repair. Staged surgical repair for large defects (abdominal contents returned gradually)
GASTROSCHISIS	1 in 30,000–50,000 live births	Herniation of abdominal contents through a hole in the abdomen often to the right of the umbilicus	Surgical repair Staged surgical repair for large defects
CLEFT LIP	1 in 1,000 live births	Failure of the mesenchymal masses of the nasal and maxillary prominences to come together	Surgical repair
CLEFT PALATE	1 in 2,500 live births	Failure of the mesenchymal masses in the palate to fuse	Surgical repair
SPINA BIFIDA: Meningocele Myelomeningocele	1 in 20,000 live births 1 in 1,000 live births	A sac with meninges and cerebrospinal fluid bulge through defect in undeveloped vertebrae A sac with meninges and nerve tissue bulge through a defect in the spinal column	Surgical repair Surgical repair
ANENCEPHALY	1 in 1,000 live births	Incomplete formation of the cranium and brain	Most babies die within a few days of birth
DEVELOPMENTAL DYSPLASIA OF THE HIP	1–2 in 1,000 live births	Dislocation of the femoral head from the acetabulum	Pavlik harness to promote abduction/flexion to stabilize hip Surgery if Pavlik harness is not successful
POLYDACTYLY		Extra digits on the hand or foot	Surgery or ligation
SYNDACTYLY	1 in 2,200 live births	Fusion of digits of hand or foot	Surgery depending on extent of anomaly
TALIPES EQUINOVARUS	1 in 1,000 live births	Sole of the foot is turned in; the back part of the foot is deformed. Also called "clubfoot," usually bilateral.	Casting/splinting Surgery Treatment depends on severity.

Sterk (2010).

Appropriate supplies and equipment based on the neonate's condition must be stocked and checked regularly. Equipment includes:

■ Monitoring devices, such as a pulse oximeter, cardiorespiratory monitor, temperature and blood pressure monitors
■ Oxygen tanks and other respiratory supplies, such as endotracheal tubes, bag and mask for resuscitation, oxygen hood, ventilator, and suctioning equipment
■ Medications
■ Intravenous therapy equipment including pumps
■ Equipment to maintain and assess thermoregulation, such as an incubator, thermometer, heat packs, chemical mattress, and blankets
■ Equipment to perform blood glucose and blood gas monitoring
■ Personal protective equipment, such as gloves and gowns

TABLE 17–14   COMMON CARDIAC ANOMALIES

TYPE OF ANOMALY	INCIDENCE	DESCRIPTION	TREATMENT
VENTRICULAR SEPTAL DEFECT (VSD)	1 in 3000 live births	Opening in the septum between the right and left ventricles of the heart.	Up to 75% of VSDs close without treatment. Treat with digoxin and diuretics if congestive heart failure is present. Surgical repair.
ATRIAL SEPTAL DEFECT (ASD)	1 in 5000 live births	Opening in the septum between the right and left atria.	ASDs may close without treatment. Treat congestive heart failure with medication. Surgical repair may be needed.
COARCTATION OF THE AORTA	1 in 10,000 live births	Narrowing of the aorta at the transverse aortic arch or in the area of the ductus arteriosus	Medical management of congestive heart failure. Surgical repair.
TETRALOGY OF FALLOT	1 in 5000 live births	Consists of four defects: 1. VSD 2. Aorta overriding VSD 3. Pulmonary stenosis 4. Hypertrophy of the right ventricle	Medical management includes propranolol for cyanotic infants. Prostaglandin E1 may be administered to maintain a patent ductus arteriosus until surgery, for infants with a severe tetralogy of Fallot. Surgical repair.
TRANSPOSITION OF GREAT VESSELS	1 in 5,000 live births	The positions of the great arteries are reversed from the normal position. Aorta emerges from the right ventricle, and the pulmonary artery emerges from the left ventricle.	This defect results in a medical emergency. Stabilization—treat acidosis. Administer prostaglandin E1 to maintain a patent ductus arteriosus until surgery is performed.

Sadowski (2010).

TABLE 17–15   COMMON GENETIC DISORDERS OF METABOLISM

TYPE OF DISORDER	INCIDENCE	DESCRIPTION	TREATMENT
PHENYLKETONURIA	1 in 10,000–15,000 live births	Lack of the enzyme needed to convert phenylalanine to tyrosine. If untreated, causes cognitive and physical problems.	Diet that restricts intake of phenylalanine.
DISORDERS OF FATTY ACID OXIDATION (e.g., medium chain acyl-CoA-deficiency)	1 in 15,000 live births	18 disorders identified. Impaired fat metabolism leads to hypoglycemia and organ failure.	Hypoglycemia is treated. Fasting is avoided.
CONGENITAL ADRENAL HYPERPLASIA	1 in 5000 live births	Cortisol production is inhibited. Adrenal hypertrophy results, with excessive production of adrenal androgens. Electrolyte imbalances common, female infants exhibit ambiguous genitalia.	Steroid administration. Corrective surgery for ambiguous genitalia.
MAPLE SYRUP URINE DISEASE	1 in 150,000	Lack of enzymes needed to metabolize leucine, valine, and isoleucine. These amino acids build up in the blood. Disease is fatal if untreated.	Peritoneal dialysis Low-protein diet

TABLE 17–15 COMMON GENETIC DISORDERS OF METABOLISM—cont'd			
TYPE OF DISORDER	INCIDENCE	DESCRIPTION	TREATMENT
GALACTOSEMIA	1 in 40,000–60,000 live births	Lack of enzyme that converts galactose to glucose. Inability to metabolize lactose. If untreated, results in liver disease, mental retardation, and cataracts.	Lactose-free or soy formula.

Strek (2010).

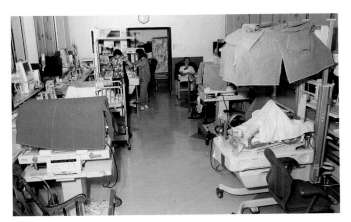

Figure 17–9   Neonatal Intensive Care Unit (NICU).

Discharge Planning

Discharge planning for high-risk neonates involves many considerations since these neonates often require special care and follow-up after release from the hospital. In some cases, infants require long-term evaluation to monitor health issues, growth, and neurodevelopment. Many high-risk conditions, such as prematurity and related complications, perinatal substance use, and congenital anomalies, may have long-term, even lifelong, physical, cognitive, and behavioral consequences. The following are critical components of the discharge process for high-risk neonates (Hummel, 2010):

■ When a high-risk neonate is admitted, planning for discharge begins. Parents should be encouraged to be involved with the care of their infant from the time of admission. Care-related teaching with parents should begin as soon after delivery as possible.
■ Interdisciplinary teams are often involved in the discharge process. The team may consist of physicians, nurse practitioners, nurses, social workers, occupational therapist, case manager, lactation consultant, respiratory therapist, nutritionist, pharmacist, and home health agency/nursing staff.
■ Readiness for discharge is assessed.
 ■ *The neonate's condition must be stable (e.g., weight gain, temperature stability, able to tolerate feedings, stable respiratory status; Fig. 17-10).*

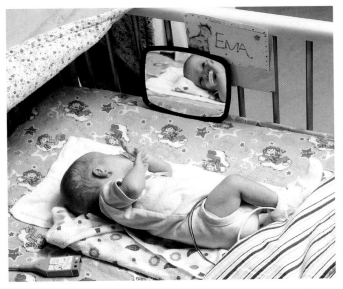

Figure 17–10   A 10-week-old neonate, born at 27 weeks' gestation, who will soon be going home.

■ *All appropriate examinations and screenings are completed, such as an eye exam, genetic disease/metabolic disease screening, and a hearing screening.*
■ *The neonate must be able to pass a car seat trial for a specified amount of time.*
 ■ Secured snugly in an appropriate size car seat at a 45-degree angle
 ■ Maintains adequate oxygenation, heart rate, and respiratory rate during trial
■ *Family's readiness to take their infant home is assessed.*
 ■ The family's willingness and ability to provide care to their infant with special needs is evaluated, as are their financial resources. In addition, the home setting is assessed for safety and adequacy.
■ *The educational needs of the family are met. Discharge teaching includes:*
 ■ General infant care, such as bathing, feeding schedule, diapering, skin care
 ■ Safety issues, such as car seat safety, positioning the infant on the back to sleep, infant CPR, baby proofing the house
 ■ Instructions on use of required equipment (e.g., apnea monitoring)

■ Information on treatments (e.g., oxygen, suctioning) and medications ordered

■ Signs and symptoms of illnesses that need to be reported to the primary care provider

■ Infant growth and developmental milestones

■ Follow-up information including visits with the pediatrician, immunization schedules, and referrals to the appropriate medical and developmental specialists

PSYCHOSOCIAL NEEDS OF PARENTS WITH HIGH-RISK NEONATES

The birth of a baby who is premature or who has conditions that place him or her at risk for illness or even death is a significant stressor for the family. Parents may grieve over the loss of an ideal baby and find the experience of having a baby with complications overwhelming. It is devastating for most parents when the woman is discharged and their baby must remain in the hospital.

Common effects on the parents and family are:

■ Delay of attachment process due to the separation of parent and newborn, which can place the newborn at risk for abuse and neglect

■ Guilt feelings by the woman, who may feel she did something wrong to cause her newborn to be ill

■ Emotional distancing of parents from their newborn as a protective mechanism due to fear of losing their child

■ Anger at the loss of control of having an ill or premature newborn

■ Disappointment at not being able to bring their newborn home

■ Disruption of family life; parents needing to return to work, caring for other child, and at the same time wanting to spend time in the hospital with their neonate

Nursing Actions

■ Orient parents to the NICU environment by explaining equipment/monitors used for their neonate.

■ Assess parents' comfort level with the NICU environment.

■ Provide opportunities for parents to share their concerns and frustrations by developing a trusting rapport with the parents and through active listening skills.

■ Provide opportunities for parents to talk about their experiences by asking parents how they are coping with the experience and by use of active listening.

■ Provide information regarding their neonate's status to both parents at a level they can understand.

■ Inform parents that they should ask any question they have regarding the condition and care of their neonate.

■ Inform parents that they can talk to their neonate's nurse at any time.

■ Assess the parents' readiness to care for their neonate and provide opportunities for them to participate in the care of their neonate.

■ Encourage parents to touch and hold their neonate as indicated by the neonate's health status.

■ Encourage the woman to pump her breast and bring the milk to the NICU to be used for feeding.
　　■ *Review breast milk storage and provide equipment as needed.*

■ Provide a private area for the woman to breastfeed when the neonate is able to nurse.

■ Encourage parents to take photos to share with their family and friends.

■ Praise parents for their involvement in the neonate's care.

■ Provide information on support groups for parents of preterm infants or infants with disabilities.

LOSS AND GRIEF

When a baby dies, parents must work through profound grief associated with the loss of their child, and the loss of their hopes and dreams for that child and their family. Grief is a process that is individual in nature. Often members of the family experience grief in different ways and in varied time lines. The stages of grief include:

■ Avoidance, disbelief, shock

■ Pain, physical discomforts, depression, difficulty concentrating, anger at self or partner, guilt

■ Acceptance and adaptation. Grief persists, but a sense of balance is achieved (Kenner, 2010).

It is important that nurses keep in mind that each person experiences and expresses grief in his or her own way. Culture, religion, and personal experience and beliefs will impact how individuals and families respond to loss. Nurses can help families that are grieving the death of their baby by carrying out various interventions including:

■ Allow parents to express their feelings by being present and listening.

■ Express empathy and condolences. Avoid clichés such as, "at least you are young; you can have another baby."

■ Refer to the baby by name, if the baby has been named.

■ Provide information about the process of grieving and what to expect physically and emotionally.

■ Provide ample opportunity for the parents and family members to spend time with the baby before and after he or she dies.

■ Provide parents with memorabilia associated with their baby, such as pictures, blankets, a cap, a lock of hair, ID bracelet, footprints, and crib card.

■ Offer to contact the hospital chaplain. Encourage the family to contact their own clergy. Explore the family's desire for baptism or other religious rites.

■ Discuss the family's plan for autopsy, a memorial or funeral, burial/cremation.

■ Encourage the family to accept help and support from others.

■ Refer parents to community services and support groups that may assist in facilitating the grief process (Kenner, 2010).

Clinical Pathway for the Preterm Infant

	Birth to First Hour	1–24 Hours of Age	24 Hours of Age to Discharge
Assessments	Review prenatal record to determine projected gestational age. Identify risk factors for premature birth. Obtain Apgar score at 1 and 5 minutes. Obtain weight, length, and head circumference. Complete neonatal assessment.	Complete gestational assessment as per hospital policy. Assess every1–2 hours or per hospital policy.	Assess every 2–4 hours or per hospital policy. Weigh the neonate every day or per hospital policy. Obtain length and head circumference weekly or per hospital policy.
Thermoregulation	Place neonate on preheated radiant warmer and dry gently immediately after birth. Cover head with warmed hat. Wrap in dry, warmed blankets for transport to NICU. Place in a radiant warmer or a thermo-regulated isolette. Assess axillary temperature every 15–30 minutes or per hospital policy.	Prevent heat loss by maintaining a NTE. Assess axillary temperature every 1–2 hours or per hospital policy. Assess for cold stress symptoms. Postpone bathing until neonate stable.	Prevent heat loss by maintaining a NTE. Encourage skin-to-skin contact or kangaroo care when neonate is stable. Dress and wrap neonate when advanced to an open crib. Assess axillary temperature every 2–4 hours or per hospital policy. Provide heat source when bathing. Assess for cold stress symptoms. Teach parents to assess temperature and signs of cold stress.
Respiratory	Clear the nose and mouth of mucus with the use of a bulb syringe. Immediately after birth, assess neonate for respiratory effort, including apnea, and provide resuscitation as needed. Apply pulse oximeter and monitor values. Assess for signs of respiratory distress: grunting, flaring, retractions. Assess lung sounds. Administer oxygen as needed. Provide respiratory support as needed. Obtain chest x-ray and blood gases as ordered.	Assess for signs of respiratory distress: grunting, flaring, retractions. Assess lung sounds. Administer oxygen as needed. Provide respiratory support as needed. Monitor pulse oximeter values. Obtain chest x-ray and blood gases as ordered. Monitor intake and output.	Assess for signs of respiratory distress: grunting, flaring, retractions. Assess lung sounds. Administer oxygen as needed. Provide respiratory support as needed. Monitor pulse oximeter values. Obtain chest x-ray and blood gases as ordered. Monitor intake and output. Obtain daily weights. Teach parents signs and symptoms of respiratory distress. Teach parents oxygen management if neonate is to be discharged with oxygen.

Continued

Clinical Pathway for the Preterm Infant—cont'd

	Birth to First Hour	1–24 Hours of Age	24 Hours of Age to Discharge
Cardiovascular	Assess skin color for cyanosis. Assess heart rate at birth, and at 1 and 5 minutes of age. Assess heart rate and rhythm every 15–30 minutes or per hospital policy thereafter. Place on cardio-respiratory monitor for continuous observation.	Assess skin color for cyanosis. Assess heart rate and rhythm every 1–2 hours or per hospital policy. Continue on cardio-respiratory monitor for continuous observation.	Assess skin color for cyanosis. Assess heart rate and rhythm every 2–4 hours or per hospital policy. Continue on cardio-respiratory monitor for continuous observation. Teach parents CPR when neonate is close to discharge.
Nutrition	Obtain and monitor blood glucose levels per hospital policy. Obtain intravenous access and administer parenteral nutrition if ordered.	Obtain and monitor blood glucose levels per hospital policy. Administer parenteral and or enteral nutrition as ordered. Encourage mother to begin pumping to supply breast milk for neonate. Encourage kangaroo care to enhance milk supply. Use non-nutritive sucking with tube feedings. Monitor for signs of feeding intolerance. Monitor intake and output.	Obtain and monitor blood glucose levels per hospital policy. Administer parenteral and or enteral nutrition as ordered. Encourage kangaroo care to enhance milk supply. Use non-nutritive sucking with tube feedings. Monitor for signs of feeding intolerance. As neonate matures, assess for signs of readiness for oral feedings. Monitor intake and output. Monitor daily weights. Teach parents proper techniques for breastfeeding or bottle feeding their neonate.
Sepsis	Obtain maternal history for risk factors. Obtain CBC and blood culture as ordered. Administer antibiotics as ordered. Assess for signs of sepsis.	Assess for signs of sepsis. Administer antibiotics as ordered.	Assess for signs of sepsis. Administer antibiotics as ordered. Teach parents strategies to prevent infection.

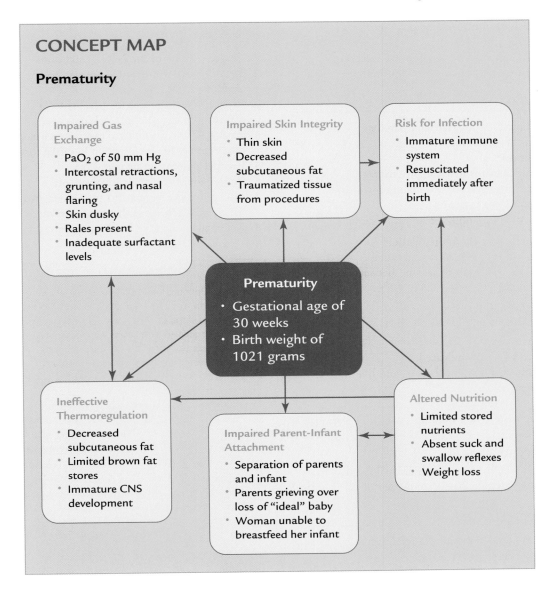

CONCEPT MAP

Prematurity

Impaired Gas Exchange
- PaO_2 of 50 mm Hg
- Intercostal retractions, grunting, and nasal flaring
- Skin dusky
- Rales present
- Inadequate surfactant levels

Impaired Skin Integrity
- Thin skin
- Decreased subcutaneous fat
- Traumatized tissue from procedures

Risk for Infection
- Immature immune system
- Resuscitated immediately after birth

Prematurity
- Gestational age of 30 weeks
- Birth weight of 1021 grams

Ineffective Thermoregulation
- Decreased subcutaneous fat
- Limited brown fat stores
- Immature CNS development

Impaired Parent-Infant Attachment
- Separation of parents and infant
- Parents grieving over loss of "ideal" baby
- Woman unable to breastfeed her infant

Altered Nutrition
- Limited stored nutrients
- Absent suck and swallow reflexes
- Weight loss

Problem No. 1: Impaired gas exchange
Goal: Adequate gas exchange
Outcome: PaO_2 is 60–70 mm Hg; $PaCO_2$ is 35–45 mm Hg; skin color is pink; lung sounds are clear; and no signs of retractions, grunting, or nasal flaring.

Nursing Actions

1. Monitor vital signs, oxygen saturation, and arterial blood gases.
2. Maintain patent airway.
3. Suction airway as indicated.
4. Administer oxygen as per orders.
5. Maintain a neutral thermal environment.
6. Cluster nursing activities.
7. Monitor for adverse effects related to surfactant replacement therapy.

Problem No. 2: Impaired skin integrity
Goal: Intact skin
Outcome: The neonate's skin will be intact and without signs of skin irritation.

Nursing Actions

1. Assess skin for redness, dryness, breakdown, and rashes.
2. Use a neutral pH cleanser and sterile water when bathing. Bathe only soiled body parts.
3. Use adhesives sparingly.
4. Apply emollient to dry areas.
5. Change diapers frequently and apply zinc-oxide.
6. Change positions frequently.
7. Use water, air, or gelled mattresses as indicated.

Problem No. 3: Risk of infection
Goal: Be free of infection
Outcome: Neonates will not exhibit signs of infection such as elevated temperature, lethargy, or purulent drainage.

Nursing Actions

1. Promote hand washing for staff and parents.
2. Assess for signs of infection.
3. Maintain intact skin.
4. Properly prepare sites for invasive procedures.
5. Properly care for invasive lines to maintain sterility.
6. Administer antibiotics as per orders.
7. Encourage use of breast milk for infant feedings.

Problem No. 4: Ineffective thermoregulation
Goal: Stable temperature within normal range
Outcome: Neonate's temperature will be between 36.4° and 37.2°C (97.5°–99°F).

Nursing Actions

1. Keep the neonate dry.
2. Use plastic barriers when indicated.
3. Prewarm radiant warmers, incubators, and linens.
4. Encourage kangaroo care.
5. Keep area free of drafts.
6. Swaddle the neonate when holding outside of warmer or incubator.

Problem No. 5: Altered nutrition
Goal: Growth and weight gain within normal ranges
Outcome: Neonate will gain 20–30 grams per day.

Nursing Actions

1. Administer parenteral nutrition, enteral feedings, or oral feedings as per orders.
2. Encourage use of breast milk.
3. Monitor weight daily.
4. Monitor length and head circumference weekly.
5. Instill breast milk or formula, when gavage feeding, over 20 minutes at a rate of 1 mL/min.
6. Monitor the neonate during feedings for signs of feeding intolerance, such as vomiting, regurgitation, and excessive gastric residual.
7. Encourage breastfeeding when indicated.
8. Monitor intake and output.

Problem No. 6: Impaired parent-infant attachment
Goal: Positive parent-infant attachment
Outcome: Parents hold the infant close to the body and the infant appears calm and relaxed; parents spend time each day with the infant and participate in care of the infant; parents respond to infant cues.

Nursing Actions

1. Orient parents to the NICU environment.
2. Provide opportunities for parents to share their concerns and frustrations.
3. Provide opportunities for parents to talk about their experiences of having a high-risk neonate.
4. Assess parents' readiness to care for their neonate and provide opportunities for participation in caring for their neonate.
5. Instruct parents on neonatal care.
6. Praise parents for their involvement.
7. Encourage the woman to pump her breast and bring her breast milk for use with infant feeding.
8. Encourage kangaroo holding by both parents.

TYING IT ALL TOGETHER

Baby girl Polk is a newly delivered 32 weeks' gestation neonate who is admitted to the NICU. Her mother, Mallory, is a 42-year-old African American single woman. Mallory is a G2 P0 who conceived after three attempts at in vitro fertilization. Mallory was admitted to the birthing unit for preterm labor. She was given magnesium sulfate, ampicillin, and two doses of betamethasone. Her labor contraction continued. When her cervix was 5 cm dilated, a decision was made to discontinue the magnesium sulfate. A few hours after the magnesium sulfate was discontinued, Mallory gave birth spontaneously to a baby girl. The 1- and 5-minute Apgar scores were 7 and 8, respectively. Baby Polk weighed 2,010 grams and was assessed at 32 weeks based on Ballard score.

Detail the aspects of your initial nursing assessment.
List the nursing diagnosis for this neonate.
What are the immediate priorities in the nursing care of Baby Polk?
Discuss the rationale for the selected priorities.
List the anticipated medical care for Baby Polk.

4 hours later:
Baby Polk is on NCPAP. There is an increase in intercostal retractions and expiratory grunting. The results of arterial blood gas (ABG) tests are Pco_2 of 70 and pH of 7.2. CBC indicates an increase in WBC.

Medical orders include initial dose of Survanta, IV of D10, glucose monitoring every 4 hours, ampicillin 50 mg/kg, and gentamicin 4 mg/kg.

Based on this additional information, list the nursing diagnosis for this neonate.
List the anticipated medical care.
Discuss the nursing care for this neonate and mother.

1 week later:
Baby Polk is extubated and is placed on high-flow nasal cannula at 1 liter. She is tolerating gavage feedings and gaining weight. She is experiencing occasional episodes of apnea and bradycardia.

Discuss the criteria for discharge from the NICU.
Describe the discharge teaching for the care of baby Polk.

■ ■ ■ Review Questions ■ ■ ■

1. A nurse is assessing a preterm baby with a gestational age of 32 weeks and birth weight of 1,389 grams. Which of the following signs if present would be a possible indication of RDS?
  A. Expiratory grunting and intercostal retractions
  B. Respiratory rate of 46 breaths per minute and presence of acrocyanosis
  C. Mild nasal flaring and heart rate of 140 beats per minute
  D. Bradycardia and bounding pulse

2. The primary risk factor for necrotizing enterocolitis (NEC) is:
  A. Early oral feedings with formula
  B. Passage of meconium during labor
  C. Prematurity
  D. Low birth weight

3. A common characteristic of a premature infant is:
  A. Absence of lanugo
  B. Dry skin
  C. Increased flexion of arms and legs
  D. Transparent and red skin

4. When gavage feeding a preterm neonate, the nurse should:
  A. Measure the tube before insertion from the mouth to the sternum.
  B. Check for placement by injecting a small amount of sterile water into the feeding tube and listen for a gurgling noise.
  C. Instill formula over a 20-minute period of time.
  D. Flush the tube at the end of feeding with dextrose water.

5. Which of the following statements is true regarding hyperbilirubinemia?
  A. Jaundice covers the entire body in pathological jaundice versus only the face in physiological jaundice.
  B. Jaundice occurs within the first 24 hours post-birth in pathological jaundice versus after 24 hours in physiological jaundice.
  C. Kernicterus only occurs in pathological jaundice.
  D. Jaundice begins to appear in term neonates when the bilirubin level is 3 mg/dL.

6. Clinical management strategies for prevention of retinopathy of prematurity (ROP) focus on targeting appropriate _____ ranges for infants at risk.
  A. Arterial pH
  B. Oxygen saturation
  C. Heart rate
  D. Core temperature

7. A neonate born at 37 weeks' gestation is determined to be small for gestational age (SGA). The most common immediate problem for this infant would be:
  A. Anemia
  B. Hypovolemia
  C. Hypoglycemia
  D. Hypocalcemia

8. Which of the following treatments is recommended for the infant experiencing drug withdrawal symptoms?
  A. Morphine
  B. Diluted formula
  C. Frequent awakening
  D. Well-lit room

9. Which is not a risk to the infant of a diabetic mother?
  A. Hyperglycemia
  B. Poor feeding
  C. Macrosomia
  D. Respiratory distress

10. If a pregnant woman is group beta strep (GBS) positive, prophylactic antibiotics should be administered if:
  A. She is a planned cesarean section
  B. The gestational age of her baby is less than 37 weeks
  C. She has vomiting and diarrhea during labor
  D. Her baby has a known congenital anomaly

References

American Academy of Pediatrics (AAP). (2012). Neonatal drug withdrawal. *Pediatrics, 129,* 540–560.

American Academy of Pediatrics (AAP). (2004). *Management of hyperbilirubinemia in the newborn infant 35 or more weeks of gestation. Pediatrics, 114,* 297–316.

Armentrout, D. (2010). Glucose management. In M. Verklan & M. Walden (Eds.), *Core curriculum for neonatal intensive care nursing.* St. Louis: Elsevier Saunders.

Askin, D. (2010). Respiratory distress. In M. Verklan & M. Walden (Eds.), *Core curriculum for neonatal intensive care nursing.* St. Louis: Elsevier Saunders.

Askin, D., & Diehl-Jones, W. (2010a). Assisted ventilation. In M. Verklan & M. Walden (Eds.), *Core curriculum for neonatal intensive care nursing.* St. Louis: Elsevier Saunders.

Askin, D., & Diehl-Jones, W. (2010b). Ophthalmologic and auditory disorders. In M. Verklan & M. Walden (Eds.), *Core curriculum for neonatal intensive care nursing.* St. Louis: Elsevier Saunders.

Association of Women's Health, Obstetric and Neonatal Nurses/ National Association of Neonatal Nurses (AWHONN/NANN). (2007). *Neonatal skin care: Evidence based clinical practice guideline.* Washington, DC: Author.

Bancalari, E., & Walsh, M. (2011). Bronchopulmonary dysplasia. In R. Martin, A. Fanaroff, & M. Walsh (Eds.), *Neonatal-perinatal medicine: Vol. 2. Diseases of the fetus and infant* (9th ed.). Philadelphia: Mosby Elsevier.

Bandstra, E., & Accornero, V. (2011). Infants of substance-abusing mothers. In R. Martin, A. Fanaroff, & M. Walsh (Eds.), *Neonatal-perinatal medicine:* Vol. 1. *Diseases of the fetus and infant* (9th ed.). Philadelphia: Mosby Elsevier.

Bellini, S. (2010). Retinopathy of Prematurity. *Improving Outcomes Through Evidence-Based Practice. Nursing for Women's Health, 14*(5), 382–9.

Blackburn, S. (2013). *Maternal, fetal, & neonatal physiology* (4th ed.). St. Louis: Elsevier.

Bradshaw, W. (2011). Gastrointestinal disorders. In M. Verklan & M. Walden (Eds.), *Core curriculum for neonatal intensive care nursing.* St. Louis: Elsevier Saunders.

Brand, M., & Boyd, H. (2010). Thermoregulation. In M. Verklan & M. Walden (Eds.), *Core curriculum for neonatal intensive care nursing.* St. Louis: Elsevier Saunders.

Bowen, S. (2010). Intrafacility and interfacility neonatal transport. In M. Verklan & M. Walden (Eds.), *Core curriculum for neonatal intensive care nursing.* St. Louis: Elsevier Saunders.

Caplan, M. (2011). Neonatal necrotizing enterocolitis. In R. Martin, A. Fanaroff, & M. Walsh (Eds.), *Neonatal-perinatal medicine:* Vol. 2. *Diseases of the fetus and infant* (9th ed.). Philadelphia: Mosby Elsevier.

Carrier, C. (2010). Developmental support. In M. Verklan & M. Walden (Eds.), *Core curriculum for neonatal intensive care nursing.* St. Louis: Elsevier Saunders.

Centers for Disease Control and Prevention (CDC). (2010). Prevention of perinatal group B streptococcal disease. *MMWR, 59,* 1–36.

Charsha, D. (2010). Care of the extremely low birth weight infant. In M. Verklan & M. Walden (Eds.), *Core curriculum for neonatal intensive care nursing.* St. Louis: Elsevier Saunders.

Dargaville, P., Copnell, B., Mills, J., & Haron, I. (2011). Randomized controlled trial of lung lavage with dilute surfactant for meconium aspiration syndrome. *The Journal of Pediatrics 158*(3), 383–389.

deVries, L. (2011). Intraventricular hemorrhage and vascular lesions. In R. Martin, A. Fanaroff, & M. Walsh (Eds.), *Neonatal-perinatal medicine:* Vol. 2. *Diseases of the fetus and infant.* (9th ed.) Philadelphia: Mosby Elsevier.

Diehl-Jones, W., & Askin, D. (2010). Hematological disorders. In M. Verklan & M. Walden (Eds.), *Core curriculum for neonatal intensive care nursing.* St. Louis: Elsevier Saunders.

Ditzenberger, G. (2010). Nutritional management. In M. Verklan & M. Walden (Eds.), *Core curriculum for neonatal intensive care nursing.* St. Louis: Elsevier Saunders.

Edwards, M. (2011). Postnatal bacterial infections. In R. Martin, A. Fanaroff, & M. Walsh (Eds.), *Neonatal-perinatal medicine:* Vol. 2. *Diseases of the fetus and infant.* (9th ed.) Philadelphia: Mosby Elsevier.

Field, P. (2011). Group B strep infection in the newborn. *Nursing, 41*(11), 62.

Furdon, S., & Benjamin, K. (2010). Physical assessment. In M. Verklan & M. Walden (Eds.), *Core curriculum for neonatal intensive care nursing.* St. Louis: Elsevier Saunders.

Goodwin, M. (2010). Apnea. In M. Verklan & M. Walden (Eds.), *Core curriculum for neonatal intensive care nursing.* St. Louis: Elsevier Saunders.

Halbardier, B. (2010). Fluid and electrolyte management. In M. Verklan & M. Walden (Eds.), *Core curriculum for neonatal intensive care nursing.* St. Louis: Elsevier Saunders.

Hamilton, B., Martin, J., & Ventura, S. (2012). Births: Preliminary data for 2011. *National Vital Statistics Reports, 61*(5). Hyattsville, MD: National Center for Health Statistics.

Hatfield, L., Chang, K., Bittle, M., Deluca, J., & Polomano, R. (2011). The Analgesic Properties of Intraoral Sucrose. *An Integrative Review. Advances in Neonatal Care, 11(2),* 83–92.

Hammerman, C., Bin-Nun, A., & Kaplan, M. (2012). Managing the patent ductus arteriosos in the premature neonate: a new look at what we thought we knew. *Seminars in Perinatology, 36,* 130–138.

Hay, W. (2012). Care of the infant of the diabetic mother. *Current Diabetes Reports, 12,* 4–15.

Hoyert, D., & Jiaquin, X. (2012). Deaths: Preliminary Data for 2011. *National Vital Statistics Reports, 61*(6). Hyattsville, MD: National Center for Health Statistics.

Hummel, P. (2010). Discharge planning and transition to home care. *Core curriculum for neonatal intensive care nursing.* St. Louis: Elsevier Saunders.

Johnston, P., Gilliam-Krakauer, M., Fuller, M., & Reese, J. (2012). Evidence-Based Use of Indomethacin and Ibuprofen in the Neonatal Intensive Care Unit. *Clinical Perinatology, 39,* 111–136.

Jones, L. (2012). Oral feeding readiness in the Neonatal Intensive Care Unit. *Neonatal Network, 31*(3), 148–154.

Kaplan, M., Wong, R., Sibley, E., and Stevenson, D. (2011). Neonatal jaundice and liver disease. In R. Martin & A. Fanaroff, *Fanaroff and Martin's neonatal-perinatal medicine (9th ed.).* St. Louis: Mosby Elsevier.

Kenner, C. (2010). Families in crisis. In M. Verklan & M. Walden (Eds.), *Core curriculum for neonatal intensive care nursing.* St. Louis: Elsevier Saunders.

Levene, M., & de Vries, L. (2011). Hypoxic-ischemic encephalopathy. In R. Martin, A. Fanaroff, & M. Walsh (Eds.), *Neonatal-perinatal medicine:* Vol. 2. *Diseases of the fetus and infant* (9th ed.). Philadelphia: Mosby Elsevier.

Lewis, D., Sanders, L., & Brockopp, D. (2011). The effect of three nursing interventions on thermoregulation in low birth weight infants. *Neonatal Network 30*(3), 160–164.

Lott, J. (2010). Immunology and infectious disease. In M. Verklan & M. Walden (Eds.), *Core curriculum for neonatal intensive care nursing.* St. Louis: Elsevier Saunders.

Ludington-Hoe, S. (2011). Thirty years of kangaroo care: Science and practice. *Neonatal Network, 30*(5), 357–362.

Lynam, L., & Verklan, M. (2010). Neurologic disorders. In M. Verklan & M. Walden (Eds.), *Core curriculum for neonatal intensive care nursing.* St. Louis: Elsevier Saunders.

Malusky, S., & Donze, A. (2011). Neutral Head Positioning in Premature Infants for Intraventricular Hemorrhage Prevention: An Evidence-Based Review. *Neonatal Network, 30*(6), 381–396.

March of Dimes. (2012). *Preterm birth: Are you at risk?* Retrieved from http://marchofdimes.com/pregnancy/pretermlabor_risk.html

McGrath, J., & Hardy, W. (2011). The infant at risk. In S. Mattson & J. Smith (Eds.), *Core curriculum for maternal newborn nursing.* St. Louis: Elsevier Saunders.

Miller, A., & Morris, L. (2011). Developmental Considerations in Working with Newborn Infants of Mothers with Diabetes. *Neonatal Network, 30*(1), 37–45.

Phelps, D. (2011). Retinopathy of prematurity. In R. Martin, A. Fanaroff, & M. Walsh (Eds.), *Neonatal-perinatal medicine:* Vol. 2. *Diseases of the fetus and infant* (9th ed.). Philadelphia: Mosby Elsevier.

Pinelli, J., & Symington, A. (2010). Non-nutritive sucking for promoting physiologic stability and nutrition in preterm infants (Review). *Cochrane Database of Systematic Reviews,* Issue 6.

Pitts, K. (2010). Perinatal substance abuse. In M. Verklan & M. Walden (Eds.), *Core curriculum for neonatal intensive care nursing.* St. Louis: Elsevier Saunders.

Sadowski, S. (2010). Cardiovascular disorders. In M. Verklan & M. Walden (Eds.), *Core curriculum for neonatal intensive care nursing.* St. Louis: Elsevier Saunders.

Sallmon H., & Sola-Visner M. (2012). Clinical research issues in neonatal anemia and thrombocytopenia. *Current Opinion in Pediatrics 24*(1), 16–22.

Steinhorn, R. (2011). Pulmonary vascular development. In R. Martin, A. Fanaroff, & M. Walsh (Eds.), *Neonatal-perinatal medicine:* Vol. 2. *Diseases of the fetus and infant.* (9th ed.) Philadelphia: Mosby Elsevier.

Sterk, L. (2010). Congenital anomalies. In M. Verklan & M. Walden (Eds.), *Core curriculum for neonatal intensive care nursing.* St. Louis: Elsevier Saunders.

Substance Abuse and Mental Health Services Administration (SAMHSA). (2010). *Results from the 2010 National Survey on Drug Use and Health: National Findings* (Office of Applied Studies, NSDUH Series H-41, DHHS Publication No. SMA 11-4658) Rockville, MD. Retrieved from www.samhsa.gov/data/NSDUH/2k10NSDUH/2k10Results.htm#4.3

Surbek, D., Drack, G., Irion, O., Nelle, M., Huang, D., & Hoesli, I. (2012). Antenatal corticosteroids for fetal lung maturation in threatened preterm delivery: indications and administration. *Archives of Gynecology and Obstetrics, 286,* 277–281.

Swartz, H., Haberman, B., & Ruddy, R. (2011). Hyperbilirubinemia. Current guidelines and emerging therapies. *Pediatric Emergency Care, 27*(9), 884–889.

Tagin, M., Woolcott, C., Vincer, M., Whyte, R., & Stinson, D. (2012). Hypothermia for neonatal hypoxic ischemic encephalopathy. An updated systematic review and meta-analysis. *Archives of Pediatric and Adolescent Medicine* 166(6):558-566. DOI: 10.1001/archpediatrics.2011.1772

Young, T., & Magnum, B. (2010). Neofax 2010. Montvale, NJ: Thomas Reuters.

Women's Health

Well Women's Health

EXPECTED STUDENT OUTCOMES

On completion of this chapter, the student will be able to:

- ☐ Define key terms.
- ☐ Identify factors that place a woman at risk for adverse health conditions.
- ☐ Discuss preventive screenings for women across the life span.
- ☐ Describe how lifestyle factors such as diet, exercise, and cigarette smoking influence the health of women.
- ☐ Discuss the effects of obesity on women's health.
- ☐ Discuss the physical and emotional changes related to perimenopause and menopause.
- ☐ Describe the health care needs of lesbians and their health care barriers.

Nursing Diagnosis

- ☐ At risk for adverse health conditions related to lack of knowledge regarding health promotion
- ☐ Knowledge deficit related to menopausal changes
- ☐ At risk for disturbed sleep pattern related to night sweats

Nursing Outcomes

- ☐ The woman will verbalize two lifestyle changes that can reduce her risk for adverse health conditions.
- ☐ The woman will verbalize changes related to menopause and methods to decrease menopausal symptoms.
- ☐ The woman will verbalize three strategies for improving disturbed sleep pattern.

HEALTH PROMOTION

Health promotion is a critical component of women's health (**Fig. 18-1**). **Health promotion** is defined by the World Health Organization as "the process of enabling people to increase control over, and to improve, their health" (WHO, 2010). Based on this definition, the focus on nursing care is directed at providing women with information and resources that enable them to increase control over and to improve their health (see Critical Component: Heart Attack and Stroke Warning Signs *and* Critical Component: HPV Vaccine).

Risk Reduction

The leading causes of death in females in the United States are:

- ■ Heart disease—24.5%
- ■ Cancer—21.7%
  - ■ *Top three cancers are breast, lung/bronchus, and colon/rectum.*
- ■ Stroke—6.5%
- ■ Chronic lower respiratory disease—5.9%
- ■ Alzheimer's disease—4.6%
- ■ Unintentional injuries—3.5%
- ■ Diabetes—2.8%

Don't have time to read this chapter? Want to reinforce your reading? Need to review for a test? Listen to this chapter on *DavisPlus*.

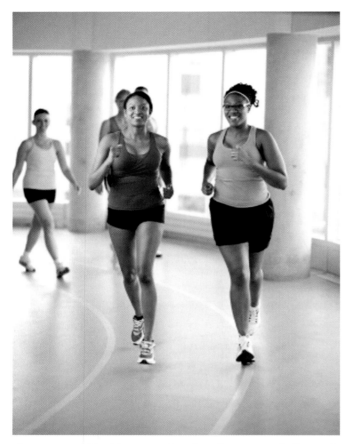

Figure 18–1   Health promotion for all women of all ages is a critical component for women's health.

- Influenza and pneumonia—2.5%
- Kidney disease—2%
- Septicemia—1.6% (CDC, 2012a)

CRITICAL COMPONENT

Heart Attack and Stroke Warning Signs

Heart Attack:

- Uncomfortable pressure, squeezing, fullness, or pain in the center of the chest
- Pain or discomfort in one or both arms, back, neck, jaw, and/or stomach
- Shortness of breath with or without chest discomfort
- Nausea
- Lightheadedness
- Sweating

Stroke:

- Sudden onset of numbness or weakness in the face, arm, and/or leg, especially on one side
- Sudden onset of trouble seeing out of one or both eyes
- Sudden onset of trouble walking, dizziness, loss of balance or coordination
- Severe headache with no known cause

(A Lifetime of Good Health, HHS, 2012)

The leading causes of death in females vary by age groups and race (**Table 18-1**). Health promotion and risk reduction can prevent or decrease the risk for many of these causes.

TABLE 18–1	TOP 3 LEADING CAUSES OF DEATH IN FEMALES BY AGE GROUP AND RACE				
	AMERICAN INDIAN/ ALASKA NATIVE	**ASIA OR PACIFIC ISLANDER**	**BLACK**	**HISPANIC**	**WHITE**
15–19	Unintentional injuries	Unintentional injuries	Unintentional injuries	Unintentional injuries	Unintentional injuries Suicide
	Suicide	Suicide	Homicide	Cancer	
	Homicide	Cancer	Cancer	Homicide	Cancer
20–24	Unintentional injuries	Unintentional injuries	Unintentional injuries	Unintentional injuries	Unintentional injuries Suicide
	Suicide	Suicide	Homicide	Homicide	
	Homicide	Cancer	Heart disease	Cancer	Cancer
25–34	Unintentional injuries	Cancer	Heart disease	Cancer	Unintentional injuries
	Chronic liver disease	Suicide	Unintentional injuries	Unintentional injuries	Cancer
	Suicide	Unintentional injuries	Cancer	Homicide	Suicide
35–44	Unintentional injuries	Cancer	Cancer	Cancer	Cancer
	Chronic liver disease	Heart disease	Heart disease	Unintentional injuries	Unintentional injuries
	Cancer	Suicide	HIV disease	Heart disease	Heart disease
45–54	Cancer	Cancer	Cancer	Cancer	Cancer
	Heart disease	Heart disease	Heart disease	Heart disease	Heart disease
	Chronic liver disease	Stroke	Stroke	Unintentional injuries	Unintentional injuries

TABLE 18–1	TOP 3 LEADING CAUSES OF DEATH IN FEMALES BY AGE GROUP AND RACE—cont'd				
	AMERICAN INDIAN/ ALASKA NATIVE	**ASIA OR PACIFIC ISLANDER**	**BLACK**	**HISPANIC**	**WHITE**
55–64	Cancer	Cancer	Cancer	Cancer	Cancer
	Heart disease	Heart disease	Heart disease	Heart disease	Heart disease
	Chronic liver disease	Stroke	Stroke	Diabetes	Chronic lower respiratory diseases
65–74	Cancer	Cancer	Cancer	Cancer	Cancer
	Heart disease	Heart disease	Heart disease	Heart disease	Heart disease
	Diabetes	Stroke	Diabetes	Diabetes	Chronic lower respiratory diseases
75–84	Heart disease	Cancer	Heart disease	Heart disease	Heart disease
	Cancer	Heart disease	Cancer	Cancer	Cancer
	Diabetes	Stroke	Stroke	Stroke	Chronic lower respiratory diseases
85+	Heart disease	Cancer	Heart disease	Heart disease	Heart disease
	Cancer	Heart disease	Cancer	Cancer	Cancer
	Alzheimer's disease	Stroke	Stroke	Alzheimer's disease	Alzheimer's disease

CDC, 2012a

Actions for Reducing Risks

■ Follow guidelines for routine screenings and immunizations (**Table 18-2**).
■ Eat a healthy diet.
■ *A healthy diet is one that is rich in vegetables, fruits, whole grains, fiber, fat-free or low-fat dairy, and fish;*
*and low in foods that are high in saturated fat and sodium (**Fig. 18-2**)*
■ *The women's diet needs to include 3 cups of low-fat or fat-free milk or low-fat yogurt and/or low-fat cheese*
■ Women who cannot get enough calcium in their diets should take a calcium supplement. This will help decrease the risk of and/or degree of osteoporosis.
■ Be physically active (see Critical Component: Physical Activity).
■ *It is recommended that women of all ages engage daily in 30 minutes of moderate physical activity such as walking briskly, swimming, bicycling, or dancing.*
■ *Physical activity/weight-bearing exercise improves bone health by slowing bone loss, improving muscle strength, and improving balance (HHS, 2012).*
■ *Women should consult with their health care provider before starting a new exercise program.*

CRITICAL COMPONENT

HPV Vaccine

■ Human papillomavirus (HPV) is the most common sexually transmitted virus in the United States.
■ HPV is the main cause of cervical cancer.
■ Gardasil and Cervarix are vaccines given to prevent most cases of cervical cancer.
■ Gardasil protects against HPV types 6 and 11, which are associated with genital warts and low-grade cervical lesions. It also protects against HPV types 16 and 18, which are associated with cervical cancer.
■ Cervarix only protects against types 16 and 18.
■ Gardasil is recommended for girls and boys 11 or 12 years of age.
■ Cervarix is recommended for girls and women 13 through 26 years of age.
■ Both vaccines are given in three doses: second dose given 1–2 months after first dose; third dose given 6 months after first dose.
■ It is most effective when given before the woman becomes sexually active.

CDC, 2012c.

CRITICAL COMPONENT

Physical Activity

Physical activity can lower the woman's risk for:

■ Heart disease
■ Colon cancer
■ Falls
■ Type 2 diabetes
■ Breast cancer
■ Depression

(HHS, 2012)

TABLE 18–2   RECOMMENDED SCREENINGS AND IMMUNIZATIONS FOR WOMEN ACROSS THE LIFE SPAN

SCREENING TESTS	AGES 19–39	AGES 40–49	AGES 50–64	AGES 65 AND OLDER
Blood pressure test	At least every 2 years	At least every 2 years	At least every 2 years	At least every 2 years
Cholesterol test	Start at age 20. Frequency is based on health history.	Frequency is based on health history.	Frequency is based on health history.	Frequency is based on health history.
Dual-energy x-ray absorptiometry scan (DXA)			Frequency is based on health history.	Frequency is based on health history.
Blood glucose test	Frequency is based on health history.	Start at age 45, then every 3 years	Every 3 years	Every 3 years
Mammogram		Every 1–2 years	Every 1–2 years	Every 1–2 years
Clinical breast exam (CBE)	Every 3 years	Every year	Every year	Every year
Pap test	Every 3 years for women ages 21–30 years Every 5 years with HPV test for women ages 30–39	Every 5 years with HPV test	Every 5 years with HPV test	Frequency based on health history
Pelvic exam	Yearly starting at age 21 or earlier if sexually active	Yearly	Yearly	Yearly
Chlamydia test	If sexually active, yearly until age 24. Yearly ages 25–39, if new partner or multiple partners	Yearly if new partner or multiple partners	Yearly if new partner or multiple partners	Yearly if new partner or multiple partners
Sexually transmitted infection (STI) tests	Frequency determined by sexual history.	Frequency determined by sexual history.	Frequency determined by sexual history.	Frequency determined by sexual history.
Colonoscopy			Every 10 years starting at age 50	Every 10 years
Eye exam	Eye exam if experiencing problems or visual changes	Baseline exam at age 40 then every 2–4 years	Every 2–4 years	Every 1–2 years
Hearing test	Every 10 years	Every 10 years	Every 3 years	Every 3 years
Skin exam	Monthly mole self-exam; every 3 years by health care provider starting at age 20	Monthly mole self-exam; yearly by health care provider	Monthly mole self-exam; yearly by health care provider	Monthly mole self-exam; yearly by health care provider
Dental and oral cancer exam	Yearly	Yearly	Yearly	Yearly
Influenza vaccine	Every fall or winter	Every fall or winter	Every fall or winter	Every fall or winter
Pneumococcal vaccine	May need one dose if a smoker or has chronic health issues	May need one dose if a smoker or has chronic health issues	May need one dose if a smoker or has chronic health issues	One dose at age 65
Human papillomavirus (HPV) vaccine	Three-dose series: given to women 19–26 years old			
Tetanus, diphtheria, pertussis (Td, Tdap) vaccine	Td every 10 years; Tdap if need a booster for whooping cough	Td every 10 years; Tdap if need a booster for whooping cough	Td every 10 years; Tdap if need a booster for whooping cough	Td every 10 years; Tdap if need a booster for whooping cough

American Cancer Society, 2012a; HHS, 2012

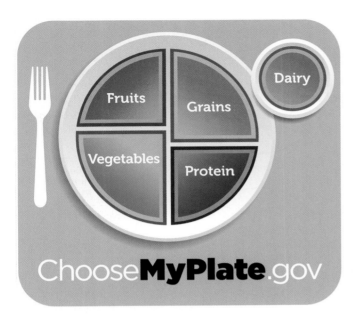

Figure 18–2 MyPlate is a tool that can be used when discussing nutrition with a client. *Source:* United States Department of Agriculture, http://ChooseMyPlate.gov

■ Maintain healthy weight.
  ■ *35.8% of women over age 20 are obese (Ogden et al., 2012).*
    ■ 31.9% of women age 30-39 are obese.
    ■ 36% of women age 40-59 are obese.
    ■ 42.3% of women age 60 and older are obese (Ogden, 2012).
  ■ *Obesity places the woman at risk for a variety of health care problems (see Critical Component: Obesity).*
■ Avoid cigarette smoking and secondhand smoke.
  ■ *Tobacco use is a leading cause of heart disease and cancer.*
  ■ *More women die from lung cancer than any other type of cancer (CDC, 2012d).*
    ■ The rate of death is 39 per 100,000 women (CDC, 2012d).
■ Limit alcohol consumption.
  ■ *Those who choose to drink alcohol should do so in moderation, which is one drink per day for women.*
  ■ *Drinking during pregnancy increases the woman's risk of having a baby with Fetal Alcohol Spectrum Disorder (CDC, 2012e).*
  ■ *Excessive drinking increases the woman's risk for infertility, miscarriages, stillbirth, and preterm birth (CDC, 2012e).*
  ■ *Excessive drinking increases a woman's risk for alcoholism, elevated blood pressure, obesity, diabetes, stroke, breast cancer, suicide, and accidents (CDC, 2012e).*

  ■ *Binge drinking increases the risk for sexual assault, especially for women in college settings (CDC, 2012e).*
■ Prevent injury from accidents.
  ■ *Motor vehicle crashes are the leading cause of death from injury among younger women.*
    ■ Risk reduction: Wear seat belts, follow speed limits, and do not drink alcohol prior to driving.
  ■ *Injury related falls are the leading cause of injury, death, and disability for women 65 years old or older.*
    ■ Risk reduction: Exercise to improve strength and balance, home modification to reduce fall hazards, and medication assessment to minimize side effects such as dizziness (Stevens & Olson, 2000).
■ Prevent sexually transmitted illnesses.
  ■ *Use condoms correctly and for all sexual contact.*
  ■ *Be in a monogamous relationship—both the woman and her partner have sex only with each other and no one else.*
  ■ *Both the woman and her partner are screened for STIs, including HIV, prior to engaging in sexual activities.*

CRITICAL COMPONENT

Obesity

Obesity is defined as a body mass index (BMI) of 30 or higher. Obesity places a woman at higher risk for:

■ Coronary heart disease
■ Type 2 diabetes
■ Cancer: endometrial, cervical, and breast
■ Low back pain
■ Knee osteoarthritis
■ Abnormal menstrual cycle and subinfertility
■ High risk pregnancies: diabetes and hypertension
■ Neonatal mortality and malformations
■ Decreased intention to breastfeed, decreased initiation of breastfeeding and decreased duration of breastfeeding

(Kulie et al., 2011)

Routine Screenings

Throughout the woman's lifetime there are screening tests that can assist the woman's health care provider in identifying potential alterations in health and in initiating early interventions (see Critical Component: Screening Mammograms). Recommended screenings and immunizations for women are presented in Table 18-2.

■ Breast cancer screening
  ■ *It is important that women know how their breasts normally look and feel and do monthly breast self-exams. They should report changes to their health care provider (**Fig. 18-3**).*

CULTURAL AWARNESS: Heath Care Beliefs And Practices

Arab Heritage	■ Disease is attributed to an inadequate diet, shifts of hot and cold, emotional or spiritual distress, and envy. ■ Risk management and preventative care are valued. ■ Women are often reluctant to seek care because of cultural emphasis placed on modesty.
Chinese Heritage	■ Older people usually try traditional Chinese medicine first and seek Western medicine when Chinese medicine does not work. ■ The balance between yin and yang is used to explain both mental and physical health. ■ Women may feel uncomfortable touching their own bodies—and they may have difficulty with breast self-exams.
Filipino Heritage	■ Some Filipinos tend to accept fate easily when they feel they cannot change a situation. ■ Individuals accept and adhere to medical recommendations, but many use alternative sources of care suggested by friends and family members. ■ Care of the body through adequate sleep, rest, nutrition, and exercise is common practice.
Hindu Heritage	■ Pap tests and mammography may be traumatic since they may not have experienced or heard of them. ■ They believe that illness attacks an individual through the mind, body, and soul. ■ Medical beliefs are a blend of modern and traditional theories and practices.
Japanese Heritage	■ Good health requires unobstructed flow of **ki** (the life force or energy) throughout the body. ■ Strategies that help restore the balance between yin and yang include use of herbal medicine, bed rest, bathing, and massage. ■ Most individuals use both modern medical and traditional providers of health care.
Mexican Heritage	■ The family is considered the most credible source of health care information. ■ Most individuals use herbal medicines and teas. ■ Many individuals practice the hot and cold theory.
Navajo Indian Heritage	■ When people are ill or out of harmony, the medicine man tells them what they did to disrupt their harmony. ■ Herbal medicine may be used without the knowledge of the health care provider. ■ Mental illness is perceived as resulting from witches or having a curse placed on them.

Source: Purnell & Paulanka (2005).

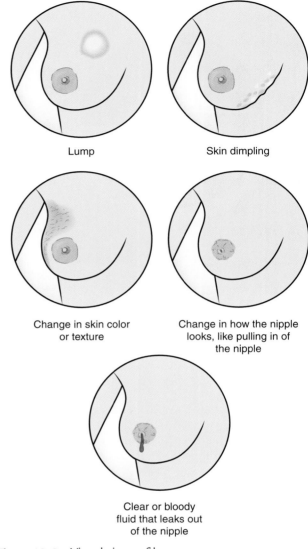

Figure 18–3   Visual signs of breast cancer.

Lump

Skin dimpling

Change in skin color or texture

Change in how the nipple looks, like pulling in of the nipple

Clear or bloody fluid that leaks out of the nipple

■ *Women who are at high risk for breast cancer (greater than a 20% lifetime risk) should be screened with MRI in addition to mammograms (American Cancer Society, 2012a).*
  ■ Lifetime risk for breast cancer can be calculated using the breast cancer risk assessment tool (www.cancer.gov/bcrisktool).
■ *Healthy People 2020 objectives:*
  ■ Increase the proportion of women who are counseled by their provider about mammograms from 69.8% to 76.8% of females ages 50–74 years (Healthy People 2012)
■ Cervical cancer screening (see Critical Component: Papanicolaou (Pap) Smear)
  ■ *Women 21–29 years of age should have a Pap test every 3 years.*

CRITICAL COMPONENT

Screening Mammograms

- Mammogram is a low-dose x-ray of the breast looking for abnormal changes.
- A specially designed x-ray machine is used.
- Each breast (one at a time) is placed between the x-ray plate and plastic plate. Pressure is gradually placed on the breast to flatten the breast. A clearer picture of the breast is obtained by flattening the breast.
- Women may experience a sense of the breast being squeezed or pinched.
- The radiologist will compare the present x-ray with previous breast x-rays, looking for changes, lumps/masses, and calcification.

- When abnormities are identified on a screening mammogram, further testing is needed, which may include a diagnostic mammogram, ultrasound, MRI, or biopsy.
- Women with breast implants need to inform the mammogram facility that they have breast implants. Implants can hide some of the breast tissue.
- Women should not wear any deodorants, perfume, lotion, or powder under their arms or on their breasts on the day of the appointment. These substances can make shadows on the x-ray.

(HHS, Office of Women's Health, 2009)

- *Women 30–65 years of age should be screened with a Pap test combined with an HPV test every 5 years.*
- *Women over 65 years of age can stop cervical cancer screening as long as they have not had any serious pre-cancers found in the previous 20 years (American Cancer Society, 2012a).*
- *Healthy People 2020 objectives:*
  - Increase the proportion of women who receive cervical cancer screening based on the most current guideline from 84.5% to 93% of females ages 21–65 years.
  - Increase the proportion of women counseled by their provider about Pap tests from 59.8% to 65.8% of females ages 21–65 years (Healthy People 2012).

CRITICAL COMPONENT

Papanicolaou (Pap) Smear

- Pap test is a microscopic examination of cells taken from the cervix.
- It is primarily used for early detection of cancerous or precancerous cells.
- It is a screening test. An abnormal result needs to be followed up with further testing.
- The best time to get a Pap test is 5 days after the menstrual period has stopped.
- The woman should not douche; use tampons; use vaginal creams, spermicide foams, creams, or jellies; use vaginal lubricants or moisturizers; or use vaginal medications for 48 hours prior to test.
- The woman should not have sexual intercourse for 48 hours prior to the test.
- A speculum is inserted in the vagina. Both cervical and vaginal specimens are obtained. A synthetic fiber brush or plastic spatula is used to obtain the specimens.

(American Cancer Society, 2012b).

REPRODUCTIVE CHANGES ACROSS THE LIFE SPAN

Throughout a woman's lifetime her body undergoes physical changes related to hormonal changes. Major reproductive changes occur during puberty and during the time before and after menopause.

Puberty

Puberty is the period of time when a person becomes sexually mature and capable of reproduction.

- Onset of puberty in girls usually occurs between the ages of 8 and 13 years.
- It is accompanied with accelerated growth of the body that usually begins with the feet and ends with the face.
- It is triggered by the production of gonadotropin-releasing hormone from the hypothalamus, which stimulates the anterior pituitary to release gonadotropins. Gonadotropins stimulate the ovaries to secrete estrogen (**Fig. 18-4**).
- Estrogen is responsible for the development of secondary sex characteristics in females. These characteristics include:
  - *Enlargement of breasts—growth of the duct system of the mammary glands and erection of nipples*
  - *Growth of body hair—axillary and pubic hair*
  - *Widening of the hips*
- **Menarche,** the initial menstrual period, usually occurs 2–2.5 years after the beginning of puberty.
- Puberty is completed when menstruation assumes a regular pattern.
- Menstrual cycle—see Chapter 3.

Menopause

Menopause is the stage of life that marks the permanent cessation of menstrual activity.

- It usually occurs between ages 35–58.
- It is a natural biological process.

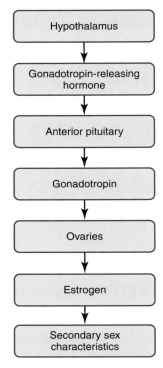

Figure 18–4   Hormonal triggers.

■ Menopause is divided into three stages:
  ■ *Perimenopause: Begins when the woman experiences menopausal signs and symptoms and ends after the first year following the last menstrual period. This stage can last several years as the woman experiences irregular menstrual cycles. It is possible for a woman to become pregnant during this stage.*
  ■ *Menopause: Occurs 12 months after a woman's last menstrual period. Average age in United States is age 51.*
  ■ *Postmenopause: Refers to the time after menopause.*

As a woman enters her late 30s, her ovaries begin to stop producing eggs and there is a decline in the production of estrogen and progesterone. The woman will begin to experience changes in her body related to the decreasing levels of estrogen. These changes are often referred to as signs and symptoms of menopause.

Signs and Symptoms of Menopause

■ Irregular periods
  ■ *Menstrual cycle may become irregular.*
  ■ *The time between cycles may become longer or shorter.*
  ■ *Menstrual flow may become heavier or lighter.*
  ■ *Cycles become anovulatory, and the woman becomes infertile.*
■ Hot flashes
  ■ *Hot flashes are the most common symptom of menopause.*
  ■ *They are caused by a vasomotor response to changes in the hormonal levels. This change triggers blood vessels near the surface of the skin to dilate, causing an increase*

of blood supply, which causes an increase in heat to the skin surface.
  ■ *When a woman experiences a hot flash, she feels a sudden sensation of warmth that spreads through her upper body and face. The woman's neck and face become red, and she begins to sweat and may feel irritable and exhausted.*
■ Night sweats
  ■ *Night sweats are hot flashes that occur while the woman is sleeping.*
  ■ *Women who experience night sweats will wake up with their bed linens and nightwear soaked from sweat.*
■ Sleep disturbances
  ■ *Women may experience altered sleep patterns related to night sweats and difficulty falling asleep and staying asleep.*
■ Vaginal dryness
  ■ *Normal vaginal mucosa and secretions are dependent on estrogen. As estrogen decreases, the vaginal tissue becomes thinner and drier.*
  ■ *Vaginal dryness can lead to discomfort during intercourse.*
■ Mood changes and trouble focusing
  ■ *These may be related more to sleep disturbances than directly to decreased estrogen.*
■ Women may also experience:
  ■ *Decreased interest in sex*
  ■ *Fatigue*
  ■ *Hair loss*
  ■ *Incontinence*
  ■ *Irregular heartbeat/palpitations*

Treating Menopausal Symptoms

There are three approaches for the treatment of menopausal symptoms: lifestyle changes, alternative medicine, and menopause hormone therapy (MHT).

■ Lifestyle changes
  ■ *Get 8 hours of sleep per night.*
  ■ *Eat a balanced diet.*
  ■ *Exercise.*
  ■ *Avoid caffeine and alcohol.*
  ■ *Avoid cigarette smoking and secondhand smoke.*
■ Alternative medicine
  ■ *Herbal supplements such as black cohosh*
  ■ *Acupuncture*
  ■ *Biofeedback*
  ■ *Hypnosis*
■ Menopausal hormone therapy (MHT).
  ■ *There are conflicting research findings on the safety of MHT. Women need to talk with their health care providers as to the benefit and risk of MHT.*
  ■ *Estrogen alone is prescribed for women who do not have a uterus.*
  ■ *Estrogen and progesterone therapy is prescribed for women who have a uterus. The use of progesterone with estrogen therapy reduces the risk of endometrial cancer.*

POSITION STATEMENT: HORMONE THERAPY

"Hormone therapy is the most effective treatment for menopausal symptoms such as hot flashes and vaginal dryness. If women have only vaginal dryness or discomfort with intercourse, the preferred treatments are low doses of vaginal estrogen. Hot flashes generally require a higher dose of hormone therapy that will have an effect on the entire body.

Women who still have a uterus need to take a progestogen (progesterone or a similar product) along with the estrogen to prevent cancer of the uterus. Five years or less is usually the recommended duration of use for this combined treatment, but the length of time can be individualized for each woman.

Women who have had their uterus removed can take estrogen alone. Because of the apparent greater safety of estrogen alone, there may be more flexibility in how long women can safely use estrogen therapy."

The North American Menopause Society, American Society of Reproductive Medicine, and The Endocrine Society (2012). Retrieved from www.endosociety.org/advocacy/policy/upload/joint-statement-the-experts-do-agree-about-hormone-therap.pdf

Treatment for Specific Menopausal Discomforts

■ Hot flashes: Avoid alcohol, hot beverages, spicy foods, warm rooms, and smoking; these can trigger hot flashes. Dress in layers, so that the woman is able to remove clothing as she becomes warm and add clothing as she cools down. Avoid wearing clothing made out of wool or synthetics. Use of fans is also helpful.
  ■ *Medications used to treat other conditions that have been shown to decrease hot flashes are: Low-dose antidepressants such as fluoxetine (Prozac); anti-seizure medication gabapentin (Neurontin); and anti-hypertensive clonidine (Catapres) (Mayo Clinic Staff, 2011).*
■ Night sweats: Sleep in cotton nightwear. Use cotton bed linens. Sleep in cool room. Sleep with fan blowing over body. Take a cool shower before bedtime.
■ Sleep disturbances: Keep the bedroom dark, quiet, and cool. Establish a regular bedtime pattern.
■ Vaginal dryness: Use water-based lubricants during sexual intercourse. Use vaginal moisturizers. Use estrogen vaginal cream. Soy flour and flaxseeds in the woman's diet may prevent or decrease the degree of vaginal dryness.

OSTEOPOROSIS

Osteoporosis is the loss of bone mass that occurs when more bone mass is absorbed than new body mass is laid down. The loss of bone mass usually occurs after the age of 35 at a rate of 0.3%–0.5%. Women who experience osteoporosis are at greater risk for vertebral and hip fractures. Osteoporosis affects both men and women, but 80% of all Americans diagnosed with osteoporosis are women.

■ Dual-energy X-ray absorptiometry scan (DXA)
  ■ *It is a diagnosis test for osteoporosis.*
  ■ *The DXA measures the bone density in the hip, the spine, and the forearm.*

■ *A T score is determined by comparing the woman's bone density to that of the average peak density of the same sex and race.*
■ *A T score of –2.5 or below is indicative of osteoporosis.*
■ *A T score of –1 to –2.5 is indicative of* **osteopenia,** *bone density between normal and osteoporosis.*

Signs and Symptoms

■ Back pain related to a fracture or collapsed vertebra
■ Loss of height related to collapsed vertebra
■ Stooped posture related to collapsed vertebra
■ Bone fractures related to bone weakness

Risk Factors for Osteoporosis

■ Caucasian women
■ Thin, small-boned women
■ Family history of osteoporosis
■ History of smoking
■ Inactivity
■ Low levels of calcium and vitamin D
  ■ *Vitamin D helps with the absorption of dietary calcium.*
■ Excessive alcohol consumption
■ Decreased levels of estrogen
■ Long-term use of steroids
■ Eating disorders such as anorexia
■ Weight loss surgery

Risk Reduction

■ Maintain a diet high in calcium and vitamin D (see Critical Component: Foods High in Calcium). This should start around 9 years of age to help form a strong bone matrix and should continue throughout the woman's life based on these guidelines:
  ■ *1,300 mg of calcium for girls 9–18 years of age*
  ■ *1,000 mg of calcium/day for women 19–50 years of age (premenopausal)*
  ■ *1,200 mg of calcium for women 51 years of age and older (menopausal)*
  ■ *600 IU of vitamin D/day for girls and women 9–70*
  ■ *800 mg/day for women older than 70 years of age (ACOG, 2012a).*
■ Engage in weight-bearing exercise.
  ■ *Walking, jogging, dancing, and weightlifting three to four times/week*

CRITICAL COMPONENT

Foods High in Calcium

■ Plain low-fat yogurt (8 oz.) – 415 mg
■ Orange juice, calcium fortified (6 oz.) – 375 mg
■ Canned sardines (3 oz.) – 325 mg
■ Cheddar cheese (1.5 oz.) – 307 mg
■ Milk, 2% milk fat (8 oz.) – 293 mg
■ Salmon (3 oz.) – 181 mg

■ Avoid smoking.
  ■ *Avoid both firsthand and secondhand smoke.*
■ Limit alcohol use.
  ■ *Heavy drinking is linked to lower bone density.*

Evidence-Based Practice: Effect of Strength Training on Bone Loss

Winters-Stone, K., Dobek, J., Nail, L., Bennett, J., Michael, L., Naik, A., & Schwartz, A. (2011). Strength training stops bone loss and builds muscle in post-menopausal breast cancer survivors: a randomized, controlled trail. *Breast Cancer Research and Treatment, 127,* 447–456.

The hypothesis of this randomized, control research study was that progressive, moderately intense resistance plus impact training would increase or maintain hip and spine bone mass, lean mass and fat mass, and reduce bone turnover compared to a control group who participated in a low-intensity, non-weight-bearing stretching program. The study included 106 women with early stage breast cancer who were greater than 1 year post radiation and/or chemotherapy; 50 years of age or greater at time of diagnosis; and free from osteoporosis and medications for bone loss. Each group participated in a 12-month program. The intervention group's program consisted of moderately-intense resistance exercises and impact training. The control group's program consisted of whole body stretching and relaxation exercises done in a seating or lying position.

The results of the study were that the women in the moderately-intense resistance plus impact training program preserved bone mineral density (BMD) at the lumbar spine to a greater degree than the women in the control group and had lower bone turnover than the control group.

Implications: Moderately-intense resistance plus impact training program can reduce risk for fracture among post-menopausal breast cancer survivors (BCS).

Pharmacotherapy

The American College of Obstetricians and Gynecologists (2012) recommends osteoporosis pharmacotherapy for the following women:

■ Women who have experienced a fragility or low-impact fracture
■ Women with a DXA T score of less than or equal to –2.5
■ Women with risk factors and with a DXA T score of less than –1.5 (ACOG, 2012a)
  ■ *The fracture risk assessment tool (FRAX) can be used to determine a 10-year risk for fractures related to osteoporosis. The tool is located at www.shef.ac.uk/FRAX/tool.jsp.*

Pharmacotherapy includes:

■ Bisphosphonates (see Critical Component: Bisphosphonates)
  ■ *Action: Inhibits resorption of bone*
    ■ **Resorption** is the process where breakdown of bone and release of minerals occurs with the resulting transfer of calcium from the bone fluid to the blood.

■ *Adverse effects: Musculoskeletal aches and pains, gastrointestinal irritation, and esophageal ulcerations.*
■ *Alendronate (Fosamax)*
  ■ Prevention: 5 mg/day or 35 mg/week
  ■ Treatment: 10 mg/day or 70 mg/week
■ *Ibandronate (Boniva)*
  ■ Prevention and treatment: 150 mg/month
  ■ Treatment: 3 mg every 3 months by I.V.
■ *Risedronate (Actonel)*
  ■ Prevention and treatment: 5 mg/day
■ *Zoledronate (Reclast)*
  ■ Prevention: 5 mg every 2 years by I.V.
  ■ Treatment: 5 mg every year by I.V.

CRITICAL COMPONENT

Bisphosphonates

To reduce side effects and to enhance absorption of the oral medication, the woman should:

■ Take the medication in the morning on an empty stomach at least 30 minutes before breakfast.
■ Take the medication with at least 8 oz. of water (do not take with juice, coffee, or tea).
■ Take the medication in a sitting or standing position.
  ■ This will decrease the risk of the pill becoming lodged in the esophagus where it can cause ulcerations and scarring.
■ Remain upright for at least 30 minutes.
  ■ This will decrease the risk of reflux of the pill into the esophagus.

(Shiel, 2012)

■ Estrogen-receptor modulators
  ■ *Action: Binds with estrogen receptors, producing estrogen-like effects on bone, and reduces resorption of bone (Vallerand & Sanoski, 2013)*
  ■ *Adverse effects: Venous thromboembolism, leg cramps, and death from stroke*
  ■ *Raloxifene (Evista)*
    ■ Prevention and treatment: 60 mg/day
■ Hormone therapy
  ■ *Conjugated estrogen + medroxyprogesterone acetate (Premphase)*
    ■ Prevention: 0.625 mg of conjugated estrogen once daily on days 1–14 and 5 mg medroxyprogesterone acetate once daily on days 15–28
    ■ Prescribed for women who have a uterus
    ■ Contraindicated for women with known or suspected estrogen-dependent neoplasia
  ■ *Conjugated estrogen (Premarin)*
    ■ Prevention: 0.3–1.25 mg/day
    ■ Prescribed for women who do not have a uterus
    ■ Contraindicated for women with known or suspected estrogen-dependent neoplasia

ADOLESCENT HEALTH

Adolescence, ages 12–19 years, is a time of physical, cognitive, and psychosocial development:

■ Physical: Biological changes that occur during this period of time include sexual maturity (development of primary and secondary sex changes), increases in height and weight (adolescent female will grow 2–8 inches and gain 15–55 pounds), and completion of skeletal growth.
■ Cognitive: The adolescent moves from being a concrete thinker to being able to think abstractly, use logic to solve problems, use deductive reasoning, and plan for the future. Adolescents begin to be concerned with moral and social issues and compare their beliefs with those of their peers.
■ Psychosocial: The adolescent is working toward role identity; who they are and who they will be in life. As they work toward role identity they develop a set of personal moral and ethical values and a greater sense of self-esteem and self-worth as well as a satisfactory sexual identity.

The majority of adolescents are physically healthy but are at risk for major health problems. Health problems and issues for female adolescents include:

■ Unintentional injuries, suicide, and homicides—these are the leading causes of death for females ages 15–19.
■ Eating disorders—obesity, anorexia, and bulimia
■ Sexually transmitted illnesses—chlamydia and gonorrhea are prevalent in adolescents.
■ Teen pregnancies—in 2011, there were 329,797 babies born to women ages 15–19 years (CDC, 2012f)
■ Issues related to self-esteem—22.1% of female adolescents report being electronically bullied, and 22% report being bullied on school property (CDC, 2010g).
■ Menstrual disorders
■ Acne

Based on the 2011 national Youth Risk Behavior Survey (YRBS), risk factors for health problems for female adolescents are (CDC, 2012g):

■ Behaviors that contribute to unintentional injury or violence
  ■ *85.95% rarely or never wear a bicycle helmet while riding a bike.*
  ■ *24.9% rode in a car driven by someone who had been drinking.*
  ■ *30.4% have texted or e-mailed while driving a car.*
  ■ *24.4% have been in a physical fight.*
  ■ *19.3% have seriously considered attempting suicide.*
  ■ *9.8% have attempted suicide.*
■ Alcohol, tobacco, and drug use
  ■ *16.1% smoke cigarettes.*
  ■ *19.8% have had five or more drinks of alcohol in a row (binge drinking).*
  ■ *37.2% have used marijuana.*
  ■ *19.8% have taken prescription drugs, such as Oxycontin, without a doctor's prescription.*

■ Unhealthy sex behaviors
  ■ *45.6% have had sexual intercourse; 34.2% are currently sexually active; 12.6% have had four or more sexual partners.*
  ■ *15.1% did not use any methods to prevent pregnancy during the last sexual intercourse.*
  ■ *18.1% have drunk alcohol or used drugs before the last sexual intercourse.*
■ Unhealthy dietary behaviors
  ■ *9.8% are obese and 15.4 are overweight.*
  ■ *17.4% have not eaten for 24 hours to lose weight or to keep weight off.*
  ■ *6% have vomited or taken laxatives to lose weight or to keep from gaining weight.*
■ Inadequate physical activity
  ■ *17.7% do not participate in at least 60 minutes of physical activity per day.*
  ■ *26.6% use computers for 3 or more hours per day.*
  ■ *31.6% watch television for 3 or more hours per day.*

Health promotion through information is an important element in assisting youth in decreasing unhealthy behaviors. Nurses working in the middle school and high school settings are in ideal positions for promoting healthy behaviors in adolescents. School nurses are often viewed by youth as safe adults to turn to when they have issues regarding health or body changes or when they are in need of sexual information. School nurses have the opportunity to provide health information and risk reduction information to large groups of adolescents and can present this information based on the needs of their school's population. School nurses can also advocate for the availability of health resources for youth in their school district.

A Healthy People 2020 goal is to increase the proportion of adolescents who annually have a wellness check-up from 68.7% to 75.6%. Wellness checkups are an ideal time to assess for risky behaviors and potential health problems and to provide health promotion information.

LESBIAN HEALTH

Lesbian, gay, bisexual, and transgender (LGBT) individuals experience health disparities related to societal stigma, discrimination, and denial of civil rights (Healthy People, 2012). Healthy People 2010's report identified the need for more research to document, understand, and address the factors that contribute to the health disparities in the LGBT communities (Healthy People, 2012). A result of this report, Healthy People 2020 has set a goal to improve the health, safety, and well-being of LGBT individuals (Healthy People, 2012).

Lesbians face barriers to quality health care. Three of these barriers are lack of health insurance, fear of negative reaction from health care provider due to sexual orientation, and lack of understanding by health care providers of lesbian health care issues. Health issues for lesbians include:

■ Cancer: Lesbians are at higher risk for breast, cervical, endometrial, and ovarian cancer due to lesbians having higher rates of smoking, alcohol use, and obesity than heterosexual women. Lesbians are also less likely to follow the recommended frequency of screening tests such as Pap test and mammograms (Gay and Lesbian Medical Association [GLMA], 2010).

■ Obesity: Lesbians have a higher body mass than heterosexual women (GLMA, 2010). This increases their risk for heart disease and cancer.

■ Polycystic ovarian syndrome (PCOS): PCOS is a common hormonal reproductive problem of all women. It appears more frequently in lesbians and increases women's risk for menstrual disorders, infertility, abnormal insulin production, and heart disease.

■ Heart disease: Lesbians are at higher risk for heart disease due to higher rates of smoking and obesity.

■ Tobacco, alcohol, and substance use: Use of these substances is higher in lesbians compared to heterosexual women.

■ Domestic violence: Domestic violence occurs in lesbian relationships, but at a lower rate than for heterosexual women. All women need to be screened for domestic violence.

■ Depression and anxiety: Lesbians report a higher rate of depression and anxiety than heterosexual women, which may be related to feelings of discrimination based on sexual orientation (HHS, 2005).

ACOG COMMITTEE OPINION

Health Care for Lesbians and Bisexual Women
"Lesbians and bisexual women encounter barriers to health care that include concerns about confidentiality and disclosure, discriminatory attitudes and treatment, limited access to health care and health insurance, and often a limited understanding as to what their health care risks may be. Health care providers should offer quality care to all women regardless of sexual orientation. The American College of Obstetricians and Gynecologists endorse equitable treatment for lesbians and bisexual women and their families, not only for direct health care needs, but also for indirect health care issues."

ACOG, (2012).

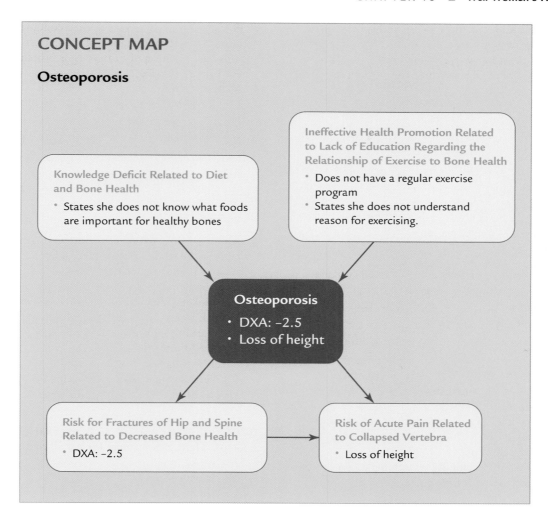

CONCEPT MAP

Osteoporosis

Knowledge Deficit Related to Diet and Bone Health
* States she does not know what foods are important for healthy bones

Ineffective Health Promotion Related to Lack of Education Regarding the Relationship of Exercise to Bone Health
* Does not have a regular exercise program
* States she does not understand reason for exercising.

Osteoporosis
* DXA: –2.5
* Loss of height

Risk for Fractures of Hip and Spine Related to Decreased Bone Health
* DXA: –2.5

Risk of Acute Pain Related to Collapsed Vertebra
* Loss of height

Problem No. 1: Knowledge deficit related to diet and bone health

Goal: Increased knowledge of the relationship of diet and bone health

Outcome: The woman's diet will include foods high in calcium and foods high in vitamin D.

Nursing Actions

1. Assess diet for calcium and vitamin D using a 24-hour food recall.
2. Explain the relationship of calcium and strong bone matrix.
3. Explain that vitamin D helps with calcium absorption.
4. Assist the woman in identifying foods she prefers that are high in calcium and foods that are high in vitamin D.

Problem No. 2: Ineffective health promotion related to lack of education regarding the relationship of exercise to bone health

Goal: Effective health promotion

Outcome: The woman will develop a regular exercise routine that includes weight-bearing and weight-lifting activities.

Nursing Actions

1. Provide information regarding the causes of osteoporosis.
2. Provide information regarding the relationship of weight-bearing exercise and improved bone mass.
3. Discuss past exercise experiences and identify previous barriers to exercising.
4. Provide information on weight-bearing exercises and weight-lifting.
5. Assist the woman in developing an exercise program that reflects her likes and meets the need for improved bone health.

Problem No. 3: Risk for fractures of hip and spine related to decreased bone health
Goal: Remains free of hip or spine fractures
Outcome: The woman will state three ways to improve bone health.

Nursing Actions

1. Explain the relationship of osteoporosis and fractures of hip and spine.
2. Assess the woman's level of knowledge regarding ways to improve bone health.
3. Provide information on nutrition and bone health.
4. Provide information on exercise and bone health.
5. Provide information on prescribed medications for treatment of osteoporosis.

Problem No. 4: Risk of pain related to collapsed vertebra
Goal: Does not experience to collapsed vertebra
Outcome: The woman will not experience pain related to osteoporosis.

Nursing Actions

1. Provide information on the benefits of calcium and vitamin D in improving bone health.
2. Provide information on the negative effects of smoking and excessive alcohol consumption on bone health.
3. Provide information on the relationship of osteoporosis and fractures of the spine.
4. Assist the woman in developing an action plan for decreasing her risk for fractures of the spine.

■ ■ ■ Review Questions ■ ■ ■

1. Based on her knowledge of the number one leading cause of death for girls/women 15–24 years of age, the clinic nurse stresses the importance of _____ with her 19-year-old client.
   A. Eating foods high in calcium and vitamin D
   B. Avoiding secondhand smoke
   C. Wearing seatbelts when traveling in an automobile
   D. Exercising daily to improve muscle strength and balance

2. In addition to being the most common sexually transmitted virus in the United States, _____ is also the main cause of cervical cancer.
   A. HIV
   B. Chlamydia
   C. Human papillomavirus
   D. Gonorrhea

3. A _____ is a screening test that involves a microscopic examination of cells taken from the cervix for early detection of cancerous or precancerous cells.
   A. Cervical biopsy
   B. Colposcopy
   C. Cervical conization
   D. Papanicolaou test

4. Lesbians are at _____ risk for breast, cervical, endometrial, and ovarian cancer than heterosexual women.
   A. higher
   B. lower
   C. the same

5. An ambulatory care nurse is discussing health promotion behaviors with her client. Her client is a 48-year-old Asian woman who has been divorced for 5 years and has a new male partner. Both the woman and her partner are smokers. The teaching plan for this client based on her risk factors include: (Select all that apply)
   A. Warning signs of heart attack and stroke
   B. Need for yearly pelvic exam that includes a chlamydia test
   C. Need for pneumococcal vaccine now and in 10 years
   D. Need for tetanus and diphtheria vaccine every 5 years

6. Obesity places women at risk for a variety of health problems. These risk include: (Select all that apply)
   A. Stroke
   B. Breast cancer
   C. Colon cancer
   D. Menstrual disorders

7. A teaching plan for a 40-year-old woman having her first mammogram should include: (Select all that apply)
   A. Informing her that she should have a mammogram every 5 years
   B. Explaining that she might experience a sensation that her breast is being squeezed or pinched
   C. Instructing her to avoid use of deodorant under her arms on the day of her appointment
   D. Explaining that this is a screening test versus a diagnostic test

8. Which of the following women are at risk for osteoporosis? Select all that apply.
   A. A 45-year-old woman with a DXA of -0.5
   B. A 25-year-old woman with anorexia
   C. A 35-year-old non-smoking woman
   D. A 30-year-old woman who had weight loss surgery

9. The ambulatory care nurse is instructing a woman regarding oral bisphosphonates in the treatment of osteoporosis. The teaching plan should include which of the following?
   A. Take the medication on a full stomach.
   B. Remain upright for 30 minutes after taking the medication.
   C. Take the medication with the evening meal.
   D. Take the medication with her calcium supplement.

10. Which of the following strategies can decrease the frequency of hot flashes related to perimenopause? Select all that apply.
    A. Avoiding alcohol drinks
    B. Avoiding hot teas
    C. Avoiding foods high in fat
    D. Avoiding cold rooms

References

American Cancer Society. (2012a). *American Cancer Society guidelines for early detection of cancer.* Retrieved from www.cancer.org/healthy/findcancer early/cancerscreeningguidelines

American Cancer Society. (2012b). Cervical cancer. Retrieved from www.cancer.org/cervical cancer/detailedguide/cervical-cancer-prevention

American College of Obstetricians and Gynecologist (ACOG). (2012a). Osteoporosis. *Obstetrics & gynecology, 120,* 718–733.

American College of Obstetricians and Gynecologist (ACOG). (2012b). Committee opinion: Health care for lesbians and bisexual women. Number 525, May 2012. Retrieved from www.acog.org/resources_and_publications/Committee_Opinions

Centers for Disease Control and Prevention. (2012a). *Leading causes of death in females United States, 2008.* Retrieved from www.cdc.gov/women/lcod/2008/htm

Centers for Disease Control and Prevention. (2012b). United States cancer statistics: 1999–2008 incidence and mortality web-based report. Retrieved from www.cdc.gov/usnc

Centers for Disease Control and Prevention. (2012c). *HPV vaccine information for young women* – fact sheet. Retrieved from www.cdc.gov/std/hpv/stdfact-vaccine-young-women.htm

Centers for Disease Control and Prevention. (2012d). *Cancer among women.* Retrieved from www.cdc.gov/cancer/dcpc/data/women/htm

Centers for Disease Control and Prevention. (2012e). *Excessive alcohol use and risk to women's health.* Retrieved from www.cdc.gov/alcohol/factr-sheets/womens-health.htm

Centers for Disease Control and Prevention. (2012f). *Teen pregnancy.* Retrieved from www.cdc.gov/Teen Pregnancy/index.htm

Centers for Disease Control and Prevention. (2012g). *Youth risk behavior surveillance system: 2011 national overview.* Retrieved from www.cdc.gov/healthyyouth/yrbs/index.htm

Gay and Lesbian Medical Association. (2010). *Ten things lesbians should discuss with their healthcare provider.* Retrieved from www.glma.org

Kulie, T., Slattengren, A., Redmer, J., Counts, H., Eglash, A., & Schrager, S. (2011). Obesity and women's health: an evidence-based review. *JABFM, 24,* 75–85.

Mayo Clinic Staff (2011). Menopause. Retrieved from www.mayoclinic.com/health/menopause

Ogden, C., Carroll, M., Kit, B., & Flegel, K. (2012). Prevalence of obesity in United States, 2009–2010. NCHS data brief. No. 82.

Purnell, L., & Paulanka, B. (2005). *Guide to culturally competent health care.* Philadelphia: F.A. Davis.

Shiel, W. (2012). Osteoporosis. Retrieved from www.medicinet.com/osteoporosis/article.htm

Stevens, J., & Olson, S. (2000). Reducing falls and resulting hip fractures among older women. Retrieved from www.cdc.gov/mmwr/preview/mmwrhtm1/rr4902a2.htm

The North American Menopause Society, American Society of Reproductive Medicine, and The Endocrine Society. (2012). The experts do agree about hormone therapy. Retrieved from www.endo-society.org/advocacy/policy/upload/joint-statement-the-experts-do-agree-about-hormone-therap.pdf

U.S. Department of Health Human Services, Office of Women's Health (HHS). (2012). *A lifetime of good health.* Retrieved from www.womenshealth.gov

U.S. Department of Health and Human Services, Office of Women's Health (HHS). (2005). *Lesbian health.* Retrieved from www.womenshealth.gov/frequentlyaskedquestions

U.S. Department of Health and Human Services, Office of Women's Health (HHS). (2009). *Mammograms.* Retrieved from www.wpmenshealth.gov

Vallerand, A., & Sanoski, C. (2013). *Davis's drug guide for nurses* (13th ed.). Philadelphia: F.A. Davis.

VanLeeuwen, A., Kranpitz, T., & Smith, L. (2010). *Davis's comprehensive handbook of laboratory and diagnostic tests with nursing implications.* Philadelphia: F.A. Davis.

World Health Organization. (2010). *Health promotion.* Retrieved from www.who.int/topics/health_promotion/en/

Alterations in Women's Health

Nursing Diagnosis

■ Knowledge deficit related to lack of information regarding menstrual disorder.
■ Anxiety related to diagnosis of breast cancer.

Nursing Outcomes

■ The woman will state causes of menstrual disorder and two possible treatments.
■ The woman will appear relaxed and report anxiety related to diagnosis of breast cancer is reduced to a manageable level.

COMMON DIAGNOSTIC PROCEDURES

Table 19-1 provides an overview of the common diagnostic procedures used in women's health care.

HYSTERECTOMY

Hysterectomy, the surgical removal of the uterus, is the second most frequently performed surgery for women in the United States (CDC, 2008). Cesarean section is the most common performed surgery.

Reasons for Hysterectomy

The top three reasons for hysterectomy are:

■ Leiomyomas—benign fibrous tumor of the uterine wall
■ Endometriosis—abnormal growth of tissue resembling the endometrium that is present outside of the uterine cavity
■ Uterine prolapse

Other reasons include:

■ Cancer—cervical, ovarian, endometrial
■ Abnormal uterine bleeding
■ Chronic pelvic pain
■ Pelvic inflammatory disease

Don't have time to read this chapter? Want to reinforce your reading? Need to review for a test?
Listen to this chapter on Davis*Plus*.

TABLE 19–1   COMMON DIAGNOSTIC PROCEDURES

TEST	INDICATION	PROCEDURE
Bone mineral densitometry (BMD)	Diagnose bone loss and osteoporosis. Assess effectiveness of osteoporosis medication therapy. Predict risk of future bone fractures.	**Dual-energy x-ray absorptiometry (DXA):** Two x-rays of different energy levels are used to measure BMD. The DXA machine (a specially designed x-ray machine) is used. X-ray is usually of the lower spine and hip. Women should not wear metal in area being x-rayed.
Breast biopsy and aspiration	Breast abnormality noted by palpation, mammography, or ultrasound. Diagnostic: To distinguish between benign and malignant tumors	**Excisional Biopsy:** The removal of the entire lump or suspicious area. This is done for lumps smaller than an inch in diameter. Tissue is examined by a pathologist to determine if cancerous cells are present. Procedure may be done using local or regional anesthesia. **Incisional Biopsy:** The removal of a portion of the tumor. Usually done with tumors larger than 1 inch in diameter. Tissue is examined by a pathologist. Procedure may be done using local or regional anesthesia. **Fine-Needle Biopsy:** A fine needle is inserted into the questionable tissue. Fluid is removed from the cyst or cells are removed from the solid mass. The fluid or cells are examined by the pathologist. Usually done as an office procedure using local anesthesia. **Core Needle Biopsy:** This procedure uses a larger-bore needle to obtain a small cylinder of tissue. Usually done as an office procedure using local anesthesia.
Cervical conization	Abnormal Pap smear Diagnostic: To detect cervical cancer Therapeutic: Treatment of cervical intraepithelial lesions	A cone-shaped portion of cervical tissue is removed. The tissue sample is removed by scalpel, CO_2 laser, or loop electrosurgical excision procedure (LEEP). Tissue is examined by a pathologist.
Colposcopy	Dysplasia, condylomas, and abnormal Pap smear Diagnostic: To rule out cancer of the cervix	The vagina and cervix are exposed with the use of a speculum. Acetic acid is placed on the cervix. A colposcope, an electric microscope with a light, is used to view the cervical area. Abnormal cervical changes are seen as white areas. A biopsy is taken from the whitest area and is evaluated by a pathologist.
Dilation and curettage	Diagnostic: To detect uterine malignancy, to evaluate fertility, and to evaluate dysfunctional uterine bleeding Therapeutic: Treat heavy uterine bleeding, dysmenorrhea, and incomplete abortion	Can be done in the doctor's office, outpatient clinic, or hospital. Metal dilators of increasing sizes are inserted into the cervical os. After the cervix is dilated, curettes are used to scrape and/or remove endometrial tissue. Tissue is evaluated by a pathologist.
Endometrial biopsy	Diagnostic: To determine cause of dysfunctional uterine bleeding and bleeding after menopause	A sample of the endometrium is obtained with the use of a Pipelle aspirator, a small hollow plastic tube, which is inserted into the uterus via the cervix. Gentle suction is applied to obtain a sample of the endometrial tissue. The sample is evaluated by a pathologist.
Laparoscopy	Diagnostic: Pelvic adhesions, infertility related to tubal or uterine causes, ectopic pregnancy, ovarian tumors or cysts, pelvic inflammatory disease, and endometriosis Therapeutic: Tubal ligation, retrieval of ova for in vitro fertilization, removal of IUD, removal of adhesions	Gynecologic laparoscopy is used to visualize the internal pelvic contents. A needle is inserted through a small incision into the peritoneal cavity, and the cavity is filled with CO_2 to enhance visualization of the organs. A laparoscope is inserted through a second incision. The laparoscope has a microscope to allow visualization, and it can be used to insert instruments required for procedures.

TABLE 19–1	COMMON DIAGNOSTIC PROCEDURES—cont'd	
TEST	INDICATION	PROCEDURE
Magnetic resonance imaging (MRI)	Use: To detect tumors of the breast, ovaries, and uterus; evaluate breast implants	MRI is a noninvasive diagnostic scanning technique using magnetic and radio waves to produce an image. The woman lies supine on a table that is slid into the MRI scanner. She must remain motionless during the scan.
Ultrasonography	Breast: Used to distinguish between solid tumors and cysts; detect very small tumors in combination with mammograms; guide interventional procedures such as cyst aspiration Pelvis: Used to detect tumors, cysts, abscesses, bleeding; distinguish between solid tumors and cysts; aid in fertility studies	High-frequency waves of different intensity are delivered by a transducer. Waves are bounced back and converted to electrical energy, which is displayed on a monitor. Breast: The woman should not apply lotion, bath powder, or other substances to the chest or breast the day of the examination. Jewelry and other metal objects must be removed from area of examination. Both breasts are usually examined. Pelvis: Can be either transabdominal or transvaginal. Transabdominal requires a full bladder. Jewelry and other metal objects must be removed from area of examination.

ACOG, 2010; VanLeeuwen, Kranpitz, & Smith, 2006; Women's Health, 2010b

Risks Related to Surgical Procedure

■ Complication related to anesthesia
■ Injury to ureters, bladder, and/or bowel
■ Hemorrhage
■ Infection
■ Deep vein thrombosis

Types of Hysterectomies

■ Total hysterectomy: Removal of the uterus and the cervix
■ Hysterectomy with salpingo-oophorectomy: Removal of the uterus, cervix, fallopian tubes, and ovaries
■ Radical hysterectomy: Removal of the uterus, cervix, fallopian tubes, ovaries, upper portion of the vagina, and lymph nodes. This is done for some cases of reproductive cancer.
■ Supracervical hysterectomy: Removal of the uterus
■ The type of hysterectomy is determined by the reason for hysterectomy and the age and health status of the woman.

Surgical and Anesthetic Techniques

■ Abdominal hysterectomy: Removal of the uterus and other structures through an abdominal incision. The external incision may be transverse (Pfannestiel), just above the pubic hairline, or vertical (low midline), below the umbilicus to just above the pubic hairline. Abdominal hysterectomy is usually the preferred technique when the reason for hysterectomy is related to a gynecologic cancer.
  ■ *General anesthesia with an endotracheal tube*
  ■ *For gynecologic cancer: in addition to general, epidural anesthesia may be used for postoperative pain management.*

■ Vaginal hysterectomy: The uterus is removed through the vagina. A pericervical incision is used. The woman is placed in a lithotomy position for the operative procedure.
  ■ *General anesthesia is most common, but also can be done with epidural or spinal anesthesia.*
■ Laparoscope-assisted vaginal hysterectomy (LAVH): The woman is placed in a steep Trendelenburg position. Laparoscope and instruments are inserted through small incisions in the abdomen (**Fig. 19-1**). The surgeon manually operates the scope and instruments. The uterus is removed through the vagina. The hysterectomy is initiated by laparoscopy and subsequent steps are performed vaginally.
  ■ *General anesthesia with endotracheal tube. This is the preferred method due to the CO_2 insufflation required for the laparoscopic procedure and the positioning of the woman during the surgical procedure.*
    ■ CO_2 insufflation causes an increase in intra-abdominal pressure that can cause intraoperative respiratory compromise. The insufflation may also cause cardiovascular compromise from decreased venous return.
    ■ The steep Trendelenburg position further increases intra-abdominal pressure and may increase risk of aspiration.
    ■ Due to the deep Trendelenburg position, the woman needs to be monitored for facial and conjunctival edema. If this occurs, extubation following surgery may need to be postponed due to increased risk of laryngeal edema.
■ Robotic-assisted laparoscopic hysterectomy: The woman is placed in a steep Trendelenburg position. Three or four small incisions are made near the umbilicus. A laparoscope and robotic instruments are inserted through the incisions into the abdomen. The laparoscope and robotic instruments are connected to the computer. The surgeon

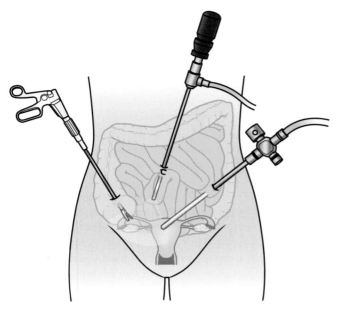

Figure 19–1 Laparoscopic hysterectomy.

controls the movements of the scope and the instruments from a computer station in the operating room.

■ *General anesthesia with an endotracheal tube and with muscle relaxation: In robotic surgery there is limited access to the patient due to the bulk of the equipment that is set over the patient. Full muscle relaxation is needed to prevent inadvertent patient movement.*

■ *Due to the deep Trendelenburg position, the woman needs to be monitored for facial and conjunctival edema. If this occurs, extubation following surgery may need to be postponed due to increased risk of laryngeal edema.*

Preoperative Care for Abdominal Hysterectomy

Medical Management

■ Physical assessment and health history
■ Laboratory tests—complete blood count, type and cross-match, urinalysis
■ Electrocardiogram
■ NPO 8 hours prior to surgery

Nursing Actions

■ Complete the appropriate admission assessments and required preoperative forms.
■ Ensure that all required documents, such as history and physical, current laboratory reports, and consent forms are in the woman's chart.
■ Verify that the woman has been NPO for 8 hours before surgery.
■ Complete the surgical checklist, which includes removal of jewelry, eyeglasses/contact lenses, and dentures.
■ Explain to the woman and family or support persons what the woman can expect before surgery and after surgery.
■ Start an IV line and IV fluid as per orders.

■ Have the woman void or insert Foley catheter as per orders.
■ Provide emotional support for the woman and her family/support persons.
■ Address the woman and/or family's questions and/or concerns.

Postoperative Care for Abdominal Hysterectomy

Medical Management

■ IV therapy
■ Medications for pain management
■ Antibiotic therapy if at risk for infection
■ Hormone replacement therapy if ovaries were removed
■ Progression of diet
■ Foley catheter for 24–48 hours post-surgery
■ Ambulate once recovered from anesthesia

Nursing Actions

■ Monitor vital signs as per protocol.
■ Monitor for blood loss—assess for blood on abdominal dressing and perineal pad.
  ■ *The woman will experience small to moderate amounts of vaginal bleeding for several days.*
■ Monitor level of consciousness and level of sensation and for side effects of anesthesia.
■ Assess lung sounds and assist the woman with deep breathing and coughing.
  ■ *Teach the woman to splint her abdomen with a pillow when she coughs.*
■ Assist the woman into a comfortable position and reposition every 2 hours.
■ Assess for pain and provide pain relief via prescribed medications, use of relaxation techniques, positioning, and/or soothing environment.
■ Assist the woman with ambulation as per orders.
  ■ *Explain to the woman that ambulation decreases her risk for deep vein thrombosis and facilitates return of intestinal peristalsis, which decreases the amount of gas build-up.*
■ Monitor intake and output.
■ D.C. IV as per orders.
■ D.C Foley catheter as per orders.
■ Assess bowel sounds and advance to a regular diet as per orders.
■ Provide opportunities for the woman to ask questions or share her concerns.
  ■ *The woman may experience emotional symptoms following surgery related to hormonal changes and loss of fertility.*
■ Provide discharge teaching:
  ■ *Keep the incision area dry, following the surgeon's instructions for bathing and dressing care.*
  ■ *Explain that walking is important in helping her to gradually return to her pre-surgery activity level.*
    ■ Instruct the woman to follow her surgeon's orders regarding level of activity and heavy lifting.
  ■ *Explain that she may experience light vaginal bleeding for several days.*

■ *Provide nutritional information—the importance of protein, iron, and vitamin C in the healing process.*
■ *Provide information on pain management techniques.*
■ *Instruct the woman not to put anything in the vagina (e.g., do not douche, use tampons, or engage in sexual intercourse) until advised by her surgeon.*
  ■ This will decrease the risk of infection.
■ *Instruct the woman to notify health care provider if:*
  ■ Increased pain or pain that is not relieved by medication
  ■ Drainage, bleeding, redness or swelling from the incisional site or increased bleeding from the vagina
  ■ Leg pain
  ■ Fever ≥ 39°C/102.2°F

MENSTRUAL DISORDERS

Menstrual disorders are the most common women's reproductive problem. These include amenorrhea, dysfunctional uterine bleeding, dysmenorrhea, and premenstrual syndrome (**Table 2**). The hypothalamus, pituitary, and ovaries are the main sites of regulation of the menstrual cycle. Normal menstrual cycles occur when the hormone levels and feedback pathway of the hypothalamus-anterior pituitary-ovaries function appropriately. (See Chapter 3 for an overview of the menstrual cycle.)

■ Hypothalamus: Secretes gonadotropin-releasing hormone (GnRH), also called luteinizing-hormone-releasing hormone (LHRH), which simulates the anterior pituitary.

■ Anterior pituitary: Secretes follicle-stimulating hormone (FSH) and luteinizing hormone (LH) that stimulates the ovaries.
■ Ovaries: The ovarian follicles respond to the increase in FSH by producing increasing amounts of estrogen. LH stimulates the ovaries to release the ova and secrete progesterone. Estrogen and progesterone influence the menstrual cycle.

CHRONIC PELVIC PAIN

Chronic pelvic pain (CPP) is pain in the pelvic region that lasts 6 months or longer and results in functional or psychological disabilities or requires treatment/intervention (Green et al., 2010). CPP is a common medical problem in women. The cause of the pain is often unknown. When the cause of the pain is known, treatment is directed at the cause. When the cause of the pain is unknown, treatment focuses on symptom management.

The woman will experience a variety of abdominal and/or pelvic pain:

■ Sharp pain
■ Uterine and/or abdominal cramping
■ Steady pain
■ Intermittent pain
■ Pressure or heaviness deep in pelvis
■ Pain during intercourse
■ Pain while having bowel movement (Mayo Clinic, 2009b)

TABLE 19–2	MENSTRUAL DISORDERS		
MENSTRUAL DISORDER	DEFINITIONS, SYMPTOMS, SIGNS	PATHOPHYSIOLOGY	MANAGEMENT
Primary amenorrhea	No menses by age 14 and no secondary sex characteristics or no menses by age 16 with secondary sex characteristics	May be related to: • Body build (i.e., minimal levels of body fat) • Heredity (family history of delayed menses) • Pituitary function (lack of secretion of FSH and LH) • Congenital absence of the vagina • 90% of cases have no identifiable cause.	Identify and treat underlying condition (e.g., hormone therapy if related to endocrine dysfunction). Provide emotional support.
Secondary amenorrhea	No menses in 6 months in a woman who has had normal menstrual cycles	May result from: • Lack of ovarian production • Pregnancy • Polycystic ovary syndrome • Nutritional disturbances • Endocrine disturbances • Uncontrolled diabetes • Heavy athletic activity • Emotional distress	Identify and treat underlying condition (e.g., correct nutritional disorder). Explain cause (e.g., heavy athletic activity).

Continued

TABLE 19–2   MENSTRUAL DISORDERS—cont'd

MENSTRUAL DISORDER	DEFINITIONS, SYMPTOMS, SIGNS	PATHOPHYSIOLOGY	MANAGEMENT
Menorrhagia	Menstrual bleeding that is excessive in number of days and amount of blood	May result from: • Anovulatory cycle with continued estrogen production • Fibroids are most common anatomic cause. • Inflammatory or infectious cause (e.g., metritis, salpingitis) • Endometrial cause (e.g., hyperplasia, polyps, cancer) • Intrauterine device (IUD)	Endometrial biopsy to assist in diagnosis of underlying cause. Identify and treat underlying condition (e.g., antibiotic therapy if related to infection). If no identifiable cause, short course of contraceptives may be prescribed. Dilation and curettage
Metrorrhagia	Bleeding between periods or after menopause	This is the most significant form of menstrual disorder and warrants immediate investigation. • Occurs with cancerous or benign tumors of the uterus • Associated with IUD and use of oral contraceptives • May be associated with trauma, cervicitis, vaginitis, polyps, ovarian cysts, cervical dysplasia	Endometrial biopsy to rule out endometrial cancer Antibiotics for infection Surgery Chemotherapy
Primary dysmenorrhea	Painful menstruation: Cramping usually begins 12–24 hours before onset of flow and lasts 12–24 hours. May experience chills, nausea, vomiting, headaches, irritability, and diarrhea	Excessive endometrial production of prostaglandin; women with primary dysmenorrhea produce 10 times the amount of prostaglandin. Prostaglandin is a myometrial stimulant and vasoconstrictor.	Explain cause. Prostaglandin inhibitors (ibuprofen) Analgesics Heat to back and lower abdomen Warm bath Exercise Oral contraceptives Diet low in fat and meat products may decrease the duration and intensity of the pain. Biofeedback Acupuncture
Secondary dysmenorrhea	Painful menstruation associated with known anatomic factors or pelvic pathology. Pain can be present at any point of the menstrual cycle.	Related to: • Endometriosis • Pelvic adhesions • Inflammatory disease • Cervical stenosis • Uterine fibroids • Adenomyoma	Identify and treat underlying condition. Same symptomatic measures as in primary dysmenorrhea.

TABLE 19–2	MENSTRUAL DISORDERS—cont'd		
MENSTRUAL DISORDER	DEFINITIONS, SYMPTOMS, SIGNS	PATHOPHYSIOLOGY	MANAGEMENT
Premenstrual syndrome (PMS)	A combination of emotional and physical symptoms that begin during the luteal phase and diminish after menstruation begins. Symptoms include (but are not limited to) lower abdominal and back pain, bloating, weight gain, breast tenderness, joint and muscle pain, oliguria, diaphoresis, diarrhea, constipation, nausea, vomiting, food cravings, acne, urticaria, headaches, vertigo, fainting, clumsiness, mood swings, depression, irritability, anxiety, lethargy, fatigue, confusion, tension, forgetfulness, sexual arousal or dysfunction.	Etiology is unknown. PMS might be related to: • Hormonal changes related the menstrual cycle • Estrogen-progesterone imbalance • Chemical changes in the brain	Limit salt intake, caffeine, animal fat, refined sugars, and alcohol. Exercise daily. Sleep 8 hours each night. Ibuprofen for physical symptoms such as cramps, backache, and breast tenderness Herbal remedies such as black cohosh, ginger, and raspberry leaf Commonly prescribed medications are antidepressants, diuretics, and oral contraceptives.

Mayo Clinic, 2009a; HHS, 2010

Causes

The causes of CPP stem from various systems, such as the reproductive, urological, and neuromuscular systems.

- Reproductive
  - *Pelvic inflammatory disease*
  - *Leiomyoma*
  - *Adhesions*
  - *Metritis*
  - *Intrauterine contraceptive device*
- Urologic
  - *Bladder neoplasm*
  - *Chronic urinary tract infection*
- Musculoskeletal
  - *Compression fracture of lumbar vertebrae*
  - *Poor posture*
  - *Fibromyalgia*
- Gastrointestinal
  - *Crohn's disease*
  - *Celiac disease*
  - *Colitis*
  - *Irritable bowel syndrome*
  - *Colon cancer*
- Neurological
  - *Shingles*
  - *Degenerative joint disease*
  - *Herniated disk*
- Psychological
  - *Personality disorders*
  - *Depression*
  - *Sleep disorders*
- Other
  - *Sexual and/or physical abuse*

Medical Management

Medical management of CPP depends on the cause. Possible treatments include:

- Pain management
  - *Physical therapy*
  - *Pain medications such as narcotics and NSAIDs*
- Hormones (for pain related to menstrual cycle and metritis)
- Antibiotics
- Steroids
- Antidepressants
- Laparoscopy surgery to release adhesions
- Nutrition (avoiding foods that can increase inflammation of colitis or irritable bowel syndrome)
- Alternative medicine

Chronic pelvic pain (CPP) is a complex disorder with multiple contributing etiologies. The treatment of women with CPP requires a multidimensional approach given the complex overlap of possible etiologies. This article reviewed recent literature in the treatment of CPP. Evidenced-based interventions are:

- NSAIDs: are the first-line treatment for CPP
- Antidepressants: used for pain and comorbidities such as depression or anxiety
- Anticonvulsants: significant pain relief with use of gabapentin either alone or with amitriptyline
- Psychotherapy: cognitive behavioral therapy has the greatest empirical evidence of success compared to counseling, group therapy, and biofeedback
- Therapies used in the treatment for endometriosis, interstitial cystitis, pelvic adhesive disease, adenomyosis, and pelvic venous congestion

Nursing Actions

- Assess and document location, characteristic, frequency, and quality of pain.
- Assess effectiveness of pain interventions.
- Assess level of knowledge regarding cause of pain.
- Provide teaching as indicated by knowledge assessment.
- Provide information regarding diagnostic tests or surgeries.
- Provide information on use of nonpharmacological techniques such as relaxation, guided imagery, hot applications, and massage.
- Teach woman to use pain-control measures before pain becomes severe.

POLYCYSTIC OVARY SYNDROME

Polycystic ovary syndrome (PCOS), also known as Stein-Leventhal syndrome, is an endocrine disorder that affects 5% to 10% of women of childbearing age. The etiology is not fully understood, but it is believed that there is a genetic component to the cause since it occurs in families (DuRant & Leslie, 2009). Women with PCOS have:

- Elevated levels of estrogen, testosterone, and LH
- Decrease in the secretion of FSH
- Multiple follicular cysts on one or both ovaries producing excess estrogen (**Fig. 19-2**)

Women with PCOS are at higher risk for:

- Type 2 diabetes
  - *Women with PCOS are at risk for insulin resistance (the body produces insulin but does not use it properly) and hyperinsulinemia (hyperglycemia present despite high levels of insulin).*
  - *Obesity increases risk for diabetes.*

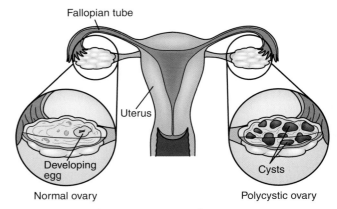

Figure 19–2 Polycystic Ovary Syndrome.

- Cardiovascular disease
  - *Insulin resistance and obesity increase the woman's risk for carotid and coronary atherosclerosis.*
  - *Endocrine changes related to PCOS increases risk for ↑low-density lipoprotein cholesterol and ↓high-density lipoprotein.*
- Hypertension
  - *Related to insulin resistance*
- Cancer—endometrial, ovarian, breast
  - *Related to high levels of continuous estrogen*
- Dyslipidemia
  - *Related to endocrine changes*
- Infertility
  - *Anovulation related to ↑androgen levels, ↑LH and ↓FSH*
- Sleep apnea
  - *Related to obesity and insulin resistance (DuRant & Leslie, 2009)*
- Metabolic syndrome (see Critical Component: Metabolic Syndrome)
  - *Endocrine changes related to PCOS increases risk of ↑low-density lipoprotein cholesterol and ↓high-density lipoprotein*

CRITICAL COMPONENT

Metabolic Syndrome

Metabolic syndrome is a group of conditions that increase an individual's risk for heart disease, stroke, and diabetes. Approximately one third of women with PCOS also have metabolic syndrome. To be diagnosed with the syndrome an individual needs to have three of the following conditions:

- Abdominal obesity: a waist circumference in women ≥ 35 inches
- High triglyceride levels: ≥ 150 mg/dL
- Low HDL cholesterol level: 50 mg/dL for women
- Increased blood pressure: Systolic ≥ 130 mm Hg and/or diastolic ≥ 85 mm Hg
- Elevated fasting blood glucose: ≥ 110 mg/dL

(National Heart Lung and Blood Institute, 2011)

Signs and Symptoms (see Critical Component: Primary Characteristics of PCOS)

- Infertility
  - *PCOS is the most common cause of female infertility; most women with PCOS do not ovulate.*
- Menstrual disorders
  - *Irregular, infrequent, and/or absent menstrual periods*
- Hirsutism
  - *Increased hair growth on face, chest, stomach, and back*
- Ovarian cysts
- Obesity
- Oily skin and acne
- Pelvic pain
- Male-pattern baldness

CRITICAL COMPONENT

Primary Characteristics of PCOS

- Ovulatory and menstrual dysfunctions
  - Anovulation
  - Amenorrhea or decreased frequency of menses
  - Menorrhagia when menses does occur
- Hyperandrogenemia
  - Excessive levels of androgens in the body
- Clinical features of hyperandrogenemia
  - Increased hair growth on face, chest, stomach, and back
  - Severe acne
  - Male-pattern baldness
- Polycystic ovaries
  - Multiple cysts on the ovaries

(Smith & Taylor, 2011)

Medical Management

- Lifestyle modifications
  - *Diet and exercise to assist in weight loss, which helps:*
    - Reduce risk for type 2 diabetes
    - Decrease levels of androgens
    - Improve the frequency of ovulation and menstruation
    - Reduce risk of cardiovascular disease (**Fig. 19-3**)
- Hormone therapy
  - *Low-dose hormonal contraceptives for women who do not wish to conceive. These contraceptives inhibit LH production, decrease testosterone levels, and reduce degree of acne and hirsutism.*
- Fertility therapy
  - *Medications that induce ovulation, such as Clomid*
  - *Assisted reproductive technology (ART), such as in vitro fertilization (IVF), may be used for women who do not respond to medications.*
- Diabetic medications
  - *Antidiabetic medications are prescribed to lower blood glucose levels. They also can lower testosterone, which reduces the degree of acne, hirsutism, and abdominal obesity and may help regulate the menstrual cycle and treat infertility.*

Nursing Actions

PCOS has both physical and psychological effects on the woman. Body image can be negatively affected by changes stemming from PCOS. Women need opportunities to share their concerns about PCOS and to receive information on methods to decrease or counteract the effects of PCOS. Areas to discuss with the woman include:

- Risk factors related to PCOS
- Weight reduction through diet and exercise
  - *Explain the benefits of weight loss on PCOS.*
  - *Provide information on healthy diet and assist the woman in developing a healthy diet plan.*
- Treatment options for hirsutism
  - *Electrolysis or laser hair removal*
- Treatment options for acne and oily skin
  - *Evaluation and treatment by dermatologist*
- Infertility issues
- Psychological effects of body changes related to PCOS such as depression and increased anxiety.

ENDOMETRIOSIS

Endometriosis is a chronic inflammatory disease in which the presence and growth of endometrial tissue is found outside the uterine cavity (see Critical Component: Endometriosis).

- The tissue responds to the changes in estrogen and progesterone levels of the menstrual cycle.
  - *Tissue is estrogen dependent; thus, it is most common during the reproductive years.*
- Tissue and/or lesions are usually found in the peritoneal surfaces of reproductive organs and adjacent structures of the pelvis, such as ovaries, fallopian tubes, bladder, bowel, and intestines.
  - *The ovaries are the most common sites.*
- Cause of endometriosis is unknown. The primary theory is that it is due to retrograde menstruation, which transports endometrial tissue outside the uterine cavity, and the tissue adheres to surrounding organs. Other theories include genetic predisposition, immunologic changes, and hormonal influences (Lentz et al., 2012).

Signs and Symptoms

One third of women with endometriosis are asymptomatic. The symptoms can vary depending on the location of the lesions. The degree of symptoms does not correlate with the size of lesions.

- Pelvic pain and dysmenorrhea
  - *Begins a few days before menses and ends at end of menstruation*
- Low back pain
- Pelvic pressure
- Dyspareunia

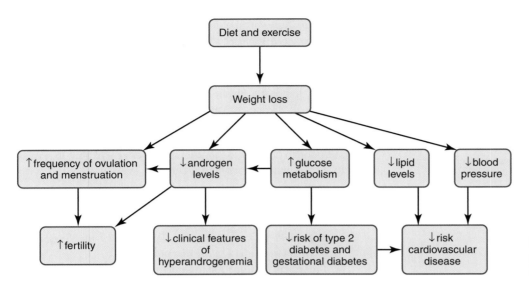

Figure 19-3 Effects of weight management in women with PCOS.

- Infertility
- Premenstrual spotting and menorrhagia
- Diarrhea, pain with defecation, and constipation (may be present with lesions of the bowel)
- Bloody urine with bladder involvement
- Fixed retroverted uterus
- Enlarged and tender ovaries

- *Common medications include:*
  - Danazol
  - GnRH agonists (Lupron, Zoladex, and Nafarelin)
  - Oral contraceptive pills
  - Progestins
- Symptoms usually return within 1–5 years after medications are stopped.

CRITICAL COMPONENT

Endometriosis

- Abnormal growth of tissue resembling the endometrium that is present outside of the uterine cavity.
- Tissue responds to changes in estrogen and progesterone levels.

  - *The tissue grows and thickens during the secretory and proliferative stages of the menstrual cycle.*
  - *The tissue breaks down and bleeds into the surrounding tissues during the menstrual phase.*

- Bleeding into surrounding tissues causes inflammation.
- Scarring, fibrosis, and adhesions can result from continued inflammation.

Medication

Nafarelin (Synarel)

- Indication: Endometriosis
- Action: A synthetic analogue of gonadotropin-releasing hormone (GnRH). Prolonged use causes a reduction in serum estrone, E_2, testosterone, and androstenedione.
- Side effects: Emotional instability, headaches, vaginal dryness, acne, cessation of menses, impaired fertility, decreased libido, hot flashes
- Route and doses: Intranasal; one spray (200 mcg) in morning in one nostril and one spray (200 mcg) in the other nostril in the evening up to a maximum of 800 mcg/day.

(Source: Vallerand & Sanoski, 2013)

Emotional Impact

The physical symptoms of endometriosis can have an effect on the woman's mental health. The woman may experience anger and grief related to loss of fertility. The pain related to endometriosis can interfere with her social activities, and dyspareunia can have an effect on intimate relationships.

Medical Management

- Analgesic therapy
  - *NSAIDs commonly used for pain management.*
- Hormonal therapy
  - *Goal is to suppress menstruation and further growth of tissue.*

- Surgical treatment
  - *Surgical removal of lesions via laparoscopy procedure and laser treatment: used for women with severe symptoms who are infertile and desire pregnancy*
  - *Hysterectomy with bilateral salpingo-oophorectomy and removal of adhesions and lesions: used for women with severe symptoms who do not desire pregnancy*
  - *Endometriosis may recur after surgical interventions.*
- Assisted reproduction
  - *Ovulation induction with intrauterine insemination or in vitro fertilization: may be used for infertile women with endometriosis who have not responded to other therapies for treatment of infertility (Lentz et al., 2012)*

Nursing Actions

- Patient education regarding endometriosis
- Patient education regarding pain management
  - *NSAIDs*
  - *Heat therapy*
  - *Biofeedback*
  - *Relaxation techniques*
- Emotional support
  - *Provide opportunities for the woman to explore her feelings related to living with endometriosis.*
- Patient education on prescribed treatment plan
  - *Information on medications, including action, side effects, and dosage*
  - *Information on surgical intervention*

INFECTIONS

Infections of the reproductive system can increase a woman's risk for cancer, chronic pain, systemic infections, and infertility. Early interventions can decrease the woman's risk for complications related to prolonged or repeated infections of the pelvic region.

Pelvic Inflammatory Disease (PID)

PID is an acute infection of the upper genital track that can involve the uterus, fallopian tubes, and ovaries, and can spread to the peritoneum.

- Both aerobic and anaerobic bacteria are causative agents with *Chlamydia trachomatis* and *Neisseria gonorrhoeae* the most common agents.
- Bacterial infections ascend from the vagina and/or cervix to uterus and fallopian tubes and then to ovaries and spread to the peritoneum.
- Consequences of acute PID are infertility, ectopic pregnancies, and chronic pelvic pain.
  - *Ectopic pregnancy is 10 times greater in women with history of PID due to the scarring and adhesions in the fallopian tubes. Scarring and adhesions are the results of the inflammatory response to the infection that destroys cells and the resulting repair of the damaged tissue.*

Risk Factors

- History of sexually transmitted infections (STI)
- Multiple sexual partners
- Under age 25 and sexually active
  - *75% of cases occur with women under 25 years of age, and it is the most common severe infection of women ages 16–25 years (Lentz et al., 2012).*
- Douching, which can push bacteria upward into uterus and through fallopian tubes
- Intrauterine devices (IUD)
  - *There is an increased risk of PID at time of placement and 3 weeks following placement of an IUD.*

Signs and Symptoms

Women with PID present with a wide range of nonspecific signs and symptoms, which increases the risk of an incorrect diagnosis.

- Women may be asymptomatic.
  - *This is referred to as atypical or silent PID (Lenza et al., 2012).*
- Severe abdominal, uterine, and ovarian pain and tenderness—most common symptom
- Irregular menses
- Abnormal vaginal discharge with foul odor
- Pain during sexual intercourse
- Fever (100.4°F or 38°C)
- Elevated white blood cell (WBC) and erythrocyte sedimentation rate (ERS)

Definitive Criteria for Diagnosing PID

- Evidence of metritis on endometrial biopsy
- Thickened fluid-filled fallopian tubes noted on transvaginal sonogram or MRI
- Abnormalities noted during laparoscopic examination

Medical Management

- Treatment is usually provided on an outpatient basis.
- Test for STI and treat as indicated.
- Oral antibiotic therapy
  - *Woman is reevaluated after 48–72 hours of antibiotic therapy.*
  - *When PID responds to treatment, the woman should be examined 4–6 weeks later for reevaluation (Lentz, 2012).*
- Treatment of sexual partner to decrease the risk of reinfection.
- Analgesia for pain management
- Hospitalization with IV antibiotic therapy for women who:
  - *are pregnant*
  - *do not respond to oral antibiotic treatment*
  - *are unable to follow or tolerate outpatient treatment plan*
  - *are severely ill*
  - *have an abscess in fallopian tube or ovaries (Women's Health, 2010a)*
- Patient education

Nursing Actions

- Patient education of risk factors for PID
- Patient education on risk reduction
  - *Be in a monogamous sexual relationship with a partner who has been screened for STI and is not infected*
  - *Use condoms correctly and each time engaged in sexual activity*
  - *Avoid douching*
- Patient education regarding proper use of antibiotics
- Patient education on signs, symptoms, and consequences of PID

VAGINITIS

Vaginitis is an inflammation of the vagina. Symptoms of vaginitis include vaginal discharge than can be malodorous depending on the causative agent, burning, irritation, or itching.

■ The vaginal flora is a delicate ecosystem primarily composed of various lactobacilli, which inhibit the growth of yeast and bacteria. Vaginitis occurs when there is a disruption of the vaginal ecosystem.
■ The most common types of vaginitis are:
   ■ *Candida vaginitis*
   ■ *Bacterial vaginosis*
   ■ *Trichomoniasis (**Table 19–3**)*

Candida Vaginitis

Candida vaginitis, also called candidiasis or a yeast infection, is caused by *Candida albicans* (see Critical Component: Candida Vaginitis). *Candida albicans* is a gram-positive fungus that lives on all surfaces of the human body. When the vaginal ecosystem is disturbed the fungus rapidly grows, causing an infection. Factors that can affect the vaginal ecosystem are:

■ Hormonal changes
   ■ *High estrogen levels during pregnancy favor growth of fungus.*
   ■ *Increased prevalence of candida vaginitis preceding and immediately following menstrual period*

TABLE 19–3 SEXUALLY TRANSMITTED INFECTIONS (STI)			
SDI	CAUSATIVE AGENT	MANIFESTATION/SYMPTOMS	TREATMENT
Acquired immune deficiency syndrome (AIDS)	Human immunodeficiency virus (HIV) (Viral)	Individual may be asymptomatic for years. Early symptoms: Sore throat, rhinitis, rash. Later symptoms: Leukopenia, idiopathic thrombocytopenia, fever, night sweats, weight loss, lymphadenopathy, dry cough. Women may also have: candidiasis, BV, PID, and menstrual cycle changes. HIV infection is usually diagnosed via the HIV-1 and HIV-2 antibody tests.	No cure for HIV currently exists. Highly active antiretroviral therapy (HAART) is the standard treatment. HAART is effective in maintaining the health of HIV-positive women and in reducing the perinatal transmission of the virus.
Chlamydia	*Chlamydia trachomatis* (Bacterial)	Most common bacterial STI in United States and the leading cause of preventable infertility and ectopic pregnancies. The majority of infected women are asymptomatic; 30% have a mucopurulent cervical discharge. Other symptoms include spotting, urethritis, lower abdominal pain, nausea, fever, pain during sexual intercourse. Chlamydia is diagnosed via cultures of cervical epithelial cells. Chlamydia can also live in the throat, rectum and urethra.	Antibiotic therapy: • Doxycycline 100 mg orally twice a day for 7 days *or* • Azithromycin 1 gm orally given in a single dose • Infected partner should also be treated to decrease risk of reinfection.
Genital warts/ condylomas	Human papilloma virus (HPV) (Viral)	Painless warty growth in the vagina or on the vulva, perineum, or anal areas	Treatment options include: • Topical application of podofilox, which can be applied by the patient • Topical application of trichloroacetic acid, which is applied by health care provider • Cryotherapy • CO$_2$ laser surgery • Electrosurgery • Surgical removal

TABLE 19–3   SEXUALLY TRANSMITTED INFECTIONS (STI)—cont'd

SDI	CAUSATIVE AGENT	MANIFESTATION/SYMPTOMS	TREATMENT
Genital herpes	Herpes simplex virus (HSV), types 1 and 2 (Viral)	Infected women may have no or minimal symptoms. Symptoms are similar to those of the flu: malaise, muscle aches, and headaches. Other symptoms can include itching and burning feeling in the genital or anal areas, vaginal discharge, feeling of pressure in pelvic area, and lymphadenopathy. Lesions (small red bumps or blisters or open sores) in area where virus entered the body-cervix, vagina. Diagnosis is usually based on patient history and examination.	There is no cure for genital herpes. Treatment plan includes: • Antiviral medications such as acyclovir • Oral analgesia for symptom management • Application of cool compresses containing peppermint oil for symptom management • Use of condoms to prevent spread of virus
Gonorrhea	*Neisseria gonorrhoeae* (Bacterial)	Women are commonly asymptomatic. Symptoms include vaginal discharge, mennorrhagia, postcoital bleeding, low backache, urinary frequency, dysuria, and pain during sexual intercourse. Gonorrhea is diagnosed via test such as cultures of the cervical discharge.	Recommended therapy is single IM dose of ceftriaxone given in combination with pro-azithromycin or doxycycline. Infected partner should be treated to decrease risk of reinfection.
Hepatitis B	Hepatitis B virus (HBV) (Viral)	HBV is found in highest concentrations in the blood and lower concentrations in semen, vaginal secretions, and wound exudates. Sexual intercourse is the most common mode of transmission. Women are often asymptomatic. Symptoms include fever, fatigue, loss of appetite, nausea, vomiting, abdominal pain, joint pain, dark-colored urine, clay-colored stools, and jaundice. Symptoms appear 60–150 days after exposure.	There is no specific treatment for acute HBV. Therapy is directed at symptom management. Antiviral medications are used for chronic HBV.
Syphilis	*Treponema pallidum* (Bacterial)	Syphilis progresses in stages: Primary syphilis symptom is a single, painless ulcer (chancre) in the genital area, mouth, or point of contact. Appears 10–90 days after contact. The chancre lasts 4–6 weeks and usually resolves without treatment. Secondary syphilis symptoms include skin rash, fever, sore throat, lymphadenopathy, muscle aches, weight loss, and fatigue. Appears 6 weeks to 6 months after the appearance of the chancre. If not treated, the symptoms resolve on own within 2–10 weeks. Tertiary syphilis: Approximately one-third of infected individuals will develop tertiary syphilis. Without treatment, the bacteria can spread throughout the body, and symptoms are related to damage of internal organs. Screening tests include rapid plasma reagin (RPR) and Venereal Disease Research Laboratory (VDRL).	Penicillin G is the treatment of choice. The specific regimen depends on the length of infection. Infected partner should be treated to decrease risk of reinfection.

Continued

| **TABLE 19–3   SEXUALLY TRANSMITTED INFECTIONS (STI)—cont'd** | | | |
SDI	CAUSATIVE AGENT	MANIFESTATION/SYMPTOMS	TREATMENT
Trichomoniasis	*Trichomonas vaginalis* (Protozoan)	Most women are asymptomatic. Symptoms appear 5–28 days after exposure. Symptoms include profuse frothy gray or yellow-green vaginal discharge with foul odor; erythema, edema, pruritus of the external genitalia, and pain during sexual intercourse. Small, red ulcerations in the vagina and/or on cervix may be observed during examination. Diagnosis: Microscopic evaluation to confirm trichomoniasis or rapid trichomoniasis test	Metronidazole (Flagyl) is medication of choice. It may be administered as a single dose of 2 grams orally or 500 mg orally twice a day for 7 days. Partner needs to be treated at same time and condoms used to prevent future infections. Women should be advised not to drink alcohol for 24 hours after completing metronidazole therapy. The combination of alcohol and medication can cause flushing, nausea, vomiting, headaches, and abdominal cramping.

■ Depressed cell-mediated immunity
■ *Women taking exogenous corticosteroids or with AIDS are at higher risk for reoccurring candida vaginitis.*
■ Antibiotic use
■ *Lactobacillus, which inhibits the growth of fungi, is part of the normal vaginal bacteria flora. Certain broad-spectrum antibiotics, such as penicillin and tetracycline, can destroy lactobacillus allowing the rapid growth of Candida albicans (Lentz, 2012).*

CRITICAL COMPONENT

Candida Vaginitis

Candida vaginitis is common in women of childbearing age. Three out of four women will experience at least one occurrence of Candida vaginitis within their lifetime.

Risk Factors

■ Suppressed immune system
■ Antibiotic therapy
■ Steroid therapy
■ Diabetes
■ Pregnancy
■ Menopause

Signs and Symptoms

■ Itching and irritation in the vulva and vagina areas are the primary symptoms.
■ White, cheesy vaginal discharge
■ Pain with sexual intercourse
■ Burning on urination
■ Vaginal pH below 4.5

Medical Management

■ Diagnosis with a wet smear of vaginal secretions
■ Most vaginal yeast infections can be treated with over-the-counter (OTC) remedies.
■ *Examples of OTC are:*
■ Miconazole (Micon-7, Monistat-3)
■ Tioconazole (Monistat-1, Vagistat-1)
■ Butoconazole (Gynazole-1)
■ Clotrimazole (Femcare)
■ *The OTC cream or suppository is placed into the vagina for 1–7 days depending on the formulation.*
■ *Health care provider needs to be contacted if symptoms continue for more than a week or if symptoms are recurrent.*
■ *Pregnant women need to consult with their health care provider before using OTC remedies.*
■ *Women with suppressed immune systems need to be treated by health care provider because candidal infections can affect various internal organs.*
■ Fluconazole (Diflucan), an antifungal prescription medication, is given when OTCs are not effective or when there is a severe infection. Treatment is a single-dose oral dose of 150 mg. The safety of use during pregnancy has not been established. It is usually compatible with women who are lactating (Vallerand & Sanoski, 2013).
■ *Women with reoccurring Candida vaginitis may be treated with a 6-month course of fluconazole.*

Nursing Actions

■ Teach the woman proper use of OTC medications.
■ Instruct the woman to notify health care provider if symptoms continue or are recurrent.
■ *Women can mistake bacteria vaginitis for Candida vaginitis, which has a different treatment plan.*

■ Instruct the woman to contact health care provider if any of the following occur:
  ■ *Bloody discharge*
  ■ *Abdominal pain*
  ■ *Fever*
■ Instruct the woman to wear cotton underwear to decrease risk of recurrent infections.

Bacterial Vaginosis

Bacterial vaginosis (BV), the most common vaginal infection, occurs when there is a disruption in the normal vaginal flora; a decrease in lactobacilli and an increase in organisms such as genital mycoplasms, peptostreptococci, and gardnerella (see Critical Component: Bacterial Vaginosis).

CRITICAL COMPONENT

Bacterial Vaginosis

■ Women who experience abnormal vaginal discharge need to be seen by their health care providers since symptoms of BV are similar to those of chlamydia, gonorrhea, candidiasis, and trichomoniasis.
■ Women with BV are at greater risk for preterm labor and metritis.
■ BV is more common in lesbians and bisexual women than in heterosexual women.

Risk Factors

■ New sexual partner—male or female
■ Multiple sexual partners
■ Lesbian couples who share sex toys without cleaning the toy between use
■ Douching
  ■ *Douching can alter the normal vaginal flora*
■ Antibiotic therapy
  ■ *Antibiotics can alter the normal vaginal flora.*

Signs and Symptoms

■ Vaginal odor, often described as fishy smelling.
■ Vaginal discharge that is often thin and white or gray; may also be described as milky

Medical Management

■ Microscopic examination of vaginal discharge to rule out other causes such as candidiasis and trichomoniasis
■ Gynecological examination to assess the appearance of the vaginal lining and the cervix
■ Pharmacological therapy:
  ■ *Metronidazole—Taken orally in pill form or inserted vaginally in a gel form*
  ■ *Clindamycin—Taken orally in pill form or inserted vaginally in gel form*
  ■ *Miconazole—Inserted vaginally in form of suppository or cream*
■ Male partner does not need to be treated.
■ Female partner may need treatment.

Nursing Actions

■ Provide education on proper administration, actions, and side effects of medications.
■ Instruct women who are taking Flagyl PO to take with meals and avoid drinking alcohol. The combination of Flagyl and alcohol can cause severe nausea and vomiting, flushing, tachycardia, and shortness of breath.
■ Provide information on signs and symptoms of possible recurrence that the woman should report to health care provider.
■ Provide information of risk factors for BV.

Sexually Transmitted Infections

The terms *sexually transmitted infections* (STIs) and *sexually transmitted diseases* (STDs) are used interchangeably in the clinical setting. STIs are primarily transmitted through vaginal intercourse, anal intercourse, and oral sex (see Critical Component: Sexually Transmitted Infections [STIs]). Table 19-3 summarizes the most common STI.

■ Chlamydia and gonorrhea are prevalent in the adolescent population and are the two most reported infectious diseases in the United States.
■ Women can have a STI and be asymptomatic.
  ■ *Women who are asymptomatic are still at risk for infecting their sexual partner.*
■ Both the woman and her partner need to be treated for the STI to decrease risk of reinfection.

CRITICAL COMPONENT

Sexually Transmitted Infections (STI)

Untreated STI places a woman at risk for:

■ Cervical cancer
■ Pelvic inflammatory disease
■ Infertility due to blocked fallopian tubes
■ Ectopic pregnancy due to blocked fallopian tubes
■ Chronic pelvic pain

Lesbians and STI

Lesbians and bisexual women are at the same risk for STI as heterosexual women. The types of sexual behavior that carry a risk for STI between women are:

■ Oral-vaginal/vulval contact: Herpes, syphilis, and gonorrhea
■ Digital-vaginal contact : HVP, bacterial vaginosis, trichomonas, chlamydia, and gonorrhea
■ Oral-anal contact: Syphilis, herpes, and hepatitis A
■ Genital-genital and genital-body contact: HPV and herpes
■ Insertive sex (use of sex toys and dildos): Trichomonas, gonorrhea, herpes, and HPV (County of Los Angeles, 2012)

Nursing Actions

- Provide information on transmission and treatment of STI.
- Provide information on methods to decrease risk of STI.
  - *Be in a monogamous sexual relationship with a partner who has been screened for STI and is not infected.*
  - *Use condoms correctly and each time engaged in sexual activity.*
  - *Talk with partner about STI and the use of condoms before engaging in sexual activities.*
  - *Talk with your health care provider and your sexual partner about any STI you or your partner presently has or had in the past.*
  - *Follow current guidelines for frequency of pelvic exams, Pap test, and HPV testing.*

Urinary Tract Infections (UTI)

- It is estimated that 20% of women will encounter a UTI during their lifetime (American College of Obstetricians and Gynecologists [ACOG], 2008).
- Women are 30 times more likely than men to develop a UTI because of the shorter length of the female urethra and proximity of urethra to rectum.
- *Escherichia coli*, which is normally found in the colon, is the most common bacteria responsible for UTI.
- Chlamydia can place a woman at risk for UTI.
- Untreated UTI places the woman at risk for pyelonephritis.
- Diagnosis of UTI is usually based on presenting symptoms and urinalysis. A urine culture and sensitivity may be required.

Risk Factors

- Young girls and menopausal women (see Critical Component: UTI and Older Women)
- Altered immunity
- Diabetes
- Urinary tract obstructions
- Pregnancy
- Sexual activity
  - *Irritation of the urethra during sexual activity can cause bacteria to migrate upward into the urinary tract.*
- Allergic reaction to certain ingredients in soaps, vaginal creams, and bubble baths

Signs and Symptoms

- Dysuria
- Urinary frequency
- Urgency
- Sensation of bladder fullness
- Suprapubic tenderness
- Cloudy, foul-smelling urine
- Backache and pelvic pain
- Fever

CRITICAL COMPONENT

UTI and Older Women

- Older women are more susceptible to UTI due to:
  - Suppressed immune system
  - Weakened muscles of the bladder that increases the risk for incomplete emptying of the bladder
  - Decreased levels of estrogen which can alter the normal vaginal flora allowing for growth of E. coli, which can spread to the urinary tract.
- Older women usually do not present with the common signs of UTI such as fever.
- When fever does occur, it is related to a serious UTI and needs immediate treatment.
- UTI places a stress on the body, and in older women the stress can cause confusion and abrupt changes in behavior.
- Symptoms of UTI in older women can include:
  - Confusion or delirium
  - Agitation
  - Hallucinations
  - Poor motor skills or dizziness
  - Falling

Medical Management

Antibiotic therapy is used for uncomplicated UTI. Medications most commonly used are:

- Trimethoprim/sulfamethoxazole (e.g., Bactrim, Septra)
- Fluoroquinolones (e.g., Cipro)
- Nitrofurantoin macrocrystals (e.g., Macrodantin)
- Amoxicillin/clavulanate (e.g., Augmentin)

Medication

Trimethoprim/Sulfamethoxazole (Bactrim)

- Indication: Urinary tract infection (also used for treatment of bronchitis, otitis media, pneumonia)
- Action: Inhibits the metabolism of folic acid in bacteria
- Common side effects: Nausea, vomiting, diarrhea, and rashes
- Route and dosage: PO; 160 mg TMP/800 mg SMX every 12 hours for 10–14 days

(Vallerand & Sanoski, 2013)

Nursing Actions

- Teach women to take full course of antibiotic therapy.
- Provide information on strategies to promote bladder health and ways to decrease risk for developing UTI.
  - *Drink 2–4 quarts of fluid each day.*
  - *Void every 2–4 hours; avoid postponing urination because when urine remains in the bladder for prolonged periods, it allows increased time for bacteria to multiply.*
  - *Empty bladder before and after intercourse to flush out bacteria in the urethra.*
  - *Remain hydrated to keep bacteria flushed out of the urinary tract system.*

■ *Drink cranberry juice to acidify the urine.*
■ *Wipe the urethral meatus and perineum from front to back after voiding.*
■ *Wear cotton underpants and change daily; avoid tight-fitting underwear and pants.*
■ *Avoid caffeine and alcohol since these can irritate the bladder.*
■ *Do not douche or use feminine hygiene products that can alter the normal vagina flora.*
■ *Avoid harsh soaps, powders, sprays; avoid bubble baths.*
■ Teach women about the signs and symptoms of UTI to be reported to their health care providers.

Leiomyoma of the Uterus

Leiomyomas of the uterus, also referred to as myomas or uterine fibroids, are benign fibrous tumors of the uterine wall. Leiomyomas:

■ Are the most common tumors in women
■ Vary in size and location
■ Are estrogen-and-progesterone sensitive
■ Growth is seen during the reproductive years due to the increase in hormone production.

Risk Factors

■ Early menarche
■ Increasing age during reproductive years—as women age, their risk for leiomyomas increases.
■ Low parity
■ Tamoxifin use
■ Obesity (Lentz, 2012)

Signs and Symptoms

Leiomyomas are usually asymptomatic. The severity of symptoms is related to the number, size, and locations of the myomas. Symptoms can include:

■ Pelvic pressure from the enlarging mass
■ Dysmenorrhea, metrorrhagia, menorrhagia
  ■ *Women are at risk for anemia due to menorrhagia.*
■ Pelvic pain
■ Urinary frequency and urgency when myomas are pressing on the bladder
■ Palpation of tumor during bimanual pelvic examination

Medical Management

■ Pelvic ultrasound to confirm diagnosis of tumors and rule out pregnancy
■ Routine pelvic examinations every 6 months to assess rate of growth
■ Blood transfusions may be needed for severe anemia related to excessive blood loss.
■ Treatment for leiomyomas is based on the size and location of the tumors, the degree to which they interfere with the woman's quality of life, and whether the woman

desires pregnancy. Most tumors will shrink after menopause. Treatment options include:
■ *GnRH agonists for three months to control bleeding and shrink tumor*
■ *Uterine artery embolization (UAE)*
  ■ Polyvinyl alcohol pellets are injected into selected blood vessels to block the blood supply to the tumor and cause it to shrink.
■ *Laser surgery:*
  ■ Laser coagulation vaporizes the fibroids and produces necrosis.
  ■ Can increase risk for infertility due to uterine scarring.
■ *Myomectomy, removal of the tumor, is common for symptomatic women who desire pregnancy.*
■ *Hysterectomy is recommended for women who do not desire pregnancy and who are experiencing excess bleeding.*
  ■ Leiomyomas are the most common indication for hysterectomy.

Nursing Actions

Nursing actions vary based on the method of medical or surgical treatment. Nurses are most likely to care for women who are being treated for myomas in the inpatient setting following a hysterectomy. (See section on hysterectomy.)

Ovarian Cysts

Ovarian cysts are enclosed sacs that contain fluid, blood, and/or cells. The cysts develop inside or on the surface of the ovaries. Ovarian cysts are often discovered during routine pelvic examinations. Two of the more common types of ovarian cysts are follicular cysts and corpus luteum cysts.

Follicular Cysts

A **follicular cyst,** a benign tumor, is the most frequent cyst that occurs on the ovary.

■ Develops during the follicular phase (first half of the menstrual cycle).
■ Forms when the dominant mature follicle fails to rupture (ovulate) and begins to fill with fluid or when an immature follicle fails to degenerate (Lentz, 2012).
■ Usually are asymptomatic.
  ■ *One-quarter of women report pain and/or sensation of heavy, achy feeling in the pelvis.*
■ Diagnosis is usually based on symptoms and bimanual examination.
  ■ *Ultrasonography may be used to aid in the diagnosis and to rule out pregnancy, but ultrasound cannot provide a definitive diagnosis.*
  ■ *CA 125 blood test: this is elevated in women with ovarian cancer, but can also be elevated in women with endometriosis, myomas, and PID.*
  ■ *Laparoscopic surgery to visualize ovaries and/or remove cyst*
    ■ Important to rule out ovarian cancer

- Most cysts spontaneously disappear either by reabsorption of the fluid within the cyst or by rupturing within 8 weeks (Lentz, 2012).
- Monitoring condition with a repeat examination in 6–8 weeks is the treatment plan of choice when the symptoms are mild.
  - *NSAIDs may be used for pain management.*
- Surgical removal if cyst:
  - *Continues to be present after several menstrual cycles*
  - *Occurs after menopause*
    - Postmenopausal women with ovarian cysts have a higher risk of ovarian cancer.
  - *Enlarges*
  - *Has an unusual appearance on the ultrasound*
  - *Causes severe pain*

Corpus Luteum Cysts

Corpus luteum cysts form from the corpus luteum during the luteal phase (second half of the menstrual cycle). Normally, the corpus luteum forms after ovulation and gradually degenerates if pregnancy does not occur. Occasionally, the corpus luteum seals and fills with fluid or blood and forms a cyst.

- The woman may experience acute lower abdominal pain and delayed menses followed by menorrhagia (Lentz, 2012).
- Diagnosis is usually based on symptoms and bimanual examination.
  - *Endovaginal ultrasound may be used to aid diagnosis and rule out pregnancy.*
  - *CA 125 blood test to aid in ruling out ovarian cancer*
- Most cysts spontaneously disappear within 1–2 menstrual cycles.
  - *Oral contraceptives may be prescribed to inhibit ovulation, which decreases risk of developing additional cysts.*
  - *Large cysts that do not resolve on own within 3 months may require surgical intervention, usually a cystectomy.*
  - *Occasionally, a cyst ruptures and causes sudden and severe abdominal pain and may require surgical intervention and blood transfusions.*
    - Rupture of the cyst can be caused by coitus, exercise, lower abdominal trauma, or pelvic exam and can cause intraperitoneal bleeding.

DISORDERS OF PELVIC SUPPORT

The most common disorders of pelvic support include pelvic organ prolapse, genital fistulas, and urinary incontinence.

Pelvic Organ Prolapse

The pelvic organs are supported by several structures:

- Pelvic floor muscles
- Pelvic ligaments
- Pelvic fascia

When these structures are weakened, a disorder referred to as pelvic organ prolapse can occur.

Pelvic organ prolapse (POP) is the descent of pelvic organs into the vagina or against the vaginal wall. Organs that can be involved are:

- Bladder
- Urethra
- Uterus
- Rectum

Risk Factors

- Childbirth trauma related to:
  - *Vaginal deliveries*
  - *Large babies*
  - *Forceps or vacuum deliveries*
  - *Poor suturing techniques with repair of episiotomies or lacerations*
- Pelvic trauma, i.e., pelvic surgery
- Stress and strain from heavy lifting
- Obesity
- Menopause
- Low levels of estrogen weaken the pelvic floor muscles.

Common disorders related to POP are uterine prolapse, cystocele, and rectocele (**Fig. 19-4**).

Uterine Prolapse

Uterine prolapse occurs when there is a weakening of the pelvic connective tissue, pubococcygeus muscle, and uterine ligaments, allowing the uterus to descend into the vagina.

Assessment Findings

- Protrusion of uterus into the vagina
- Low backache
- Sensation of heaviness in the pelvis or vagina
- Sensation that the uterus is falling out
- Difficult or painful intercourse

Medical Management

- Vaginal pessary: A rubber or silicone-based ring that is placed in the vagina and supports the uterus; is used in a mild degree of prolapse (**Fig. 19-5**).
- Surgery, which may include hysterectomy

Nursing Actions

- Explain the importance of Kegel exercises for improving pelvic muscle strength and teach the woman how to do Kegel exercises.
- Instruct the woman on the treatment and prevention of constipation, such as a high-fiber diet and increased fluid intake. This will help in reducing straining during defecation and decrease stress on existing POP.
- Instruct the woman to avoid heavy lifting to decrease stress on pelvic organs.
- Explain the relationship between increased weight and increased risk of prolapsed uterus and discuss weight reduction strategies.
- Provide post-operative care for women having a hysterectomy.

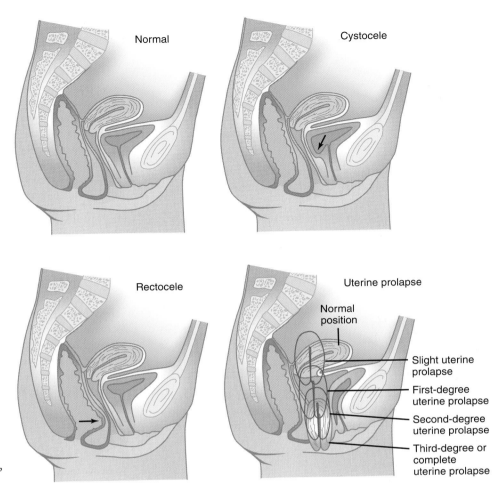

Figure 19-4 Cystocele, rectocele, and uterine prolapse.

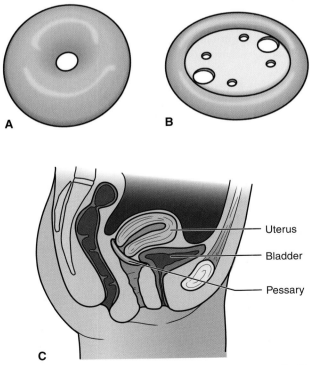

Figure 19-5 Vaginal pessary A. Doughnut pessary, B. Ring pessary, C. Inserted pessary.

Cystocele and Rectocele

■ **Cystocele:** Bulging of the bladder into the vagina. This occurs when the wall between the vagina and bladder weakens and stretches.

■ **Rectocele:** Bulging of the rectum into the vagina. This occurs when the wall between the vagina and the rectum weakens and stretches.

Assessment Findings for Cystocele

■ Bulging mass in the anterior vaginal wall
■ Sense of fullness or pressure in the vaginal area
■ Straining, coughing, bearing down, lifting, or standing for a prolonged period of time increases the degree of bulging
■ Stress incontinence
■ Bladder infections
■ Urine leakage during intercourse
■ Sexual dysfunction such as dyspareunia, vaginal dryness, and irritation (Lentz, 2012)

Assessment Findings for Rectocele

■ Bulging mass in the posterior vaginal wall
■ Straining and prolonged standing can increase the degree of the bulging.
■ Irritation of the vaginal mucosa
■ Constipation

Medical Management

Medical management is based on degree of bulging, effects on the woman's quality of life, and health of the woman. Treatment options include:

- Pessary
- Hormone replacement therapy
- Surgery

Nursing Actions

- Explain the importance of Kegel exercises for improving pelvic muscle strength and teach the woman how to do Kegel exercises.
- Instruct the woman on the treatment and prevention of constipation, such as a high-fiber diet and increased fluid intake. This will help in reducing straining during defecation and decrease stress on existing POP.
- Instruct the woman to avoid heavy lifting to decrease stress on pelvic organs.
- Explain the relationship between increased weight and increased risk of cystoceles/rectoceles and discuss weight reduction strategies.

Genital Fistulas

Genital fistulas are abnormal connections between the vagina and bladder, vagina and urethra, and/or vagina and rectum. The fistula provides a pathway for fecal material or urine to enter the vagina.

Risk Factors

- Trauma of tissue related to childbirth
- Hysterectomy—injury to surrounding tissue
- Pelvic radiotherapy—radiation can damage and weaken pelvic tissue
- Violent coitus or sexual abuse—perforation of tissue caused by forced intercourse
- Crohn's disease—weakening of tissue related to inflammation

Assessment Findings

- Leakage of urine or fecal material from the vagina
- Foul vaginal odor
- Irritation of the vaginal mucosa

Medical Management

- Pelvic, rectal, and perineal skin exams to determine the location and severity of fistula.
- Small fistulas may resolve on their own if tissue is allowed to rest.
- Larger fistulas may require surgical repair.

Nursing Actions

- Reinforce teaching and clarify information provided by the primary health care provider.
- Postoperative care:
  - *Assess vital signs as per protocol.*
  - *Assess perineal area for increased bleeding.*

- *Assess for pain and use appropriate pain management techniques.*
- *Provide post-operative teaching:*
  - Instruct the woman with rectal fistula repair to increase fiber in her diet and increase fluid intake to decrease risk of constipation. Maintaining soft stool decreases trauma to the site and promotes healing.
  - Explain the importance of sitz baths to promote healing and comfort. Sitz baths are usually prescribed.
  - Provide medication information. Antibiotics are usually prescribed.
  - Instruct to notify surgeon when there is an elevated temperature, increased bleeding, or increased pain.

Urinary Incontinence

Urinary incontinence is the loss of bladder control. Urinary incontinence can range from stress urinary incontinence to sudden urge to void followed by uncontrolled voiding. **Stress incontinence** is leakage of urine when there is an increase in intra-abdominal pressure related to such events as coughing, sneezing, and laughing. Urinary incontinence can have a profound effect on the woman's quality of life by limiting her activities due to the embarrassment of uncontrolled urination.

Risk Factors

- Childbirth
- Aging, which leads to a decrease in estrogen and a weakening of muscles, which decreases the ability of the urethra to remain closed
- Obesity—the risk increases for every 5 units of body mass index increase (Lentz, 2012).
- Smoking, which causes chronic coughing and places stress on the urinary sphincters
- Diabetes—neuropathy

Assessment Findings

- Leakage of urine when coughing, sneezing, laughing, or lifting
- Sudden and intense urge to void followed by uncontrolled voiding

Medical Management

- Treatment is based on the degree of incontinence and the effect it has on quality of life.
- Behavioral techniques
  - *Bladder training: Waiting 5 minutes from feeling the urge to void to urinating and gradually increasing the time between urge to voiding*
  - *Scheduled toilet trips: Developing a schedule for voiding and not waiting to feel the urge to void*
  - *Limiting alcohol and caffeine use: These act as a bladder stimulant and as a diuretic.*
  - *Losing weight*
- Pelvic floor exercises
  - *Kegel exercises: Improve pelvic floor muscle strength*

- Medications
  - *Anticholinergic drugs (Detrol): Used for overactive bladders*
  - *Estrogen cream applied to the genital tissues: Improves the tone and tissue in the urethral and vaginal areas*
- Medical devices
  - *Pessary: Inserted in the vagina; helps hold the bladder in place*
  - *Urethral insert: A small tampon-like disposable plug that the woman inserts into urethra prior to activities that can cause stress incontinence, such as sport activity or exercise. The plug is removed after the activity and prior to voiding.*
- Surgery

Medication

Tolterodine (Detrol)

- Action: Inhibits cholinergic mediated bladder contractions.
- Common side effects: Dry mouth, headache, and dizziness
- Route and dosage: PO; 2 mg twice daily

(Data from Vallerand & Sanoski, 2013)

Nursing Actions

- Instruct the woman on the importance of Kegel exercises and teach her how to do Kegel exercises.
- Instruct the woman on the treatment and prevention of constipation by increasing fiber in the diet and increasing fluid intake.
- Instruct her to avoid heavy lifting.
- Explain the relationship between increased weight and increased risk of urinary incontinence and discuss weight reduction strategies.
- Maintain skin integrity by instructing the woman to keep the area clean and dry.
- Encourage the woman to decrease alcohol and caffeine intake, as both cause an increase in urination.
- Provide strategies for retraining the bladder, such as scheduling toileting times and gradually increasing the wait time after she feels the urge to void.

BREAST DISORDERS

Breast disorders include both benign and malignant diseases. Discovery of a breast mass or changes in the breast can evoke a woman's feelings of fear and anxiety that she may have cancer. The three most common breast symptoms are:

- Pain
  - *Pain is usually related to hormonal changes and is most common in perimenopausal women. Pain can also be associated with cysts of the breast. Less than 10% of women with breast cancer will present solely with pain.*
- Discharge
  - *Nipple discharge is not a frequent symptom of breast cancer.*
  - *Discharge from the nipple is classified as spontaneous or elicited. Elicited discharge is discharge that is the result of nipple compression or stimulation.*
  - *Elicited discharge from both nipples that is milky in color and nonbloody is considered normal.*
  - *Spontaneous discharge or elicited discharge from one nipple or discharge that is bloody needs further evaluation.*
- Breast mass
  - *Palpable breast masses are common and are usually benign, but all breast masses need to be evaluated to rule out malignancy.*

Breast self-examination (BSE), clinical breast examinations, and mammography are important in the early detection and treatment of benign and cancerous tumors of the breast (see Chapter 18 for recommended screening and testing).

Fibrocystic Changes

Fibrocystic changes, also known as benign breast disease (BBD), are fluid-filled cysts and are the most common benign breast condition.

- Fibrocystic changes occur in over 50% of women and more often in women in their 20s and 30s.
- The cysts are often tender to touch and fluctuate in size in response to the menstrual cycle.
- Fibrocystic development may be related to an imbalance of estrogen and progesterone.
- Caffeine intake may exacerbate the condition.

Evidence-Based Practice: Incontinence

Spencer, J. (2012). Continence promotion. *Nursing of women's health, 16*, 327–340.

Urinary incontinence is common in women ages 35 and older, yet it often goes untreated due to underreporting by women to their health care provider.

The author reports on the results of a program designed to improve women's knowledge and perspective on urinary incontinence and to encourage care-seeking behaviors. The continence promotion program was an hour-long session that provided information on the prevalence and types/causes of incontinence and the different methods to promote continence. Each participant received a "toolkit" that included a PowerPoint presentation, education video, knowledge questionnaire, and a brochure addressing incontinence issues. Pretest and posttest along with a one

month follow-up phone call were used to evaluate the program. There were measureable changes in the participants' knowledge level at the end of the session, and participants reported behavior changes during the one month follow-up phone call.

Implications:

It is important that women understand that incontinence does not have to be an inevitable part of aging and that there are treatment options. Nurses can have a major role in continence promotion through community educational programs addressing urinary incontinence.

"Toolkit" can be accessed at www.continenceconversation.com

Signs and Symptoms

- Cyclic bilateral breast pain—pain is usually in the upper, outer quadrants of the breasts.
- Increased engorgement and density of the breasts
- Increased nodularity of the breasts
- Fluctuation in the size of the cystic areas

Medical Management

- Differentiate between fibrocystic changes and breast cancer using mammogram and ultrasound. Health care provider may also aspirate the cyst for evaluation of fluid.
- Management centers on symptom relief
- *Diuretics during the premenstrual phase of cycle*
- *Supportive bra—wearing a sports bra day and night*
- *Oral contraceptives—symptoms return in 40% of the women after they discontinue the therapy (Lentz, 2012)*
- *Danazol may be prescribed for severe symptoms.*
- *Avoidance of caffeine, smoking, and alcohol*
- *NSAIDs*
- *Application of heat to the breast*

Nursing Actions

- Teach the woman BSE and changes that need to be reported to her health care provider.
- Provide information on methods of symptom relief, such as heat to breast and supportive bra.

Breast Cancer

Breast cancer is the most common cancer in women in the United States. One in eight women will have breast cancer at some point in her life. Breast cancer in early stages usually produces no symptoms and cannot be felt on palpation. The woman's prognosis improves with early detection and treatment (see Critical Component: Breast Cancer Screening Tool).

Risk Factors

The major risk factors are:

- Increasing age:
  - *Age is the main risk factor.*
  - *85% of breast cancers occur in women after age 40; this increases into the 70s and then decreases.*
- Geographic
  - *Women in the United States, Western Europe, and Australia have the highest rates of breast cancer compared with other countries (Lentz, 2012).*
- Defects in breast cancer gene 1 *(BRCA1)* or breast cancer gene 2 *(BRCA 2)*
- Biopsy-confirmed atypical hyperplasia (ACS, 2012)
- Mammographically dense breasts (ACS, 2012)
- Personal history of breast cancer in at least one breast

Additional factors include:

- High endogenous estrogen or testosterone levels
- High bone density (ACS, 2012)

- Family history of breast cancer
- Exposure to chest radiation
- Excess weight
- Exposure to estrogen: Early onset of menarche, late menopause, or use of hormone therapy
- Smoking
- Exposure to carcinogens
- Excessive use of alcohol
- Exposure to diethylstilbestrol (DES)

Diagnosis

The screening and diagnostic procedures/tests used in the diagnosis of breast cancer may include (**Fig. 19-6**):

- Diagnostic mammograms—images of the area of concern that provide additional information on size and character of the mass
- Breast ultrasounds—assist in determining if the area of concern is a fluid-filled cyst or solid mass
- Magnetic resonance imaging (MRI)—useful in differentiating benign from malignant tissue, especially in women with dense, fibroglandular breasts and from scar tissue and new tumors in women who have had previous lumpectomy (Lentz, 2012)
- Breast biopsy—diagnostic test that can distinguish between benign and malignant tissue

Indicators of Disease Prognosis

- Stage of cancer (**Table 19-4**)
  - *Type and tumor size*
  - *Presence of lymph node involvement*
- Presence of hormone receptor levels
- Presence of HER2/neu (human epidermal growth factor receptor 2) in the tumor tissue

---

CRITICAL COMPONENT

Breast Cancer Screening Tool

- A breast cancer screening tool developed by the National Cancer Institute (NCI) and National Surgical Adjuvant Breast and Bowel Project (NSABP) estimates a woman's risk of developing invasive breast cancer in 5 years and up to age 90.
- It considers data such as the woman's age, family history of breast cancer, and previous breast biopsies.
- It can be accessed at www.cancer.gov/bcrisktool

(National Cancer Institute [NCI], 2011)

Medical Management

Treatment is determined by stage of cancer. The breast cancer staging system goes from stage 0 (ductal carcinoma in situ, the earliest form of breast cancer) to stage IV (the cancer has metastasized to distant organs or to distant lymph nodes).

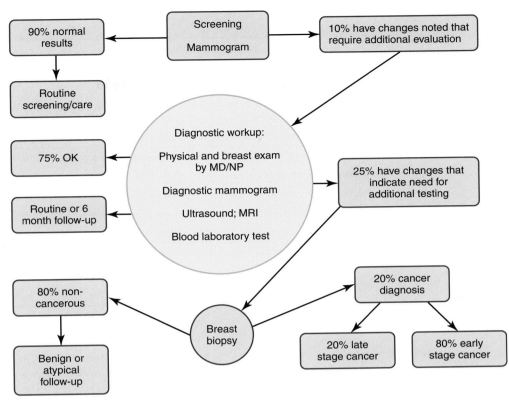

Figure 19–6 Breast cancer diagnosis process.

Source: Imaginis, 2002

TABLE 19–4	STAGING OF BREAST CANCER
STAGE 0	Ductal carcinoma in situ—cancer cells are limited to a duct and have not invaded into surrounding tissue; this is the earliest form of breast cancer.
STAGE IA	The tumor is 2 cm or less in size, and it has not spread to the lymph nodes or distant sites.
STAGE IB	The tumor is 2 cm or less. There is evidence of micrometastases in one to three axillary lymph nodes. It has not spread to distant sites.
STAGE IIA	The cancer has not spread to distant sites, and one of the following applies: • The tumor is larger than 2 cm and less than 5 cm across; it has not spread to the lymph nodes. • The tumor is 2 cm or less; it has spread to one to three axillary nodes with cancer in the lymph nodes larger than 2 mm across. • The tumor is 2 cm or less, and tiny amounts of cancer are found in the internal mammary lymph nodes. • The tumor is 2 cm or less and has spread to one to three axillary lymph nodes and to internal mammary lymph nodes.
STAGE IIB	The cancer has not spread to a distant site, and one of the following applies: • The tumor is larger than 2 cm and less than 5 cm across; it has spread to one to three axillary lymph nodes, and/or tiny amounts of cancer are found in the internal mammary lymph nodes. • The tumor is larger than 5 cm; it has not grown into the chest wall and has not spread to the lymph nodes.
STAGE IIIA	The tumor has not spread to distant sites, and one of the following applies: • The tumor is 5 cm or less. It has spread to four to nine axillary lymph nodes, or it has enlarged the internal mammary lymph nodes. • The tumor is more than 5 cm but has not invaded the chest wall or skin. It has spread to one to nine axillary nodes or to internal mammary nodes.

Continued

TABLE 19–4	STAGING OF BREAST CANCER—cont'd
STAGE IIIB	The cancer has not spread to distant sites. The tumor has grown into the chest wall or skin, and one of the following applies: • It has not spread to lymph nodes. • It has spread to one to three axillary lymph nodes, and/or tiny amounts of cancer are found in internal mammary lymph nodes. • It has spread to four to nine axillary lymph nodes, or it has enlarged the internal mammary lymph nodes.
STAGE IIIC	The cancer has not spread to distant sites. The tumor is any size, and one of the following applies: • It has spread to 10 or more axillary lymph nodes. • It has spread to lymph nodes under or above the clavicle. • It involves axillary lymph nodes and has enlarged the internal mammary lymph nodes. • It has spread to four or more axillary nodes, and tiny amounts are found in internal mammary lymph nodes.
STAGE IV	The cancer has spread to distant organs or lymph nodes distant from the breast. The most common sites are the bone, liver, brain, or lung.
ACS, 2009b	

Medical management requires a multitreatment approach of surgery, radiation, chemotherapy, and hormone therapy.

■ Surgical interventions
  ■ *Lumpectomy: The lump and an area of surrounding normal tissue are removed. This procedure is usually followed by radiation therapy.*
  ■ *Partial or segmental mastectomy: The tumor, the surrounding breast tissue, a portion of the lining of the chest wall, and some of the axillary lymph nodes are removed. This procedure is usually followed by radiation therapy.*
  ■ *Simple mastectomy: All the breast tissue along with the area surrounding the nipple and areola are removed. This procedure may be followed by radiation therapy, chemotherapy, or hormone therapy.*
  ■ *Modified radical mastectomy: The entire breast and several axillary lymph nodes are removed; the chest wall is left intact.*
  ■ *Some women who have mastectomies choose to undergo breast reconstruction. Breast reconstruction, when desired, is performed by a plastic surgeon at the same time as the mastectomy.*
■ Radiation therapy
  ■ *Two types of radiation therapy*
    ■ External radiation: A radiation therapy machine aims radiation toward the tumor. Treatments are given 5 days a week for 5-6 weeks.
    ■ Internal radiation (mammo site): A radioactive substance sealed in needles, seeds, wires, or a catheter are placed directly into or near the tumor. Treatments are given twice a day for 5 days for a total of 10 sessions.
  ■ *Radiation therapy usually begins 3–4 weeks after surgery.*
■ Chemotherapy
  ■ *Oncotype DX test may be performed to determine if the woman is likely to benefit from chemotherapy (see Critical Component: Oncotype DX Test).*

  ■ *Chemotherapy is most commonly used to treat advanced metastatic cancer or to prevent recurrence of cancer.*
  ■ *Usually, a combination of two or more drugs is used.*
  ■ *Chemotherapy agents may be administered orally or intravenously.*
  ■ *Generally, four to eight treatments are given over 6–8 months.*
■ Hormone therapy
  ■ *Some breast cancer cells require estrogen to grow and are classified as estrogen-receptor positive. This means that the cancer cells have a protein to which estrogen binds.*
  ■ *Antiestrogen medications such as tamoxifen (Nolvadex-D) bind to these protein receptors, blocking estrogen binding and reducing the influence of estrogen on the tumor.*
  ■ *Fulvestrant (Faslodex) given by injection reduces the number of estrogen receptors on breast tumors.*
  ■ *Aromatase inhibitors such as anastrozole (Arimidex) may be used in postmenopausal women whose cancer is classified as estrogen-receptor positive. Aromatase inhibitors interfere with the amount of estrogen produced by the woman's body tissue (not the ovaries) by blocking the conversion of androgens into estrogens.*
■ Targeted therapy
  ■ *Tratuzumab (Herceptin), a monoclonal antibody that directly targets the HER2 protein of breast tumors, is a treatment option for women with breast cancer that overproduce HER2 (ACS, 2012).*

Nursing Actions

■ Provide emotional support to the woman and family.
  ■ *Provide opportunities for the woman and family to share their feeling and concerns.*

■ Provide current, evidence-based information to the woman and family regarding treatment options.

  ■ *Encourage the woman to consider all options and seek other opinions or other professionals if she is not comfortable with recommendations.*

■ Provide information on methods that address side effects from treatment (**Tables 19-5** and **19-6**)

■ Provide information on nutrition that promotes healing and enhances the immune system.

■ Provide information on complementary modalities such as imagery, journal writing, and hypnosis that can be used to diminish side effects from cancer treatment therapies.

■ Provide information regarding community resources.

  ■ *Look Good .... Feel Better is a free program that helps women learn beauty techniques to restore their self-image and cope with appearance-related side effects of cancer treatment (ACS, 2012).*

  ■ *Breast cancer support such as American Cancer Society Reach to Recovery Program*

CRITICAL COMPONENT

Oncotype DX Test

■ Oncotype DX test is a genomic assay that assesses the activity of 21 different genes taken from a tissue sample of the cancer tumor.

■ The Oncotype DX test assists the health care provider in determining if the cancer is:

  ■ likely to recur

  ■ likely to benefit from chemotherapy

■ Women with stage I or II, estrogen-receptor-positive (ER+) breast cancer that has not spread to the lymph nodes may benefit from this test in determining type of cancer treatment.

(Breastcancer.org, 2010)

Medication

Tamoxifen (Nolvadex-D)

■ Indications: Reduces risk of breast cancer in women who are at increased risk for developing breast cancer; treatment of breast cancer

■ Action: Competes with estrogen for binding sites in the breast

■ Serious side effects: Pulmonary embolism, stroke, uterine malignancies

■ Common side effects: Vaginal dryness, hot flashes, joint pain, leg cramps, nausea

■ Route and dose: PO; 10–20 mg twice daily or 20 mg daily for 5 years

(Vallerand, & Sanoski, 2013; NCI, 2008)

Gynecological Cancers

Cervical Cancer

Forty years ago, cervical cancer was the leading cause of cancer-related deaths in women. It is now rated as the 14th leading cause of cancer related deaths (Eheman et al., 2012). This decrease in cervical cancer–related death can be attributed to women getting Pap tests, which aids in detecting cervical cancer at an early stage.

■ The human papillomavirus (HPV) is the primary cause of cervical cancer.

  ■ *50% of all sexually active men and women will get HPV at some point in their lives (CDC, 2009).*

■ Pap test is used for cervical cytological screening (see recommended screenings and immunizations for women across the life span in Chapter 18).

  ■ *Women with abnormal cervical cytology screening need further evaluation, since the Pap test is a screening test*

TABLE 19–5	MANAGEMENT OF RADIATION SIDE EFFECTS

Side effects, except for fatigue, are directly related and limited to the site being treated with radiation therapy, e.g., radiation therapy for breast cancer does not cause diarrhea.

SIDE EFFECT	WAYS TO MANAGE

Diarrhea: Related to damage of healthy cells in large and small intestine	• Drink 8–12 cups of clear liquids.
	  • Gatorade or Pedialyte for electrolyte replacement
	 • Eat small frequent meals.
	  • Five to six small meals rather than three large meals
	 • Eat foods that provide nourishment without increasing risk for diarrhea.
	  • Foods that are low in fiber, fat, and lactose
	  • Fresh fruit
	  • Cooked vegetables
	 • Take antidiarrheal medications such as Imodium A-D.
	 • Take care of rectum
	  • Use baby wipes instead of toilet paper
	  • Take sitz baths

Continued

TABLE 19–5   MANAGEMENT OF RADIATION SIDE EFFECTS—cont'd

SIDE EFFECT	WAYS TO MANAGE
Fatigue: Related to anemia, depression, infection, and medications	• Get 8 hours of sleep per night. 　• The woman may need more sleep per night than she needed before radiation therapy • Plan time to rest. 　• Take 10- to 15-minute rest breaks throughout the day. 　• Take several naps during the day. • Decrease daily activities 　• The woman may not have enough energy for all the activity she used to do. She should select the activities that are most important to her and limit those that are less important. • Exercise 　• 15–30 minutes of daily exercise improves overall feeling of well-being. • Change work schedule. 　• May need to decrease work hours for a few weeks. • Ask family and friends for help at home.
Sexual and fertility changes: Related to damage to healthy tissue of the vagina and ovaries	• Fertility 　• Women desiring future pregnancies need to talk with health care provider about ways to preserve fertility, such as preserving eggs for future use. • Sexual difficulties 　• Use water or mineral-based lubricant if experiencing vaginal dryness. • Vaginal stenosis 　• Discuss use of vaginal dilators with health care provider.
Skin changes: Related to damage of healthy tissue	• Skin care 　• Gently wash area; do not rub, scrub, or scratch. • Avoid heat and cold. 　• Wash in lukewarm water. 　• Do not use heating pads or ice packs. • Wear soft and loose-fitting cloths around treatment area. • Protect skin from sun.
Urinary and bladder changes: Related to damage of healthy cells of bladder and urinary tract, causing inflammation, ulcers, and infections	• Drink 6–8 cups of fluid per day. • Avoid coffee, black tea, alcohol, and spices. • Report changes to health care provider. 　• May require antibiotic therapy.

NCI, 2007

TABLE 19–6   MANAGEMENT OF CHEMOTHERAPY SIDE EFFECTS

ANEMIA	• Eat high-protein foods such as meat, peanut butter, and eggs. • Eat foods high in iron, such as red meats, leafy greens, and cooked dried beans.
APPETITE CHANGES	• Eat five or six small meals per day. • Try new food to keep up interest in foods. • Eat with friends and family. • Eat with plastic forks and spoons and use glass pots if food tastes like metal. • Drink milkshakes or eat soup because these are easier to swallow.
BLEEDING PROBLEMS	• Use electric shaver instead of a razor. • Wear shoes all the time (except when sleeping). • Brush teeth with soft toothbrush. • Avoid being constipated.

TABLE 19–6 MANAGEMENT OF CHEMOTHERAPY SIDE EFFECTS—cont'd	
CONSTIPATION	• Eat high-fiber foods such as whole-grain bread, fruits, and vegetables. • Increase fluid intake. • Exercise 15–30 minutes per day.
MOUTH AND THROAT CHANGES	• Brush teeth and tongue with soft toothbrush after each meal. • Rinse mouth with solution prescribed. • Use lip balm. • Choose foods that are soft, wet, and easy to swallow.

Cancer Care, 2012

and not a diagnostic test. A cervical conization is done for definitive diagnosis.

- Most women who are diagnosed with cervical cancer have not had regular Pap tests or have not followed up on abnormal results.
- Cervical cancer is typically slow growing and begins with dysplasia, a precancerous condition.
  - *Dysplasia is 100% treatable and may resolve on its own.*
- Undetected or untreated precancerous changes can develop into cervical cancer and spread to the bladder, intestines, lungs, and liver.

Risk Factors

- HPV infection (most important risk factor)
- Early onset of sexual activity (before 16 years)
- Cigarette smoking
- STI
- Inadequate cervical screening
- Multiple sex partners
- In utero exposure to DES
- Use of birth control pills for 5 or more years
- Given birth to three or more children

Risk Reduction

See Chapter 18.

Signs and Symptoms

Early cervical cancer usually does not produce symptoms. Signs and symptoms that may indicate early cervical cancer are:

- Continuous vaginal discharge that may be watery, pink, brown, bloody, or foul smelling
- Abnormal vaginal bleeding between periods, after intercourse, or after menopause
- Menstrual period that becomes heavier and lasts longer

Sign and Symptoms of Advanced Cervical Cancer:

- Loss of appetite
- Loss of weight
- Fatigue
- Pelvic, back, and/or leg pain
- Leaking of urine or feces from vagina

Medical Management

- Cervical cone biopsy to establish diagnosis
- Additional testing to determine if cancer is confined to the cervix or if it has spread to other organs:
  - *Computed tomography (CT) scan*
  - *Magnetic resonance imaging (MRI)*
  - *Positron emission tomography (PET) scan*
  - *Intravenous pyelography (IVP)*
  - *Chest x-ray*
  - *Cystoscopy*
  - *Blood studies*
- Staging of cervical cancer (**Table 19-7**)
- Treatment depends on stage of cancer and the woman's desire for pregnancy (Table 19-7).
- Chemotherapy is used for cervical cancer that has either metastasized or recurred.
- Target drug therapy
  - *Drugs that have an effect on cancer cells while having little effect on healthy cells*
  - *They block the growth of cancer cells by preventing the cancer cells from dividing or by distorting them.*
  - *Avastin (beracizumab) is one such drug that is given in combination with chemotherapy drugs.*

Nursing Actions

Patient education and support are critical nursing actions for women with cervical cancer.

- Provide emotional support to the woman and her family.
- Provide information on nutrition that promotes healing.
- Explain the importance of rest and sleep in the promotion of healing.
- Provide information on community support services.
- Care for women undergoing surgical treatment:
  - *Address the woman's and family's questions regarding surgical procedure.*
  - *Provide preoperative and postoperative care.*
- Care for woman undergoing radiation therapy:
  - *Provide information on ways to manage side effects related to external radiation (Table 19-5) (see Critical Component: Complications of External Radiation).*

- *Teach the importance of skin care in decreasing risk of tissue breakdown.*
- *Instruct the woman to check with health care provider regarding types of lotions and creams to use.*
- *Instruct the woman to avoid the use of adhesive tape on the treatment area.*
- *Recommend exposing the treatment area to air whenever possible to promote skin integrity.*
- Care for woman undergoing chemotherapy:
  - *Administer chemotherapy as per orders.*
  - *Provide information on the management of side effects related to chemotherapy (Table 19-6).*

CRITICAL COMPONENT

Complications of External Radiation

- Proctitis
- Cystitis
- Vaginal scarring and stenosis
- Anemia
- Bruising
- Increased risk for infection
- Skin rash
- Sexual difficulties
- Premature menopause
- Vesicovaginal fistulas

(NCI, 2010)

Endometrial Cancer

Endometrial cancer is cancer that forms in the tissue lining of the uterus. It is the fourth leading cause of cancer-related death in women (Eheman et al., 2012). Diagnosis is established by histologic examination of endometrial tissue.

Risk Factors

- Menopausal hormone therapy (MHT): Unopposed estrogen therapy in women with a uterus. This can cause endometrial hyperplasia, an increased number of cells in the lining of the uterus.
- Menopause after age 52
- Obesity: Obesity affects the synthesis and metabolism of sex hormones and insulin. Obese women tend to have higher levels of estrogen related to the body making additional estrogen in fatty tissue.
- Tamoxifen: Drug used to treat breast cancer
- Nulliparity
- Diabetes
- Polycystic ovarian syndrome

Signs and Symptoms

- Postmenopausal bleeding or abnormal premenopausal bleeding (most common symptom)
- Abnormal vaginal discharge
- Difficult or painful urination
- Pain during intercourse
- Pelvic pain or pressure

TABLE 19–7 STAGING AND TREATMENT OF CERVICAL CANCER	
STAGES	TREATMENT OPTIONS
Stage 0: Abnormal cells are in the epithelium. These cells may become cancer. Also called carcinoma in situ	• Loop electrosurgical excision procedure (LEEP) • Laser surgery • Conization • Cryosurgery • Total hysterectomy • Internal radiation
Stage I: Cancer has invaded the cervix and is confined to the cervix. Stage IA$_1$: Cancer is ≤ 3 mm deep and ≤ 7 mm wide. Stage IA$_2$: Cancer is 3 mm but ≤ 5 mm deep and ≤ 7 mm wide. Stage IB$_1$: Cancer can only be seen with a microscope and is ≥ 5 mm deep and ≤ 7 mm wide or can be seen without a microscope and is ≤ 4 cm. Stage IB2: Cancer is seen without microscope and is 4 cm.	• Total hysterectomy with or without bilateral salpingo-oophorectomy • Conization • Modified radical hysterectomy and removal of lymph nodes • Internal radiation therapy • Combination of internal and external radiation therapy • Radical hysterectomy and removal of lymph nodes • Radical hysterectomy with removal of lymph nodes followed by radiation therapy and chemotherapy • Combination of radiation therapy and chemotherapy

TABLE 19-7 STAGING AND TREATMENT OF CERVICAL CANCER—cont'd

STAGES	TREATMENT OPTIONS
Stage II: Cancer has extended beyond the cervix but not into the pelvic wall. It has invaded the upper but not lower portion of the vagina. Stage IIA: Cancer has spread to the upper two-thirds of the vagina but not to the tissues around the uterus. Stage IIA$_1$: Cancer can be seen without a microscope and is ≤ 4 cm. Stage IIA$_2$: Cancer can be seen without a microscope and is >4 cm. Stage IIB: Cancer has spread beyond the cervix to the tissues around the uterus.	• Internal and external radiation therapy and chemotherapy • Radical hysterectomy and removal of lymph nodes • Radical hysterectomy and removal of lymph nodes followed by radiation therapy and chemotherapy
Stage III: Cancer has extended to the lower one-third of the vagina and/or to the pelvic wall and/or has caused kidney problems (may block the flow of urine). Stage IIIA: Cancer has spread to lower one-third of the vagina but not into the pelvic wall. Stage IIIB: Cancer has spread into the pelvic wall and/or has become large enough to block the ureters.	• Radical hysterectomy and removal of lymph nodes followed by internal and external radiation therapy and chemotherapy
Stage IV: Cancer has spread to the bladder, rectum, or other parts of the body. Stage IVA: Cancer has spread to nearby organs such as bladder or rectum. Stage IVB: Cancer has spread to other parts of the body such as liver, lungs, bones, or distant lymph nodes.	• Radical hysterectomy and removal of lymph nodes followed by internal and external radiation therapy and chemotherapy

NCI, 2012

Stages

■ Stage I: Tumor confined to uterine corpus.
■ Stage II: Tumor invades cervical stroma but does not extend beyond the uterus.
■ Stage III: Tumor has spread outside of uterus but confined to pelvis.
■ Stage IV: Tumor has spread outside the pelvis or into the mucosa of the bladder or rectum or distant metastasis (Lentz, 2012).

Medical Management

■ Treatment is based on size of tumor, stage of tumor, tumor grade, and whether tumor is effected by estrogen.

■ Treatment options
   ■ *Abdominal hysterectomy along with removal of fallopian tubes, ovaries, and local lymph nodes—stage I*
   ■ *Radical hysterectomy—stage II, III, IV*
   ■ *Radiation therapy*
   ■ *Chemotherapy*
   ■ *Hormonal therapy (progesterone)*

Nursing Actions

■ Provide emotional support to the woman and her family.
■ Provide information on nutrition that promotes healing.
■ Explain the importance of rest and sleep in the promotion of healing.

- Provide preoperative and postoperative care.
- Administer chemotherapy as per orders.
- Provide information on management of side effects from radiation and/or chemotherapy as it applies to the woman (Tables 19-5 and 19-6).

Ovarian Epithelial Cancer

Ovarian epithelial tumor is the most common type of ovarian cancer and the third leading cause of cancer related deaths in women (Eheman et al., 2012). Symptoms of ovarian cancer are often vague, making it difficult to diagnose the disease during early stages. Diagnosis is established by histologic examination of the tumor usually at time of surgery.

Risk Factors

- Family history of a first-degree relative with the disease; the most important risk factor (Lentz, 2012)
- Personal history of cancer
- Age over 55
- Eastern European Jewish background
- Never given birth
- Have endometriosis
- Tested positive for *BRCA1* or *BRCA2*

Signs and Symptoms

- Early stages are often asymptomatic or the woman will have vague abdominal, genitourinary, or reproductive symptoms (see Critical Component: Ovarian Cancer Symptom Diary):
  - *Pressure or pain in the abdomen, pelvis, back, or leg*
  - *Swollen or bloated abdomen*
  - *Urinary urgency and frequency*
  - *Difficulty eating or feeling full quickly (Cesario, 2010)*

CRITICAL COMPONENT

Ovarian Cancer Symptom Diary

The four most common occurring early warning signs of ovarian cancer are:

- Bloating
- Pelvic/abdominal pain
- Difficulty eating or feeling full quickly
- Urinary symptoms

To assist in early detection of ovarian cancer, women may be asked to keep a log of their symptoms for one month. They are instructed to record when they experienced any of the four common symptoms. They record the day of the week and the specific symptom.

Women who experience any of these symptoms more than 12 times in one month and these symptoms first appeared within the past 12 months should be evaluated for possible ovarian cancer (Cesario, 2010). An example of the log is located at www.ovarian.org.uk

---

Stages

- Stage I: Cancer cells are found in one or both ovaries.
- Stage II Cancer cells have spread to other tissue in the pelvis.
- Stage III: Cancer cells have spread outside the pelvis or to the regional lymph nodes.
- Stage IV: Cancer cells have spread to tissue outside the abdomen and pelvis (Lentz, 2012).

Medical Management

- Tests and procedures
  - *Transvaginal ultrasound to identify changes in ovaries*
  - *CT scan and MRI to confirm presence of pelvic mass*
  - *PET scan to assess for metastasis to other body organs*
  - *Barium enema x-ray to determine if there is colon and/or rectal involvement*
  - *OVA1: A multivariate index that examines 5 serum biomarkers: CA-125, A-1, transthyretin, Beta2-Microglulin, and transferrin*
    - Premenopausal women: Score of 5.0 or higher—strong probability of ovarian cancer
    - Postmenopausal women: Score of 4.4 or higher—strong probability of ovarian cancer (Li, 2012)
  - *Risk of ovarian malignancy algorithm (ROMA) classifies patients into high-risk and low-risk groups for having epithelial ovarian cancer. HE4, human epididymis protein 4, in combination with CA-125 are used in the algorithm.*
    - A ROMA score of ≥12.5% is considered high risk for premenopausal women.
    - A ROMA score of ≥14.4% is considered high risk for postmenopausal women (Li, 2012).
- Stage I—Total abdominal hysterectomy and bilateral salpingo-oophorectomy, omentectomy, and biopsy of lymph nodes and other pelvic and abdominal tissues and chemotherapy when high grade tumors are present
- Stages II and III—Total abdominal hysterectomy and bilateral salpingo-oophorectomy, omentectomy, and biopsy of lymph nodes and other pelvic and abdominal tissues and chemotherapy with or without radiation therapy
- Stage IV—Surgery to remove as much of tumor as possible followed by chemotherapy

Nursing Actions

- Provide preoperative and postoperative care.
- Administer chemotherapy as per orders.
- Provide information on management of chemotherapy side effects (Table 19-7).
- Provide emotional support to the woman and her family.

*I*NTIMATE PARTNER VIOLENCE

Intimate partner violence (IPV), also called domestic violence, is physical, sexual, and/or psychological harm by a current or former intimate partner or casual dating partner (see Critical Component: Signs of Intimate Partner Violence).

- IPV is a complex health and social issue affecting women around the world (Magnussen et al., 2011).

■ Approximately 1.3 million women per year are physically assaulted by an intimate partner (National Institute of Justice [NIJ], 2007).

■ IPV occurs across all socioeconomic, religious, and ethnic groups.

■ Approximately 50% of children living in homes of IPV are also abused.

■ IPV is associated with 40%–50% of all murdered women (NIJ, 2007).

■ IPV during pregnancy is associated with increased incidence of low-birth-weight infants, preterm birth, and neonatal death.

■ Physical violence includes, but is not limited to, slapping, shaking, choking, burning, and use of weapons.

■ Sexual violence includes, but is not limited to, forcing a partner to engage in sexual activity against her will; trading sex for food, money, or drugs.

■ Psychological/emotional violence includes, but is not limited to, humiliating the woman, controlling what the woman can and cannot do, isolating the woman from family and friends, and denying access to money.

CRITICAL COMPONENT

Signs of Intimate Partner Violence

■ Repeated nonspecific complaints
■ Overuse of health care system
■ Hesitancy, embarrassment, or evasiveness in relating history of injury
■ Time lag between injury and presentation for care
■ Untreated serious injuries
■ Overly solicitous partner who stays close to the woman and attempts to answer questions directed at her
■ Injuries of head, neck, face, and areas covered by a one-piece bathing suit; during pregnancy, the breasts and abdomen are particular targets of assault
■ Presence of bruises at various stages of healing

(Krieger, 2008)

Nursing Actions

■ The American Nurses Association (ANA) advocates for:
  ■ *Universal screening: All patients are screened for IPV.*
  ■ *Routine assessment: A detailed assessment when screening suggests that the woman is at risk for abuse.*
  ■ *Documentation of abuse: Documentation is essential for providing a record of abuse and facilitating communication among health professionals.*
  ■ *Reporting IPV: Nurses need to be aware of laws regarding mandatory reporting. California, Colorado, Kentucky, New Hampshire, New Mexico, and Rhode Island have laws that require reporting of IPV.*

■ Common questions asked in an IPV screening tool are:
  ■ *Has your partner ever hit you?*
  ■ *Do arguments with your partner result in you feeling bad about yourself?*
  ■ *Do you ever feel frightened by what your partner says or does?*
  ■ *Do you feel safe in your current relationship?*

■ When a woman discloses IPV, the nurse should assess to determine urgent safety needs and assist with developing plan of care.

■ Provide information regarding IPV and safe shelters.

■ Assist the woman in developing strategies to protect herself from harm.

CONCEPT MAP

Polycystic Ovary Syndrome (PCOS)

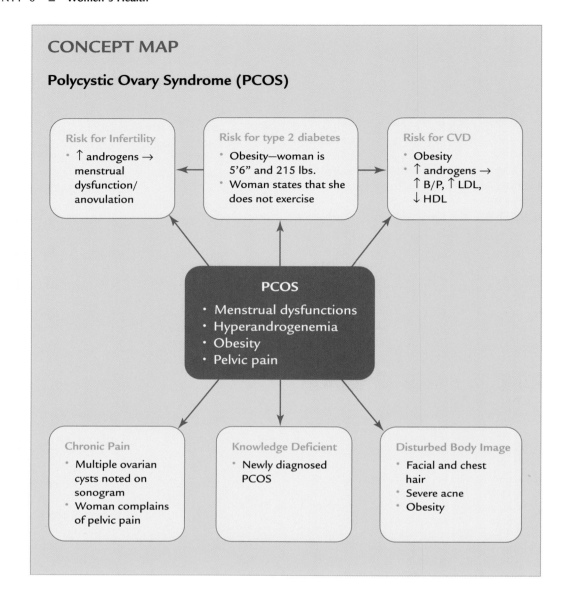

Risk for Infertility
- ↑ androgens → menstrual dysfunction/ anovulation

Risk for type 2 diabetes
- Obesity—woman is 5'6" and 215 lbs.
- Woman states that she does not exercise

Risk for CVD
- Obesity
- ↑ androgens → ↑ B/P, ↑ LDL, ↓ HDL

PCOS
- Menstrual dysfunctions
- Hyperandrogenemia
- Obesity
- Pelvic pain

Chronic Pain
- Multiple ovarian cysts noted on sonogram
- Woman complains of pelvic pain

Knowledge Deficient
- Newly diagnosed PCOS

Disturbed Body Image
- Facial and chest hair
- Severe acne
- Obesity

Problem No. 1: Risk for infertility

Goal: Increased knowledge regarding relationship of PCOS and infertility

Outcome: The woman verbalizes causes of infertility and methods to improve fertility.

Nursing Actions

1. Provide the woman with information on the causes of infertility related to PCOS—anovulation related to increased androgen levels, increased LH, and decreased FSH.
2. Inform the woman that weight loss can improve fertility— weight loss is the first-line treatment for infertility (Smith & Taylor, 2011).
   a. Assist woman in developing a weight management program that includes diet and physical activities.

3. Explain medical options for treating infertility
   a. Treat type 2 diabetes—maintaining normal ranges of serum glucose can regulate menstrual cycle and increase ovulation rates.
   b. Ovulation inducing medications

Problem No. 2: Risk for type 2 diabetes

Goal: Serum glucose levels within normal ranges

Outcome: The woman exercises 3 days a week for 30 minutes and eats foods low in carbohydrates and fats.

Nursing Actions

1. Explain that weight loss and exercise improve insulin resistance (the body produces insulin but does not use it properly) and hyperinsulinemia (hyperglycemia present despite high levels of insulin).

2. Explain the other benefits of a weight management program that include diet and exercise:
   a. Improves fertility
   b. Decreases androgen levels
   c. Decreases lipid levels
   d. Decreases blood pressure
3. Assist the woman in developing a weight management program by:
   a. Asking the woman to identify the types of physical activities she enjoys and how these can be used in a weight management program.
   b. Asking her to identify the foods she enjoys and incorporate them into weight reduction diet.
   c. Teaching the woman food groups important in a healthy diet.

Problem No. 3: Risk for CVD
Goal: ↓B/P; ↓LDL & ↑HDL
Outcome: The woman exercises 3 days a week for 30 minutes and eat foods low in carbohydrates and fats.

Nursing Actions

1. Explain the importance of weight loss through diet and exercise in decreasing risk for CVD.
   a. Exercise improves cardiopulmonary function, insulin sensitivity, and a decreased BMI (Smith & Taylor, 2011)
2. Assist the woman in developing a weight management program with realistic weight loss and exercise goals.
3. Provide information on prescribed medications for decreasing risk of CVD.

Problem No. 4: Chronic pain
Goal: Decreased pain
Outcome: The woman states her pelvic pain has decreased in frequency and intensity.

Nursing Actions

1. Assess level of pain, location of pain, and frequency of pain.
2. Ask about past pain management techniques and their effectiveness in treating pain related to PCOS.
3. Ask the woman to identify factors that increase or decrease the pain, e.g., lack of sleep, lifting objects.
   a. Discuss ways to decrease factors that increase pain.
4. Assist woman in developing a pain management program that includes:
   a. Pain diary: List when pain occurs, intensity of pain, how long it lasted, pain management measures used, and effectiveness of pain management. Instruct her to share this with her health care provider.
   b. Pharmacological: medications—Take medication at start of pain and use adequate amounts as prescribed.
   c. Non-pharmacological: relaxation techniques, massage, acupressure

Problem No. 5: Knowledge deficit
Goal: Increased knowledge regarding PCOS
Outcome: The woman develops a plan of action for living with PCOS.

Nursing Actions

1. Ensure that the environment is conducive for learning—quiet room free of distractions.
2. Assess the woman's level of knowledge regarding PCOS.
3. Assist the woman in identifying priority learning needs and address these needs such as:
   a. Causes of PCOS
   b. Effect of PCOS on her body and mind
   c. Treatment options
   d. Ways to cope with changes related to PCOS
4. Assist the woman in developing a plan of action for living with PCOS.

Problem No. 6: Disturbed body image
Goal: Improved body image
Outcome: The woman verbalizes methods to decrease degree of acne and methods to decrease facial and chest hair.

Nursing Actions

1. Sit with the woman and through active listening, encourage the woman to express her thoughts and concerns regarding facial and chest hair and acne.
2. Provide information on causes of body changes due to PCOS.
3. Provide information on treatment for acne, i.e., dermatological assessment and prescribed medications.
4. Provide information on hair removal.
5. Refer the woman to PCOS support groups.

■ ■ ■ **Review Questions** ■ ■ ■

1. Factors that can contribute to chronic pelvic pain (CPP) include (select all that apply):
   A. Crohn's disease
   B. Celiac disease
   C. Sleep disorders
   D. Intrauterine contraceptive device

2. During a teaching session, the nurse explains that women with polycystic ovary syndrome (POS) have:
   A. Decreased levels of luteinizing hormone (LH)
   B. Increased levels of testosterone
   C. Increased secretion of follicle-stimulating hormone (FSH)
   D. Decreased levels of estrogen

3. Risk factors for bacterial vaginosis (BV) include (select all that apply):
   A. Poor hygiene
   B. Poor nutrition
   C. Antibiotic therapy
   D. Smoking

4. Chemotherapy is commonly used in the treatment plan of:
   A. All who have breast cancer
   B. Women who have stage 0 breast cancer
   C. Women who have stage II breast cancer with low risk of recurrence
   D. Women who have stage IV breast cancer

5. Instruction to a patient experiencing diarrhea related to radiation therapy includes (select all that apply):
   A. Drink 8–12 cups of clear liquid per day
   B. Eat three large meals per day
   C. Eat foods high in fiber
   D. Use baby wipes instead of toilet paper

6. A medical work-up for a 28-year-old woman presenting with chronic pelvic pain with normal menstrual cycles would include (select all that apply):
   A. Laparoscopy
   B. Colposcopy
   C. Urinalysis
   D. Endometrial biopsy

7. A definition of menorrhagia is:
   A. Bleeding that is excessive in number of days and amount of bleeding
   B. Bleeding between periods or after menopause
   C. Painful menstruation
   D. Bleeding related to cervical dysplasia

8. A 45-year-old woman present at the women's health clinic complains of a foul vaginal odor and leakage of fecal material from her vagina. This is most likely related to:
   A. Rectocele
   B. Bacterial vaginitis
   C. Genital fistulas
   D. Endometrial cancer

9. During a routine assessment of a 60-year-old woman in the women's health clinic, the nurse notes numerous bruises at various stages of healing on the woman's chest and abdomen. The first nursing action is:
   A. Complete a fall risk assessment
   B. Question the woman about her relationship with her partner
   C. Question her about medications that can cause bruising
   D. Assess for vertigo

10. Which woman is at highest risk for ovarian cancer?
    A. A 60-year-old Jewish woman who recently emigrated from Israel and has never been pregnant
    B. A 40-year-old African-American woman who has four children and history of PID
    C. A 55-year-old woman who recently emigrated from China and whose sister received treatment for stage I ovarian cancer
    D. A 30-year-old obese woman with history of endometriosis

References

American Cancer Society. (2012). *Breast cancer facts and figures 2011–2012*. Retrieved December 11, 2012, from www.cancer.org/acs/groups/content/@epidemiologysurveilence/document/acspc-030975.pdf

American Cancer Society. (2009b). *How is breast cancer staged?* Retrieved from www.cancer.org/cancer/breatcancer/detailerguide/breast-cancer-staging

American College of Obstetricians and Gynecologists. (2008). *Treatment of urinary tract infections in non-pregnant women* (Practice Bulletin No. 91, pp. 10–12). Washington DC: Author.

American College of Obstetricians and Gynecologists. (2010). *Dilation and curettage*. Retrieved from www.acog.org/publications/patient_education/bp062.cfm

Breastcancer.org. (2010). *Oncotype DX test*. Retrieved from www.breastcancer.org/symptoms/testing/types/oncotype_dx.jsp

Cancer Care (2012) *Understanding and managing chemotherapy side effects*. Retrieved from www.media.cancercare.org/publication/original/24-ccc_chemo_side_effect.pdf?1330707352

Centers for Disease Control and Prevention (CDC). (2009). *Genital HPV infection: CDC fact sheet*. Retrieved from www.cdc.gov/STD/HPV/STDFact-HPV

Centers for Disease Control and Prevention (CDC). (2008). Women's reproductive health: hysterectomy fact sheet. Retrieved from www.cdc.gov/reproductivehealth/WomensRH/00-040FS_Hysterectome.htm

Cesario, S. (2010). Advances in early detection of ovarian cancer. *Nursing for women's health, 14*, 223–234.

County of Los Angeles Public Health. (2012). *Resources for lesbian and bisexual women*. Retrieved from www.publichealth.lacounty.gov/std/lesbian_bi.htm

DuRant, M., & Leslie, N. (2009). Ovary syndrome: A cognitive behavioral strategy. *Nursing of women's health, 13*, 293–300.

Eheman, C., Henley, J., Ballard-Barbash, R., Jacobs, E., Schymura, M., Noone, A., Pan, L., Anderson, R., Fulton, J., Kohler, B., Jemal, A., Ward, E., Plescia, M., Ries, L., & Edwards, B. (2012). Annual report to the nation on the status of cancer, 1975–2008, featuring association with excess weight and lack of sufficient physical activity. *Cancer, 118*, 2338–2366.

Green, I., Cohen, L., Finkenzeller, D., & Christo, P. (2010). Interventional therapies for controlling pelvic pain: What is the evidence? *Current pain and headache reports, 14,* 22–32.

Krieger, C. (2008). Intimate partner violence: A review for nurses. *Nursing for Women's Health, 12,* 226–234.

Lentz, G., Roger, L., Gerhenson, D., & Katz, V. (2012). Comprehensive gynecology (6th ed.). Philadelphia, PA: Elsevier.

Li, A. (2012). *New biomarkers for ovarian cancer: OVA1 and ROMA in diagnosis.* Retrieved from www.modernmedicine.com/modernmedicine/article/articleDetail.jsp?id=769662

Mayo Clinic. (2009a). *Premenstrual syndrome* (PMS). Retrieved from www.mayoclinic.com/health/ptrmenstrual-syndrome/DS00134

Mayo Clinic. (2009b). *Chronic pelvic pain.* Retrieved from www.mayoclinic.com/health/chronic-pelvic-pain/DS00571/MRTOD

National Cancer Institute. (NCI). (2007). *Radiation therapy and you: Support for people with cancer.* Retrieved from www.cancer.gov/cancertopics/coping/radiation-therapy-and-you/page8

National Cancer Institute. (2008). *Tamoxifen: Questions and answers.* Retrieved from www.cancer.gov/cancertopics/factsheet/Therapy/tamoxifem

National Cancer Institute. (2011). *Breast cancer risk assessment tool.* Retrieved from www.cancer.gov/brisktool/

National Cancer Institute. (2012). *Cervical cancer treatment.* Retrieved from www.cancer.gov/cancertopics/pdq/treatment/cervical/Patient/page2

National Heart Lung and Blood Institute. (2011). *What is metabolic syndrome?* Retrieved from www.nhlbi/nih.gov/health/health-topics/topics

National Institute of Justice (NIJ). (2007). *How widespread is intimate partner violence?* Retrieved from www.ojp.usdoj.gov/nij/topics/crime/intimate-partner-violence/extent.htm

Smith, J., & Taylor, J. (2011). Polycystic ovary syndrome. *Nursing for women's health, 15,* 403–410.

Spencer, J. (2012). Continence promotion. *Nursing for women's health, 16,* 327–340.

U.S. Department of Health and Human Services (HHS), Office of Women's Health. (2010). *Premenstrual syndrome.* Retrieved from www.womenhealth.gov

Vallerand, A., & Sanoski, C. (2013). *Davis's drug guide for nurses (13th ed.).* Philadelphia, PA: F.A. Davis.

VanLeeuwen, A., Kranpitz, T., & Smith, L. (2010). *Davis's comprehensive handbook of laboratory and diagnostic tests with nursing implications* (3rd ed.). Philadelphia: F.A. Davis.

Women's Health (2010a). Pelvic inflammatory disease fact sheet. Retrieved from www.womenshealth.gov/publications/factsheet/pelvic-inflammatory-disease.cfm

Women's Health (2010b). *What is a colposcopy?* Retrieved from www.womenshealth.aboutcom//cs/cervicalconditions/a/colposcopy.htm

Answers to Chapter Review Questions

Chapter 1
1. C
2. D
3. A
4. D
5. B
6. B
7. A
8. C
9. C
10. A

Chapter 2
1. D
2. C
3. B
4. C
5. B
6. D
7. C
8. C
9. A
10. B

Chapter 3
1. A, B, C
2. B
3. B
4. C
5. D
6. A, C, D
7. A
8. A
9. A, D
10. B

Chapter 4
1. D
2. B
3. C
4. B
5. C
6. C
7. C
8. D
9. A
10. B
11. B
12. C
13. C
14. D

Chapter 5
1. A
2. B
3. B
4. B
5. A
6. C
7. B
8. A
9. B
10. C

Chapter 6
1. B
2. C
3. B
4. A
5. A
6. C
7. D
8. D
9. B
10. B

Chapter 7
1. C
2. D
3. D
4. C
5. B
6. A
7. C
8. B
9. A
10. D
11. B
12. A

Chapter 8
1. C
2. B
3. D
4. B
5. B
6. C
7. D
8. C
9. C
10. A

Chapter 9
1. B
2. C
3. A
4. A
5. D
6. A
7. A

Chapter 10
1. C
2. A
3. B
4. C
5. B
6. B
7. D
8. B
9. D
10. A

Chapter 11
1. C
2. A
3. B
4. D
5. C
6. A
7. D
8. B
9. A
10. A

Chapter 12
1. B, C
2. A
3. C
4. B, C, D
5. A, D
6. A, C, D
7. B
8. C
9. D
10. A, B, C

Chapter 13
1. C
2. B
3. D
4. A, B, C, D
5. A, B, C
6. B, C, D
7. A, B, C, D
8. A
9. C
10. B, C, D

Chapter 14
1. B
2. A, B, C, D
3. C
4. B
5. A, B, D
6. D
7. A, B
8. A, B, C, D
9. A
10. B

Chapter 15
1. B
2. D
3. C
4. B

5. C
6. C, D
7. B, C
8. C
9. D
10. C

5. A
6. C
7. A, B, C, D
8. B
9. C
10. B, D

5. B
6. B
7. C
8. A
9. A
10. B

4. A
5. A, B. C
6. B, D
7. B, C, D
8. B, D
9. B
10. A, B

3. C
4. D
5. A, D
6. A, C
7. A
8. C
9. B
10. C

Chapter 16

1. A
2. C
3. A
4. C

Chapter 17

1. A
2. C
3. D
4. C

Chapter 18

1. C
2. C
3. D

Chapter 19

1. A, B, C, D
2. B

Appendices

ASSOCIATION OF WOMEN'S HEALTH, OBSTETRIC AND NEONATAL NURSING

QUICK CARE GUIDE

Breastfeeding Support: Prenatal Care Through The First Year, Second Edition

This Quick Care Guide is based on AWHONN's Breastfeeding Support: Prenatal Care Through the First Year Evidence-Based Clinical Practice Guideline, second edition; it is meant to serve as a quick reference for the clinician. Detailed clinical practice guidelines, referenced rationales and evidence ratings are included in the Guideline. Evidence supporting the benefits of breastfeeding, critical messages, responsibilities and key assessment and teaching points summarized herein are presented in the Guideline.

BENEFITS OF BREASTFEEDING

Discussions with women who are considering or are undecided about breastfeeding should include description of the following benefits:

For infants:
- Natural source of nutrients necessary for optimal growth and development during the first 6 months
- Decreased incidence or severity of infections such as GI and respiratory infections, otitis media, necrotizing enterocolitis, gastroenteritis, meningitis and urinary tract infections
- Potential protective effect against sudden infant death syndrome (SIDS)
- Potential protective effect against childhood and adult-onset diseases such as insulin-dependent diabetes, allergies, asthma, lymphoma, ulcerative colitis, and adult-onset hypertension
- Less gastric reflux and constipation than formula feeding
- Potential for enhanced cognitive development

For women:
- Enhanced uterine involution resulting in less postpartum blood loss and reduced risk of infection
- Delayed resumption of ovulation that may facilitate family planning
- Association between earlier return to pre-pregnancy weight compared with women who do not breastfeed
- Reduced risk of osteoporosis, ovarian cancer and premenopausal breast cancer, and rheumatoid arthritis
- Enhanced mother-infant attachment, maternal role attainment and self-esteem

Breastfeeding is less expensive than formula feeding and can contribute to significant health care cost savings.

CRITICAL MESSAGES TO SHARE WITH WOMEN AND THEIR PARTNERS

- Breastfeeding is the optimal method of infant feeding.
- Most women can breastfeed successfully when they are given consistent information and support.
- Breastfeeding can be sustained upon return to work or school.
- Ideally, infants should breastfeed exclusively for the first year of life, i.e., during the first 6 months, the infant receives only breast milk; during the second 6 months, as other foods are introduced, the only source of milk given to the infant is breast milk.

RESPONSIBILITIES AND OPPORTUNITIES

- Deliberate integration of breastfeeding information into academic and professional education programs will help ensure that health care professionals gain the knowledge needed to promote and support breastfeeding.
- Nurses working with breastfeeding women should maintain current, evidence-based knowledge of breastfeeding practice and can be instrumental in initiating or participating in lactation research.
- Breastfeeding support programs should be culturally sensitive and age- and community-appropriate.
- Nurses and other health care professionals should relay consistent, supportive messages about breastfeeding.
- Nurses can be instrumental in promoting breastfeeding as our cultural norm by supporting legislation that promotes breastfeeding and educating society about the benefits of breastfeeding.

ASSOCIATION OF WOMEN'S HEALTH, OBSTETRIC AND NEONATAL NURSING QUICK CARE GUIDE
Breastfeeding Support: Prenatal Care Through The First Year

Key Assessment Parameters	Key Teaching Points
Preconception and Prenatal Care	
• During the first preconception or prenatal visit, ask the woman whether anyone has explained to her the benefits of breastfeeding for herself and her infant. Assess the woman's knowledge of and experiences with breastfeeding.	• Educate women about maternal and neonatal benefits of breastfeeding. • Previous breastfeeding experiences, positive or negative, influence choice of feeding method. Some factors, such as perceived insufficient milk supply, can be addressed by education and support that continue throughout pregnancy and the early postpartum period.
• Explore the woman's beliefs and attitudes about breastfeeding.	• Discuss and correct misconceptions about breastfeeding. Address concerns or ambivalence.
• For the woman who is undecided about breastfeeding, continue to explore her concerns and desires during subsequent contacts.	• Continue targeted, culturally appropriate education throughout pregnancy. Culture and beliefs can positively or negatively influence the woman's decision to initiate or continue breastfeeding.
• If the woman plans to breastfeed, ask how long she plans to do so and how long she plans to breastfeed exclusively.	• Suggest that return to work or school does not mean that the woman must stop breastfeeding. Benefits continue as long as the infant is breastfeeding, even when the infant is being partially breastfed.
• Verify presence of support for the woman's decision to breastfeed.	• Discuss community resources that are available to the woman such as support groups, lactation consultants and La Leche League. • Explain that family, friends and health care providers (including peer counselors) can help a woman meet her breastfeeding goals.
• Review the woman's history. Assess her breasts and nipples for risk factors and physical characteristics that may affect breastfeeding.	• Explain that many physical characteristics do not preclude breastfeeding. Share interventions to address indentified problem(s). For example, infants are often able to grasp and pull out inverted nipples during early feedings at the breast. • Some women who have had previous breast surgery are able to exclusively breastfeed their infants. Regardless of the amount of breast milk received by the infant, both mother and infant benefit.
Postpartum Care—First Two Weeks	
• Assess parental knowledge and ability to establish correct infant latch onto the breast.	• Instruct parents how to correctly position infant at breast. • Facilitate uninterrupted skin-to-skin contact at birth and during hospitalization. Ideally, the first feeding should occur within 1 hour of birth if mother and infant are stable. • Instruct mother how to identify a correct latch: infant's nose, cheeks and chin should touch the breast. The woman should feel tugging, not pinching or pain, when the infant sucks. The infant is usually held tummy-to-tummy with the mother, and the mother positions her fingers to ensure the lactiferous sinuses are not blocked.
• Assess parental knowledge of infant states and ability to demonstrate caring for the infant as the infant transitions between states.	• Teach parents that infant may be sleepy for the first 24 hours. Try to wake the infant every 2–3 hours for feeding. Assure them that waking and feeding the infant should get progressively easier throughout the first 24 hours. • Teach parents about infant states and help parents identify how their infant transitions between states.
• Assess parental knowledge of and ability to respond to infant feeding cues.	• Teach early infant feeding cues: rooting, hand-to-mouth movements, sucking movement and sounds, mouth opening in response to tactile stimulation and quietly alert state. Crying is a late feeding cue.
• Assess parent's ability to identify signs of adequate milk intake.	• Educate parents that infant should have at least one stool and one void in the first 24 hours, three or more voids and one to two stools per day by day 3 and six or more voids and three or more stools per day by day 4. Other signs include light colored urine, audible swallows and appropriate weight gain; a maternal sign of adequate intake is full breasts at the start of a feeding that become soft by the end.

ASSOCIATION OF WOMEN'S HEALTH, OBSTETRIC AND NEONATAL NURSING
QUICK CARE GUIDE
Breastfeeding Support: Prenatal Care Through The First Year

Key Assessment Parameters	Key Teaching Points
• Assess parents' ability to identify and respond to infant cues of satiety. • Assess parental knowledge about ways to support the mother-infant dyad in a successful breastfeeding experience.	• Teach parents infant cues of satiety: a gradual decrease in the number of sucks, pursed lips, pulling away from breast and releasing the nipple, relaxed body, leg extension, absence of hunger cues, sleep and contented state. • Parental education should include the following: - Discourage the use of pacifiers until the baby is able to latch on and breastfeed successfully. - The infant should receive only breast milk unless medically indicated. - Discourage routine distribution of formula sample packs. • Provide parents with resources to contact after discharge, such as a lactation consultant, La Leche League or a breast-feeding support group. • Recommend follow up with a health care provider within 3–5 days after discharge, or within 48 hours of discharge for infants discharged from the hospital prior to 48 hours of age.
Postpartum Care—Two Weeks Through First Year • Discuss how long the woman intends to breastfeed.	• Describe the association between an infant's age when first given formula and time of weaning. • Explain that internationally, many professional organizations agree that exclusive breastfeeding during the first 6 months of life (except when medical contraindications exist) provides adequate nutrition to facilitate optimal growth and development and protection against diarrhea and respiratory tract infections. • Define exclusive breastfeeding: the infant receives only breast milk and no other liquid or solid supplements except vitamins, minerals and medications. • Discuss feeding after 6 months, when other foods are introduced into the infant's diet. Exclusive breastfeeding during this time means that the only source of milk given to the infant continues to be breast milk. If a mother and infant desire, breastfeeding may continue for the first year of life and beyond.
• Assess for the presence of individuals in the woman's life who support her decision to breastfeed.	• Describe the influence that support from partners, maternal grandmother, employers and fellow employees may have on the duration of breastfeeding.
• Identify factors that may decrease duration of breast-feeding.	• Discuss factors that may negatively influence duration of breastfeeding: - Perceived insufficient milk supply - Returning to work before 2 months postpartum - Wanting to leave the infant or have someone else feed - Born outside the United States - Postpartum depression • Engage adolescent women in discussions about unique concerns, e.g., relatives' advice to quit, embarrassment, modesty and concern about breastfeeding in public. • Explain that early introduction of pacifiers may be associated with decreased duration of breastfeeding. As an intervention to decrease the risk of SIDS, pacifiers should be introduced to breastfeeding infants after 1 month of age when breastfeeding is well established.
• Identify challenges to breastfeeding.	• Discuss challenges to breastfeeding, including lack of support and returning to work. • Provide the breastfeeding woman with resources for her employer that describe how the employer and the work environment can support breastfeeding. • Describe periods of rapid infant growth (2 weeks, 6 weeks and 3 months) when women may perceive that their milk supply has decreased because their infant is breastfeeding more often. • Explain that "stabbing" or "burning" pain or pruritus on the surface of the breast may be associated with a fungal infection such as Candida albicans. Should these occur, consultation with a health care provider is important to rule out other sources of infection and to treat both the mother and the infant as indicated.

ASSOCIATION OF WOMEN'S HEALTH, OBSTETRIC AND NEONATAL NURSING
QUICK CARE GUIDE
Breastfeeding Support: Prenatal Care Through The First Year

Key Assessment Parameters	Key Teaching Points
• Assess the woman's knowledge of available professional and community resources.	• Encourage participation in breastfeeding support groups, regular visits to Women, Infants, and Children (WIC) program office (if the mother participates in WIC) and follow-up phone calls to registered nurses, lactation consultants or the primary health care provider, all of which may help increase the duration of breastfeeding.
• Discuss options to support continued breastfeeding after returning to work.	• Encourage use of a double rather than a single pump to decrease the length of time needed to pump. • Encourage women to begin pumping before returning to work. The more experience a woman has with pumping the more efficient she becomes and the less time pumping will take.
• Assess the breastfeeding woman's understanding of techniques to wean her infant.	• Describe weaning techniques, such as replacing one feeding during the day with solid food, a bottle or cup depending on the infant's age and stage of development. After the infant has adjusted, replace a second feeding at the opposite time of day. Generally, the first morning and last evening feedings are the last to be stopped.
Vulnerable and Preterm Infants	
• Assess woman's beliefs, attitudes and knowledge about providing own mother's milk for her vulnerable/preterm infant.	• Explain that human milk affords unique advantages for the vulnerable/preterm infant (such as protection from necrotizing enterocolitis, better gastric function and reduced incidence of infection), as well as for the woman. • Teach the woman to optimize milk yield using the following suggested techniques: - Begin milk expression within 6 hours after delivery, using an electric, hospital-grade breast pump with double collection kit whenever possible. - Express milk at the infant's bedside. - Engage in skin-to-skin contact at least 30 minutes daily, whenever feasible. - Mechanically express approximately 8–10 times daily during the first week to 10 days postpartum. - Individualize the frequency of mechanical expression on the basis of milk output. - Continue mechanical expression for 2 minutes after milk droplets cease flowing.
• Determine woman's willingness to provide human milk via various options.	• Instruct that human milk may be provided to the infant via tube feeding (gavage), cup- or finger-feedings, as well as by bottle. • Instruct parents how to properly collect, store and transport human milk to the hospital. • Assist parents to identify resources necessary to collect, store and transport milk.
• Assess woman's and infant's readiness for oral feeding at breast.	• When the infant is medically stable, teach mothers who desire to transition the infant to feeding at breast to put the infant to breast following milk expression to help him or her acclimate to sucking. • Demonstrate positions that provide head and shoulder support of the infant, such as the football hold, when infant suction if compromised. • Remind the mother to express remaining milk after each breastfeeding session. • Suggest that thin silicone nipple shields may increase milk transfer with this infant population. • Explain that infant test-weighing provides an accurate estimate of infant milk intake.
• Assess parental knowledge related to the vulnerable/preterm infant's milk intake after discharge.	• Discuss that modified demand feedings will likely be needed, coupled with infant test-weighing for a period of time. • Emphasize the difference between insufficient milk supply and the infant's ability to consume adequate milk volume. • Teach that appropriate follow-up after discharge is critical for the mother of a vulnerable/preterm infant.

Appendix B

Laboratory Values

LABORATORY VALUE	NONPREGNANT	PREGNANT	NEWBORN
Hemoglobin, g/dL	12–16	11–13	13.5–20.5
Hematocrit, %	37–47	33–39	45–65
Red cell count, 10^6cells/mm^3	4.2–5.4	3.8–4.4	5.33–5.47
White blood cell count, 10^3cells/mm^3	4.5–11.0	5.0–12.0	9.4–34.0
Platelets, mm^3	150,000–400,000	No significant change	150,000–450,000
Fibrinogen, mg/dL	200–400	↑ levels late in pregnancy	125–300
Serum cholesterol, total, mg/dL	150–199	↑ 60%	Rises rapidly after birth, reaching adult levels by day 1
Blood glucose, mg/dL	80–120	↓ 10–20%	≥40
Fasting	65–99	≤ 95	
2-hour postprandial	≤ 105	≤ 120	
Total bilirubin, mg/dL	0.3–1.2	No significant change	<24 hours: <6.0 1–2 days: <10 3–5 days: <12

Conversions: Approximate Temperature Equivalents

CONVERSIONS: Approximate Temperature Equivalents			
°C	°F	°C	°F
35.5	95.9	37.8	100.04
35.6	96.08	37.9	100.22
35.7	96.26	38.0	100.4
35.8	96.44	38.1	100.58
35.9	96.62	38.2	100.76
36.0	96.8	38.3	100.94
36.1	96.98	38.4	102.12
36.2	97.16	38.5	101.3
36.3	97.34	38.6	101.48
36.4	97.52	38.7	101.66
36.5	97.7	38.8	101.84
36.6	97.88	38.9	102.02
36.7	98.06	39.0	102.2
36.8	98.24	39.1	102.38
36.9	98.42	39.2	102.56
37.0	98.6	39.3	102.74
37.1	98.78	39.4	102.92
37.2	98.96	39.5	103.1
37.3	99.14	39.6	103.28
37.4	99.32	39.7	103.46
37.5	99.5	39.8	103.64
37.6	99.68	39.9	103.82
37.7	99.86	40.0	104.0

$$°C = (°F - 32) \times 5/9$$
$$°F = (°C \times 1.8) + 32$$

Appendix D

Cervical Dilation Chart

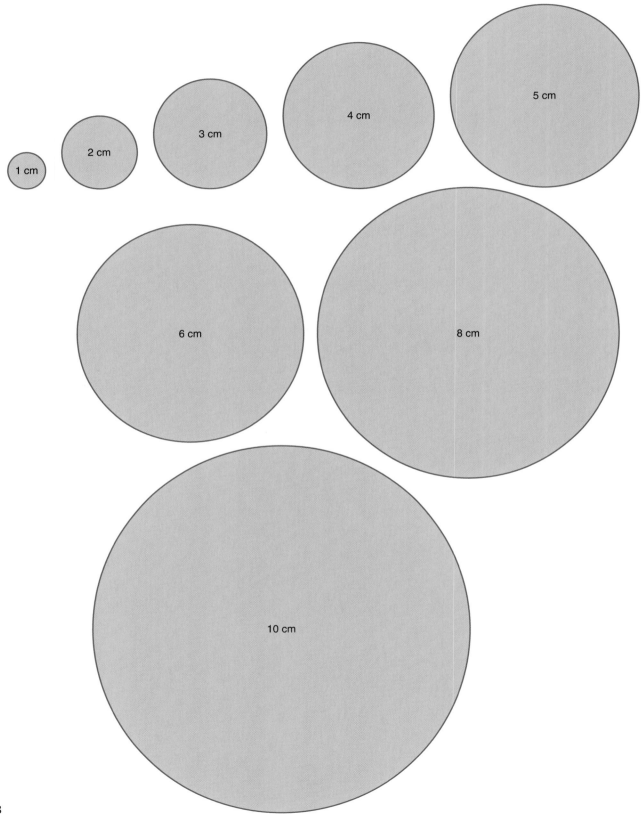

Newborn Weight Conversion Chart

NEWBORN WEIGHT CONVERSION CHART
Pounds and Ounces to Grams

Ounces	Pounds												
	0	1	2	3	4	5	6	7	8	9	10	11	12
0	0	454	907	1361	1814	2268	2722	3175	3629	4082	4536	4990	5443
1	28	482	936	1389	1843	2296	2750	3203	3657	4111	4564	5019	5471
2	57	510	964	1417	1871	2325	2778	3232	3685	4139	4593	5046	5500
3	85	539	992	1446	1899	2353	2807	3260	3714	4167	4621	5075	5528
4	113	567	1021	1474	1928	2381	2835	3289	3742	4196	4649	5103	5557
5	142	595	1049	1503	1956	2410	2863	3317	3770	4224	4678	5131	5585
6	170	624	1077	1531	1984	2438	2892	3345	3799	4252	4706	5160	5613
7	198	652	1106	1559	2013	2466	2920	3374	3827	4281	4734	5188	5642
8	227	680	1134	1588	2041	2495	2949	3402	3856	4309	4763	5216	5670
9	255	709	1162	1616	2070	2523	2977	3430	3884	4337	4791	5245	5698
10	284	737	1191	1644	2098	2551	3005	3459	3912	4366	4819	5273	5727
11	312	765	1219	1673	2126	2580	3034	3487	3941	4394	4848	5301	5755
12	340	794	1247	1701	2155	2608	3062	3515	3969	4423	4876	5330	5783
13	369	822	1476	1729	2183	2637	3091	3544	3997	4451	4904	5358	5812
14	397	850	1304	1758	2211	2665	3119	3572	4026	4479	4933	5386	5840
15	425	879	1332	1786	2240	2693	3147	3600	4054	4508	4961	5415	5868

1 kg = 2.2046 lbs
1 lb = 454 g
1 oz = 28.3 g

Immunization and Pregnancy

Immunization & Pregnancy

Vaccines help keep a pregnant woman and her growing family healthy.

Vaccine	Before pregnancy	During pregnancy	After pregnancy	Type of Vaccine	Route
Hepatitis A	Yes, if at risk	Yes, if at risk	Yes, if at risk	Inactivated	IM
Hepatitis B	Yes, if at risk	Yes, if at risk	Yes, if at risk	Inactivated	IM
Human Papillomavirus (HPV)	Yes, if 9 through 26 years of age	No, under study	Yes, if 9 through 26 years of age	Inactivated	IM
Influenza TIV	Yes	Yes	Yes	Inactivated	IM, ID (18-64 years)
Influenza LAIV	Yes, if less than 50 years of age and healthy; avoid conception for 4 weeks	No	Yes, if less than 50 years of age and healthy; avoid conception for 4 weeks	Live	Nasal spray
MMR	Yes, avoid conception for 4 weeks	No	Yes, give immediately postpartum if susceptible to rubella	Live	SC
Meningococcal: • polysaccharide • conjugate	If indicated	If indicated	If indicated	Inactivated Inactivated	SC IM
Pneumococcal Polysaccharide	If indicated	If indicated	If indicated	Inactivated	IM or SC
Tetanus/Diphtheria Td	Yes, Tdap preferred	Yes, Tdap preferred if 20 weeks gestational age or more	Yes, Tdap preferred	Toxoid	IM
Tdap, one dose only	Yes, preferred	Yes, preferred	Yes, preferred	Toxoid/ inactivated	IM
Varicella	Yes, avoid conception for 4 weeks	No	Yes, give immediately postpartum if susceptible	Live	SC

CS226523B   10/2011

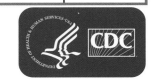

Glossary

Abortion (AB)   The spontaneous or induced termination of a pregnancy prior to 20 weeks' gestation

Abruptio placenta   The separation of the placenta from its site of implantation before delivery

Abusive head trauma (AHT)   Also referred to as shaken baby syndrome, is a traumatic brain injury that occurs when an infant is violently shaken.

Accelerations   Visually apparent, abrupt increase in FHR above the baseline

Acme phase   The peak of intensity of a contraction

Acrocyanosis   Cyanosis of hands and feet in newborn

Active phase   Second phase of labor; cervical dilation from 4 to 7cm

Advocacy   An action taken in response to our ethical responsibility to intervene on behalf of those in our care

Afterpains   Moderate to severe cramp-like pains caused by uterine contractions during the first few postpartum days

Alcohol related birth defects (ARBD)   Congenital anomalies associated with alcohol use during pregnancy

Alcohol related neurodevelopmental disorder (ARND)   Refers to abnormalities of the central nervous system that are associated with prenatal alcohol exposure

Alpha-Fetoprotein (AFP)/ α_1-Fetoprotein/ Maternal serum alpha fetoprotein (MSAFP)   A glycoprotein produced by the fetus used for assessing for the levels of AFP in the maternal blood as a screening tool for certain developmental defects in the fetus such as fetal neural tube defects (NTDs) and ventral abdominal wall defects

Amenorrhea   Absence of menstruation

Amniocentesis   Diagnostic procedure in which a needle is inserted through the maternal abdominal wall into the uterine cavity to obtain amniotic fluid

Amniotic fluid   Fluid contained within the amniotic sac

Amniotic fluid embolism (AFE)/Anaphylactoid syndrome   A rare, but often fatal complication that occurs during pregnancy, labor and birth, or postpartum in which amniotic fluid which contains fetal cells, lanugo, and vernix enters the maternal vascular system and initiates a cascading process that leads to maternal cardio respiratory collapse and disseminated intravascular coagulation (DIC)

Amniotic fluid index (AFI)   Screening tool that measures the volume of amniotic fluid with ultrasound to assess fetal well-being and placental function

Amniotomy (AROM)   The artificial rupture of membranes

ANA Code of Ethics   Makes explicit the primary goals, values, and obligations of the profession of nursing

Antepartum/antepartal   The time period beginning with conception and ending with the onset of labor

Anticipatory guidance   The provision of information and guidance to women and their families that promotes being informed about and prepared for events to come

Apgar score   A rapid assessment of five physiological signs that indicate the physiological status of the newborn at birth

Assessment   A systematic, dynamic process by which the nurse, through interaction with women, newborns and families, significant others, and health care providers, collects, monitors, and analyzes data; data may include the following dimensions: psychological, biotechnological, physical, sociocultural, spiritual, cognitive, developmental, and economic, as well as functional abilities and lifestyle

Assisted reproductive technologies (ART)   Treatments for infertility that involve the surgical removal of the oocytes and combining them with sperm in a laboratory setting.

Asymmetric intrauterine growth restriction   A disproportional reduction in the size of structures and organs; results from maternal or placental conditions that occur later in pregnancy related to impeded placental blood flow

Attachment   Emotional connection that forms between the infant and his or her parents; it is bi-directional from parent to infant and infant to parent

Auscultation   When the Doppler or fetoscope (a listening devise) is used to assess the fetal heart rate by listening

Autonomy   Refers to two concepts that operate as a whole; one is the right of self-determination or the right of the individual to make his or her own choice to accept or reject treatment; the ability to exercise autonomous rights requires and is related to elements in informed consent; the second aspect is concerned with respect of persons, that is, to respect the patient's decision irrespective of the nurses' own values

Ballard maturational score (BMS)   Standardized test to calculated the gestational age of the neonate

Baseline FHR   The average fetal heart rate (FHR) rounded to increments of 5 beats per minute (bpm) during a 10-minute segment between uterine contractions, accelerations, or decelerations

Baseline variability   The fluctuations or variations of the fetal heart rate (FHR) of 2 cycles/min or greater during a steady state in the absence of contractions, accelerations, or decelerations

Beneficence   The obligation to do good; beneficence is concerned not only with doing good but also with removing harm and preventing harm

Bilirubin   Is the yellow pigmentation derived from the breakdown of red blood cells

Biochemical assessment   Involves biological examination and chemical determination

Biophysical profile (BPP) biophysical assessment (BPA)   An ultrasound assessment of fetal status along with a NST

Biophysical risk factors   Factors that originate from the mother or fetus and impact the development or function of the mother or fetus; these risk factors include genetic, nutritional, medical, and obstetric issues.

Biparietal diameter (BPD)   The largest transverse measurement and an important indicator of head size; 9.25 cm

Birth rate   Number of live births per 1,000 people

Bishop's score   An assessment of the cervix to assess cervical ripeness

Blastocyst   Stage of embryo development that follows the morula stage; the blastocyst is composed of an inner cell mass referred to as the embryoblast and an outer cell layer referred to as the trophoblast

Bloody show Brownish or blood-tinged cervical mucus discharge

Body Mass Index (BMI) A tool for determining appropriate body weight compared to height

Bonding Emotional feelings between parent and newborn that begin during pregnancy or shortly after birth; it is unidirectional from parent to newborn

Bradycardia Baseline FHR of less than 110 bpm lasting for 10 minutes or longer

Braxton-Hicks contractions Intermittent, painless, and physiological uterine contractions occurring in some pregnancies in the second and third trimesters that do not result in cervical change and are associated with false labor

Breech presentation The presenting part of the fetus is the buttocks and/or feet.

Breast engorgement Distention of milk glands

Bronchopulmonary dysplasia (BPD) A chronic lung condition that affects neonates that have been treated with mechanical ventilation and oxygen for problems such as respiratory distress syndrome

Brow presentation When the fetal head presents in a position midway between full flexion and extreme extension

Brown adipose tissue Also referred to as brown fat or non-shivering thermogenesis; a highly dense and vascular adipose tissue that is unique to neonates

Caput succedaneum A localized soft tissue edema of the scalp

Cardinal movements of labor The positional changes that the fetus goes through to best navigate the birth process

Cephalic presentation The presenting part is the head.

Cephalhematoma Hematoma formation between the periosteum and skull with unilateral swelling

Cephalopelvic disproportion (CPD) A condition in which the size, shape, or position of the fetal head prevents it from passing through the lateral aspect of the maternal pelvis or when the maternal pelvis is of a size or shape that prevents the decent of the fetus through the pelvis; term used when the maternal bony pelvis is not large enough or appropriately shaped to allow for fetal decent

Cervical dilation This measurement estimates the dilation of the cervical opening by sweeping the examining finger from the margin of the cervical opening on one side to that on the other.

Cervical effacement This measurement estimates the shortening of the cervix from 2 cm to paper thin measured by palpation of cervical length with fingertips.

Cervical ripening The process of physical softening and opening of the cervix in preparation for labor and birth

Cervix The neck or lowest part of the uterus; interfaces with the vagina

Cesarean birth Also referred to as cesarean section or c-section (C/S); an operative procedure in which the fetus is delivered through an incision in the abdominal wall and the uterus

Cesarean delivery on maternal request (CDMR) A cesarean section that is performed at the request of the woman prior to labor beginning and in the absence of maternal or fetal medical condition that presents a risk for labor

Chadwick's sign Bluish-purple coloration of the vagina and cervix evident in the first trimester of pregnancy

Childbearing and newborn health care A model of care addressing the health promotion, maintenance, and restoration needs of women from the preconception through the postpartum period; and low-risk, high-risk, and critically ill newborns from birth through discharge and follow-up, within the social, political, economic, and environmental context of the mother's, her newborn's, and the family's lives

Cholelithiasis Presence of gallstones in the gallbladder

Chronic pelvic pain (CPP) Pain in the pelvic region that lasts 6 months or longer and results in functional or psychological disabilities or requires treatment/intervention

Chorionic villi Projections from the chorion that embed into the decidua basalis and later form the fetal blood vessels of the placenta

Chorionic villus sampling (CVS) Aspiration of a small amount of placental tissue (chorion) for chromosomal, metabolic, or DNA testing

Circumcision An elective surgery to remove the foreskin of the penis

Circumoral cyanosis A benign localized transient cyanosis around the mouth

Classical cesarean delivery A vertical midline incision made into the abdominal wall with a vertical incision in the upper segment of the uterus performed for cesarean births

Cleavage Mitotic cell division of the zygote, fertilized oocyte

Clinical pelvimetry Measurements of the dimensions of the bony pelvis during an internal pelvic examination for determination of adequacy of the pelvis for a vaginal birth

Cold stress A term used when there is excessive heat loss that leads to hypothermia and results in the utilization of compensatory mechanisms to maintain the neonate's body temperature

Colic A term used to describe uncontrollable crying in healthy infants under the age of 5 months

Collaborative working relationships Working together with mutual respect for the accountability of each profession to the shared goal of quality patient outcomes

Colostrum Clear, yellowish breast fluid, which precedes milk production; it contains proteins, nutrients, and immune globulins; produced prenatally as early as the second trimester and prior to lactation in the first days after birth

Combined decelerations A deceleration pattern that has combined features, such as a variable deceleration that is also a late deceleration

Combined spinal epidural analgesia (CSE) Involves the injection of local anesthetic and/or analgesic into the subarachnoid space

Complete abortion Products of conception are totally expelled from uterus

Complete breech A fetal presentation where there is complete flexion of thighs and legs and a buttocks presentation of the fetus

Compound presentation The fetus assumes a unique posture usually with the arm or hand presenting alongside the presenting part.

Conception Also known as fertilization; occurs when a sperm nucleus enters the nucleus of the oocyte

Conduction Transfer of heat to cooler surface by direct skin contact such as cold hands of caregivers or cold equipment

Conjugated bilirubin The conjugated form of bilirubin (direct bilirubin) is soluble and excretable.

Contraction stress test (CST) Screening tool to assess fetal well-being with EFM in women with nonreactive NST at term gestation; the purpose of the CST is to identify a fetus that is at risk for compromise through observation of the fetal response to intermittent reduction in utero placental blood flow associated with stimulated uterine contractions (UCs)

Convection   Loss of heat from the neonate's warm body surface to cooler air currents such as air conditioners or oxygen masks

Coparenting   A conceptual term that refers to the ways that parents and/or parental figures relate to each other in the role of parents

Cotyledons   Rounded portions, lobes, of the maternal side of the placenta

Couvade syndrome   The occurrence in the mate of a pregnant woman of symptoms related to pregnancy, such as nausea, vomiting, and abdominal pain

Cultural stereotyping   The practice of making generalizations about a person based on his or her culture

Culturally competent care   Providing care to patients and their families that is effective, understandable, and respectful care in a manner that is compatible with their cultural beliefs, practices, and preferred language

Cystitis   Infection of the bladder

Cystocele   Bulging of the bladder into the vagina

Daily fetal movement count (kick counts)   Maternal assessment of fetal movement by counting fetal movements in a period of time to identify potentially hypoxic fetus

Decidua basalis   The portion of the decidua that forms the maternal portion of the placenta

Decrement phase   The descending or relaxation of the uterine muscle

Descent   The movement of the fetus through the birth canal during the first and second stage of labor

Diabetes mellitus (DM)   A chronic metabolic disease characterized by hyperglycemia as a result of limited or no insulin production

Diagnosis   A clinical judgment about the patient's response to actual or potential health conditions or needs; diagnoses provide the basis for determination of a plan of nursing care to achieve expected outcomes

Diagnostic tests   Tests that help to identify a particular disease or provide information which aids in the making of a diagnosis

Diastasis recti/Diastasis recti abdominis   A separation of the two rectus abdominis muscle bands at the midline

Dilation   The enlargement or opening of the cervical os

Direct bilirubin   Conjugated bilirubin

Direct obstetric death   Death of a woman resulting from complications during pregnancy, labor/birth, and/or postpartum, and from interventions, omission of interventions, or incorrect treatment

Disseminated intravascular coagulation (DIC)   Syndrome in which the coagulation pathways are hyperstimulated; occurs when the body is breaking down blood clots faster than it can form a clot, thus quickly depleting the body of clotting factors and leading to hemorrhage

Diversity   A quality that encompasses acceptance and respect related to but not limited to age, class, culture, disability, education level, ethnicity, family structure, gender, ideologies, political beliefs, race, religion, sexual orientation, style, and values

Doula   A Greek word meaning "woman's servant"; an assistant hired to give the woman support during pregnancy, labor and birth, and postpartum

Dubowitz neurological exam   Standardized tool to assess gestational age of neonate

Ductus arteriosus   Structure in fetal circulation that connects the pulmonary artery with the descending aorta; the majority of the oxygenated blood is shunted to the aorta via the ductus arteriosus with smaller amounts going to the lungs

Ductus venosus   Structure in fetal circulation that connects the umbilical vein to the inferior vena cava. This allows the majority of the high levels of oxygenated blood to enter the right atrium.

Duration of contractions   Length of a contraction measured by counting from the beginning to the end of one contraction and measured in seconds

Dysfunctional labor   Abnormal uterine contractions that prevent the normal progress of cervical dilation or descent of the fetus

Dystocia   A long, a difficult, or an abnormal labor

Early decelerations   A gradual decrease in FHR, 20–30 bpm below baseline; generally the onset, nadir, and the recovery mirror the contraction

Eclampsia   Preeclampsia with the onset of tonic clonic seizure/convulsions which place the mother and fetus at risk for death

Ectoderm   The outer layer of cells in the developing embryo

Ectopic pregnancy   A pregnancy that develops as a result of the blastocyst implanting somewhere other than the endometrial lining of the uterus; implantation of a fertilized ovum outside the uterus

Effacement   The shortening and thinning of the cervix

Effleurage   A massage technique using a very light touch of the fingers in two repetitive circular patterns over the gravid abdomen; done by lightly stroking the abdomen in rhythm with breathing during contractions

Elective abortion (EAB)   Termination of pregnancy before viability at the request of the woman but not for reasons of the impaired health of the maternal health or fetal disease

Electronic fetal monitoring (EFM)   A technique for fetal assessment based on the fact that the FHR reflects fetal oxygenation

Embryo   Term used for the developing human from the time of implantation through 8 weeks of gestation

Embryoblast   The inner cell mass of the blastocyst which develops into the embryo

Embryonic membranes   Two membranes, amnion and chorion, which form the amniotic sac; the chorionic membrane (outer membrane) develops from the trophoblast; the amniotic membrane (inner membrane) develops from the embryoblast; the embryo and amniotic fluid are contained within the amniotic sac

En face   Position in which the mother and newborn are face-to-face with eye contact

Endoderm   The inner layer of cells in the developing embryo

Endometrial biopsy   A biopsy of the endometrial tissue of the uterus to assess for the response of the uterus to hormonal signals that occur during the menstrual cycle

Endometrial cycle   Pertains to the changes in the endometrium of the uterus in response to the hormonal changes that occur during the ovarian cycle; this cycle consist of three phases: proliferative phase, secretory phase, and menstrual phase

Endometriosis   A chronic inflammatory disease in which the presence and growth of endometrial tissue is found outside the uterine cavity

Endometritis/Metritis   An infection of the endometrium that usually starts at the placental site and can spread to encompass the entire endometrium

Endometrium   The mucous membrane lining the interior of the uterus

Engagement   Occurs when the greatest diameter of the fetal head passes through the pelvic inlet

Engrossment   Phenomenon experienced by new fathers who have an intense preoccupation about and interest in their newborn

Entrainment   Phenomenon in which the newborn and infant moves his or her arms and legs in rhythm with speech patterns of an adult

Environmental risk factors   Risks in the workplace or the general environment that impact pregnancy outcomes; various environmental substances can effect fetal development; examples include exposure to chemicals, radiation, and pollutants

Epidural anesthesia   Involves the placement of a very small catheter and injection of local anesthesia and or analgesia between the 4th and 5th vertebrae into the epidural space

Epidural block   An anesthetic injected in the epidural space; located outside the dura mater between the dura and spinal canal via an epidural catheter

Episiotomy   An incision in the perineum to provide more space for the fetal presenting part at delivery

Epstein's pearls   White, pearl-like epithelial cysts on neonate's gum margins and palate

Epispadias   An abnormality in which urethral opening is on dorsal side of penis

Erythemia toxicum   A rash with red macules and papules (white to yellowish-white papule in center surrounded by reddened skin) that appear in different areas of the body, usually the trunk area. Can appear within 24 hours of birth and up to 2 weeks.

Ethical dilemma   A choice that has the potential to violate ethical principles

Ethics   Based in philosophical discussions of ancient Greek scholars about the nature of good and evil or right and wrong.

Ethnocentrism   The belief that the customs and values of the dominant culture are preferred or superior in some way

Evaluation   The process of determining the patient's progress toward attainment of expected outcomes and the effectiveness of nursing care

Evaporation   Loss of heat that occurs when water on neonate's skin is converted to vapors such as during bathing or directly after birth

Evidence based nursing (EBN)   Combining the best research evidence with clinical expertise while taking into account the patients' preferences and their situation in the context of the available resources part of nursing practice

Evidenced-based practice (EBP)   The integration of best research evidence, clinical expertise, and patient values in making decisions about the care of patients

Expulsion   During this cardinal movement the shoulders and remainder of the body are delivered.

Extension   This cardinal movement, which is facilitated by resistance of the pelvic floor, causes the presenting part to pivot beneath the pubic symphysis and the head to be delivered; occurs during the second stage of labor.

External rotation   During this cardinal movement the sagittal suture moves to a transverse diameter and the shoulders align in the anteroposterior diameter; the sagittal suture maintains alignment with the fetal trunk as the trunk navigates through the pelvis.

Extremely low birth weight infant (ELBW)   An infant who weighs less than 1,000 grams at birth

Face presentation   When the fetal head is in extension rather than flexion as it enters the pelvis

False labor   Irregular contractions with little or no cervical changes

Family-centered maternity care   A model of obstetric care that views pregnancy and childbirth as a normal life event or life transition that is not primarily medical but rather developmental; health care is provided in an inclusive manner, with family and significant others, including children, as an active part of the process; the emphasis is on holistic care, with the focus on the pregnant woman and her well-being, including emotional and psychosocial considerations

Ferguson's reflex   A physiological response of the woman, activated when the presenting part of the fetus is at least at +1 station; it is usually accompanied by spontaneous bearing-down efforts

Ferning   When a sample of fluid in the upper vaginal area is obtained, the fluid is placed on a slide and assessed for "ferning pattern" under a microscope to confirm rupture of membranes.

Fertility rate   Total number of live births, regardless of age of mother, per 1,000 women of reproductive age, 15–44 years

Fetal alcohol syndrome (FAS)   Refers to a wide array and spectrum of physical, cognitive, and behavioral abnormalities associated with maternal alcohol use during pregnancy

Fetal attitude or posture   The relationship of the fetal parts to one another; this is noted by the flexion or extension of the fetal joints

Fetal bradycardia   Baseline FHR of less than 110 bpm lasting for 10 minutes or longer

Fetal dystocia   May be caused by excessive fetal size, malpresentation, multifetal pregnancy, or fetal anomalies

Fetal fibronectin (fFN)   A protein detected via immunoassay; a positive test is >50 ng/mL.

Fetal heart rate accelerations   The visually abrupt, transient increases (onset to peak <30 sec) in the FHR above the baseline, 15 beats above the baseline and last from 15 seconds to less than two minutes

Fetal heart rate decelerations   Transitory decreases in the FHR baseline; they are classified as early, variable, or late decelerations

Fetal lie   Refers to the long axis (spine) of the fetus in relationship to the long axis (spine) of the woman

Fetal position   Location of the presenting part and specific fetal structures to determine fetal position in relation to maternal pelvis; relation of the denominator or reference point to the maternal pelvis

Fetal presentation   Determined by the part, or pole, of the fetus that first enters the pelvic inlet

Fetoscope   Stethoscope used to auscultate fetal heart rate

Fetus   Term used for the developing human from 9 weeks' gestation to birth

Fidelity   Refers to the faithfulness or obligation to keep promises

First-degree laceration   A laceration that involves the perineal skin and vaginal mucous membrane

First stage of labor   Begins with onset of labor and ends with complete cervical dilation

Flexion   When the chin of the fetus moves toward the fetal chest; flexion occurs when the descending head meets resistance from maternal tissues

Follicular phase   Part of the ovarian cycle; it begins the first day of menstruation and last 12–14 days; during this phase, the graafian follicle is maturing

Footling breech   When either one (single footling) or both (double footling) feet of the fetus present first in the pelvis

Foramen ovale   A structure in fetal circulation; it is an opening between the right and left atria; blood high in oxygen is shunted to the left atrium via the foramen ovale

Forceps   An instrument used to assist with delivery of the fetal head, typically done to improve the health of the woman or the fetus

Foremilk   The milk that is produced and stored between feedings and released at the beginning of the feeding session; it has higher water content

Fourth degree laceration   A laceration that extends into the rectal mucosa and to expose the lumen of the rectum

Fourth stage of labor   Begins with the delivery of the placenta and typically ends within 4 hours or with the stabilization of the mother postpartum

Frank breech   A fetal presentation where there is complete flexion of the thighs and the legs extend over the anterior surfaces of the body

Frequency of contractions   Determined by counting number of contractions in a 10-minute period, counting from the start of one contraction to the start of the next contraction in minutes

Fundus   The upper portion of the uterus

Gate control theory of pain   States that sensation of pain is transmitted from the periphery of the body along ascending nerve pathways to the brain; due to the limited number of sensations that can travel along these pathways at any given time, an alternate activity can replace travel of the pain sensation; thus closing the gate control at the spinal cord and reducing pain impulses traveling to the brain

General anesthesia   The use of IV injection and/or inhalation of anesthetic agents that render the woman unconscious

Genital fistulas   An abnormal connection between the vagina and bladder, rectum, and/or urethra; the fistula provides a pathway for fecal material and/or urine to enter the vagina

Genome   An organism's complete set of DNA

Genotype   Refers to a person's genetic makeup

Gestational diabetes mellitus (GDM)   Any degree of glucose intolerance with the onset or first recognition in pregnancy

Gestational hypertension   A relatively benign disorder without underlying physiological changes in the mother; high blood pressure detected for the first time after mid-pregnancy, without proteinuria; diagnosis is made postpartum

Glans penis   Tip of the penis

Gonadotoxins   Factors, such as drugs, infections, illness, and heat exposure, that can have an adverse effect on spermatogenesis

Goodell's sign   The softening of the cervix in the first trimester of pregnancy

Gravida   A pregnant woman; also, the number of times a woman has been pregnant (Gravida/Para notation)

Harlequin sign   One side of body is pink and the other side is white.

Hegar's sign   The softening of the lower uterine segment (isthmus) in the first trimester of pregnancy

HELLP syndrome   (Hemolysis, Elevated Liver enzymes, and Low Platelets) Acronym used to designate the variant changes in laboratory values that is a complication of severe preeclampsia

Hematomas   A collection of blood within the connective tissues; common sites in the postpartum woman are the vagina and perineal areas

Hind milk   The milk produced during the feeding session and released at the end of the session; it has a higher fat content

Hydatiform mole   A benign proliferate growth of the trophoblast in which the chorionic villi develop into edematous, cystic, vascular transparent vesicles that hang in grapelike clusters without a viable fetus

Hydrocele   Enlarged scrotum due to excess fluid

Hyperbilirubinemia   Term used when there is a high level of unconjugated bilirubin in the neonate's blood

Hyperemesis Gravidarum   Vomiting during pregnancy that is so severe it leads to dehydration, electrolyte and acid base imbalance, and starvation ketosis.

Hyperstimulation   Excessive uterine activity

Hypertonic uterine dysfunction   Uncoordinated uterine activity

Hypospadias   An abnormality in which the urethral opening is on ventral surface of penis

Hypotonic uterine dysfunction   Occurs when the pressure of the UC is insufficient (<25 mmHg) to promote cervical dilation and effacement

Hysterectomy   The surgical removal of the uterus

Hysterosalpingogram   A radiological examination that provides information about the endocervical canal, uterine cavity, and the fallopian tubes

Implantation   The embedding of the blastocyst into the endometrium of the uterus

Implementation   The process of taking action by intervening, delegating, and/or coordinating; women, newborns, families, significant others, or health care providers may direct the implementation of interventions within the plan of care

Inadequate expulsive forces   Occurs in the second stage of labor when the woman is not able to push or bear down

Incompetent cervix   A mechanical defect in the cervix that results in painless cervical dilation and ballooning of the membranes into the vagina followed by expulsion of an immature fetus in the second trimester

Incomplete abortion   Fragments of products of conception are expelled and tissue parts are retained in the uterus.

Increment phase   The ascending or buildup of the contraction which begins in the fundus and spreads throughout the uterus

Indirect bilirubin   Unconjugated bilirubin

Indirect obstetrical death   Death of a woman that is due to a preexisting disease or a disease that develops during pregnancy that is not directly related to obstetrical cause but is aggravated by the changes of pregnancy

Induced abortion   The medical or surgical termination of pregnancy prior to viability

Induction   The deliberate stimulation of uterine contractions before the onset of spontaneous labor

Inevitable abortion   Termination of pregnancy is in progress.

Infant mortality   Infant death prior to the first birthday

Infertility   The inability to conceive and maintain a pregnancy after 12 months (6 months for women over 35 years old age) of unprotected sexual intercourse

Intensity   Strength of the contraction and measure by palpation, or internally by an intrauterine pressure catheter (IUPC) in mmHg

Interconceptional interval   The period of time in between pregnancies

Internal rotation   This cardinal movement, the rotation of the fetal head, aligns the long axis of the fetal head with the long axis of the maternal pelvis; occurs mainly during second stage of labor.

Internal uterine pressure catheter (IUPC)   This monitoring provides an objective measure of the pressure of contractions expressed as mmHg

Intrapartum period   Begins with the onset of regular uterine contractions and lasts until the expulsion of the placenta

Intrauterine growth restriction (IUGR)   A decrease rate of fetal growth usually due to a decrease in cell production related to chronic malnutrition; there are two types of IUGR, symmetric and asymmetric

Involution   The process by which the uterus returns to a prepregnant size, shape, and location; and the placental site heals

Isthmus   The narrower, lower segment of the uterus

Justice   The principle of fairness, that others are entitled to equal treatment or to be treated fairly

Kernicterus   An abnormal accumulation of unconjugated bilirubin in the neonate's brain cells

Labor   The process in which the fetus, placenta, and membranes are expelled through the uterus

Labor augmentation   The stimulation of ineffective uterine contractions after the onset of spontaneous labor to manage labor dystocia

Lacerations   Tears in the perineum that may occur at delivery

Lactation   The production of breast milk

Lanugo   Fine, downy hair that develops after 16 weeks of gestation

Large for gestational age (LGA)   Term used for neonates whose weight is above the 90th percentile for gestational age

Latching-on   Refers to the newborn's ability to grasp the breast and to effectively suckle

Late deceleration   A visually apparent gradual decrease of FHR below the baseline. Lowest part of the deceleration occurs after the peak of the contraction

Late maternal death   Death of a woman that occurs more than 42 days after termination of pregnancy from a direct or indirect obstetrical cause

Late premature/late preterm   Neonate born between 34 and 37 weeks' gestation

Latent phase   First phase of labor; the early and slower part of labor with cervical dilation from 0–3 cm

Leiomyomas of the uterus   Also referred to as myomas or uterine fibroids; benign fibrous tumor of the uterine wall

Leopold's maneuvers   A series of four maneuvers used to palpate a gravid uterus to determine fetal position, presentation, and size

Let-down reflect   Also referred to as milk ejection reflex; results in milk being ejected into and through the lactiferous duct system

Leukorrhea   A white, odorless, physiological vaginal discharge; increases in pregnancy due to increased mucus secretion by cervical glands

Lightening   Term used to describe the descent of the fetus into the true pelvis ,which occurs approximately 2 weeks before term in first-time pregnancies

Local   An anesthetic injected into perineum at episiotomy site

Lochia   Bloody discharge from the uterus that contains sloughed off tissue; it undergoes changes that reflect the healing stages of the uterine placental site

Long term variability (LTV)   The changes in FHR range or fluctuations in the FHR baseline

Low birth weight infant (LBW)   An infant who weighs less than 2,500 grams but greater than 1,500 grams at birth, regardless of gestational age

Low lying placenta   The placenta is implanted in the lower uterine segment in close proximity to the internal cervical os.

Luteal phase   Part of the ovarian cycle; it begins after ovulation and last approximately 14 days

Macrocephaly   Head circumference greater than the 90th percentile

Macrosomia   Birth weight above 4,000–4,500 grams

Magnetic resonance imaging (MRI)   Diagnostic radiological evaluation of tissue and organs from multiple planes

Mammogram   A low-dose x-ray of the breast

Marginal placenta previa   The placenta is at the margin of the internal cervical os

Mastitis   Inflammation/infection of the breast

Maternal death   Death of a woman during pregnancy or within 42 days of termination of pregnancy; the death is related to the pregnancy or aggravated by pregnancy, or management of the pregnancy; it excludes death from accidents or injuries

Maternal phases   A process, defined by Reva Rubin, that occurs during the first few weeks of the postpartum period; this process includes three phases: Taking-in, Taking-hold, and Letting-go

Maternal tasks of pregnancy   Psychological work done by the pregnant woman toward the development of a positive adaptation to pregnancy and the establishment of a maternal identity

Maternal touch   A process, described by Reva Rubin, that new mothers transition through beginning with the first physical contact with their newborns

Meconium stool   The first stool eliminated by the neonate; it is sticky, thick, black, and odorless

Medical nutritional therapy (MNT)   A cornerstone of diabetes management for all diabetic women; the goal is to provide adequate nutrition, prevent diabetic ketoacidosis, and postprandial euglycemia

Meiosis   A process of two successive cell divisions that produces cells that contain half the number of chromosomes (haploid).

Menarche   The initial menstrual period

Menopause   The permanent cessation of menstrual activity; *occurs 12 months after a woman's last menstrual period*

Menstrual phase   Part of the endometrial cycle; it occurs in response to hormonal changes and results in the sloughing off of the endometrial tissue

Mesoderm   The middle layer of cells in the developing embryo

Metritis/Endometritis   An infection of the endometrium that usually starts at the placental site and can spread to encompass the entire endometrium

Microcephaly   Head circumference below the 10th percentile of normal for newborns gestational age

Milia   White papules on the neonate's face; more frequently seen on the bridge of the nose and chin

Missed abortion   Embryo or fetus dies during first 20 weeks of gestation but is retained in uterus

Mitotic cell division or mitosis   Occurs when a cell (parent cell) divides and forms two daughter cells that contain the same number of chromosomes as the parent cell

Moderately premature   Neonate born between 32 and 34 weeks' gestation

Modified BPP   Combines a non-stress test with an amniotic fluid index (AFI) as an indicator of short-term fetal well-being and AFI as an indicator of long-term placental function to evaluate fetal well-being

Molding   The ability of the fetal head to change shape to accommodate/fit through the maternal pelvis

Mongolian spots   Flat bluish discolored areas on the lower back and/or buttock. Seen more often in African American, Asian, Latin, and Native American infants

Morula   16-cell solid sphere that forms three days following fertilization as a result of mitotic cell division of the zygote

Mottling   A benign transient pattern of pink and white blotches on the skin

Multigravida   A woman who has been pregnant multiple times

Multipara   A woman who has given birth after 20 weeks' gestation multiple times

Multiple gestation   A pregnancy with more than one fetus

Myomectomy   Surgical removal of fibroids

Myometrium   The smooth muscle layer of the uterus

Nadir   The lowest point of the deceleration; occurs at the peak of the contraction

Naegele's rule   The standard formula for calculating an estimated date of birth based on an LMP (LMP minus 3 months plus 7 days)

Natal teeth   Immature caps of enamel and dentin with poorly developed roots

Necrotizing enterocolitis (NEC)   A gastrointestinal disease that affects neonates; this disease results in inflammation and necrosis of the bowel, usually the proximal colon or terminal ileum

Neonatal abstinence syndrome   Also referred to as neonatal withdrawal; may result from intrauterine exposure to various substances, including opioids such as heroin, methadone, oxycodone, and Demerol; alcohol; Valium; caffeine; and barbiturates

Neonatal period   The time period from birth through the first 28 days of life

Neutral thermal environment (NTE)   Refers to an environment that maintains body temperature with minimal metabolic changes and/or oxygen consumption

Non-stress test (NST)   Screening tool that uses electronic fetal monitoring to assess fetal well-being

Nonmaleficence   The obligation to do no harm

Nonreassuring FHR   An abnormal FHR pattern that reflects an unfavorable physiological response to the maternal-fetal environment, this term is no longer in common use

Nulligravida   A woman who has never been pregnant

Nullipara   A woman who has never given birth after 20 weeks' gestation

Obstetrical emergency   An urgent clinical situation that places either the maternal or fetal status at risk for increased morbidity and mortality

Occiput posterior   When the occiput of the fetus is in the posterior portion of the pelvis rather than the anterior

Occult prolapse   When the cord is palpated through the membranes but does not drop into the vagina

Oligohydramnios   Decreased amounts of amniotic fluid (less than 500 mL at term or 50% reduction of normal amounts) during pregnancy

Ominous FHR patterns   Fetal heart rates associated with increased risk of fetal acidemia

Oogenesis   The formation of a mature ovum (egg)

Open glottis   Refers to spontaneous, involuntary bearing down accompanying the forces of the uterine contraction and is usually characterized by expiratory grunting or vocalizations by a woman during pushing

Operative vaginal delivery   A vaginal birth that is assisted by a vacuum extraction or forceps

Organogenesis   The formation and development of body organs that occurs during the first trimester of pregnancy

Orthostatic hypotension   A sudden drop in the blood pressure when the woman stands up from a sitting or lying position

Osteoporosis   The loss of bone mass that occurs when more bone mass is absorbed than new body mass is laid down

Outcome   A measurable individual, family, or community state, behavior, or perception that is responsive to nursing interventions

Ovarian cycle   Pertains to the maturation of ova and consist of three phases: follicular phase, ovulatory phase, and luteal phase

Ovulatory phase   Part of the ovarian cycle; it begins when estrogen levels peak and ends with the release of the oocyte (egg)

from the mature graafian follicle; the release of the oocyte is referred to ovulation

Oxytocin induction   Pharmacological method for induction of labor with oxytocin

Papanicolaou smear   A screening test used to identify cervical cancer

Para   A woman who has given birth to an infant after 20 weeks' gestation; also, the number of births that occurred after 20 weeks' gestation (Gravida/Para notation) or the number of infants born after 20 weeks' gestation (TPAL notation)

Partial placenta previa   The placenta partially covers the internal cervical os.

Parturition   (or labor) The process in which the fetus, placenta, and membranes are expelled through the uterus

Passage   Includes the bony pelvis and the soft tissues of cervix, pelvic floor, vagina, and introitus (external opening to the vagina)

Passenger   The fetus

Patent ductus arteriosus (PDA)   Occurs when the ductus arteriosus remains open or remains open after birth

Peak pressure   The maximum uterine pressure during a contraction measured with an IUPC

Pelvic dystocia   Related to the contraction of one or more of the three planes of the pelvis

Pelvic inflammatory disease (PID)   A general term that refers to an infection of the uterus, fallopian tubes, and other reproductive organs

Pelvic organ prolapse (POP)   The descent of pelvic organs into the vagina or against the vaginal wall

Percutaneous umbilical blood sampling (PUBS)   The removal of fetal blood from umbilical cord for fetal blood sampling; also referred to as cordocentesis

Perinatal   The time period "around" the birth of a baby; generally refers to the weeks before and after a baby is born, from 28 weeks' gestation to 28 days after birth

Periodic and nonperiodic changes   Accelerations or decelerations in the FHR that are related to uterine contractions and persist over time

Persistent pulmonary hypertension (PPHN)   Results when the normal vasodilation and relaxation of the pulmonary vascular bed does not occur

Pfannenstiel incision or "bikini cut"   A transverse skin incision at the level of the mons pubis with a transverse incision in the lower uterine segment performed for cesarean births

Phenotype   Refers to how the genes are outwardly expressed (i.e., eye color, hair color, height)

Phenylketonuria (PKU)   An inborn error of metabolism that affects the neonate's ability to metabolize phenylalanine, an amino acid commonly found in many foods such as breast milk and formula

Physiological anemia of pregnancy   A relative anemia in mid to late pregnancy due to physiological hypervolemia without a correspondingly proportionate increase in erythrocytes in the maternal system

Pica   A craving for and consumption of non-food substances such as starch and clay; can result in toxicity due to ingested substances or malnutrition from replacing nutritious foods with non-food substances

Pilonidal dimple   A small pit or sinus in the sacral area at top of crease between the buttocks

Placenta accreta   An abnormality of implantation defined by degree of invasion into uterine wall of trophoblast of placenta, invasion of trophoblast beyond the normal boundary

Placenta increta   Invasion of trophoblast that extends into myometrium

Placenta percreta   Invasion of trophoblast beyond the serosa

Placenta previa   Occurs when the placenta attaches to the lower uterine segment of the uterus, near or over the internal cervical os, instead of in the body or fundus of the uterus

Placental reserve   Describes the reserve oxygen available to the fetus to withstand the transient changes in blood flow and oxygen during labor

Polycystic ovary syndrome (PCOS)   Also known as Stein-Leventhal syndrome, is an endocrine disorder that affects 5%–10% of women of childbearing age that involves multiple follicular cysts on one or both ovaries

Polydactyly   Extra digits of hands or feet

Polyhydramnios or hydramnios   Increased amounts of amniotic fluid (1,500–2,000 mL)

Position   Maternal position during labor and birth

Position of cervix   Relationship of the cervical os to the fetal head and is characterized as posterior, mid position, or anterior

Post term pregnancy   One that has a gestational period of 42 completed weeks

Postpartum   The 6-week period of time following childbirth

Postpartum blues   Also known as baby blues; occurs during the first few weeks postpartum and lasts for a few days; it is a time of heightened maternal emotions with the woman being tearful and irritable with emotional swings

Postpartum chills   Episode of shaking and feeling cold that is experienced by most women during the first few hours following birth

Postpartum depression (PPD)   A mood disorder characterized by severe depression that occurs within the first 6–12 months postpartum

Postpartum psychosis (PPP)   A variant of bipolar disorder and is the most serious form of postpartum mood disorders

Postterm   Born after completion of 41 weeks' gestation

Powers   Refer to the involuntary uterine contractions of labor and the voluntary pushing or bearing down powers that combine to propel and deliver the fetus and placenta from the uterus

Practice standards   Standards that help to guide professional nursing practice; they summarize the nursing profession's best judgment and optimal practice based on current research and clinical practice

Precipitous labor   Labor that lasts less than 3 hours from onset of labor to birth

Preconception care   Well-woman health care focusing on preparation for and anticipation of a pregnancy, including health promotion, risk screening, and implementation of interventions prior to pregnancy, the goal being to modify risk factors that could negatively impact a pregnancy in order to optimize perinatal outcomes

Preeclampsia   Hypertension accompanied by underlying systemic pathology that can have severe maternal and fetal impact; a systemic disease with hypertension accompanied by proteinuria after 20th week of gestation.

Preeclampsia superimposed on chronic HTN   Occurs with hypertensive women who develop new onset proteinuria; proteinuria before 20th week gestation or sudden uncontrolled hypertension

Prenatal   The entire time period during which a woman is pregnant; includes the antepartum/antepartal and the intrapartal periods

Prenatal care   Health care relating to pregnancy that a woman receives during the pregnancy and prior to the onset of labor

Prescriptive behavior   Expected behavior of the pregnant woman during the childbearing period

Presenting part   The specific fetal structure lying nearest to the cervix

Preterm birth   Any birth that occurs after 20 weeks and before 37 completed weeks of pregnancy

Preterm premature rupture of membranes (PPROM)   Rupture of membranes with a premature gestation (<37 weeks).

Premature rupture of membranes   Rupture of the chorioamniotic membranes before the onset of labor.

Prolonged rupture of membranes   Rupture of the membranes for greater than 24 hours

Preterm/premature infant   An infant born after 20 weeks and before 37 completed weeks of gestation

Primary engorgement   An increase in the vascular and lymphatic system of the breasts, which precedes the initiation of milk production; the woman's breasts become larger, firm, warm, and tender and woman may feel a throbbing pain in the breasts

Primigravida   A woman who is pregnant for the first time

Primipara   A woman who has given birth after 20 weeks' gestation one time

Prodromal labor   When contractions are frequent and painful in early labor but ineffective in promoting dilation and effacement

Prolactin   The primary hormone responsible for lactation

Prolapse of the umbilical cord   When the cord lies below the presenting part of the fetus

Proliferative phase   Part of the endometrial cycle; it follows menstruation and ends with ovulation; during this phase the endometrium is preparing for implantation by becoming thicker and more vascular

Prolonged deceleration   A visually apparent abrupt decrease in FHR below baseline that last >2 minutes and <10 minutes

Prolonged rupture of membranes (PROM)   Rupture of membranes longer than 24 hours

Psychosocial risk factors   Maternal behaviors or lifestyles that have a negative response to the mother or fetus; examples include: smoking, caffeine, alcohol/drugs, and psychological status

Pudendal block   An anesthetic injected in the pudendal nerve (close to the ischial spines) via needle guide known as "trumpet"

Pulmonary surfactant   A substance that is composed of 90% phospholipids and 10% proteins that is used in the treatment of respiratory distress syndrome of the neonate

Quad screen   Adds inhibin-A to the triple marker screen to increase detection of Trisomy 21 to 80%

Quickening   A woman's first awareness/perception of fetal movement within her uterus

Radiation   Transfer of heat from neonate to cooler objectives that are not in direct contact with neonate such as cold walls of isolate or cold equipment near neonate

Reassuring FHR   Normal FHR pattern that reflects a favorable physiological response to maternal-fetal environment this term is no longer in common use

Rectoceles   Bulging of the rectum into the vagina

Recurrent abortion   Condition in which two or more successive pregnancies have ended in spontaneous abortion

Respect for others   The principle that all persons are equally valued

Respiratory distress syndrome (RDS)   A life-threatening lung disorder that results from underdeveloped and small alveoli, and insufficient levels of pulmonary surfactant

Resting tone   The pressure in the uterus between contractions

Restrictive behavior   Activities during the childbearing period which are limited for the woman based on cultural practices

Review of systems (ROS)   A component of the health history that includes systematic questioning about health status by body system, typically in a head-to-toe sequence, in order to gather information about current and past medical experiences.

Rh factor   A type of antigen on the surface of red blood cells; if a woman's RBCs have the antigen, she is Rh positive, and if they do not have the antigen, she is Rh negative; this is significant and can cause isoimmunization from blood incompatibility if fetal blood enters the maternal system in an Rh positive fetus and an Rh negative mother

Rights approach   The focus is on the individual's right to choose; includes the right to privacy, to know the truth, and to be free from injury or harm

Risk management   A systems approach to the prevention of litigation; it involves the identification of systems problems, and analysis and treatment of risks before a suit is brought

Rupture of the uterus   When there is a partial or complete tear in the uterine muscle

Screening test   A test designed to identify those who are not affected by a disease or abnormality

Second-degree laceration   A laceration that involves skin, mucous membrane, and fascia of perineal body

Second stage of labor   Begins at complete dilation of cervix and ends with delivery of the neonate

Secretory phase   Part of the endometrial cycle; it begins after ovulation and ends with the onset of menstruation; during this phase the endometrium continues to thicken

Septic abortion   A condition in which products of conception become infected during abortion process

Shaken baby syndrome   Also referred to **as abusive head trauma (AHT);** a traumatic brain injury that occurs when an infant is violently shaken

Short-term variability (STV)   The changes in the FHR from one beat to the next; is measured with a fetal scalp electrode; this term is no longer used

Shoulder dystocia   Refers to difficulty encountered during delivery of the shoulders after the birth of the head

Shoulder presentation   The presenting part is the shoulder; when the fetal spine is vertical to the maternal pelvis

Small for gestational age (SGA)   A term used for neonate whose weight is below the 10th percentile for gestational age

Social support   Support given by someone with whom the expectant mother has a personal relationship, involving the primary groups of most importance to the individual woman

Sociodemographic risk factors   Variables that pertain to the woman and her family and place an increased risk to the mother and the fetus; examples include income, access to prenatal care, age, parity, marital status, and ethnicity

Sperm antibodies   An immunological reaction against the sperm that causes a decrease in sperm motility

Spermatogenesis   The process in which mature functional sperm are formed

Spinal block   An anesthetic injected in the subarachnoid space

Spontaneous abortion (SAB)   Abortion occurring without medical or mechanical means; also called miscarriage

Spontaneous rupture of the membranes (SROM)   Rupture of the membranes that occurs naturally

Standard   An authoritative statement enunciated and promulgated by the profession and by which the quality of practice, service, or education can be judged

Standards of care   Authoritative statements that describe competent clinical nursing practice for women and newborns demonstrated through assessment, diagnosis, outcome identification, planning, implementation, and evaluation

Standards of nursing practice   Authoritative statements that describe the scope of care or performance common to the profession of nursing and by which the quality of nursing practice can be judged; standards of nursing practice for women and newborns include both standards of care and standards of professional performance

Standards of professional performance   Authoritative statements that describe competent behavior in the professional role, including activities related to quality of care, performance appraisal, resource utilization, education, collegiality, ethics, collaboration, research, and research utilization

Station   The level of the presenting part in the birth canal in relationship to the ischial spines; refers to the relationship of the ischial spines to the presenting part of the fetus and assists in assessing for fetal descent during labor

Striae   A band of depressed tissue most commonly seen on abdomen, thighs, buttocks, or breasts due to stretching of the skin; synonymous with stretch marks

Stripping the membranes   Digital separation of the chorionic membrane from the wall of the cervix and lower uterine segment during a vaginal exam done by a primary care provider to stimulate labor

Subinvolution of the uterus   A term used when the uterus does not decrease in size and does not descend into the pelvis

Supine hypotensive syndrome   Hypotension resulting from compression of the vena cava when a woman lies supine and the gravid uterus exerts pressure on the inferior vena cava

Symmetric intrauterine growth restriction   A generalized proportional reduction in the size of all structures and organs except for heart and brain

Syndactyly   Webbed digits of hands or feet

Taboos   Cultural restrictions believed to have serious consequences

Tachycardia   Baseline FHR of greater than 160 bpm lasting 10 minutes or longer

Tachysystole   Abnormally frequent contractions, 5 or more contractions in 10 minutes

Teratogens   are any drug, virus, infection, or other exposures that can cause embryo/fetal developmental abnormality

Term birth   A birth that occurs after 37 completed weeks of gestation

Therapeutic abortion (TAB)   Termination of pregnancy for serious maternal medical indications or serious fetal anomalies

Third-degree laceration   A laceration involves skin, mucous membrane, muscle of perineal body, and extends to the rectal sphincter

Third stage of labor   Begins immediately after the delivery of the fetus and involves separation and expulsion of the placenta and membranes

Threatened abortion   Continuation of pregnancy is in doubt as symptoms indicate termination of pregnancy is in progress

Thrombosis   Blood clot within the vascular system

Tocodynamometer   An external uterine monitor to measure contractions

TORCH   An acronym that stands for Toxoplasmosis, Other (hepatitis B), Rubella, Cytomegalovirus, and Herpes Simplex virus

Total placenta previa   The placenta completely covers the internal cervical os.

Toxoplasma   A protozoan parasite found in cat feces and uncooked or rare beef and lamb

Transepidermal water loss (TEWL)   Water loss that can occur through the neonate's immature skin

Transition phase   Third phase of labor; dilation to 10 cm

Transitional stool   Neonatal stools that begin around the 3rd day and can continue for 3 or 4 days; the stool transitions from black to greenish black, to greenish brown, to greenish yellow

Transverse presentation   The presenting part is usually the shoulder

Trial of labor after cesarean (TOLAC)   When a trial of labor and vaginal birth is attempted in a woman who has had a prior cesarean birth

Triple marker   A screening that combines all three chemical markers (AFP, hCG, and estriol levels) with maternal age to detect some trisomies and neural tube defects

Trophic feedings   Small volume enteral feedings that are administered to neonates

Trophoblast   Outer cell mass of the blastocyst which assists in implantation and becomes part of the placenta

True labor   Contractions occur at regular intervals and increase in frequency, duration, and intensity; true labor contractions bring about changes in cervical effacement and dilation

Turtle sign   The retraction of the fetal head against the maternal perineum after delivery of the head

Type 1 diabetes mellitus   A result of autoimmunity of beta cells of the pancreas resulting in absolute insulin deficiency

Type 2 diabetes mellitus   Characterized by insulin resistance and inadequate insulin production

Ultrasonography   The use of high-frequency sound waves to produce an image of an organ or tissue

Umbilical artery doppler flow   Studies assess the rate and volume of blood flow through placenta and umbilical cord vessels using ultrasound

Umbilical cord   The structure that connects the fetus to the placenta; it consists of 2 arteries and 1 vein and is surrounded by Wharton's Jelly

Unconjugated bilirubin   A relatively insoluble bilirubin and mostly bound to albumin; also called indirect bilirubin

Undescended testes   An abnormality in which testes are not in the scrotum

Urinary incontinence   Loss of bladder control

Uterine atony   A decreased tone of the uterine muscle postpartum that is the primary cause of immediate postpartum hemorrhage

Uterine fibroids   Benign growths of the muscular wall of the uterus

Uterine hypertonus   An increasing resting tone >20–25 mmHg, peak pressure >80 mmHg or Montevideo units >400

Uterine prolapse   Occurs when there is a weakening of the pelvic connective tissue, pubococcygeus muscle, and uterine ligaments which allows the uterus to descend into the vagina

Uterus   The muscular reproductive organ that contains and supports a pregnancy

Utilitarian approach   This approach suggests that ethical actions are those that provide the greatest balance of good over evil and provides for the greatest good for the greatest number

Utility   The greatest good for the individual or an action that is valued; utility is concerned with the evaluation of risk and benefit or benefit versus burden

Vacuum assisted delivery   A birth involving the use of a vacuum cup on the fetal head to assist with delivery of the fetal head

Vaginal birth after a cesarean (VBAC)   When a trial of labor and vaginal birth is attempted in a woman who has had a prior cesarean birth

Vaginitis   An inflammation of the vagina

Valsalva maneuver   the method of breath holding, closed-glottis pushing

Variable deceleration   A visually apparent abrupt decrease in the FHR below baseline; the decrease is ≥15 bpm lasting ≥15 seconds and <2 minutes in duration

Veracity   The obligation to tell the truth

Vernix caseosa   A protective substance secreted from sebaceous glands that covered the fetus during pregnancy

Very low birth weight infant (VLBW)   An infant who weighs less than 1,500 grams at birth

Very premature/preterm   Neonate born at less than 32 weeks' gestation

Vibroacoustic stimulation (VAS)   Screening tool that uses auditory stimulation (using an artificial larynx) to assess fetal well being with electronic fetal monitoring when NST is non-reactive

Wharton's Jelly   A collagen substance which surrounds of vessels of the umbilical cord and protects the vessels from compression

Zygote   A fertilized oocyte which contains the diploid number of chromosomes (46)

Photo and Illustration Credits

Roberta Durham author photo by James Edwards

Chapter 2

Figure 2-1. Chapman, L. and Durham, R. *Maternal–Newborn Nursing: The Critical Components of Nursing Care*. 2010. Philadelphia: F.A. Davis.

Figure 2-2. Chapman, L. and Durham, R. *Maternal–Newborn Nursing: The Critical Components of Nursing Care*. 2010. Philadelphia: F.A. Davis.

Chapter 3

Figure 3-1. Scanlon, V. and Sanders, T. (2007). *Essentials of Anatomy and Physiology* (5th ed., p. 469). Philadelphia: F.A. Davis.

Figure 3-2. Scanlon, V. and Sanders, T. (2007). *Essentials of Anatomy and Physiology* (5th ed., p. 478). Philadelphia: F.A. Davis.

Figure 3-3. Scanlon, V. and Sanders, T. (2007). *Essentials of Anatomy and Physiology* (5th ed., p. 479). Philadelphia: F.A. Davis.

Figure 3-4. Scanlon, V. and Sanders, T. (2007). *Essentials of Anatomy and Physiology* (5th ed., p. 305). Philadelphia: F.A. Davis.

Figure 3-5. Scanlon, V. and Sanders, T. (2007). *Essentials of Anatomy and Physiology* (5th ed., p. 484). Philadelphia: F.A. Davis.

Figure 3-6. Scanlon, V. and Sanders, T. (2007). *Essentials of Anatomy and Physiology* (5th ed., p. 485). Philadelphia: F.A. Davis.

Figure 3-7. Scanlon, V. and Sanders, T. (2007). *Essentials of Anatomy and Physiology* (5th ed., p. 485). Philadelphia: F.A. Davis.

Figure 3-8. Scanlon, V. and Sanders, T. (2007). *Essentials of Anatomy and Physiology* (5th ed., p. 485). Philadelphia: F.A. Davis.

Figure 3-9. Scanlon, V. and Sanders, T. (2007). *Essentials of Anatomy and Physiology* (5th ed., p. 485). Philadelphia: F.A. Davis.

Figure 3-10. Scanlon, V. and Sanders, T. (2007). *Essentials of Anatomy and Physiology* (5th ed., p. 485). Philadelphia: F.A. Davis.

Figure 3-11. Scanlon, V. and Sanders, T. (2007). *Essentials of Anatomy and Physiology* (5th ed., p. 485). Philadelphia: F.A. Davis.

Figure 3-12. Scanlon, V. and Sanders, T. (2007). *Essentials of Anatomy and Physiology* (5th ed., p. 485). Philadelphia: F.A. Davis.

Chapter 4

Figure 4-1. Ward, S.L. and Hisley, S: *Maternal-Child Nursing: Optimizing Outcomes for Mothers, Children and Families*, Enhanced Revised Reprint. 2009. Philadelphia: F.A. Davis.

Figure 4-3. Scanlon, V. and Sanders, T. (2007). *Essentials of Anatomy and Physiology* (5th ed., p. 485). Philadelphia: F.A. Davis.

Figure 4-4. Ward, S.L. and Hisley, S: *Maternal-Child Nursing: Optimizing Outcomes for Mothers, Children and Families*, Enhanced Revised Reprint. 2009. Philadelphia: F.A. Davis.

Figure 4-5. Ward, S.L. and Hisley, S: *Maternal-Child Nursing: Optimizing Outcomes for Mothers, Children and Families*, Enhanced Revised Reprint. 2009. Philadelphia: F.A. Davis.

Figure 4-6. Ward, S.L. and Hisley, S: *Maternal-Child Nursing: Optimizing Outcomes for Mothers, Children and Families*, Enhanced Revised Reprint. 2009. Philadelphia: F.A. Davis.

Figure 4-7 Chapman, L. and Durham, R. *Maternal–Newborn Nursing: The Critical Components of Nursing Care*. 2010. Philadelphia: F.A. Davis.

Figure 4-8. Chapman, L. and Durham, R. *Maternal–Newborn Nursing: The Critical Components of Nursing Care*. 2010. Philadelphia: F.A. Davis.

Figure 4-9. U.S. Department of Agriculture. MyPyramid.gov Website. Washington, DC. *What Should I Eat? MyPyramid For Moms* http://www.choosemyplate.gov/food-groups/downloads/resource/pregnancyposter.pdf. Accessed August 13, 2013.

Figure 4-10. Chapman, L. and Durham, R. *Maternal–Newborn Nursing: The Critical Components of Nursing Care*. 2010. Philadelphia: F.A. Davis.

Chapter 5

Figure 5-1. Chapman, L. and Durham, R. *Maternal–Newborn Nursing: The Critical Components of Nursing Care*. 2010. Philadelphia: F.A. Davis.

Figure 5-2. Chapman, L. and Durham, R. *Maternal–Newborn Nursing: The Critical Components of Nursing Care*. 2010. Philadelphia: F.A. Davis.

Figure 5-3. Chapman, L. and Durham, R. *Maternal–Newborn Nursing: The Critical Components of Nursing Care*. 2010. Philadelphia: F.A. Davis.

Chapter 6

Figure 6-1. Chapman, L. and Durham, R. *Maternal-Newborn Nursing: The Critical Components of Nursing Care.* 2010. Philadelphia: F.A. Davis.

Figure 6-2. Chapman, L. and Durham, R. *Maternal-Newborn Nursing: The Critical Components of Nursing Care.* 2010. Philadelphia: F.A. Davis.

Figure 6-4. Chapman, L. and Durham, R. *Maternal-Newborn Nursing: The Critical Components of Nursing Care.* 2010. Philadelphia: F.A. Davis.

Figure 6-7. Chapman, L. and Durham, R. *Maternal-Newborn Nursing: The Critical Components of Nursing Care.* 2010. Philadelphia: F.A. Davis.

Chapter 7

Figure 7-1. Chapman, L. and Durham, R. *Maternal-Newborn Nursing: The Critical Components of Nursing Care.* 2010. Philadelphia: F.A. Davis.

Figure 7-2. Chapman, L. and Durham, R. *Maternal-Newborn Nursing: The Critical Components of Nursing Care.* 2010. Philadelphia: F.A. Davis.

Figure 7-3. Chapman, L. and Durham, R. *Maternal-Newborn Nursing: The Critical Components of Nursing Care.* 2010. Philadelphia: F.A. Davis.

Figure 7-4. Chapman, L. and Durham, R. *Maternal-Newborn Nursing: The Critical Components of Nursing Care.* 2010. Philadelphia: F.A. Davis.

Figure 7-6. Chapman, L. and Durham, R. *Maternal-Newborn Nursing: The Critical Components of Nursing Care.* 2010. Philadelphia: F.A. Davis.

Figure 7-7. Chapman, L. and Durham, R. *Maternal-Newborn Nursing: The Critical Components of Nursing Care.* 2010. Philadelphia: F.A. Davis.

Figure 7-8. Chapman, L. and Durham, R. *Maternal-Newborn Nursing: The Critical Components of Nursing Care.* 2010. Philadelphia: F.A. Davis.

Figure 7-9. Dillon, P. (2007). *Nursing Health Assessment: A Critical Thinking, Case Studies Approach* (2nd ed.) Philadelphia: F.A. Davis.

Figure 7-10. Ward, S.L. and Hisley, S: *Maternal-Child Nursing: Optimizing Outcomes for Mothers, Children and Families,* Enhanced Revised Reprint. 2009. Philadelphia: F.A. Davis.

Figure 7-11. Holloway, B., Moredich, C., and Aduddell, K. (2006). *OB Peds Women's Health Notes: Nurse's Clinical Pocket Guide,* p. 45. Philadelphia: F.A. Davis.

Figure 7-12. Chapman, L. and Durham, R. *Maternal-Newborn Nursing: The Critical Components of Nursing Care.* 2010. Philadelphia: F.A. Davis.

Figure 7-13. Ward, S.L. and Hisley, S: *Maternal-Child Nursing: Optimizing Outcomes for Mothers, Children and Families,* Enhanced Revised Reprint. 2009. Philadelphia: F.A. Davis.

Chapter 8

Figure 8-2. Ward, S.L. and Hisley, S: *Maternal-Child Nursing: Optimizing Outcomes for Mothers, Children and Families,* Enhanced Revised Reprint. 2009. Philadelphia: F.A. Davis.

Figure 8-4. Ward, S.L. and Hisley, S: *Maternal-Child Nursing: Optimizing Outcomes for Mothers, Children and Families,* Enhanced Revised Reprint. 2009. Philadelphia: F.A. Davis.

Figure 8-5. Ward, S.L. and Hisley, S: *Maternal-Child Nursing: Optimizing Outcomes for Mothers, Children and Families,* Enhanced Revised Reprint. 2009. Philadelphia: F.A. Davis.

Figure 8-6. Ward, S.L. and Hisley, S: *Maternal-Child Nursing: Optimizing Outcomes for Mothers, Children and Families,* Enhanced Revised Reprint. 2009. Philadelphia: F.A. Davis.

Figure 8-8B. Chapman, L. and Durham, R. *Maternal-Newborn Nursing: The Critical Components of Nursing Care.* 2010. Philadelphia: F.A. Davis.

Figure 8-9. Ward, S.L. and Hisley, S: *Maternal-Child Nursing: Optimizing Outcomes for Mothers, Children and Families,* Enhanced Revised Reprint. 2009. Philadelphia: F.A. Davis.

Figure 8-10. Ward, S.L. and Hisley, S: *Maternal-Child Nursing: Optimizing Outcomes for Mothers, Children and Families,* Enhanced Revised Reprint. 2009. Philadelphia: F.A. Davis.

Figure 8-11. Ward, S.L. and Hisley, S: *Maternal-Child Nursing: Optimizing Outcomes for Mothers, Children and Families,* Enhanced Revised Reprint. 2009. Philadelphia: F.A. Davis.

Figure 8-12. Ward, S.L. and Hisley, S: *Maternal-Child Nursing: Optimizing Outcomes for Mothers, Children and Families,* Enhanced Revised Reprint. 2009. Philadelphia: F.A. Davis.

Figure 8-15. Chapman, L. and Durham, R. *Maternal-Newborn Nursing: The Critical Components of Nursing Care.* 2010. Philadelphia: F.A. Davis.

Figure 8-16. Chapman, L. and Durham, R. *Maternal-Newborn Nursing: The Critical Components of Nursing Care.* 2010. Philadelphia: F.A. Davis.

Figure 8-17. Ward, S.L. and Hisley, S: *Maternal-Child Nursing: Optimizing Outcomes for Mothers, Children and Families,* Enhanced Revised Reprint. 2009. Philadelphia: F.A. Davis.

Figure 8-20. Ward, S.L. and Hisley, S: *Maternal-Child Nursing: Optimizing Outcomes for Mothers, Children and Families,* Enhanced Revised Reprint. 2009. Philadelphia: F.A. Davis.

Figure 8-22. Adapted from Chapman, L. and Durham, R. *Maternal-Newborn Nursing: The Critical Components of Nursing Care.* 2010. Philadelphia: F.A. Davis.

Figure 8-23. Adapted from Chapman, L. and Durham, R. *Maternal-Newborn Nursing: The Critical Components of Nursing Care*. 2010. Philadelphia: F.A. Davis.

Figure 8-24. Chapman, L. and Durham, R. *Maternal-Newborn Nursing: The Critical Components of Nursing Care*. 2010. Philadelphia: F.A. Davis.

Figure 8-25. Chapman, L. and Durham, R. *Maternal-Newborn Nursing: The Critical Components of Nursing Care*. 2010. Philadelphia: F.A. Davis.

Figure 8-26. Ward, S.L. and Hisley, S: *Maternal-Child Nursing: Optimizing Outcomes for Mothers, Children and Families*, Enhanced Revised Reprint. 2009. Philadelphia: F.A. Davis.

Figure 8-27. Ward, S.L. and Hisley, S: *Maternal-Child Nursing: Optimizing Outcomes for Mothers, Children and Families*, Enhanced Revised Reprint. 2009. Philadelphia: F.A. Davis.

Figure 8-28. Chapman, L. and Durham, R. *Maternal-Newborn Nursing: The Critical Components of Nursing Care*. 2010. Philadelphia: F.A. Davis.

Figure 8-29. Chapman, L. and Durham, R. *Maternal-Newborn Nursing: The Critical Components of Nursing Care*. 2010. Philadelphia: F.A. Davis.

Figure 8-30. Chapman, L. and Durham, R. *Maternal-Newborn Nursing: The Critical Components of Nursing Care*. 2010. Philadelphia: F.A. Davis.

Figure 8-31. Chapman, L. and Durham, R. *Maternal-Newborn Nursing: The Critical Components of Nursing Care*. 2010. Philadelphia: F.A. Davis.

Figure 8-32. American Heart Association, 2010.

Figure 8-33. Chapman, L. and Durham, R. *Maternal-Newborn Nursing: The Critical Components of Nursing Care*. 2010. Philadelphia: F.A. Davis.

Figure 8-34. Dillon, P. (2007). *Nursing health assessment: A critical thinking, case, studies approach* (2nd ed.) Philadelphia: F.A. Davis.

Figure 8-35. Ward, S.L. and Hisley, S: *Maternal-Child Nursing: Optimizing Outcomes for Mothers, Children and Families*, Enhanced Revised Reprint. 2009. Philadelphia: F.A. Davis.

Figure 8-37. Ward, S.L. and Hisley, S: *Maternal-Child Nursing: Optimizing Outcomes for Mothers, Children and Families*, Enhanced Revised Reprint. 2009. Philadelphia: F.A. Davis.

Figure 8-38. Ward, S.L. and Hisley, S: *Maternal-Child Nursing: Optimizing Outcomes for Mothers, Children and Families*, Enhanced Revised Reprint. 2009. Philadelphia: F.A. Davis.

Chapter 8 concept map created by Sylvia Fisher.

Chapter 9

Figure 9-1. Dillon, P. (2007). *Nursing health assessment: A critical thinking, case, studies approach* (2nd ed., p. 837). Philadelphia: F.A. Davis.

Figure 9-2. Ward, S.L. and Hisley, S: *Maternal-Child Nursing: Optimizing Outcomes for Mothers, Children and Families*, Enhanced Revised Reprint. 2009. Philadelphia: F.A. Davis.

Figure 9-3. Ward, S.L. and Hisley, S: *Maternal-Child Nursing: Optimizing Outcomes for Mothers, Children and Families*, Enhanced Revised Reprint. 2009. Philadelphia: F.A. Davis.

Figure 9-4. Chapman, L. and Durham, R. *Maternal-Newborn Nursing: The Critical Components of Nursing Care*. 2010. Philadelphia: F.A. Davis.

Figure 9-5. Lyndon A., and Ali L. U. (2009). *Fetal heart rate monitoring: Principles and practice* (4th ed.). Dubuque, IA: Kendal/Hunt.

Figure 9-6. Holloway, B., Moredich, C., and Aduddell, K. (2006). *OB Peds Women's Health Notes: Nurse's Clinical Pocket Guide* (p. 57). Philadelphia: F.A. Davis.

Figure 9-9. Chapman, L. and Durham, R. *Maternal-Newborn Nursing: The Critical Components of Nursing Care*. 2010. Philadelphia: F.A. Davis.

Figure 9-10. Chapman, L. and Durham, R. *Maternal-Newborn Nursing: The Critical Components of Nursing Care*. 2010. Philadelphia: F.A. Davis.

Figure 9-11. Chapman, L. and Durham, R. *Maternal-Newborn Nursing: The Critical Components of Nursing Care*. 2010. Philadelphia: F.A. Davis.

Figure 9-12. Chapman, L. and Durham, R. *Maternal-Newborn Nursing: The Critical Components of Nursing Care*. 2010. Philadelphia: F.A. Davis.

Figure 9-13. Holloway, B., Moredich, C., and Aduddell, K. (2006). *OB Peds Women's Health Notes: Nurse's Clinical Pocket Guide*, p. 59. Philadelphia: F.A. Davis.

Figure 9-14. Holloway, B., Moredich, C., and Aduddell, K. (2006). *OB Peds Women's Health Notes: Nurse's Clinical Pocket Guide*, p. 59. Philadelphia: F.A. Davis.

Figure 9-15. Chapman, L. and Durham, R. *Maternal-Newborn Nursing: The Critical Components of Nursing Care*. 2010. Philadelphia: F.A. Davis.

Figure 9-16. Holloway, B., Moredich, C., and Aduddell, K. (2006). *OB Peds Women's Health Notes: Nurse's Clinical Pocket Guide*, p. 61. Philadelphia: F.A. Davis.

Figure 9-19. Chapman, L. and Durham, R. *Maternal-Newborn Nursing: The Critical Components of Nursing Care*. 2010. Philadelphia: F.A. Davis.

Figure 9-21. Chapman, L. and Durham, R. *Maternal-Newborn Nursing: The Critical Components of Nursing Care*. 2010. Philadelphia: F.A. Davis.

Chapter 10

Figure 10-1. Chapman, L. and Durham, R. *Maternal-Newborn Nursing: The Critical Components of Nursing Care*. 2010. Philadelphia: F.A. Davis.

Figure 10-2. Chapman, L. and Durham, R. *Maternal-Newborn Nursing: The Critical Components of Nursing Care*. 2010. Philadelphia: F.A. Davis.

Figure 10-3. Chapman, L. and Durham, R. *Maternal-Newborn Nursing: The Critical Components of Nursing Care*. 2010. Philadelphia: F.A. Davis.

Figure 10-4. Chapman, L. and Durham, R. *Maternal-Newborn Nursing: The Critical Components of Nursing Care*. 2010. Philadelphia: F.A. Davis.

Figure 10-9. Chapman, L. and Durham, R. *Maternal-Newborn Nursing: The Critical Components of Nursing Care*. 2010. Philadelphia: F.A. Davis.

Figure 10-10. Ward, S.L. and Hisley, S: *Maternal-Child Nursing: Optimizing Outcomes for Mothers, Children and Families*, Enhanced Revised Reprint. 2009. Philadelphia: F.A. Davis.

Figure 10-11. Ward, S.L. and Hisley, S: *Maternal-Child Nursing: Optimizing Outcomes for Mothers, Children and Families*, Enhanced Revised Reprint. 2009. Philadelphia: F.A. Davis.

Figure 10-12. Chapman, L. and Durham, R. *Maternal-Newborn Nursing: The Critical Components of Nursing Care*. 2010. Philadelphia: F.A. Davis.

Figure 10-14. Chapman, L. and Durham, R. *Maternal-Newborn Nursing: The Critical Components of Nursing Care*. 2010. Philadelphia: F.A. Davis.

Figure 10-16. Ward, S.L. and Hisley, S: *Maternal-Child Nursing: Optimizing Outcomes for Mothers, Children and Families*, Enhanced Revised Reprint. 2009. Philadelphia: F.A. Davis.

Figure 10-17. Ward, S.L. and Hisley, S: *Maternal-Child Nursing: Optimizing Outcomes for Mothers, Children and Families*, Enhanced Revised Reprint. 2009. Philadelphia: F.A. Davis.

Figure 10-18. Ward, S.L. and Hisley, S: *Maternal-Child Nursing: Optimizing Outcomes for Mothers, Children and Families*, Enhanced Revised Reprint. 2009. Philadelphia: F.A. Davis.

Figure 10-19. Ward, S., and Hisley, S. (2009). *Maternal-Child Nursing Care: Optimizing Outcomes for Mothers, Children, and Families*, (p. 454), Philadelphia: F.A. Davis.

Occiput posterior. Chapman, L. and Durham, R. *Maternal-Newborn Nursing: The Critical Components of Nursing Care*. 2010. Philadelphia: F.A. Davis.

Face presentation. Chapman, L. and Durham, R. *Maternal-Newborn Nursing: The Critical Components of Nursing Care*. 2010. Philadelphia: F.A. Davis.

Brow presentation. Chapman, L. and Durham, R. *Maternal-Newborn Nursing: The Critical Components of Nursing Care*. 2010. Philadelphia: F.A. Davis.

Shoulder presentation. Chapman, L. and Durham, R. *Maternal-Newborn Nursing: The Critical Components of Nursing Care*. 2010. Philadelphia: F.A. Davis.

Frank breech. Chapman, L. and Durham, R. *Maternal-Newborn Nursing: The Critical Components of Nursing Care*. 2010. Philadelphia: F.A. Davis.

Complete breech. Chapman, L. and Durham, R. *Maternal-Newborn Nursing: The Critical Components of Nursing Care*. 2010. Philadelphia: F.A. Davis.

Footling breech (single). Chapman, L. and Durham, R. *Maternal-Newborn Nursing: The Critical Components of Nursing Care*. 2010. Philadelphia: F.A. Davis.

Footling breech (double). Chapman, L. and Durham, R. *Maternal-Newborn Nursing: The Critical Components of Nursing Care*. 2010. Philadelphia: F.A. Davis.

Chapter 11

Figure 11-1. Chapman, L. and Durham, R. *Maternal-Newborn Nursing: The Critical Components of Nursing Care*. 2010. Philadelphia: F.A. Davis.

Figure 11-2. Chapman, L. and Durham, R. *Maternal-Newborn Nursing: The Critical Components of Nursing Care*. 2010. Philadelphia: F.A. Davis.

Figure 11-4. Chapman, L. and Durham, R. *Maternal-Newborn Nursing: The Critical Components of Nursing Care*. 2010. Philadelphia: F.A. Davis.

Chapter 12

Figure 12-3. Dillon, P. (2007). *Nursing health assessment: A critical thinking, case, studies approach* (2nd ed., p. 844). Philadelphia: F.A. Davis.

Figure 12-4. Chapman, L. and Durham, R. *Maternal-Newborn Nursing: The Critical Components of Nursing Care*. 2010. Philadelphia: F.A. Davis.

Figure 12-5. United States Department of Agriculture. www.ChooseMyPlate.gov. Accessed August 13, 2013.

Chapter 13

Figure 13-1. Chapman, L. and Durham, R. *Maternal-Newborn Nursing: The Critical Components of Nursing Care*. 2010. Philadelphia: F.A. Davis.

Figure 13-2. Chapman, L. and Durham, R. *Maternal-Newborn Nursing: The Critical Components of Nursing Care*. 2010. Philadelphia: F.A. Davis.

Figure 13-3. Chapman, L. and Durham, R. *Maternal-Newborn Nursing: The Critical Components of Nursing Care*. 2010. Philadelphia: F.A. Davis.

Figure 13-4. Chapman, L. and Durham, R. *Maternal-Newborn Nursing: The Critical Components of Nursing Care*. 2010. Philadelphia: F.A. Davis.

Chapter 14

Figure 14-2. Holloway, B., Moredich, C., and Aduddell, K. (2006). *OB Peds Women's Health Notes: Nurse's Clinical Pocket Guide*, p. 83. Philadelphia: F.A. Davis.

Figure 14-3. Chapman, L. and Durham, R. *Maternal-Newborn Nursing: The Critical Components of Nursing Care*. 2010. Philadelphia: F.A. Davis.

Chapter 15

Figure 15-2. Chapman, L. and Durham, R. *Maternal-Newborn Nursing: The Critical Components of Nursing Care*. 2010. Philadelphia: F.A. Davis.

Figure 15-3. Chapman, L. and Durham, R. *Maternal-Newborn Nursing: The Critical Components of Nursing Care.* 2010. Philadelphia: F.A. Davis.

Figure 15-4. Chapman, L. and Durham, R. *Maternal-Newborn Nursing: The Critical Components of Nursing Care.* 2010. Philadelphia: F.A. Davis.

Figure 15-5. Ward, S.L. and Hisley, S: *Maternal-Child Nursing: Optimizing Outcomes for Mothers, Children and Families,* Enhanced Revised Reprint. 2009. Philadelphia: F.A. Davis.

Figure 15-6. Chapman, L. and Durham, R. *Maternal-Newborn Nursing: The Critical Components of Nursing Care.* 2010. Philadelphia: F.A. Davis.

Figure 15-8. Reprinted from Journal of Pediatrics, 119:418, Ballard, J et al. Copyright 1991, with permission from Elsevier.

Figure 15-10. Chapman, L. and Durham, R. *Maternal-Newborn Nursing: The Critical Components of Nursing Care.* 2010. Philadelphia: F.A. Davis.

Figure 15-11. Chapman, L. and Durham, R. *Maternal-Newborn Nursing: The Critical Components of Nursing Care.* 2010. Philadelphia: F.A. Davis.

Neonatal posture. Chapman, L. and Durham, R. *Maternal-Newborn Nursing: The Critical Components of Nursing Care.* 2010. Philadelphia: F.A. Davis.

Measuring head circumference. Dillon, P. (2007). *Nursing Health Assessment: A Critical Thinking, Case Studies Approach* (2nd ed., p. 856). Philadelphia: F.A. Davis.

Measuring chest circumference. Dillon, P. (2007). *Nursing Health Assessment: A Critical Thinking, Case Studies Approach* (2nd ed., p. 856). Philadelphia: F.A. Davis.

Measuring length. Dillon, P. (2007). *Nursing Health Assessment: A Critical Thinking, Case Studies Approach* (2nd ed., p. 857). Philadelphia: F.A. Davis.

Weighing neonate. Dillon, P. (2007). *Nursing Health Assessment: A Critical Thinking, Case Studies Approach* (2nd ed., p. 864). Philadelphia: F.A. Davis.

Taking axillary temperature. Chapman, L. and Durham, R. *Maternal-Newborn Nursing: The Critical Components of Nursing Care.* 2010. Philadelphia: F.A. Davis.

Auscultating heart. Dillon, P. (2007). *Nursing Health Assessment: A Critical Thinking, Case Studies Approach* (2nd ed., p. 864). Philadelphia: F.A. Davis.

Stork bite. Dillon, P. (2007). *Nursing Health Assessment: A Critical Thinking, Case Studies Approach* (2nd ed., p. 859). Philadelphia: F.A. Davis.

Palpating fontanels. Dillon, P. (2007). *Nursing Health Assessment: A Critical Thinking, Case Studies Approach* (2nd ed., p. 860). Philadelphia: F.A. Davis.

Assessing neck. Chapman, L. and Durham, R. *Maternal-Newborn Nursing: The Critical Components of Nursing Care.* 2010. Philadelphia: F.A. Davis.

Normal eye line. Dillon, P. (2007). *Nursing Health Assessment: A Critical Thinking, Case Studies Approach* (2nd ed., p. 861). Philadelphia: F.A. Davis.

Hearing test. Chapman, L. and Durham, R. *Maternal-Newborn Nursing: The Critical Components of Nursing Care.* 2010. Philadelphia: F.A. Davis.

Flatten nose. Chapman, L. and Durham, R. *Maternal-Newborn Nursing: The Critical Components of Nursing Care.* 2010. Philadelphia: F.A. Davis.

Thrush. Dillon, P. (2007). *Nursing Health Assessment: A Critical Thinking, Case Studies Approach* (2nd ed., p. 862). Philadelphia: F.A. Davis.

Auscultating lungs posteriorly. Dillon, P. (2007). *Nursing Health Assessment: A Critical Thinking, Case Studies Approach* (2nd ed., p. 863). Philadelphia: F.A. Davis.

Auscultating lungs anteriorly. Dillon, P. (2007). *Nursing Health Assessment: A Critical Thinking, Case Studies Approach* (2nd ed., p. 863). Philadelphia: F.A. Davis.

Auscultating heart. Dillon, P. (2007). *Nursing Health Assessment: A Critical Thinking, Case Studies Approach* (2nd ed.). Philadelphia: F.A. Davis.

Inspection of cord. Chapman, L. and Durham, R. *Maternal-Newborn Nursing: The Critical Components of Nursing Care.* 2010. Philadelphia: F.A. Davis.

Female genitalia. Chapman, L. and Durham, R. *Maternal-Newborn Nursing: The Critical Components of Nursing Care.* 2010. Philadelphia: F.A. Davis.

Palpating the scrotum. Dillon, P. (2007). *Nursing Health Assessment: A Critical Thinking, Case Studies Approach* (2nd ed., p. 865). Philadelphia: F.A. Davis.

Checking gluteal folds. Dillon, P. (2007). *Nursing Health Assessment: A Critical Thinking, Case Studies Approach* (2nd ed.). Philadelphia: F.A. Davis.

Barlow-Ortolani maneuver #1. Dillon, P. (2007). *Nursing Health Assessment: A Critical Thinking, Case Studies Approach* (2nd ed., p. 866). Philadelphia: F.A. Davis.

Barlow-Ortolani maneuver #2. Dillon, P. (2007). *Nursing Health Assessment: A Critical Thinking, Case Studies Approach* (2nd ed., p. 866). Philadelphia: F.A. Davis.

Barlow-Ortolani maneuver #3. Dillon, P. (2007). *Nursing Health Assessment: A Critical Thinking, Case Studies Approach* (2nd ed., p. 866). Philadelphia: F.A. Davis.

Acrocyanosis. Chapman, L. and Durham, R. *Maternal-Newborn Nursing: The Critical Components of Nursing Care.* 2010. Philadelphia: F.A. Davis.

Mongolian spot. Chapman, L. and Durham, R. *Maternal-Newborn Nursing: The Critical Components of Nursing Care.* 2010. Philadelphia: F.A. Davis.

Milia. Chapman, L. and Durham, R. *Maternal-Newborn Nursing: The Critical Components of Nursing Care.* 2010. Philadelphia: F.A. Davis.

Lanugo. Chapman, L. and Durham, R. *Maternal-Newborn Nursing: The Critical Components of Nursing Care.* 2010. Philadelphia: F.A. Davis.

Jaundice. Chapman, L. and Durham, R. *Maternal-Newborn Nursing: The Critical Components of Nursing Care.* 2010. Philadelphia: F.A. Davis.

Molding. Chapman, L. and Durham, R. *Maternal-Newborn Nursing: The Critical Components of Nursing Care.* 2010. Philadelphia: F.A. Davis.

Caput succedaneum. Ward, S.L. and Hisley, S: *Maternal-Child Nursing: Optimizing Outcomes for Mothers, Children and Families*, Enhanced Revised Reprint. 2009. Philadelphia: F.A. Davis.

Cephalohematoma. Ward, S.L. and Hisley, S: *Maternal-Child Nursing: Optimizing Outcomes for Mothers, Children and Families*, Enhanced Revised Reprint. 2009. Philadelphia: F.A. Davis.

Epstein's pearls. Dillon, P. (2007). *Nursing health assessment: A critical thinking, case, studies approach* (2nd ed., p. 862). Philadelphia: F.A. Davis.

Natal teeth. Dillon, P. (2007). *Nursing Health Assessment: A Critical Thinking, Case Studies Approach* (2nd ed., p. 861). Philadelphia: F.A. Davis.

Moro reflex. Dillon, P. (2007). *Nursing Health Assessment: A Critical Thinking, Case Studies Approach* (2nd ed., p. 868). Philadelphia: F.A. Davis.

Startle reflex. Dillon, P. (2007). *Nursing Health Assessment: A Critical Thinking, Case Studies Approach* (2nd ed., p. 868). Philadelphia: F.A. Davis.

Tonic neck reflex. Dillon, P. (2007). *Nursing Health Assessment: A Critical Thinking, Case Studies Approach* (2nd ed., p. 868). Philadelphia: F.A. Davis.

Rooting reflex. Dillon, P. (2007). *Nursing Health Assessment: A Critical Thinking, Case Studies Approach* (2nd ed., p. 870). Philadelphia: F.A. Davis.

Sucking reflex. Chapman, L. and Durham, R. *Maternal-Newborn Nursing: The Critical Components of Nursing Care*. 2010. Philadelphia: F.A. Davis.

Palmar grasp reflex. Dillon, P. (2007). *Nursing Health Assessment: A Critical Thinking, Case Studies Approach* (2nd ed., p. 869). Philadelphia: F.A. Davis.

Plantar grasp reflex. Dillon, P. (2007). *Nursing Health Assessment: A Critical Thinking, Case Studies Approach* (2nd ed., p. 869). Philadelphia: F.A. Davis.

Babinski. Dillon, P. (2007). *Nursing Health Assessment: A Critical Thinking, Case Studies Approach* (2nd ed., p. 869). Philadelphia: F.A. Davis.

Stepping/Dancing reflex. Dillon, P. (2007). *Nursing Health Assessment: A Critical Thinking, Case Studies Approach* (2nd ed., p. 870). Philadelphia: F.A. Davis.

Heel stick. Ward, S.L. and Hisley, S: *Maternal-Child Nursing: Optimizing Outcomes for Mothers, Children and Families*, Enhanced Revised Reprint. 2009. Philadelphia: F.A. Davis.

Intramuscular injection. Chapman, L. and Durham, R. *Maternal-Newborn Nursing: The Critical Components of Nursing Care*. 2010. Philadelphia: F.A. Davis.

Chapter 16

Figure 16-1. Chapman, L. and Durham, R. *Maternal-Newborn Nursing: The Critical Components of Nursing Care*. 2010. Philadelphia: F.A. Davis.

Figure 16-2. Scanlon, V. and Sanders, T. (2007). *Essentials of Anatomy and Physiology* (5th ed., p. 467). Philadelphia: F.A. Davis.

Figure 16-3. Ward, S.L. and Hisley, S: *Maternal-Child Nursing: Optimizing Outcomes for Mothers, Children and Families*, Enhanced Revised Reprint. 2009. Philadelphia: F.A. Davis.

Figure 16-4. Ward, S.L. and Hisley, S: *Maternal-Child Nursing: Optimizing Outcomes for Mothers, Children and Families*, Enhanced Revised Reprint. 2009. Philadelphia: F.A. Davis.

Figure 16-5. Chapman, L. and Durham, R. *Maternal-Newborn Nursing: The Critical Components of Nursing Care*. 2010. Philadelphia: F.A. Davis.

Figure 16-6. Chapman, L. and Durham, R. *Maternal-Newborn Nursing: The Critical Components of Nursing Care*. 2010. Philadelphia: F.A. Davis.

Figure 16-7. Chapman, L. and Durham, R. *Maternal-Newborn Nursing: The Critical Components of Nursing Care*. 2010. Philadelphia: F.A. Davis.

Figure 16-8. Chapman, L. and Durham, R. *Maternal-Newborn Nursing: The Critical Components of Nursing Care*. 2010. Philadelphia: F.A. Davis.

Figure 16-9. Chapman, L. and Durham, R. *Maternal-Newborn Nursing: The Critical Components of Nursing Care*. 2010. Philadelphia: F.A. Davis.

Figure 16-10. Chapman, L. and Durham, R. *Maternal-Newborn Nursing: The Critical Components of Nursing Care*. 2010. Philadelphia: F.A. Davis.

Figure 16-11. Chapman, L. and Durham, R. *Maternal-Newborn Nursing: The Critical Components of Nursing Care*. 2010. Philadelphia: F.A. Davis.

Figure 16-12. Chapman, L. and Durham, R. *Maternal-Newborn Nursing: The Critical Components of Nursing Care*. 2010. Philadelphia: F.A. Davis.

Figure 16-13. Chapman, L. and Durham, R. *Maternal-Newborn Nursing: The Critical Components of Nursing Care*. 2010. Philadelphia: F.A. Davis.

Figure 16-14. Chapman, L. and Durham, R. *Maternal-Newborn Nursing: The Critical Components of Nursing Care*. 2010. Philadelphia: F.A. Davis.

Figure 16-15. Chapman, L. and Durham, R. *Maternal-Newborn Nursing: The Critical Components of Nursing Care*. 2010. Philadelphia: F.A. Davis.

Chapter 17

Figure 17-1. Chapman, L. and Durham, R. *Maternal-Newborn Nursing: The Critical Components of Nursing Care*. 2010. Philadelphia: F.A. Davis.

Figure 17-2. Chapman, L. and Durham, R. *Maternal-Newborn Nursing: The Critical Components of Nursing Care*. 2010. Philadelphia: F.A. Davis.

Figure 17-3. Chapman, L. and Durham, R. *Maternal-Newborn Nursing: The Critical Components of Nursing Care*. 2010. Philadelphia: F.A. Davis.

Figure 17-4. Chapman, L. and Durham, R. *Maternal-Newborn Nursing: The Critical Components of Nursing Care*. 2010. Philadelphia: F.A. Davis.

Figure 17-6. Chapman, L. and Durham, R. *Maternal-Newborn Nursing: The Critical Components of Nursing Care*. 2010. Philadelphia: F.A. Davis.

Figure 17-7. Chapman, L. and Durham, R. *Maternal-Newborn Nursing: The Critical Components of Nursing Care*. 2010. Philadelphia: F.A. Davis.

Figure 17-8. Chapman, L. and Durham, R. *Maternal-Newborn Nursing: The Critical Components of Nursing Care*. 2010. Philadelphia: F.A. Davis.

Figure 17-9. Chapman, L. and Durham, R. *Maternal-Newborn Nursing: The Critical Components of Nursing Care*. 2010. Philadelphia: F.A. Davis.

Figure 17-10. Chapman, L. and Durham, R. *Maternal-Newborn Nursing: The Critical Components of Nursing Care*. 2010. Philadelphia: F.A. Davis.

Gavage feeding. Chapman, L. and Durham, R. *Maternal-Newborn Nursing: The Critical Components of Nursing Care*. 2010. Philadelphia: F.A. Davis.

Care of Neonate Receiving Phototherapy. Chapman, L. and Durham, R. *Maternal-Newborn Nursing: The Critical Components of Nursing Care*. 2010. Philadelphia: F.A. Davis.

Chapter 18

Figure 18-2. United States Department of Agriculture. www.ChooseMyPlate.gov. Accessed August 13, 2013.

Figure 18-3. US Department of Health and Human Services (2012).

Figure 18-4. Chapman, L. and Durham, R. *Maternal-Newborn Nursing: The Critical Components of Nursing Care*. 2010. Philadelphia: F.A. Davis.

Chapter 19

Figure 19-4. Chapman, L. and Durham, R. *Maternal-Newborn Nursing: The Critical Components of Nursing Care*. 2010. Philadelphia: F.A. Davis.

Note: Illustrations are indicated by f, tables by t and boxes by b.